Richard S. Pavelec, S.R.A.
Department of Medicine (M-013)
University of California, San Diego
La Jolla, California 92093

Techniques in Extracorporeal Circulation

docendo discimus

To Mr Bernard G. S. Cayzer, who has continuously promoted medical research through his great support and generosity

By the same editor

Biological Tissue in Heart Valve Replacement
Current Techniques in Extracorporeal Circulation
Tissue Heart Valves

TECHNIQUES IN EXTRACORPOREAL CIRCULATION

Second Edition

Edited by

Marian I. Ionescu, MD, FACS

Consultant Cardiothoracic Surgeon,
The General Infirmary at Leeds,

Senior Clinical Lecturer in Cardiothoracic Surgery
at Leeds University, Leeds, England

Butterworths

London Boston Durban Singapore Sydney Toronto Wellington

First published 1976
Second edition 1981
Reprinted 1982

British Library cataloguing in Publication Data

Techniques in extracorporeal circulation. – 2nd ed.
1. Cardiovascular system – Surgery
2. Blood – Circulation, Artificial
I. Ionescu, Marian I.
617'.41 RD598

ISBN 0-407-00173-5

Typeset by Butterworths Litho Preparation Department
Printed in England by Butler & Tanner Ltd, London and Frome

Foreword

The field of extracorporeal circulation is still advancing rapidly, with many new techniques in patient management, as well as operative procedures. It is therefore fitting that this knowledge be brought together in a new edition.

Clinical and experimental studies have encouraged the widespread adoption of myocardial preservation techniques. Similarly, coronary artery surgery, which, a few years ago, was viewed with scepticism in many centres, has now found a secure position. Improvements in bubble oxygenators have made this the most generally used device, although there are a growing number of surgeons who prefer to use a membrane oxygenator. The ideal form of this device may soon be realized.

This edition, like the first, contains excellent chapters by the world's leading cardiac surgeons. A new generation is emerging through the sponsorship of these pioneers, so we are finding new names assuming prominent roles.

It is evident that experimental and clinical research are behind the improvements, and so long as they are being supported, we may expect advances to be made.

Readers will find this to be the best contemporary publication on extracorporeal cardiac surgery techniques.

Frank A. Gerbode

Preface to Second Edition

The preface to the first edition of this book was preceded by Michelangelo's humble remark 'ancora imparo'. Even for the contents of this small book on techniques in extracorporeal circulation it proved its timeless veracity as we 'continue to learn'.

The first edition however, despite many shortcomings, has fulfilled its role.

During the past few years the energetic clinical and research activities have led to many advances and have further broadened the concept of artificial circulation and oxygenation so that an increasing number of subspecialities are now attaining a certain contour.

In recent years, several areas of extracorporeal circulation have assumed increasing importance. The progress made in the field of ischaemic heart disease and the major impact of myocardial protection through cardioplegia are only two of the most obvious examples. Refinements in the construction and performance of bubble oxygenators and the introduction of disposable membrane oxygenating systems have changed the techniques of heart-lung bypass and broadened its scope.

Many pioneers in these fields have discovered and rediscovered noteworthy features of great clinical significance.

This second edition attempts to summarize the major technical problems and touches on some of the more theoretical aspects of extracorporeal circulation but does not necessarily provide final answers.

In an effort to keep abreast of the many advances which have occurred, a number of additional topics have been included in this present edition. Several new, outstanding contributors have participated, whilst the great majority of those chapters which appeared in the first edition have been updated or augmented.

Despite the awareness of discontinuity and reiteration, this second edition of *Techniques in Extracorporeal Circulation* retains the structure of most modern books by being comprised of a series of individual chapters.

I wish to express my enthusiasm for the privilege of editing this text and gratefully acknowledge the outstanding contributions of the authors who have joined in this endeavour.

I should like to thank Miss Wendy Lawrence for the complex and seemingly endless secretarial work.

My sincere appreciation is extended to Messrs Butterworths for their unfailing attention to detail and for the maintenance of the high standards for which they are known.

Marian I. Ionescu

Preface to First Edition

ancora imparo
Michelangelo Buonarotti

Extracorporeal circulation with an artificial heart-lung machine has established itself as the routine adjunct to intracardiac and vascular surgery. Since its introduction in 1953 this method has been progressively improved by development and simplification of the equipment and by better understanding of the body response to the alterations induced by the use of artificial perfusions.

The method, established in the experimental laboratory, has been perfected by clinical use. For many poorly understood aspects the method has continued to be investigated in the laboratory, where answers and solutions have been found for innumerable bewildering and knotty clinical problems.

A superficial look at today's methods would give the uninformed the general impression that no substantial progress has been made in the past ten years. For example, the same principle of bubble oxygenation used at the beginning of the open-heart surgery era is almost universally employed today. The same may be said for metallic prosthetic valves with a ball or disc occluder mechanism. The best method for 'myocardial preservation' during open-heart surgery is yet to be established and the Montagues of hypothermia still have to convince the Capulets of coronary perfusion of the veracity and superiority of their principle just as much as they had to ten years ago.

On closer examination, one realizes that during the past ten years an enormous wealth of data and knowledge has been accumulated and the application of this knowledge has made clinical perfusions incomparably better and safer. The results of cardiovascular surgery obtained today, whether in the newborn or the elderly, for great arteries or coronary arteries, in routine cases or in emergencies, when compared with the results obtained only ten years ago, are the best proof of progress and continuous improvement in extracorporeal circulation.

During the past few years many new and exciting principles and techniques based on extracorporeal circulation have been brought into clinical use. Deep hypothermia for heart surgery in the newborn, prolonged extracorporeal oxygenation–perfusion for pulmonary insufficiency and intra-aortic balloon pumping for circulatory assistance are some of the major achievements of the past decade.

The paucity of books devoted exclusively to extracorporeal circulation has prompted us to bring together in a single volume standard *current techniques in extracorporeal circulation* along with the more recent developments in this field. This is an attempt to answer some of the innumerable practical problems associated with the routine use of artificial circulation and oxygenation and to present some models of standardized techniques.

A major problem with such a book is to decide what to include and what to omit. We are aware that omissions have been made but we have aimed to keep the subject matter strictly circumscribed in the interest of text size and readability. The esoteric has been omitted on purpose and emphasis is placed on the current practical methodology.

Advances in modern surgical and perfusion techniques have been developed to such a degree that an entirely new spectrum of problems evolves with each new development. Such rapid changes and imrpovements will certainly call for another publication in the near future and this is another reason for limiting the size of this book.

Since this is a multi-authored book and the chapters are designed to be read separately, some reiteration has been inevitable, although an attempt was made to avoid repetition.

Major attention has been focused on the cardiovascular system, the lung, the renal function and haematological changes. Clearly the brain, liver, gut, muscle masses and reticuloendothelial system are of great importance in the body response to extracorporeal circulation but the measurement of their function in the cardiovascular patient is at the moment largely in the realm of the investigator. Although the principles and techniques described have become routine for practical purposes, they are by no means beyond challenge. As William Hazlitt put it 'when a thing ceases to be a subject of controversy, it ceases to be a subject of interest'.

The Editors join the contributors in hoping that this volume will be of interest to those active in the field of cardiovascular surgery.

We take great pleasure in expressing our thanks to Dr Frank Gerbode for kindly writing the Foreword of this work. We are grateful to Miss Nancy Evans for her continuous and enthusiastic help.

Completion of this book within a few months was promised, but it has taken almost two years and we appreciate the forbearance and continuous help of our publishers, Butterworth and Co. Ltd.

M. I. Ionescu

Contributors

conjunctis viribus

Brian G. Barratt-Boyes, KBE, MB, ChM, FRACS, FACS, FRSNZ,
Surgeon-in-Charge,
Cardiothoracic Surgical Unit,
Green Lane Hospital,

Hon. Professor of Surgery,
University of Auckland,
Auckland,
New Zealand

Robert H. Bartlett, MD,
Professor of General and Thoracic Surgery,
University of Michigan,
Ann Arbor,
Michigan,
USA

William A. Baumgartner, MD,
Chief Resident,
Department of Cardiovascular Surgery,
Stanford University School of Medicine,

Former Chief Resident,
Cardiac Transplantation Service,
Stanford,
California,
USA

Lawrence I. Bonchek, MD,
Professor and Chairman,
Department of Thoracic and Cardiovascular Surgery,
The Medical School of Wisconsin,
Milwaukee,
Wisconsin,
USA

Harvey S. Borovetz, PhD,
Research Assistant Professor,
Department of Surgery and Civil Engineering,
University of Pittsburgh,
School of Medicine,
Pittsburgh,
Pennsylvania,
USA

M. L. Bramson, MLB, ACGI, FRAeS,
Consulting (Biomedical) Engineer,
Institutes of Medical Sciences,
Pacific Medical Center,
San Francisco,
California,
USA

David Bregman, MD,
Assistant Professor of Surgery,
Chest Surgical Service,
College of Physicians and Surgeons of Columbia University,

The Surgical Service of Presbyterian Hospital,
New York,
New York,
USA

Gerald D. Buckberg, MD,
Professor of Surgery,
University of California Medical Center,

UCLA Hospital and Clinics,
The Center for the Health Sciences,
Los Angeles,
California,
USA

Lawrence H. Cohn, MD,
Professor of Surgery,
Harvard Medical School,

Cardiovascular Surgeon,
Brigham and Women's Hospital,
Boston,
Massachusetts,
USA

John J. Collins, Jr., MD,
Professor of Surgery,
Harvard Medical School,

Chief,
Cardiothoracic Surgery,
Brigham and Women's Hospital,
Boston,
Massachusetts,
USA

Delos M. Cosgrove, MD,
Department of Thoracic and Cardiovascular Surgery,
Cleveland Clinic,
The Clinic Centre,
Cleveland,
Ohio,
USA

G. Michael Deeb, MD,
Senior Resident,
General and Thoracic Surgery,
University of Pittsburgh,
School of Medicine,
Pittsburgh,
Pennsylvania,
USA

Marc R. de Leval, MD,
Consultant Cardiothoracic Surgeon,
The Hospital for Sick Children,
Great Ormond Street,
London,
England

Richard N. Edie, MD,
Assistant Professor of Surgery,
College of Physicians and Surgeons of Columbia University,

Hospital of the University of Pennsylvania
Philadelphia,
USA

E. G. V. Evans, BSc, PhD, MI Biol,
Senior Lecturer in Medical Mycology,
University Departments of Microbiology and Dermatology,
The General Infirmary,
Leeds,
England

Anna Mae Fosberg, BS,
Chief Extracorporeal Perfusionist,
Brigham and Women's Hospital,

Associate in Surgery,
Harvard Medical School,
Boston,
Massachusetts,
USA

Roger Freeman, MB, ChB, MRCPath,
Consultant Microbiologist,
Freeman Hospital,
Newcastle-upon-Tyne,
England

Alan B. Gazzaniga, MD,
Professor of Surgery,
Department of Surgery,
University of California at Irvine,
Irvine,
California,
USA

Frank Gerbode, MD,
President of the Board,
The Institutes of Medical Sciences,
Pacific Medical Center,
San Francisco,

Clinical Professor of Surgery Emeritus,
Stanford University School of Medicine,
Stanford,
California,
USA

Colin G. Green,
Extracorporeal Circulation Specialist,
Polystan A/S,
Copenhagen,
Denmark

Bartley P. Griffith, MD,
Senior Resident,
Department of General and Thoracic Surgery,
University of Pittsburgh,
School of Medicine,
Pittsburgh,
Pennsylvania,
USA

V. Antony Grimshaw, MA, MB, BChir, FFARCS,
Consultant Anaesthetist,
The General Infirmary at Leeds,
Leeds,
England

Robert L. Hardesty, MD,
Assistant Professor,
Department of Surgery,
University of Pittsburgh,
School of Medicine,
Pittsburgh,
Pennsylvania,
USA

Michael D. Hargreaves, MB, ChB, FFARCS (Eng),
Consultant Anaesthetist,
The General Infirmary at Leeds,
Leeds,
England

Susan M. Haubert, RN,
Head Perfusionist,
Surgical Service,
Columbia Presbyterian Medical Center,
New York,
New York,
USA

J. Donald Hill, MD,
Chairman,
Department of Cardiovascular Surgery,
Presbyterian Hospital of Pacific Medical Center,
San Francisco,
California,
USA

Tin-Kan Hung, PhD,
Research Professor of Civil Engineering and Neurosurgery,
University of Pittsburgh,
School of Medicine,
Pittsburgh,
Pennsylvania,
USA

Marian I. Ionescu, MD, FACS,
Consultant Cardiothoracic Surgeon,
The General Infirmary at Leeds,

Senior Clinical Lecturer in Cardiothoracic Surgery at Leeds University,
Leeds,
England

Robert B. Karp, MD,
Professor of Surgery,
School of Medicine and the Medical Center,
The University of Alabama in Birmingham,
Birmingham,
Alabama,
USA

Earle B. Kay, MD,
Cleveland,
Ohio,
USA

Willem J. Kolff, MD, PhD,
Professor of Surgery,
Head of Division of Artificial Organs,
Department of Surgery,
College of Medicine,

Research Professor of Engineering,
College of Engineering,

Director,
Institute for Biomedical Engineering,
University of Utah,
Salt Lake City,
Utah,
USA

Nicholas T. Kouchoukos, MD,
Professor of Surgery,
School of Medicine and the Medical Center,
The University of Alabama in Birmingham,
Birmingham,
Alabama,
USA

Stanley Lee-Son, MD,
Assistant Professor of Anaesthesia,
Harvard Medical School,

Anaesthesiologist,
Brigham and Women's Hospital,
Boston,
Massachusetts,
USA

Floyd D. Loop, MD,
Chief,
Department of Thoracic and Cardiovascular Surgery,
Cleveland Clinic,
The Clinic Center,
Cleveland,
Ohio,
USA

James R. Malm, MD,
Director,
Chest Surgical Service,
Presbyterian Hospital,

Professor of Clinical Surgery,
College of Physicians and Surgeons of Columbia University,

Attending Surgeon,
Presbyterian Hospital,
New York,
New York,
USA

Charles A. S. Marrin, MD,
Resident in Chest Surgery,
Columbia Presbyterian Medical Center,
New York,
New York,
USA

David A. S. Mary, MB, ChB, MRCP, PhD,
Senior Lecturer,
Department of Cardiovascular Studies,
University of Leeds,
Leeds,
England

David Mendelsohn, MD,
Cleveland,
Ohio,
USA

C. Harold Mielke, Jr., MD,
Chief of Haematology and Director of Haematology Research,
Presbyterian Hospital,
Pacific Medical Center,
San Francisco,
California,
USA

Hossein Naraghipour, MD,
Cleveland,
Ohio,
USA

J. J. Osborn, MD,
Director,
Intensive Care Services,
Pacific Medical Center,
San Francisco,
California,
USA

Derek T. Pearson, MB, FRCP, FFARCS,
Consultant Anaesthetist,
Regional Cardiothoracic Centre,
Freeman Hospital,
Newcastle-upon-Tyne,
England

Bruce A. Reitz, MD,
Assistant Professor of Cardiovascular Surgery,
Department of Cardiovascular Surgery,
Stanford University,
School of Medicine,
Stanford,
California,
USA

Michele F. Roesler, MD, FRCS(Ed),
Registrar in Cardiothoracic Surgery,
The General Infirmary at Leeds,
Leeds,
England

Inge H. Rygg, MD,
Associate Professor of Cardiac Surgery,
Department of Thoracic Surgery,
Division of Cardiac Surgery,
Righospitalet,
University of Copenhagen,
Copenhagen,
Denmark

Harris B. Shumacker, Jr., MD,
Distinguished Professor of Surgery Emeritus,
Indiana University Medical Center,

Senior Surgical Consultant,
St. Vincent Hospital and Health Center,
Indianapolis,
Indiana,
USA

Henry M. Spotnitz, MD,
Assistant Professor of Surgery,
Chest Surgical Service,
College of Physicians and Surgeons of Columbia University,

The Surgical Service of Presbyterian Hospital,
New York,
New York,
USA

Albert Starr, MD,
Professor and Chief,
Cardiopulmonary Surgery,
Division of Cardiopulmonary Surgery,
University of Oregon,
Health Sciences Center,
Portland,
Oregon,
USA

Edward B. Stinson, MD,
Associate Professor,
Department of Cardiovascular Surgery,
Stanford University School of Medicine,
Stanford,
California,
USA

Anand P. Tandon, MD, MRCP,
Consultant Physician,
The Royal Halifax Infirmary and Halifax General Hospital,
Halifax,
England

Hans H. J. Zwart, MD, PhD,
Cardiovascular Surgeon,
Kettering Medical Center, Cox Heart Institute, Miami Valley Hospital,
St. Elizabeth Medical Center, Good Samaritan Hospital,

Associate Clinical Professor,
Wright State University Medical School,
Dayton,
Ohio,
USA

Contents

1

Physiology and Pathophysiology of Extracorporeal Circulation

Robert H. Bartlett and Alan B. Gazzaniga

omnem movere lapidem

Introduction

The term 'physiology' was coined by the great Dutch physician Boerhaave to describe the study of interdependent organ function under normal conditions. Extracorporeal circulation (ECC) imposes several abnormal conditions which lead to a series of changes in normal organ function. The physiology of ECC, for purposes of this discussion, refers to interdependent organ function during conditions of venoarterial cardiopulmonary bypass with an extracorporeal device. Physiological function under these conditions differs considerably from normal physiology. The changes occurring with ECC are outlined in *Table 1.1*. The normal functions of blood flow, gas exchange, blood surface interface effects and reticuloendothelial function are the physiologic functions which are replaced in total or in part by the extracorporeal device. Subsequent changes in neurological, renal, hepatic and other functions are secondary to these substitutions. The mechanical and pharmacological factors which are inherent in the design of the device (and hence are responsible for physiologic changes) are also listed in *Table 1.1*.

Abnormal, deteriorating, or inadequate organ function associated with extracorporeal circulation is the pathophysiology of ECC. It is difficult, if not impossible, to separate uniform and ubiquitous changes in organ

TABLE 1.1

The physiology and pharmacology of extracorporeal circulation compared to normal circulation and pulmonary function

Normal function	*Physiological changes with ECC*	*Mechanical factors*	*Pharmacological factors*
	↓ Total flow Negative venous P	Venous cannula size	Steroids
	↑ Adrenergic response		Adrenergic blockers
	↑ Renin-angiotensin	Arterial cannula site	
	Abnormal distribution		Diuretics
Blood flow	Non-pulsatile Non-servo	Pump characteristics	Volume expanders
	↓ Tissue washout		
	↓ Oxygen delivery Acidosis	Heat exchanger	Hypothermia Buffers-tris HCO_3^-
Gas exchange	O_2 - CO_2 exchange requires large blood volume	Oxygenator Disc Bubble Membrane	
	Microbubbles		Defoamer
	Emboli and aggregates	Reservoirs, connectors, tubing	? Platelet-active drugs
Blood-endothelial interface	Stagnant zones Anticoagulation	Surface coating	Heparin
	↑ Fibrinolytic activity		Priming solutions
	↓ Platelet function	Coronary suction	
Reticuloendothelial function	Blood dilution		Haemodilution
	Tissue histiocytes loaded	Filters	
	Phagocytosis ↓		

function associated with ECC from specific organ damage or deteriorating function due to our imperfect attempts to substitute devices for the heart and lungs. Hence, while some aspects of ECC can be clearly identified as pathophysiology (gross air embolism for example), in the current state of the art other aspects cannot be separated from normal function of the apparatus (platelet aggregate formation for example). In this sense *Table 1.1* represents both the physiology of ECC and the inherent pathophysiology.

Haemodynamics, blood volume and endocrine response to cardiopulmonary bypass

With the blood heparinized and venous and arterial cannulae in place, venoarterial bypass is instituted by draining venous blood via siphon into the extracorporeal device and returning a like amount of blood into the arterial circulation. As heart-lung bypass is gradually begun, flow through the pulmonary artery falls off faster than bypass flow increases, hence total flow in the systemic circulation decreases. These phenomena are diagrammed in *Figure 1.1*. Peripheral and pulmonary hypotension occur, and the final flow on total bypass may be less than the original baseline flow at the same blood volume. Hypotension is probably due to the haemodilution of the oxygenator priming solution[82]. Haemodilution reduces blood viscosity and secondarily systemic vascular resistance. Hypotension may occur when

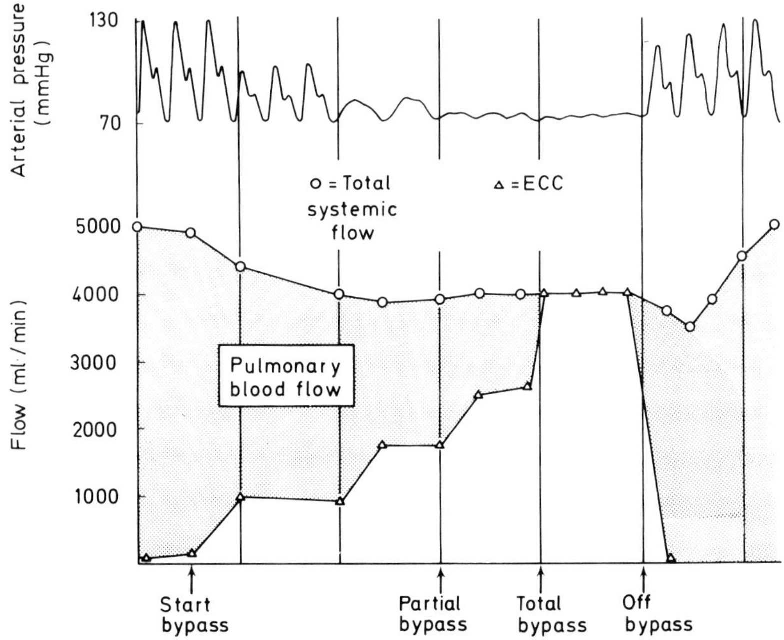

Figure 1.1 Changes in pulmonary and systemic haemodynamics as cardiopulmonary bypass is instituted

whole blood prime is used and therefore changes in viscosity do not fully explain the phenomenon. Others have felt that release of vasoactive substances occurs when bypass is begun and this produces hypotension[118].

If blood flow is held constant during perfusion, there will be a gradual decrease in the venous reservoir which requires transfusion replacement. The loss in blood volume might be explained by loss at the surgical site as well as sequestration into dissected tissues. Another factor is that oxygenator-priming solutions are usually haemodiluted to a varying degree depending on the surgical team's preference and particular case involved. Breckenridge, Digerness and Kirklin[30] and Cohn, Angell and Shumway[39] noted as much as a 20 per cent increase in extracellular fluid space following cardiopulmonary bypass. During the early experience with clinical perfusion, it was felt that a 'hidden reduction' in blood volume was due to sequestration secondary to homologous transfusion reaction or due to stagnant areas in the circulation[116]. Studies by Giannelli *et al.*[70] seem to eliminate this as a cause for alterations in blood volume during ECC. Plasma volume loss may also result from diuresis induced by adding mannitol or a potent diuretic to the oxygenator-priming solution. If blood volume replacement does not occur, perfusion of tissues is not optimal and metabolic acidosis follows.

As bypass is continued, there is generalized increase in sympathetic tone due to release of epinephrine from the adrenal medulla and norepinephrine from sympathetic nerve endings[154, 181]. This release of catecholamines is a result of stimulation of both the carotid sinus and aortic baroreceptors[84]. These receptors appear to respond to low-pulse amplitude which occurs during non-pulsatile perfusion[176], when total flow is decreased. Renin secretion from the kidney is increased in response to the decrease in mean arterial pressure and reduction in left atrial pressure. The increase in sympathetic tone results in arteriolar constriction, returning the arterial pressure toward normal.

If total flow remains constant, with the increase in pressure blood is preferentially directed to organs which are more responsive to increased perfusion pressure and least dependent on arteriolar tone. This includes the two most important organs – the brain and the heart. At the same time blood flow is most decreased in organs in which the vasculature is sensitive to an increased arteriolar tone and least sensitive to increased perfusion pressure such as skin and skeletal muscle. The resulting redistribution of blood flow under these circumstances has been studied by several investigators[113, 160, 161]. The results indicate that during cardiopulmonary bypass there is a redistribution of blood flow that results from factors other than alterations in pulse pressure or the use of non-pulsatile perfusion. The factors include anaesthesia, peripheral emboli, amount of haemodilution, effects on blood elements, etc. This neuroendocrine response and redistribution phenomenon may be diminished by alpha-adrenergic blocking anaesthetic drugs, such as halothane, in which case the arterial pressure remains relatively low under conditions of constant flow. Adding to the blood volume causes an increase in perfusion pressure if flow is held constant. Occasionally the neuroendocrine sympathetic response will dominate the haemodynamics, creating the syndrome of hypertension at constant flow with poor organ perfusion which may be serious enough to require definite alpha-adrenergic pharmacologic blockade[35, 65, 114, 122]. Usually at a constant but less than normal flow, the pressure will reflect a balance of increased sympathetic tone and alpha blockade induced by anaesthesia.

The haemodynamics of ECC have been evaluated by Gazzaniga *et al.*[64, 65] who utilized the method of skeletal muscle surface pH measurement to evaluate the perfusion metabolism relationship in that specific tissue. Since the arterial blood under conditions of anaesthesia or bypass is completely saturated with oxygen, decreasing muscle surface pH is a direct reflection of decreasing capillary flow. An initial decrease in muscle surface pH occurs with the induction of anaesthesia and its attendant minor myocardial depressant effects, demonstrating the sensitivity of the measurement. With the institution of cardiopulmonary bypass, muscle surface pH drops remarkably and then gradually continues to fall during the period of ECC, indicating inadequate tissue perfusion. The addition of blood volume results in an increase in arterial pressure at constant flow and minimizes to some extent the decreased organ perfusion resulting in a low plateau of muscle surface pH rather than a continuing fall. Preloading with volume can further minimize the low flow. The addition of alpha-adrenergic blockade reverses or nearly eliminates the muscle surface acidosis, indicating the major role of alpha-adrenergic stimulation during ECC[65]. Venous pH, as a more general and less sensitive measure of organ

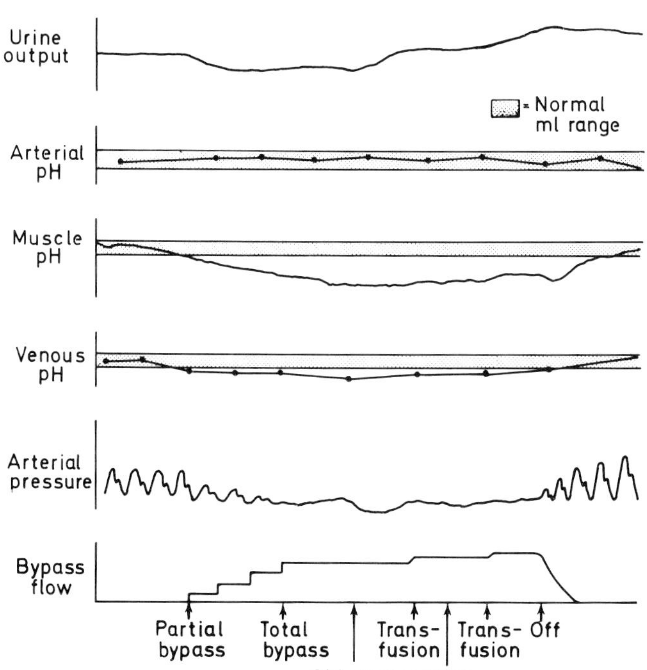

Figure 1.2 Muscle surface pH during extracorporeal circulation, as a measure of the tissue perfusion. Increasing blood volume and decreasing arteriolar sympathetic tone resulted in improved perfusion

perfusion, falls during bypass at a constant P_{CO_2}. More specifically, a condition of metabolic acidosis can be detected by measurement of pH and P_{CO_2}[114]. Urine output usually falls during bypass, although the concomitant effects of antidiuretic endocrine stimuli and pharmacologically induced diuresis by haemodilution, mannitol, or diuretics, make observation of the urine output a questionable indicator of perfusion in a clinical situation. These effects are summarized in *Figure 1.2*.

Mechanical limitations to physiological cardiopulmonary bypass

Even with conditions of alpha-blockade and volume loading, can normal peripheral blood flow of 3.1 ℓ/min per m^2 be achieved with an artificial device? Probably so, but at the expense of somewhat increased risk due to increased flow in the extracorporeal circuit (i.e. high arterial line pressure, faster pumping rates, more surface exposure per minute, more chance of micro-air embolism, possibly greater chance of aggregate embolism). With the current state of the art, bypass flow of 2.2 to 2.4 ℓ/min per m^2 is generally considered an adequate and safe compromise[153, 182]. The resulting moderate flow state is well tolerated for the one to two hours required for most intracardiac operations and this does not result in any permanent sequelae. Hence flow levels of 2.4 ℓ/min per m^2 have come to be considered 'normal' physiology of extracorporeal circulation during condition of total cardiopulmonary bypass, although this need not necessarily be the case.

Mechanical factors affecting bypass flow rates include the size and position of venous and arterial cannulae, the nature of the pump and type of oxygenator. The flow obtained in total bypass is a function of the blood volume and the diameter of the venous lines. Assuming that 100 cmH_2O of siphon suction is applied to the venous cannulae, the maximal possible flow increases linearly with tubing size until high flow rates are achieved[143]. Under conditions of inadequate venous return, whether due to low blood volume or low arterial perfusion with sequestration, the flow through the venous line is regulated by the collapsing of vena cavae around the venous cannulae. Under conditions of adequate venous return the bypass flow is limited by the size and length of the venous drainage lines. The resistance to flow is directly related to the length of tubing and inversely related to the fourth power of the radius of the tubing[18].

Under the conditions of non-pulsatile flow the size of the arterial cannula is not a major consideration. If 5 ℓ/min is pumped 5 ℓ/min will emanate from the cannula orifice. If the cannula is long and narrow, high pressure in the arterial perfusion line will result, with the possibility of tubing separation or rupture, but adequate flow is still delivered. The jet effects imposed by such an arterial constriction are generally not significant enough to cause blood damage and they become important only if the jet is directed at the left subclavian or carotid orifice, or at a specific atherosclerotic plaque[106]. Whether arterial perfusion is provided retrograde via a femoral or iliac artery or prograde via the aortic arch or subclavian artery, it appears to have no effect on the physiology of ECC under conditions of total bypass or under conditions of partial bypass when lung function is normal.

Resistance to flow in the arterial cannula does become an important factor if pulsatile flow is desired in the extracorporeal circuit. Under conditions of pulsatile pumping, flow rates during the systolic phase may be five to ten times the baseline minute flow rate. Resistance in a small arterial cannula may become a critical limiting factor by damping the pulse contour and reaching the point of significant jet effect, causing red cell damage.

Pulsatile flow during ECC has been a controversial subject. Since blood flow is normally pulsatile it would seem desirable to try to emulate this pulse contour with a mechanical device. There is universal agreement that the kidney 'interprets' non-pulsatile flow as inadequate flow, resulting in renin production and antidiuresis. This phenomenon, first described over 25 years ago, has been found by all investigators[76, 103, 121, 183, 196]. Several groups could find no other effects of non-pulsatile total body perfusion[28, 83, 161, 200]. However, equally competent researchers have reported a syndrome of high systemic vascular resistance, high blood catecholamine levels and poor tissue perfusion, resulting in cerebral changes, renal failure and severe lactic acidosis[50, 154, 165]. Trinkle *et al.* found this syndrome during non-pulsatile perfusion in animals[186], but found an equal incidence of the poor perfusion syndrome in both pulsatile and non-pulsatile flow during cardiac surgery in man[185]. These apparent contradictions can be resolved by careful examination of the experimental methods correlated with the classic studies of Harrison *et al.*[84, 85].

Normally, blood flow is approximately 110 ml/kg body weight with a pulse amplitude of 20–40 mmHg (with some species variations). The studies that demonstrated acidosis and organ failure during non-pulsatile flow were all conducted at flow rates ranging from 60 to 100 ml/kg[50, 154, 165, 172, 183, 186]. Those investigators who found no difference between pulsatile and non-pulsatile flow used total perfusion rates of 130–200 ml/kg[28, 83, 161, 200]. This relationship could have been predicted from the studies of Harrison *et al.*[84, 85] who showed that adrenal catecholamine secretion is regulated in part by carotid sinus baroreceptors. Decreased pulse amplitude caused maximal catecholamine output when total flow was less than normal, but minimal catecholamine output during normal and above normal flow rates. From Harrison's findings, one might expect no difference between normal flow, pulsatile perfusion and non-pulsatile perfusion at flow rates over 110 ml/kg. The high-resistance-acidosis syndrome would occur during non-pulsatile perfusion only at flow rates of 80–110 ml/kg, and the high-resistance-acidosis syndrome during both pulsatile and non-pulsatile perfusion at flow rates less than 70 ml/kg. This corresponds almost exactly to the reports listed above. Harrison's studies and most of the comparative studies listed above were carried out at 37°C. The effects of hypothermia and its relationship to normal blood flow requirement of the carotid sinus adrenal axis have not been thoroughly studied. This probably accounts for some of the variations seen during clinical cases[139, 185].

The implications of these studies for total cardiopulmonary bypass in cardiac surgery are significant as total perfusion is usually carried out at flow rates of 70–100 ml/kg. At this abnormally low flow rate the adrenal catecholamine secretion is increased by the decreased pulse amplitude, hence pulsatile flow[31] or alpha-blockade should be used to ameliorate the systemic effects of the altered flow pattern. During partial cardiopulmonary bypass for life support, total flow should be maintained as near normal as possible, and should be regulated by whatever means necessary to assure a pulse amplitude of 15 mmHg or more.

Gas exchange and oxygen delivery

Gas exchange has proved to be the easiest problem of ECC. Flowing blood is exposed to oxygen either directly or through a gas-permeable membrane. Oxygen diffuses into the blood plasma because of a gradient between high $P\text{O}_2$ in the gas phase and the low $P\text{O}_2$ in mixed venous blood. Oxygen then diffuses from the plasma through the red cell membrane to combine with unsaturated haemoglobin. The chemical binding of oxygen to haemoglobin proceeds very rapidly and the limiting factor in oxygenation of flowing blood is the rate of oxygen diffusion through plasma[15]. Hence, the thickness of the blood film between gas bubbles or surfaces, or between gas exchange membranes becomes the rate-limiting factor. CO_2 diffuses out of the flowing blood in the gas exchange device because of the gradient between the $P\text{CO}_2$ in mixed venous blood and the partial pressure of CO_2 in the ventilating gas. Although the gradient for CO_2 exchange is relatively low and can never be greater than the mixed venous $P\text{CO}_2$, the rate of diffusion of CO_2 through plasma is so rapid that CO_2 removal always proceeds more efficiently than oxygenation. Hence, to avoid excess CO_2 removal with its attendant alkalosis, the gradient is diminished by adding CO_2 to the ventilating gas or by reducing the gas flow.

Oxygenator performance

The performance characteristics of the gas exchange device must be thoroughly documented to plan the best extracorporeal circuit for any given patient. Since CO_2 removal is almost invariably greater than oxygenation, it is sufficient to describe the performance of gas exchange devices in terms of their oxygenating efficiency. The following factors must be known about the gas exchange device. How much oxygen can actually be supplied per minute? How much oxygen can be supplied under conditions of variable blood flow and variable mixed venous saturation? How much O_2 can be supplied at flow rates which are compatible with adequate perfusion for the patient in question (i.e. at least 2.4 ℓ/min per m^2)? What flow of ventilating gas is required? How much foreign surface is exposed to the flowing blood (this number is easy to derive for membrane oxygenators, but much more difficult for gas interface oxygenators)? What effects does the gas exchange device have on the components of flowing blood, if any?

Many of these factors have been conveniently combined into a single expression of oxygenator performance defined as *rated flow*[60]. The rated flow is the flow at which blood leaving the oxygenator is 95 per cent saturated, under the conditions of normal mixed venous blood inflow. In other words, when venous blood (haemoglobin 15 g/100 ml $P\text{O}_2$, 40 mmHg, saturation 65 per cent, O_2 content 15ml/100 ml) is pumped through a gas exchange device at 100 ml/min, the outflow blood will be 100 per cent saturated (Po_2 150mmHg, O_2 content 20 ml/100 ml). The amount of O_2 actually delivered by the device is determined by the flow rate and the arteriovenous (AV) difference. In this example the O_2 delivery is 5 ml/100 ml blood × 100 ml/min = 5 ml O_2 delivery/min. As blood flow through the device is increased, a point is reached at which the limiting factor is the thickness of the blood film and the rate at which O_2 diffuses through that particular film. When that point is exceeded, the outflow blood will exit at less than 100 per cent saturation. The rated flow for a given device is that flow at which this limitation is reached. The *rated O_2 delivery* is the amount of O_2 that can be taken up by the blood at the rated flow. The upper limit of O_2 delivery is related to the flow and to the amount of unsaturated haemoglobin presented to the oxygenator per minute. If total bypass flow is decreased at a constant level of tissue oxygen consumption, venous saturation must decrease as more oxygen is extracted from the flowing blood. As long as this does not exceed the oxygenating capability of the gas exchange device, the oxygenator will compensate and function at a wider arteriovenous (AV) difference. Some of these variables are outlined in *Figure 1.3*, in which the oxygen delivery per minute is

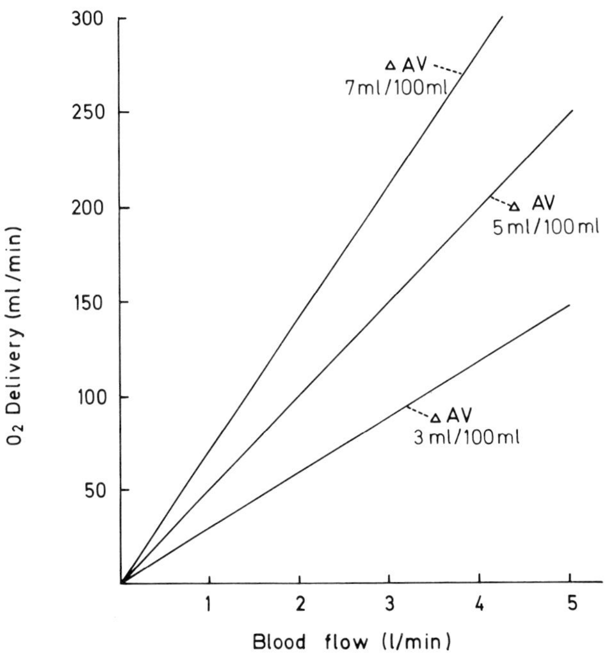

Figure 1.3 Oxygen delivery is directly related to blood flow and arteriovenous difference. The maximum oxygen that can be delivered for a given blood flow at a given venous saturation is shown here. This represents the maximum amount of oxygen delivery that could be accomplished by a gas exchange device under a given set of flow and inlet conditions

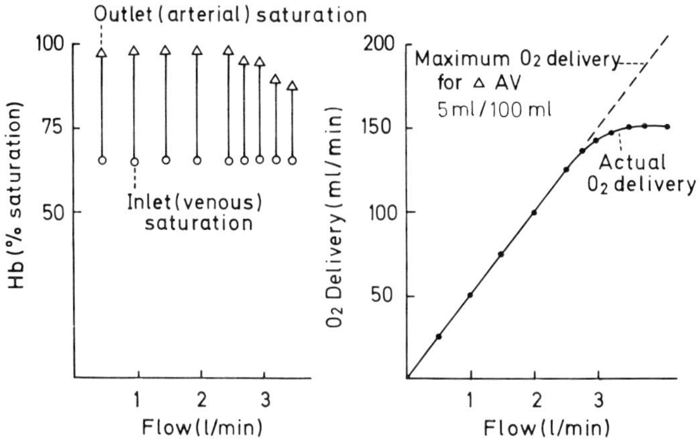

Figure 1.4 The concept of rated flow. A hypothetical gas exchange device has a maximum oxygen transfer capability of 150 ml/min based on the surface area and blood flow characteristics. As long as the oxygen transport capability of flowing blood is less than 150 ml/min fully saturated blood leaves the oxygenator. When the oxygen transport capability of flowing blood exceeds this amount, desaturated blood results. Under normal venous blood conditions this occurs at a flow rate of 3 ℓ/min, the rated flow for this device. At flow rates in excess of 3 ℓ/min, the outlet blood is desaturated, the AV difference is narrow, and the actual oxygen transferred reaches a plateau

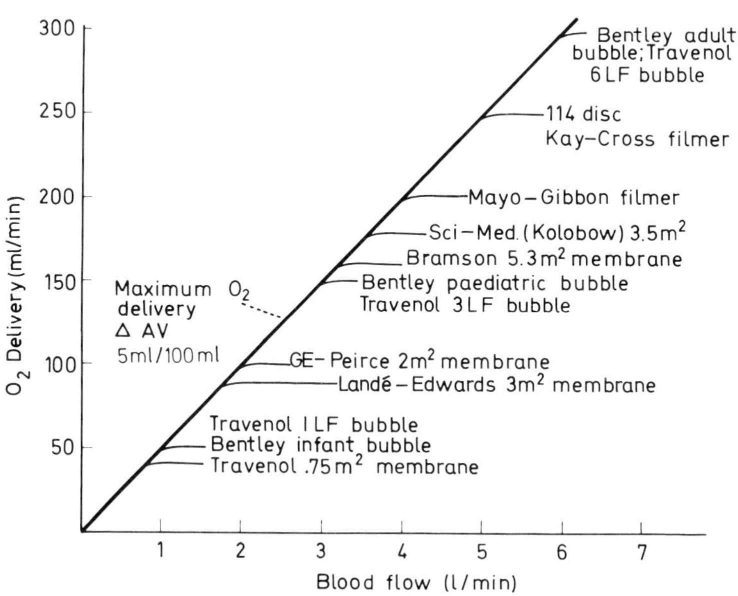

Figure 1.5 Rated flow under normal venous inlet conditions for a variety of commercial oxygenators. (Data based on publications cited in text or manufacturer's data sheet.) When modular units are used in parallel the rated flow becomes the sum of rated flows of all units in the circuit

related to the flow in ℓ/min for different levels of venous saturation or arteriovenous difference. Notice that oxygen delivery is entirely dependent on flow. Decreasing flow severely decreases oxygen delivery, although fully saturated blood with a high P_{O_2} will be perfused into the arterial system.

Reports on oxygenating performance of gas exchange devices must include at least enough data to calculate inflow and outflow O_2 content and rated flow. These data are available in most recent experimental studies[11, 38, 53, 60, 130, 142] but are not available for some of the older established oxygenators[45, 201]. In planning the components of an extracorporeal circuit the oxygen requirement of the patient at normothermia is calculated (150 ml/min per m^2). The blood flow which will deliver this amount of oxygen with an AV difference of 5 ml/100 ml, is calculated or determined from a graph (*Figure 1.3*). The cannulae, tubing and pump are chosen to provide the desired flow. An oxygenator is selected which has a rated flow at or above the desired flow.

The concept of rated flow is demonstrated again in *Figure 1.4* and the rated flow for several oxygenators is outlined in *Figure 1.5*. If a gas exchange device is operated at flow rates higher than its rated flow, desaturated blood will be perfused and the actual O_2 delivery per minute reaches a fairly level plateau regardless of the flow rate.

Types of oxygenators

Assuming that the oxygenator will be used at appropriate flow rates below the rated flow, the choice of an oxygenator must be related to the ease of use and the possible damage to blood components. Two basic types of gas exchange devices are used in extracorporeal circuits: a *direct gas interface oxygenator* in which O_2 is bubbled, filmed, or foamed directly through blood and blood is then defoamed or debubbled through some type of settling or filtering chamber, or a *membrane oxygenator* in which a gas exchange membrane is interposed between the gas phase and the blood phase. Membranes may be silicone 'rubber' or microporous materials. Gas interface oxygenators have the advantage of simplicity, disposability and relatively low cost. Disadvantages include the possibility of gross or microscopic air embolism, relatively large priming volumes (although if the priming volume remains constant its exact volume is not important), variable reservoir level resulting in potential shifts in blood volume between the intracorporeal and extracorporeal circuit and the effects of direct gas interface including protein denaturation[48, 112], increased fragility of red cells[20], susceptibility to haemolysis, denaturation of platelet membrane materials resulting in platelet aggregation, clumping and removal from circulation[52, 57]. The effects of gas interface oxygenators may be caused more by the repeated renewal of the interface[13] than by the nature of the interface itself[100, 144]. Membrane oxygenators have the advantage of eliminating blood-gas interface effects, constant blood volume and ease of operation. The disadvantages of membrane oxygenators include expense, potential difficulty in eliminating all bubbles during priming and moderately large, although constant, priming volumes in some instances. Changes in plasma proteins, lipoproteins and red cells surfaces, which occur with gas interface oxygenators, appear not to occur with membrane oxygenators[48, 112]. However, some degree of platelet surface modification with resultant aggregation occurs with the membrane oxygenator[52, 57].

Many of the published reports on pump or membrane oxygenator characteristics have included an open gas interface reservoir in the experimental design[21, 52, 55]. Data from these studies are applicable to ECC for cardiac surgery, as coronary suction will always require some of the blood exposed to a direct gas interface. However, characterization of physiological changes of ECC or blood surface exposure should be done in experimental models which specifically exclude any gas interface to eliminate variables caused by that non-physiological condition.

Microporous membranes are made of non-wettable substances such as Teflon perforated with multiple small holes which permit gas transfer but preclude blood leakage because of surface tension effects. Laboratory and clinical results with microporous oxygenators are encouraging[55, 71, 131]. Oxygen and CO_2 transfer in a gas-to-gas test system are virtually unlimited with this type of membrane, but the plasma oxygen diffusion limitations still exist when blood is applied to the membrane. Hence, microporous membranes will have oxygen transfer characteristics similar to other membrane oxygenators of similar flow design. CO_2 transfer will be significantly better, however. The latter consideration is important only in oxygenators where mixing is intense[11] and CO_2 transfer is the limiting design variable. Haematologic studies indicate that the blood interface effects are more similar to a membrane device than a gas interface device[71]. Specific types of gas interface and membrane oxygenators and performance data are discussed in subsequent chapters of this book. Of the gas interface oxygenators, bubble oxygenators are most widely used because of the ease of assembly and priming and the low expense. Similar physiological effects are induced by all blood-gas interface oxygenators, whether of bubble, filming or foaming type. Membrane oxygenators can be characterized as sandwich type,[91, 104, 108, 166, 187], capillary type or induced mixing type[11]. Physiological effects on flowing blood appear to be the same between different types of membrane oxygenators. The reader interested in membrane oxygenator design, development and use is referred to an excellent review by Drinker[49]. Clinical use of membrane oxygenators for prolonged ECC has been reviewed by Peirce[141], Zapol and Qvist[205] and Bartlett and Gazzaniga[13].

Blood surface interface effects

The effects of prolonged (more than 6 hours) direct gas exposure on plasma proteins and formed blood elements discussed above are so obvious and lethal that the more subtle changes due to the prosthetic vascular interface have been masked in many studies. This aspect of ECC is recently coming under more careful scrutiny. Normally flowing blood is continuously exposed to endothelial cells. Fibrin formation probably takes place continuously on the endothelial surface balanced exactly by plasmin formation and concomitant fibrinolysis. Both of these reactions proceed at a very slow and balanced rate so that the end effect is a slow but definitely measurable gradual fibrinogen-to-fibrin conversion, an identical rate of fibrin degradation and elimination of fibrin degradation products. This delicate balance is abruptly upset by exposure of blood to collagen fibres underlying endothelial cells, tissue collagen, tissue thromboplastin, air, necrotic tissue or disrupted cells and to some extent foreign material in the bloodstream itself such as endotoxin. Under these circumstances the conversion of fibrinogen to fibrin is grossly exaggerated and proceeds to clotting much faster than fibrinolysis takes place. Concomitantly, platelet surfaces are altered, platelet adhesion and aggregation occur, platelets release platelet factor III, stimulating further formation of fibrin clot. The fact that this chain of events occurs results in normal haemostasis. If serious deficiencies occur in any of the various protein enzymes which constitute the coagulation mechanism, or if any of these enzyme steps are inhibited by a drug or by lack of a catalyst such as calcium, or if platelet numbers or function are severely decreased, then haemostasis is disordered. (Presumably a state of excess plasmin formation with fibrinolysis could also account for disordered coagulation, although the actual clinical occurrence of this phenomenon is rare.) The enzymes of the protein coagulation system (clotting factors) have received appropriate interest and study over the past two decades in relationship to ECC[12, 57]. The number and quality of platelets[44, 51, 88, 164] and the status of the plasminogen–plasmin system[62, 63] with the production of fibrin degradation products (FDP) are equally as important when considering surface interface effects.

Fibrin formation and lysis

In the process of ECC the blood is suddenly exposed to various types of plastic, glass, metal, cloth, direct gas bubble interfaces and a variety of foreign chemicals used for coating and priming the device. During cardiac surgery, blood is aspirated from the field ('coronary' suction) and mixed with the perfusate. This blood may include tissue thromboplastin, clots, lysed clots, serum, gross particles of fat and muscle and bone, suture and other foreign material all mixed together with large amounts of air to the point of being frothy[135, 137]. In addition to all these abnormal circumstances, the extracorporeal circuit contains innumerable flat edges, right-angle turns, totally stagnant zones, recirculating zones, jet zones—in short, flow characteristics unlike anything found in conditions of normal physiology. All of these factors have the effect of stimulating both the protein and the platelet arms of the clotting system. Considering the magnitude of forces which combine to stimulate clotting in the extracorporeal system, it seems incredible that this complex system can be held totally in abeyance by a single drug–heparin. Understanding and controlling coagulation and anticoagulants is the major thrust of research in prolonged ECC. However, for cardiac surgery it is apparent that effective total anticoagulation, presumably with heparin, will always be a central part of this technique because of the problems of coronary suction and low pulmonary and atrial flow.

The physiological changes associated with ECC must include those associated with heparinization as part of the normal baseline. To measure clotting accurately by any of the many tests which require a fibrin clot as an end point, the amount of heparin in the blood must be measured or estimated and inactivated with the appropriate amount of hexadimethrine bromide (Polybrene)[57]. For intracardiac surgery it is desirable to maintain a prolonged clotting time with excessive amounts of heparin during the period of bypass. This requires at least 200 units/kg of patient weight and 200 units/ℓ of blood in the priming solution. To provide an extra margin of safety most teams infuse 300 units/kg into the patient and 150 units/kg at 30 minute intervals during the entire period of bypass. (Since heparin activity is measured by bioassay, activity is standardized in units of anticoagulant activity. Most heparin preparations are considered to contain 100 units/mg, although this may be technically incorrect.) Heparin is derived from animal tissues by various manufacturers. Heparin can be derived from any tissue where mast cells exist. The lung of most species is uniquely deficient in the enzyme heparinase; hence, heparin derived from animal lungs has been said to be the most stable and reliable[73]. This has been questioned by Jaques[96]. Heparin carries a very strong negative charge and will become bonded to positive charges wherever they occur on glass or plastic

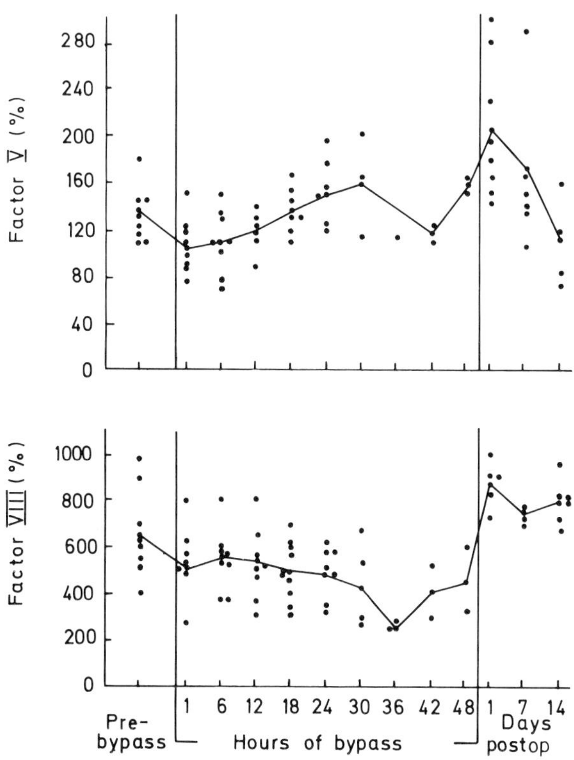

Figure 1.6 Changes in clotting factors during prolonged ECC in the sheep. (Reproduced from Fong *et al.*[57] by courtesy of *Transactions of the American Society for Artificial Internal Organs*)

surfaces; therefore, care must be taken when adding small amounts of heparin to fluids which are exposed to a large surface area. Fletcher *et al.*[56] have reported a series of studies showing that ECC can be carried out in dogs and monkeys without heparin. These provocative studies deserve careful scrutiny.

Changes that occur in the coagulation platelet system during prolonged ECC (24–48 hours) without gas interfaces are outlined in *Figures 1.6* and *1.7*. These studies are used as examples of extensive blood surface contact. Changes during the first few hours are typical of those seen during cardiac surgery. In these studies partial (60–80 per cent) venoarterial bypass was carried out in awake lambs and the heparin dose regulated at a low level. The initial changes are due to surface absorption and dilution with the prime. These data indicate coagulation changes due to ECC alone without a gas interface. In *Figure 1.8* the changes are compared to a 24 hour bypass with the bubble oxygenator. Changes are exaggerated after 4–6 hours.

Several of the many steps between activation of surface factor (factor XII) and fibrin formation are inhibited by heparin. There is good evidence that many proteins are absorbed on foreign surfaces within seconds of exposure to flowing blood[192]. One of these proteins is fibrinogen; in fact fibrinogen may have the greatest affinity for protein binding sites on plastic and glass and metal[119]. In the absence of anticoagulant this fibrinogen is

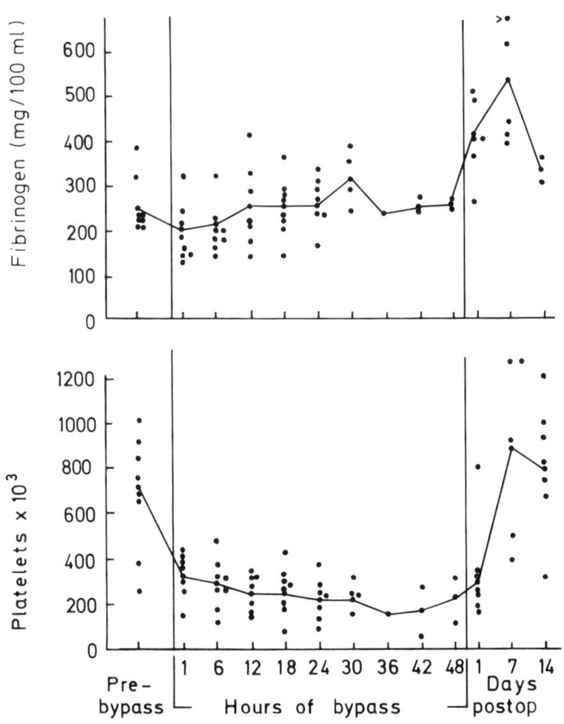

Figure 1.7 Changes in clotting factors during prolonged ECC in the sheep. (Reproduced from Fong *et al.*[57] by courtesy of *Transactions of the American Society for Artificial Internal Organs*)

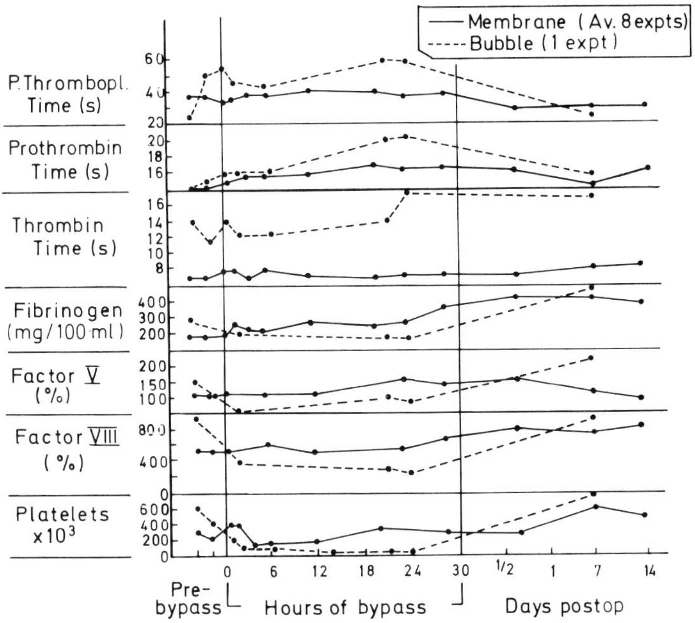

Figure 1.8 Changes in clotting factors during prolonged extracorporeal circulation in the sheep. Eight sheep perfused with membrane oxygenators are compared to values for one sheep perfused with a bubble oxygenator. The major differences between the bubble and membrane oxygenators become apparent after 4–6 hours of ECC. (Reproduced from Fong *et al.*[57] by courtesy of *Transactions of the American Society for Artificial Internal Organs*)

then converted into fibrin within minutes, leading to clot formation. With heparin present this fibrinogen is not converted and clotting does not occur.

The other protein clotting factors are similarly absorbed to some extent by foreign surface exposure so that the actual amount of clotting factors drops significantly with the initiation of bypass. At the same time synthesis of fibrinogen and other clotting factors by the liver increases, so that the concentration of these proteins returns to pre-bypass levels within a period of hours and remains normal throughout a prolonged bypass period. Excessive synthesis continues so that these proteins may be present in greater than normal amounts after bypass, creating a hypercoagulable state[10, 57]. During the 1–3 hour period of ECC required for most intracardiac operations this compensation has not had time to proceed to completion, hence levels of protein clotting factors including fibrinogen are generally normal or slightly decreased at the time when bypass is discontinued and heparin is inactivated[61].

Activation of circulating plasminogen to plasmin invariably occurs as fibrinogen is activated to fibrin; hence any clot contains the enzymatic means for its own self-destruction. Evidence of active circulating plasmin can be detected whenever gross clotting is present. Measurements of fibrinolytic activity indicate increased circulating plasmin during thoracotomy prior to heparinization[102]. These levels remain constant or decrease during the period of heparinization and ECC.

Plasmin is destroyed in the reticuloendothelial (RE) cells in the liver. Decreased RE function post-bypass[178] leads to higher blood levels of plasmin. There is no evidence to indicate that this circulating plasmin is harmful; specifically it is not associated with abnormal bleeding following a period of ECC. This delicate balance between fibrin formation and fibrinolysis and the potential for abrupt increase in fibrin formation upon reversal of heparin in a patient where all of the protein factors have been stimulated by foreign surface exposure, has led some investigators to propose that heparin should not be inactivated at the end of bypass but rather be allowed to gradually metabolize over a period of 1–4 hours[61]. This suggestion is valuable in theory although it has not been extensively adopted clinically. Brooks and Bahnson[33] described excessive fibrinolysis after ECC associated with a plasminogen activator contaminating reused portions of a pump oxygenator. In that instance, excess fibrinolytic activity *was* associated with abnormal bleeding.

Platelet activity during extracorporeal circulation

Platelet physiology has gained the spotlight for ECC research in this decade. It is of such importance that Chapter 14 of this book is devoted primarily to that subject. The concentration of platelets drops abruptly with the onset of ECC and continues to fall as long as bypass continues[57].

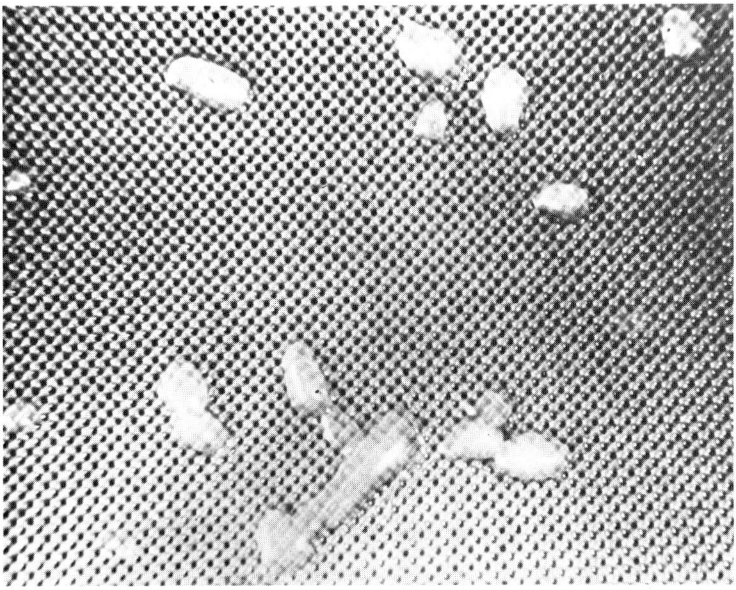

Figure 1.9 Platelet aggregates trapped on a 25 μm filter during ECC. (Reproduced from Dutton *et al.*[52] by courtesy of *Journal of Thoracic and Cardiovascular Surgery*)

This is due in part to platelets adhering directly to the foreign surfaces but to a greater extent to platelets adhering to each other and to white cells, forming platelet aggregates of 10–200 μm which are infused into the patient[44, 51]. These aggregates circulate widely and would appear to become emboli in capillary beds. Dutton *et al.*[52] have shown that even the best designed extracorporeal circuit generates platelet aggregate 'emboli' (*Figure 1.9*). Since all platelets do not disappear during ECC either platelet formation must be greatly increased or the platelet aggregate 'emboli' must break down into individual platelet components. Evidence favouring the latter has been presented in an elegant study by Hicks *et al.*[88]. They demonstrated that during venovenous partial bypass, radioactively tagged platelets were not trapped in the lung (the target capillary bed); rather they appear in the reticuloendothelial system, particularly in the spleen and the liver, for a period of time and reappear in the circulating blood. Further evidence that platelet aggregates do not form significant microvascular emboli is available from prolonged venoarterial bypass carried out for severe pulmonary insufficiency. If platelet aggregates caused true emboli and disrupted the microcirculation, tissue damage would result. However, during prolonged ECC we have perfused patients on near total bypass (5ℓ/min) for 3 to 16 days without evidence of systemic organ damage and without embolization, infarcts, or aggregates found in tissue at autopsy.

Ubiquitous thrombocytopenia associated with ECC has led to investigation of inhibition of platelet function by drugs, to determine the effect on that phenomenen[124, 155, 191]. These studies have shown that drugs which decrease platelet adhesiveness (dipyridamole, Pluronic F68) minimize the platelet loss, with prompt return to normal levels post-bypass, whereas aspirin, which affects platelet factor III release only and Syndoxicon, a drug which affects aggregation only, do not influence platelet count during or after bypass. These studies suggest that the mechanism of thrombocytopenia is platelet aggregation with removal of the aggregates by the reticuloendothelial cells, particularly in the spleen and liver. These aggregates are reversible and the same platelets recirculate, perhaps after regaining adequate amounts of ADP. Some of this effect can be prevented by dipyridamole administration, although the value of maintaining a higher platelet count by inhibiting adhesion has not yet been demonstrated. Becker, Smith and Dobell[16] have shown evidence of improved tissue perfusion and less metabolic acidosis during bypass conducted in dipyridamole-treated animals. Addonizio *et al.*[3] have reported that platelet numbers and function are preserved during ECC with prostaglandin E_1. Normal function (as measured by bleeding time) returns after ECC. In the future the combination of heparin with short-acting platelet function inhibitors will probably be a routine technique in ECC. The relationships of platelet count, function tests and drugs are discussed in detail in Chapter 14.

Haemodynamic and flow factors in relation to surface effects

Stagnant blood will clot even in undamaged endothelial-lined surfaces. Correspondingly, areas with very low flow in an extracorporeal circuit will form thrombus even when the patient is completely heparinized. Scientific validity was lent to this empirical observation recently by Spaeth *et al.*[174]

who demonstrated the formation of fibrin and platelet deposits on surfaces where flow was stagnant. It is equally important to avoid right-angled turns and eddy current areas in extracorporeal circuits. Thrombus begins to form at the downstream right-angled edge of anticoagulant-coated plastic rings placed in the venous circulation[23]. A 2 mm step-off between a connector and a piece of tubing in the bypass circuit would seem insignificant with 5 or 6 ℓ/min of blood lavaging its surface. However, a non-circulating area many microns in diameter will exist in the corner of such a junction where platelets and white cells may lie relatively still for long periods of time. Here, heparin may be metabolized and thrombus formation occurs. The fewer connections and access sites and the simpler the extracorporeal circuit, the less the problem of thrombus formation and direct embolization will be. The interested reader is referred to a detailed symposium summarizing the state of knowledge in flowing blood surface interface effects[190, 193].

Use of filters

Because of the evidence presented above that platelet aggregate formation is not necessarily detrimental to microcirculation it appears unnecessary to attempt to filter out aggregates which form during a single pass through the extracorporeal circuit. The observation that significant amounts of material can be removed from the circulation by filters[69] does not necessarily mean that filtration is beneficial. However, it is of extreme importance to filter out aggregates that are glued together with fibrin which will not break up when they arrive at a capillary bed. For these reasons careful filtration of the coronary aspirate and of transfused blood is mandatory, whereas on-line filtration of the entire arterial perfusion is not. In fact total perfusion filtration may be detrimental, as platelet aggregates will be removed from the circulation and may disassemble more slowly in a prosthetic filter than in the spleen, liver or lymph nodes. Dacron wool filters of 20–30 μm pore size have the overall effect of removing large numbers of platelets from the circulation. Polyurethane 50 μm filters do not have this effect but may let small fibrin particles get by. Guidoin *et al.*[78] have recently published comparative studies of commonly used filters. It should be noted that filters do serve as excellent microbubble traps and 50 μm filters may be recommended for the main arterial line when a bubble oxygenator is used [37]. The problem of on-line filtration will be solved when membrane oxygenators are generally available at a cost sufficiently low to warrant their use for intracardiac operations. Most membrane oxygenators are, by nature of their construction, also excellent filters with pore sizes ranging from 100 to 200 μm.

Interface effects on other formed elements

There are few reports on haemolysis and blood cell survival which do not involve a blood-gas interface somewhere in the study system. However, studies of prolonged partial ECC in normal animals[12, 80, 104] and in patients[90] and prolonged intracorporeal implantation of pumping devices with prosthetic linings[19] all indicate that haemolysis is negligible and the survival of radioactive-labelled red blood cells is not altered by prolonged exposure to the prosthetic interfaces in systems without a gas interface. This is true regardless of the oral intake of the animal or patient studied. Since ECC for cardiac surgery will usually involve a direct gas interface and coronary suction, the haemolysis which occurs after the red cells have been exposed to a gas interface will always be a part of ECC for cardiac surgery. Several investigators have studied the mechanical and chemical factors affecting red cell fragility and haemolysis under circumstances of gas exposure[20, 23, 145]. Indeglia *et al.*[93] studied red cell lysis under controlled conditions and found that haemolysis increased dramatically in lipaemic plasma and decreased with decreasing temperature in normal and lipaemic plasma. They concluded that the factors which predispose sensitized red cells to haemolysis are more chemical than mechanical, and pointed out the importance of avoiding lipaemic blood for transfusion or priming for ECC.

All types of white blood cells decrease in concentration with the initiation of ECC. This may be explained partly on the basis of simple dilution but aggregation and embolization may also occur. These effects can be inhibited by prostaglandin E_1[26].

White blood cell concentration returns to normal or above normal levels in 2 to 4 hours after institution of bypass. This occurs primarily in the granulocytic series[23, 57]. Although the actual number of white cells is increased, phagocytic function is decreased, as pointed out by Silva, Hoeksema and Fekety[173]. Changes in phagocytic activity and other reticuloendothelial functions are discussed in the next section.

Clinical significance of blood surface interface effects

Coagulation during bypass is prevented with heparin although many surface effects occur. The important clinical problem is returning to normal haemostasis and prevention of bleeding after ECC. First of all the heparin effect must be neutralized. This is generally done by adding an equal dose of protamine sulphate. Clot in the operative field is evidence of adequate heparin reversal. If bleeding persists, the heparin effect should be measured by some accelerated clotting time technique[8, 129, 147]. If the heparin effect persists more protamine is given and the measurements repeated. Deheparinization was studied by Jaberi, Bell and Benson[94] who reported better heparin control with accelerated blood recalcification time, and more accurate protamine administration. These results were confirmed by Bull *et al.*[34], Babka *et al.*[7] and Friesen and Clement[59]. Activated clotting time (ACT) must be measured in whole blood (rather than plasma) because the heparin effect is inversely related to platelet count. We have found that kaolin-activated clotting (as in most commercial systems) is satisfactory when the platelet count is normal, but inadequate during thrombocytopenia. This may account for erratic results reported by some[6]. For measuring ACT during ECC, therefore, the reagent should contain fresh thromboplastins[129]. Routine use of accelerated clotting time measurements when reversing heparin should become a routine aspect of clinical ECC. Protamine is a moderate peripheral vasodilator and will cause hypotension when infused rapidly. It has a positive inotropic effect and peripheral flow appears to increase with protamine[77]. Despite evidence of increased fibrinolytic activity and altered platelet function with ECC, postoperative bleeding which requires reoperation is almost always related to specific bleeding vessels[74]. If the patient is allowed to bleed but transfused to the point of near total blood volume, then a coagulopathy associated with platelet-poor bank blood will be produced, requiring fresh platelet transfusion. The indication for reoperation should be precise and conservative (for example, cumulative chest drainage of 15 per cent of the blood volume any time within the first 12 hours after bypass requires reoperation). When a significant coagulopathy occurs, it is associated with prolonged bypass with gas interface oxygenation, low platelet count, and multiple transfusions. This coagulopathy is not reversed by epsilon aminocaproic acid, hence it is not due to excessive fibrinolysis[67]. The defect is in platelet quantity and quality, and must be treated by fresh platelet concentrate or fresh blood. This fact establishes a good rationale for drawing off 500 ml of the patient's blood with exchange replacement immediately prior to bypass. This blood is then reinfused at the end of bypass, as has been suggested by Hallowell *et al*[79]. A rapidly metabolized drug which would inhibit platelet adhesiveness during bypass (such as dipyridamole[16] or PGE_1[3]) may have a similar effect of returning healthy 'protected' platelets to the circulation after bypass.

Patients with platelet function defects prior to bypass will present severe bleeding problems after operation despite normal 'screen' tests of coagulation. These rare disorders are suggested by a history of bleeding with minor trauma and are detected by bleeding time or *in vitro* platelet function tests. A recent review of the subject is that of Deykin[46]. Ekert and Sheers[54] have recently demonstrated abnormal platelet function in children with cyanotic congenital heart disease which returned to normal after correction of the cardiac defect. This may explain the propensity to bleeding which occurs after bypass in cyanotic heart disease[102] and which improves with platelet transfusion[202].

After ECC, clotting factors and platelets return to normal or above normal levels[57]. In occasional cases where abnormal coagulation occurs 24 hours or more after bypass it is usually due to consumption coagulopathy associated with low cardiac output[29].

Organ function and damage during extracorporeal circulation

As noted in the preceding section, total cardiopulmonary bypass, as usually carried out, invokes a moderate low flow state. Changes in organ function which occur following ECC are those of one to two hours of relatively inadequate perfusion for metabolic demands, rather than specific effects of the bypass. Studies of prolonged near-total bypass in awake alert animals and patients without significant metabolic or functional sequelae substantiate this observation. The changes that do occur in heart, liver, lung, renal and brain function are discussed below.

Central nervous system

Cerebral effects of ECC may be minor and transient or major and permanent. When neurological findings do occur they suggest a microembolic or macroembolic cause[4]. Carlson *et al.*[37] have reported results comparing bubble and membrane oxygenators combined with ultrasonic detection of microbubbles in the arterial circuit. A high correlation was found between bubble oxygenator use, microbubble embolism, and minor cerebral dysfunction following operation. Brain function by psychological testing was more nearly normal and returned to normal more quickly in the patients perfused with the membrane oxygenator, in whom no microbubbles were present in the arterial circuit. The use of a filter as a microbubble trap diminished particles and improved central nervous system (CNS) function with the bubble oxygenator. This finding appears to be a consequence of the type of oxygenator used rather than a physiological effect of ECC *per se*. It provides strong clinical evidence that filters should be used with bubble oxygenators for the purpose of serving as a microbubble trap. Similar findings have been reported by others[101, 115, 140].

Organic brain damage was detectable in 4 per cent of 96 patients undergoing ECC reported by Frank *et al.*[58] and non-specific delirium occurred in an additional 20 per cent. The occurrence of brain dysfunction is related to the duration of ECC, as clearly shown by Lee *et al.*[111].

The percentage of patients with central nervous system damage was 10 per cent after 1 hour ECC, 25 per cent after 2 hours and 35 per cent after 3 hours. Similar data were reported by Tufo, Ostfeld and Shekelle[188], Gilman[72], Sveinsson[179] and Kornfeld *et al.*[105]. Most of this central nervous system damage is manifested as delirium or disorientation and the disturbance returns to normal in 1–4 weeks. Follow-up tests of intellectual functioning showed improvement compared to preoperative studies[58]. This delirium syndrome, which is reversible, related to the duration of bypass with gas interface oxygenators, and minimized by the use of membrane oxygenators or microbubble filters, is probably due to microbubble embolism. One would suspect that transient minor damage to all organs must occur in the same patients. Brain damage which is not reversible is usually lethal[89, 203] and is detectable during operations by electroencephalography (EEG)[162, 203]. It is due to gross embolism of fat or other particles[89], or to hypotension during or after bypass in older patients[188]. Timmis *et al.*[184] showed that the intracranial pressure increased above 35cmH_2O is associated with CNS damage during high flow bypass, but the cause of such intracranial hypertension was not identified. This may also be related to microbubble emboli occurring at high-flow rates. Geha *et al.*[68] documented normal brain metabolism during ECC even with alkalosis and hypocapnia, eliminating inadequate perfusion and abnormal oxygenation as causes for this syndrome.

In summary, transient brain dysfunction is common and increases in incidence with the duration of bypass. It appears to be due to microbubble embolism, is most common with bubble oxygenators and can be minimized with microbubble filters. Major brain damage is usually due to particulate embolism or hypotension superimposed on atherosclerosis. Scrupulous attention to cleaning the field prior to coronary suction and filtration of coronary suction will help to prevent particulate embolism. Maintenance of adequate perfusion pressure before and after ECC is recommended in patients with atherosclerosis.

Hepatic, renal, pulmonary and myocardial function

Liver damage is detectable by isoenzyme determination within minutes of the institution of bypass, but this is generally clinically insignificant. In approximately 10 per cent of patients (almost always in adults[166]) jaundice occurs following bypass. When liver damage does occur it appears as cholestatic jaundice which regresses spontaneously. Rarely, massive central centrilobular necrosis occurs in patients with very low cardiac output postoperatively[166]. The reported incidence of serum hepatitis after open-heart surgery has ranged from 0 to 51 per cent depending on the source of the transfused blood[195]. Rosenblum and Heidenburg[157] have presented a compelling argument suggesting that hepatosplenomegaly after bypass in children (postperfusion syndrome) is a variant of posttransfusion hepatitis.

Gastrointestinal complications are rare. Upper gastrointestinal bleeding occurred in 0.22 per cent of 7333 patients operated upon at the Mayo Clinic[199]. Katz *et al.*[99] reported an incidence of 10 per cent. Pancreatitis has also been reported[138]. Moores *et al.*[126] found elevated blood and urine amylase after ECC, particularly with non-pulsatile flow.

Renal failure of some degree occurred in 1 to 3 per cent of patients on cardiopulmonary bypass reported by Norman, McDonald and Sloan[133], 7 per cent reported by Abel *et al.*[1,2] and 12 per cent reported by Bhat *et al.*[22]. This would be expected from the effects of renin and angiotensin on renal cortical flow, related, at least in part, to the non-pulsatile pulse contour. When renal failure does occur it is usually a manifestation of acute tubular necrosis and is reversible. If excessive haemolysis occurs through malfunction of a device or an excessively long perfusion period with a gas interface oxygenator, renal failure from haemoglobin casts may occur. This may be minimized by alkalinizing the urine during bypass with bicarbonate and inducing osmotic diuresis with mannitol. Selmonosky[169] studied the renal function in 63 patients who underwent ECC for intracardiac surgery. He found the blood urea nitrogen concentration and the urine volume to be unreliable indicators of renal function. However, the urinary-urea concentration, and, more specifically, the urinary-urea : blood-urea ratio proved to be very valuable parameters indicating renal failure early in the postperfusion course. For example, on the first postoperative day patients who developed significant renal failure all had urine-to-blood-urea ratios less than 20 whereas patients who did not develop renal failure had ratios of 20 to 100. This test can be done rapidly in the laboratory and will indicate incipient renal failure, alerting the physician to a much more cautious management of fluid infusion in that group of patients. Mortality of acute renal failure is high (88 per cent in Abel's series).

Lung damage following heart-lung bypass used to be common enough to be described as 'pump lung'. Pulmonary insufficiency is now unusual following bypass of 2 hours or less but invariably occurs to some degree when perfusion is carried out longer. This effect is not related to lung perfusion[1] or lack of perfusion[171] via the pulmonary artery or to primary increased pulmonary extravascular water[134]. The lung, more than any other organ, displays the effects of denatured proteins, cellular breakdown or microembolism. Any particulate material occurring in the blood before or after bypass will manifest itself as pulmonary damage. The decrease in pulmonary insufficiency in the last decade is related to at least two important factors: (1) Prepackaged, sterile, single-use, easily primed circuits, which can be prepared immediately before instituting bypass rather than requiring long periods or recirculation and blood interface exposure prior to bypass; (2) A better understanding of pulmonary physiology and management after operation, particularly the use of prolonged (24 hours) intubation and mechanical ventilation assuring good alveolar inflation in patients who did not ventilate well by themselves. There is ample evidence that the well inflated alveolus is less susceptible to humoral damage than the collapsed alveolus[9]. The same principle holds true during ECC. Weedn, Coalson and Greenfield[196] demonstrated that lung dysfunction was least in a group of dogs managed with static inflation during ECC, rather than static deflation or conventional ventilation. The lungs should be managed by static inflation during ECC unless this interferes with cardiac exposure. The humoral factors which damage pulmonary capillaries may be lysosomal enzymes from poor peripheral perfusion[65, 152] but also include aggregated polymorphonuclear leukocytes from homologous blood, as demonstrated independently by Rabelo *et al.*[148] and Ratliff *et al.*[149]. White cell aggregates and lung dysfunction were decreased with the use of blood filtration[40], or membrane oxygenators[36]. These studies further emphasize the potential problems of homologous blood interaction and suggest that pulmonary complications can best be minimized by reducing the amount of transfused blood, in addition to maximum inflation ventilation, careful attention to pulmonary haemodynamics and minimum blood-gas exposure time.

Cardiopulmonary bypass by itself does not affect *myocardial function*. Many changes occur in myocardial function after operation, related to the type of operation, the valve, the cardiac chamber being repaired, or the amount of coronary perfusion during bypass. These considerations will be discussed in detail in subsequent chapters.

Reticuloendothelial function changes

Silva, Hoeksema and Fekety[173] have reported an elegant study of phagocytosis and bacterial killing of circulating leukocytes during ECC. Using the nitroblue-tetrazolium test for phagocytosis, they found a significantly decreased phagocytic activity in the circulating white cells in 12 ECC patients. They postulated that these changes were due to derangements in oxidative metabolism of these circulating white cells and supported this hypothesis by demonstrating that the bactericidal activity was decreased in two of four patients in whom it was measured. This clinical study supported the laboratory work of Kusserow and Larrow[107] in which decreased phagocytic activity during ECC in dogs was demonstrated. Decreased activity in fixed tissue phagocytes has been demonstrated by

Subramanian *et al.*[177, 178]. They conducted ECC and isolated liver perfusion in rats and demonstrated that the clearance of radioactive gold by Kupfer cells in the liver was significantly impaired with ECC. In a later study this same group demonstrated that blood which was recirculated *ex vivo* for 30 minutes caused the same effect when perfused through a rat liver. They concluded from these studies that the decreased reticuloendothelial (RE) function was due to mechanical or chemical effects of the extracorporeal circuit on blood rather than the effect on the liver itself. The reason for this impaired RE function of circulating and fixed phagocytes has not been identified, but these observations correlate very nicely with the studies of platelet aggregation and uptake in RE organs as described earlier. If circulating and fixed phagocytes become loaded with platelet aggregates or other microparticles and debris from coronary suction or the extracorporeal circuit, then the ability of these cells to further phagocytize radioactive gold or bacteria would be reduced. If this hypothesis is proven to be true, it affords further evidence that avoiding platelet aggregation by platelet-active drugs or surface modification may be important not only in haemostasis but in maintenance of normal RE function after ECC. It should be briefly pointed out however that the relationship of this impaired RE function to significant clinical infection has yet to be demonstrated.

Metabolism and pharmacology related to extracorporeal circulation

Hypothermia

Aside from the moderate low flow state imposed by most cardiopulmonary bypass as mentioned above, there are no specific metabolic sequelae of extracorporeal circulation. One appropriate method to compensate for the moderate low flow is the use of moderate hypothermia which decreases oxygen requirement and CO_2 production so that the lower flow can be matched to specific metabolic requirements. The use of moderate hypothermia (to 30°C) is widely carried out, although the effects of skin and perhaps muscle ischaemia related to this cold temperature and the increased sympathetic effects may balance out any possible advantages. In addition, the blood viscosity increases as the temperature drops so that use of haemodilution to lower the haematocrit is required in order to decrease blood viscosity.

The major advantage of hypothermia is to allow a safety factor to the surgeon. Faced with excessive bleeding, the entire bypass circuit can be turned off safely and the brain protected by hypothermia for periods from 10 minutes at 30°C to 60 minutes at 4°C. Even more important than this life-saving manoeuvre is the possibility afforded by moderate hypothermia of cross-clamping the aorta, eliminating coronary perfusion and providing a dry field at 32°C. This can be carried out safely for 20 to 30 minutes, can be repeated at regular intervals if necessary, and extended longer with cardioplegic techniques. These techniques are discussed in detail by subsequent authors. Reviews of hypothermia have been published by two pioneers in the field: Swan[180] and Blair[24].

Haemodilution and priming

The priming volume of the circuit depends on the gas exchange device, the venous reservoir volume and the blood volume of the patient. It is feasible to avoid blood transfusion altogether at the expense of oxygen-carrying capacity. A high haematocrit and excellent oxygen-carrying capacity can be achieved with an all-blood prime, but at the expense of increased viscosity, haemolysis and potential for transfusion reaction, hepatitis and blood interactions. These factors balance out at a bypass haematocrit of 25 to 30 per cent which generally requires 500 to 1000 ml of blood in the prime or to be infused during the bypass. Blood should be less than 24 hours old to maintain adequate levels of active blood platelets; otherwise fresh components should be used. The type of anticoagulant is not particularly important but heparin should be added to the primed bypass circuit before it comes in contact with calcium ion if citrate is used as the original anticoagulant[97, 170]. The remainder of the prime can be 5 per cent glucose, saline or any isotonic crystalloid or colloid solution. When non-blood prime is used the resultant 'exchange transfusion' and rapid haemodilution will result in equilibration of priming solution into ,the appropriate body fluid space causing hypovolaemia as referred to earlier in this chapter. Saline or saline-like crystalloid solutions will equilibrate into the extracellular fluid, requiring volume supplement to return blood volume to normal. Prime with crystalloid solutions necessarily expands the total body water and the extracellular fluid compartments more than is actually necessary. Hence, if non-blood priming fluid is to be used, protein or dextran solutions are theoretically, and actually, more appealing. The ideal non-blood priming solution would contain albumin and larger protein molecules such as globulins and would facilitate oxygen transport. Stroma-free haemoglobin solution is such a material which can be manufactured from outdated bank blood and has ideal characteristics as a priming solution for ECC or a blood substitute in general[146, 151]. The theoretical advantage of including some albumin in the circulating prime before any blood is added has been suggested by Landé *et al.*[109]. Exposing the foreign surface to albumin first allows albumin to align on any exposed, charged binding sites, decreasing the likelihood of fibrinogen attachment with later platelet deposition. Six per cent dextran (either 70 000 or 40 000 molecular weight) is useful as a priming solution and may decrease platelet aggregation[87]. The entire prime is recirculated, brought to an appropriate temperature, and buffered to pH 7.4 with tris buffer (THAM). Blood should be added last, as close to bypass time as possible.

Several investigators have studied the effect of eliminating blood transfusion for the cardiac surgical patient altogether. The reasons for wishing to do this include lack of expense, simplicity, saving, vital blood bank stores, and, more importantly, avoiding the possible effects of microembolism from platelet fibrin aggregates in stored blood, interactions between donor blood from different sources (the homologous blood syndrome) and the recent evidence showing possible transfused white cell damage to lung and other organs. The problem of platelet fibrin aggregate formation in banked blood has been clearly identified by the studies of McNamara *et al.*[123]. These aggregates do occur and are characterized by fibrin formation presumably as small areas of clotting take place where citrate has been metabolized in the stored blood. All blood transfused to patients on ECC (or for that matter to any patient) which is more than 5 days old should be filtered through fine mesh filters which will remove these aggregates and diminish the possibility of transfusing them into patients where they might form microemboli. However, viable or non-viable white cells are still transfused into the patient even with filters. This is a significant consideration in ECC patients where several units of blood may be required and justifies the use of packed red cells, washed red cells, or frozen reconstituted red cells[81] in that circumstance. Litwack *et al.*[117] who originally proposed the homologous blood syndrome have recently reported experience with 29 patients who underwent ECC and cardiac surgery without donor blood, or with minimal blood. The conduct of ECC in these patients proceeded without particular difficulty and a cogent argument can be made for avoiding blood transfusion as much as possible during ECC. The use of blood salvage and autotransfusion before and after ECC[98, 167] and reinfusion of washed cells from the used circuit[127] are major advances which save blood bank resources.

Electrolyte and metabolic changes

Fluid and electrolyte disorders following ECC for cardiac surgery are major clinical considerations. Sodium retention, expanded extracellular fluid (ECF) and decreased total body potassium are characteristic of the patient with some degree of cardiac failure preoperatively, particularly if the patient had been treated with diuretics. Inadequate postoperative myocardial function as a result of hypothermia, anoxia, or the cardiac lesion itself may cause similar problems. A sophisticated study of fluid compartment composition and electrolyte status was reported by Pacifico, Digerness and Kirklin[136]. They used moderate haemodilution and found a significant increase in extracellular fluid and exchangeable sodium with a significant decrease in total body potassium in response to ECC. The increased ECF would be expected from the equilibration of a saline type of haemodilution priming solution, plus the effects of gas interface exposure of platelets, white cells and proteins which might increase capillary permeability. The decreased total body potassium is explained on the basis of kaluresis, and anticipated maximal aldosterone response associated with maximum stress. Similar changes in blood potassium concentration were reported by Dieter, Neville and Pifarré[47]. Hypokalaemia is the only major electrolyte abnormality of significance and is important because of the potential of developing digitalis-induced arrhythmias. Hypokalaemia should be avoided by including potassium chloride in the priming solution[86, 136]. Extensive studies on calcium[43, 125, 156] and magnesium[156, 168, 189] show that these cations decrease initially with dilution at the onset of bypass and remain somewhat low throughout ECC. The levels can be maintained at normal by addition of moderate amounts of magnesium chloride or calcium at the end of ECC. Although some authors have presented evidence suggesting that hypomagnesaemia may predispose to arrhythmia in ECC patients[189] it appears that these minor variations in calcium and magnesium do not commonly cause significant clinical abnormalities.

Glucose metabolism in relation to pancreatic blood flow and insulin secretion during ECC had been studied and reported by Mandelbaum and Morgan[120]. They found that the insulin secretion rate remained normal during ECC, although the splanchnic flow increased so that portal venous levels of insulin decreased during ECC. Pancreatic islets responded normally to hypertonic glucose and tolbutamide stimulation during ECC. No major alterations in glucose utilization or oxygen consumption due to insulin abnormalities *per se* have been demonstrated with ECC. Protein denaturation and presumed catabolism related to ECC have been discussed earlier in relationship to blood-gas interface effects. Wallace, Mooz and Blakemore[194] undertook a study of protein metabolism in ECC patients to evaluate the importance of this phenomenon. They found a uniform and significant increase in plasma amino acids which were demonstrated to be arising from the liver. They postulated that the origin of these amino acids may be caused by a block in enzymatic protein synthesis in the liver with free amino acid 'spilling over' into the peripheral circulation. It is also possible that denatured protein with or without associated platelets could be phagocytized in the reticuloendothelial cells of the liver, broken down and released as amino acids. This interesting area of metabolism during ECC deserves further study.

Pathophysiology of extracorporeal circulation

It is noted in the introduction that pathophysiology of ECC refers to malfunction of this extracorporeal artificial organ. This may be due to a mechanical defect or failure in the system itself, or due to improper regulation of the device by the operator.

Mechanical failure should be avoided by a preventative maintenance programme of replacing elements of the bypass circuit at regular intervals. The use of single-use, disposable, presterilized items for all blood contact has largely eliminated failures in this area. Careful attention to roller pump settings and continuous monitoring of flow and pressure in the arterial line during bypass will minimize mechanical complications. The pump team should rehearse rapid replacement of any part of the bypass circuit as well as drills to deal with man-made problems of air embolism, thrombosis in the oxygenator, aortic dissection, improper venous cannulation, etc. Attention to these details in avoiding pathophysiological function of the extracorporeal circuit will be discussed by other authors in this book.

Components of the extracorporeal circuit must be absolutely clean, inert, sterile and non-toxic. Mechanical cleaning may not be adequate to remove all foreign proteins and pyrogens from reused portions of the circuit. Such a foreign protein was acting as a plasminogen activator and causing abnormal bleeding in open-heart patients in a recent study. Cleaning in 20 per cent sodium hydroxide removed the offending material[33]. Prepackaged single-use components should be clean but may not be necessarily so. Systemic emboli of particles of Dacron and nylon thread, antifoam, or other materials may originate from components which are allegedly clean for single use. Some extracorporeal components may contain plasticizers or solvents which could leak out into the circulating blood during ECC. All plastic materials which are used for contact with human blood must meet USP standards for biomedical plastics. These standards involve injecting extracts of the material into animals and subcutaneous implantation of the material in animals. All medical plastics undergo this testing procedure. Designations such as 'medical grade' or 'implant tested' do not connote any specific standard or unique characteristic. An excellent review of biomedical plastics and polymers, including safety and standardization procedures, was recently published by Boretos[27].

The fact that plastic raw materials have successfully undergone conventional USP testing does not mean that a finished product will be non-toxic. Adhesive used in construction, heat sealing, radiation or gas sterilization may alter the characteristics of the material or add new materials which are potentially damaging to the patient. A tragic experience with toxicity of ethylene oxide sterilization of an extracorporeal circuit resulting in fatality and clearly identified later in dogs was reported by Stanley *et al.*[175].

This lethal toxicity associated with ethylene oxide has now been described from several sources; however virtually nothing is known of the interactions of drugs such as halothane, penthrane, nitrous oxide, narcotics, antibiotics and analgesics with prolonged exposure to various plastic surfaces. Clinical experience would indicate that minimal interaction takes place although we have all seen clear polyvinyl chloride tubing become turbid and white silicone tubing become yellow with prolonged blood exposure. The interrelationships of these types of plastics with blood components for long periods of time deserve further study.

Antifoam is coated on some part of all gas interface oxygenators. When present in excessive amounts or when incompletely adhered to the surface, particles of this material may break loose and embolize[150]. The plastic material itself can erode on the inside of the extracorporeal circuit. Polyvinyl chloride tubing in the roller pump usually deteriorates by cracking and breaking from the outer edge in; however, prolonged pumping with a roller pump on silicone rubber tubing results in crumbling away from the inside out[92].

If air is trapped in the extracorporeal circuit and suddenly enters the arterial perfusion line, systemic air embolism will result. The possibility of this occurring from the arterial line filters has recently been demonstrated by Wellons and Nolan[197] who showed that air could be trapped in the arterial line filter. This problem was solved by ventilating the filter with carbon dioxide prior to priming. Carbon dioxide is much more soluble than oxygen or nitrogen in priming solution and bubbles could be completely removed in this fashion. The same procedure is helpful in priming membrane oxygenators. Prevention of air embolism from intracardiac chambers has been emphasized by many authors[75,110]. Techniques to avoid air embolism from cardiac chambers while ECC is turned on and off for various manoeuvres are described in other chapters.

Finally, *infection* occurring as a result of contamination of the extracorporeal circuit is another form of pathophysiology associated with ECC.

Blakemore *et al.*[25] have shown that the extracorporeal circuit becomes contaminated from the coronary suction line although the ventilation gas fed to the oxygenator itself may be contaminated from the tubing or from nebulizing or humidification devices. Appropriate use of air filters wherever possible and meticulous attention to avoiding air contamination in the field of the cardiotomy coronary suction will help minimize this contamination. However, bloodstream contamination, particularly in the face of decreased phagocytic and bactericidal RE function, as mentioned previously, predispose the ECC patient to infection. The possibility of infection and contamination during ECC has prompted most surgeons to add prophylactic antibiotics to the perfusion system or to the patient during ECC, although their value is not well demonstrated[17, 41, 158, 163].

Drugs and extracorporeal circulation

Since neuroendocrine regulation of cardiac output is absent during total heart-lung bypass, vasoactive drugs are often necessary to balance peripheral vascular resistance and flow to the pump. High arterial pressure and poor venous return, if not due to mechanical problems, are treated with alpha-adrenergic blockade (Rogitine or chlorpromazine). Low pressure and low flow are managed with volume replacement but may be supplemented with phenylephrine or epinephrine. Heparin is given on schedule and buffers are added as needed. Useful adjuncts to the management of bypass include mannitol to induce osmotic diuresis[133], antibiotics[41, 158], steroids for their protective effect against lysosomal disruption in the low flow state[65, 152] and possibly dipyridamole to decrease platelet adhesiveness[124]. Pluronic F68, a non-ionic detergent, has been proposed to diminish fat embolism[198] but it was proven ineffective by Danielson, Dubilier and Bryant[42]. Although Pluronic appears to diminish haemolysis associated with the gas interface oxygenator, its safety has not been completely established.

Conclusions

Extracorporeal circulation involves the use of a prosthetic device to totally replace the function of the heart and lungs and partially replace the blood endothelial interface and reticuloendothelial system. Properly used, it allows the function of the other organs of the body to remain unchanged during the conduct of this procedure.

Moderate hypovolaemia due to haemodilution and hypotension usually accompany ECC, with systemic flow maintained at an adequate but barely normal level. Gas exchange is easily accomplished by any of a variety of devices. The major physiological alterations caused by ECC are related to prosthetic surface exposure, and manifested primarily by platelet aggregation.

References

1. Abel, R. M., Buckley, M. J., Austen, W. G., Barnett, G. O., Beck, C. H. and Fischer, J. E. 'Acute post-operative renal failure in cardiac surgical patients.' *Journal of Surgical Research*, **20,** 341 (1976)
2. Abel, R. M., Buckley, M. J., Austen, W. G., Barnett, G. O., Beck, C. H. and Fischer, J. E. 'Aetiology, incidence, and prognosis of renal failure following cardiac operations. Results of a prospective analysis of 500 consecutive patients.' *Journal of Thoracic and Cardiovascular Surgery*, **71,** 323 (1976)
3. Addonizio, V. P., Strauss, J. F., Macarak, E. J., Colman, R. W. and Edmunds, L. H. 'Preservation of platelet number and function with Prostaglandin E_1 during total cardiopulmonary bypass in rhesus monkeys.' *Surgery*, **83,** 619 (1978)
4. Allardyce, D. B., Yoshida, S. H. and Ashmore, P. G. 'The importance of microembolism in the pathogenesis of organ dysfunction caused by prolonged use of the pump oxygenator.' *Journal of Thoracic and Cardiovascular Surgery*, **52,** 706 (1966)
5. Anderson, N. B. and Jawahar, G. 'Pulmonary function, cardiac status, and post-operative course in relation to cardiopulmonary bypass.' *Journal of Thoracic and Cardiovascular Surgery*, **59,** 474 (1970)
6. Arkin, C. F., Shahsavari, M., Copeland, B. E. and Kim, A. 'Evaluation of the activated clotting time to control heparin and protamine dosage in open-heart surgery.' *Journal of Thoracic and Cardiovascular Surgery*, **75,** 790 (1978)
7. Babka, R., Colby, C., El-Etr, A. and Pifarré, R. 'Monitoring of intra-operative heparinization and blood loss following cardiopulmonary bypass surgery.' *Journal of Thoracic and Cardiovascular Surgery*, **73,** 780 (1977)
8. Baden, J. P., Sonnenfield, M., Ferlic, R. M. and Sellers, R. D. 'The bason test: a rapid bedside test for control of heparin therapy.' *Surgical Forum*, **22,** 172 (1971)
9. Bartlett, R. H. 'Post traumatic pulmonary insufficiency.' In *Surgery Annual.* Cooper, ch. 1. New York: Appleton-Century-Crofts (1971)
10. Bartlett, R. H., Burns, N. E., Fong, S. W., Gazzaniga, A. B., Achauer, B. M. and Fraille, J. 'Prolonged partial veno-arterial bypass: physiologic, biochemical and haematologic response.' *Surgical Forum*, **23,** 178 (1972)
11. Bartlett, R. H., Drinker, P. A., Burns, N. E., Fong, S. W. and Hyans, T. 'The toroidal flow membrane oxygenator: design, performance, and prolonged bypass testing of clinical model.' *Transactions of the American Society for Artificial Internal Organs*, **18,** 369 (1972)
12. Bartlett, R. H., Fong, S. W., Burns, N. E. and Gazzaniga, A. E. 'Prolonged partial veno-arterial bypass: physiologic, biochemical and haematologic responses.' *Annals of Surgery*, **180,** 850 (1974)
13. Bartlett, R. H. and Gazzaniga, A. B. 'Extracorporeal circulation for cardiopulmonary failure.' *Current Problems in Surgery*, **15,** 5 (1978)
14. Bartlett, R. H., Isherwood, J., Moss, R. A., Olszewski, W. L., Polet, H. and Drinker, P. A. 'A toroidal flow membrane oxygenator: four day partial bypass in dogs.' *Surgical Forum*, **20,** 152 (1969)
15. Bartlett, R. H., Kittredge, D., Noyes, B. S., Willard, R. H. and Drinker, P. A. 'Development of a membrane oxygenator: overcoming blood diffusion limitation.' *Journal of Thoracic and Cardiovascular Surgery*, **58,** 795 (1969)
16. Becker, R. M., Smith, M. R. and Dobell, A. R. C. 'Effect of platelet inhibition on platelet phenomena in cardiopulmonary bypass in pigs.' *Annals of Surgery*, **52,** 179 (1972)

17. Benner, J. E. 'Metabolism of antibiotics during cardiopulmonary bypass for open-heart surgery.' *American Society of Microbiology*, **92,** 373 (1969)
18. Berne, R. M. and Levy, M. N. *Cardiovascular Physiology*. St. Louis; C. V. Mosby Co. (1972)
19. Bernhard, W. F., Hussain, M., Robinson, T., Button, L., Frieze, S. and Curtis, G. W. 'An appraisal of blood trauma and the blood material interface following prolonged assisted circulation.' *Journal of Thoracic and Cardiovascular Surgery*, **58,** 801 (1969)
20. Bernstein, E. F., Blackshear, P. L. Jr. and Keller, K. H. 'Factors influencing erythrocyte destruction in artificial organs.' *American Journal of Surgery*, **114,** 126 (1967)
21. Bernstein, E. F. and Gleason, L. R. 'Factors influencing haemolysis with roller pumps.' *Surgery*, **61,** 432 (1967)
22. Bhat, J. G., Gluck, M. C., Lowenstein, J., Baldwin, D. S. 'Renal failure after open-heart surgery.' *Annals of Internal Medicine*, **84,** 677 (1976)
23. Blackshear, P. L., Jr. 'Summation: flow-related surface phenomena.' *Federation Proceedings*, **30,** 1709 (1971)
24. Blair, E. 'Recent advances in surgery. A physiologic classification of clinical hypothermia.' *Surgery*, **58,** 607 (1965)
25. Blakemore, W. S., McGarrity, G. J., Thiurer, R. J., Wallace, H. W., MacVaugh, H., III, Coriell, L. L. 'Infection by air-borne bacteria with cardiopulmonary bypass.' *Surgery*, **70,** 830 (1971)
26. Bolanowski, P. J. P., Bauer, J., Machiedo, G. and Neville, W. E. 'Prostaglandin influence on pulmonary intravascular leukocytic aggregation during cardiopulmonary bypass.' *Journal of Thoracic and Cardiovascular Surgery*, **73,** 221 (1977)
27. Boretos, J. W. *Concise Guide to Biomedical Polymers; Their Design, Fabrication and Moulding*. Springfield: Thomas (1973)
28. Boucher, J. K., Rudy, L. W. and Edmunds, L. H. 'Organ blood flow during pulsatile cardiopulmonary bypass.' *Journal of Applied Physiology*, **36,** 86 (1974)
29. Boyd, A. D., Engelman, R. M., Beaudet, R. L. and Lackner, H. 'Disseminated intravascular coagulation following extracorporeal circulation.' *Journal of Thoracic and Cardiovascular Surgery*, **64,** 685 (1972)
30. Breckenridge, I. M., Digerness, S. B. and Kirklin, J. W. 'Validity of concept of increased extracellular fluid after open-heart surgery.' *Surgical Forum*, **20,** 169 (1969)
31. Bregman, D. 'Mechanical support of the failing heart'. (*Current Problems in Surgery*, vol. 13, no. 12.) Chicago: Year Book Medical Publishers (1976)
32. Brinsfield, D. E., Hopf, M. A., Geering, R. B. and Galletti, P. M. 'Haemotological changes in long-term perfusion.' *Journal of Applied Physiology*, **17,** 531 (1962)
33. Brooks, D. H. and Bahnson, H. T. 'An outbreak of haemorrhage following cardiopulmonary bypass. Epidemiologic studies.' *Journal of Thoracic and Cardiovascular Surgery*, **63,** 449 (1971)
34. Bull, B. S., Korpman, R. A., Huse, W. M. and Briggs, D. B. 'Heparin therapy during extracorporeal circulation. 1. Problems inherent in existing heparin protocols.' *Journal of Thoracic and Cardiovascular Surgery*, **69,** 674 (1975)
35. Burack, B., Marcus, D., Miyamoto, A., Escher, D. J. W. and Robinson, G. 'Response of class IV patients to alpha blockade prior to open-heart surgery.' *American Heart Journal*, **84,** 456 (1972)
36. Byrick, R. J. and Noble, W. H. 'Post-perfusion lung syndrome. Comparison of Travenol bubble and membrane oxygenators.' *Journal of Thoracic and Cardiovascular Surgery*, **76,** 685 (1978)

37. Carlson, R. G., Landé, A. J., Landis, B., Rogoz, B., Baxter, J., Patterson, R. H., Jr., Stenzel, K. and Lillehei, C. W. 'The Landé–Edwards membrane oxygenator during heart surgery.' *Journal of Thoracic and Cardiovascular Surgery*, **66,** 894 (1973)
38. Clark, R. E. and Mills, M. 'The infant temptrol oxygenator.' *Journal of Thoracic and Cardiovascular Surgery*, **60,** 54 (1969)
39. Cohn, L. H., Angell, W. W. and Shumway, N. E. 'Body fluid shifts after cardiopulmonary bypass. 1. Effects of congestive heart failure and haemodilution.' *Journal of Thoracic and Cardiovascular Surgery*, **62,** 423 (1971)
40. Connell, R. S., Page, U. S., Bartley, T. D., Bigelow, J. C. and Webb, M. C. 'The effect on pulmonary ultrastructure of Dacron-wool filtration during cardiopulmonary bypass.' *Annals of Thoracic Surgery*, **15,** 217 (1973)
41. Conte, J. E., Jr., Cohen, S. N., Roe, B. B. and Elashoff, R. M. 'Antibiotic prophylaxis and cardiac surgery: a prospective double-blind comparison of single-dose versus multiple-dose regimens.' *Annals of Internal Medicine*, **76,** 943 (1972)
42. Danielson, G. K., Dubilier, L. D. and Bryant, L. R. 'Use of pluronic F-68 to diminish fat emboli and haemolysis during cardiopulmonary bypass.' *Journal of Thoracic and Cardiovascular Surgery*, **59,** 178 (1970)
43. Das, J. B., Eraklis, A. J., Adams, J. G., Jr. and Gross, R. E. 'Changes in serum ionic calcium during cardiopulmonary bypass with haemodilution.' *Journal of Thoracic and Cardiovascular Surgery*, **62,** 449 (1971)
44. de Leval, M., Hill, J. D., Mielke, H., Bramson, M. L., Smith, C. and Gerbode, F. 'Platelet kinetics during extracorporeal circulation.' *Transactions of the American Society for Artificial Internal Organs*, **18,** 355 (1972)
45. DeWall, R. A., Bentley, D. J., Hirose, M., Battung, V., Najafi, H. and Roden, T. 'A temperature controlling (omnithermic) disposable bubble oxygenator for total body perfusion.' *Chest*, **49,** 207 (1966)
46. Deykin, D. 'Emerging concepts of platelet function.' *New England Journal of Medicine*, **290,** 144 (1974)
47. Dieter, R. A., Neville, W. E. and Pifarré, R. 'Hypokalaemia following haemodilution cardiopulmonary bypass.' *Annals of Surgery*, **171,** 17 (1969)
48. Dobell, A. R. C., Mitri, M., Galva, R., Sarkozy, E. and Murphy, D. 'Biologic evaluation of blood after prolonged recirculation through film and membrane oxygenators.' *Annals of Surgery*, **161,** 617 (1965)
49. Drinker, P. A. 'Progress in membrane oxygenator design.' *Anaesthesiology*, **37,** 242 (1972)
50. Dunn, J., Kirsch, M., Harness, J., Carroll, M., Straker, J. and Sloan, H. 'Haemodynamic, metabolic, and haematologic effects of pulsatile cardiopulmonary bypass.' *Journal of Thoracic and Cardiovascular Surgery*, **68,** 138 (1974)
51. Dutton, R. C. and Edmunds, L. H., Jr. 'Measurement of emboli in extracorporeal perfusion system.' *Journal of Thoracic and Cardiovascular Surgery*, **65,** 523 (1973)
52. Dutton, R. C., Edmunds, L. H., Jr., Hutchinson, J. C. and Benson, B. R. 'Platelet aggregate emboli produced in patients during cardiopulmonary bypass with membrane and bubble oxygenators and blood filters.' *Journal of Thoracic and Cardiovascular Surgery*, **67,** 258 (1973)
53. Dutton, R. C., Mather, F. W., III, Walker, S. N., Lipps, B. J., Jr., Rudy, L. W., Severinghaus, J. W. and Edmunds, L. H., Jr. 'Development and evaluation of a new hollow-fibre membrane oxygenator.' *Transactions of the American Society for Artificial Internal Organs*, **17,** 331 (1971)
54. Ekert, H. and Sheers, M. 'Preoperative and post-operative platelet function in cyanotic congenital heart disease.' *Journal of Thoracic and Cardiovascular Surgery*, **68,** 184 (1974)

55. Eiseman, B., Birnbaum, D., Leonard, R. and Martinez, F. J. 'A new gas permeable membrane for blood oxygenators.' *Surgery, Gynecology and Obstetrics*, **135,** 732 (1972)
56. Fletcher, J. R., McKee, A. E., Watson, L. P. and Anderson, R. D. 'Veno-arterial cardiopulmonary bypass without heparin in the baboon.' *ASAIO Journal*, **2,** 17 (1979)
57. Fong, S. W., Burns, N. E., Williams, G., Woldanski, C., Gazzaniga, A. B. and Bartlett, R. H. 'Changes in coagulation and platelet function during prolonged extracorporeal circulation (ECC) in sheep and man.' *Transactions of the American Society for Artificial Internal Organs*, **20,** 229 (1974)
58. Frank, K. A., Heller, S. S., Kornfeld, D. S. and Malm, J. R. 'Long-term effects of open-heart surgery on intellectual functioning.' *Journal of Thoracic and Cardiovascular Surgery*, **64,** 811 (1972)
59. Friesen, R. H. and Clement, A. J. 'Individual responses to heparinization for extracorporeal circulation.' *Journal of Thoracic and Cardiovascular Surgery*, **72,** 875 (1976)
60. Galletti, P. M., Richardson, P. D., Snider, M. T. and Friedman, L. I. 'A standardized method for defining the overall gas transfer performance of artificial lungs.' *Transactions of the American Society for Artificial Internal Organs*, **18,** 359 (1972)
61. Gans, H. and Castaneda, A. R. 'Problems in haemostasis during open-heart surgery. VII. Changes in fibrinogen concentration during and after cardiopulmonary bypass with particular reference to the effect of heparin in neutralization of fibrinogen.' *Annals of Surgery*, **165,** 551 (1967)
62. Gans, H., Castaneda, A. R., Subramanian, V. A., John, S. and Lillehei, C. W. 'Problems in haemostasis during open-heart surgery. IX. Changes observed in the plasminogen-plasma system and their significance for therapy.' *Annals of Surgery*, **166,** 980 (1967)
63. Gans, H., Subramanian, V. A., Lillehei, C. W. and Castaneda, A. R. 'Problems in haemostasis during open-heart surgery. VIII. On the *in vivo* turnover rate of plasminogen activator after cardiopulmonary bypass.' *Surgery*, **62,** 292 (1967)
64. Gazzaniga, A. B., Byrd, C. L. and Gross, R. E. 'The use of skeletal muscle surface hydrogen ion concentration to monitor peripheral perfusion: experimental and clinical results.' *Surgical Forum*, **21,** 147 (1970)
65. Gazzaniga, A. B., Byrd, C. L., Stewart, D. R. and Gross, R. E. 'Effects of dexamethasone and chlorpromazine on skeletal muscle surface hydrogen ion concentration during cardiopulmonary bypass.' *Annals of Surgery*, **176,** 757 (1972)
66. Gazzaniga, A. B., Byrd, C. L., Stewart, D. R. and O'Connor, N. E. 'Evaluation of central venous pressure as a guide to volume replacement in children following cardiopulmonary bypass.' *Annals of Thoracic Surgery*, **13,** 148 (1972)
67. Garcia, J. B., Pakrashi, B. C., Mary, D. A., Tandon, R. K. and Ionescu, M. I. 'Postoperative blood loss after extracorporeal circulation for heart valve surgery.' *Journal of Thoracic and Cardiovascular Surgery*, **65,** 487 (1972)
68. Geha, A. S., Malt, S. H., Nara, Y. and Baue, A. E. 'Effect of cardiopulmonary bypass on cerebral metabolism.' *Journal of Thoracic and Cardiovascular Surgery*, **61,** 200 (1969)
69. Gervin, A. S., McNeer, J. F., Wolfe, W. G., Puckett, C. L. and Silver, D. 'Ultrapore haemofiltration during extracorporeal circulation.' *Journal of Thoracic and Cardiovascular Surgery*, **67,** 237 (1974)
70. Giannelli, S., Ayres, S. M., Fleming, P., Conrad, W., Schwartz, M. D. and Gould, H. 'Peripheral vascular volumes and whole body haematocrit during human heart lung bypass.' *Circulation*, **41,** 629 (1970)

71. Gille, J. P., Trudell, L., Snider, M. T., Borsanyi, A. S. and Galletti, P. M. 'Capability of the microporous, membrane-lined, capillary oxygenator in hypercapneic dogs.' *Transactions of the American Society for Artificial Internal Organs*, **16,** 365 (1970)
72. Gilman, S. 'Cerebral disorders after open-heart operations.' *New England Journal of Medicine*, **272,** 489 (1965)
73. Goldberg, E., O'Reilly, M. and Chaithiraphan, S. 'Prevention of post-brachial arteriotomy thrombosis.' *Lancet*, **1,** 789 (1972)
74. Gomes, M. M. R. and McGoon, D. C. 'Bleeding patterns after open-heart surgery.' *Journal of Thoracic and Cardiovascular Surgery*, **60,** 87 (1969)
75. Gomes, O. M., Pereira, S. N., Castagna, R. C., Bittencourt, D., Amaral, R. V. G. and Zerbini, E. J. 'The importance of the different sites of air injection in the tolerance of arterial air-embolism.' *Journal of Thoracic and Cardiovascular Surgery*, **65,** 563 (1973)
76. Goodman, T. A., Gerard, D. F., Bernstein, E. F. and Dilley, R. B. 'The effects of pulseless perfusion on the distribution of renal cortical blood flow and on renin release.' *Surgery*, **80,** 31 (1976)
77. Gourin, A., Streisand, R. L. and Stuckey, J. H. 'Total cardiopulmonary bypass, myocardial contractility, and the administration of protamine sulfate.' *Journal of Thoracic and Cardiovascular Surgery*, **61,** 160 (1970)
78. Guidoin, R., Laperche, Y., Martin, L., Awad, J. and Winchester, J. 'Disposable filters for microaggregate removal from extracorporeal circulation.' *Journal of Thoracic and Cardiovascular Surgery*, **71,** 502 (1976)
79. Hallowell, P., Bland, J. H. L., Chir, B., Buckley, M. J. and Lowenstein, E. 'Transfusion of fresh autologous blood in open-heart surgery.' *Journal of Thoracic and Cardiovascular Surgery*, **64,** 941 (1972)
80. Hanson, E. L., Bartlett, R. H., Burns, N. E., Shultz, M. C., LaCava, E. J., Polet, H. and Drinker, P. A. 'Prolonged use of a membrane oxygenator in air-breathing and hypoxic lambs. I: venovenous bypass.' *Surgery*, **73,** 284 (1973)
81. Hanson, E. L., Fosberg, A. M., LaCava, E. J., Steitz, C. W. and Collins, J. J., Jr. 'Studies with frozen blood for oxygenator priming.' *Journal of Thoracic and Cardiovascular Surgery*, **64,** 87 (1972)
82. Hardesty, R. L., Baker, L. D., Gall, D. A. and Bahson, H. T. 'Systemic resistance during cardiopulmonary bypass.' *Surgical Forum*, **20,** 185 (1969)
83. Harken, A. H. 'The influence of pulsatile perfusion on oxygen uptake by the isolated canine hind limb.' *Journal of Thoracic and Cardiovascular Surgery*, **70,** 237 (1975)
84. Harrison, T. S., Chawla, R. C., Seton, J. F. and Robinson, B. H. 'Carotid sinus origin of adrenergic responses compromising the effectiveness of artificial circulatory support.' *Surgery*, **68,** 20 (1970)
85. Harrison, T. S. and Seton, J. F. 'An analysis of pulse frequency as an adrenergic excitant in pulsative circulatory support.' *Surgery*, **73,** 868 (1973)
86. Henney, P. R., Riemenschneider, T. A., DeLand, E. C. and Maloney, J. V., Jr. 'Prevention of hypokalaemic cardiac arrhythmias associated with cardiopulmonary bypass and haemodilution.' *Surgical Forum*, **21,** 145 (1971)
87. Hepps, S. A., Roe, B. B., Wright, R. R. and Gardner, R. C. 'Amelioration of the pulmonary post perfusion syndrome with haemodilution and low molecular weight dextran.' *Surgery*, **54,** 232 (1963)
88. Hicks, R. E., Dutton, R. C., Ries, C. A., Price, D. C. and Edmunds, L. J., Jr. 'Production and fate of platelet aggregate emboli during venovenous perfusion.' *Surgical Forum*, **24,** 250 (1973)
89. Hill, J. D., Aguilar, M. J., Baranco, A. and Gerbode, F. 'Neuropathological manifestations of cardiac surgery.' *Annals of Thoracic Surgery*, **7,** 409 (1969)

90. Hill, J. D., de Leval, M. R., Fallat, R. J., Bramson, M. L., Eberhart, R. C., Schmult, H. D., Osborn, J. J., Barber, R. and Gerbode, F. 'Acute respiratory insufficiency: treatment with prolonged extracorporeal oxygenation.' *Journal of Thoracic and Cardiovascular Surgery*, **64,** 551 (1972)
91. Hill, J. D., de Leval, M. R., Mielke, C. H., Jr., Branson, M. L. and Gerbode, F. 'Clinical prolonged extracorporeal circulation for respiratory insufficiency: haematological effects.' *Transactions of the American Society for Artificial Internal Organs*, **18,** 546 (1972)
92. Hyans, T. Personal communication. Edwards Laboratories (1973)
93. Indeglia, R., Shea, M. A., Varco, R. L. and Bernstein, E. F. 'Mechanical and biological considerations in erythrocyte damage.' *Surgery*, **62,** 47 (1967)
94. Jaberi, M., Bell, W. R. and Benson, D. W. 'Control of heparin therapy in open-heart surgery.' *Journal of Thoracic and Cardiovascular Surgery*, **67,** 133 (1973)
95. Jacobs, L. A., Klopp, E. H., Seamone, W., Topaz, S. R. and Gott, V. L. 'Improved organ function during cardiac bypass with a roller pump modified to deliver pulsatile flow.' *Journal of Thoracic and Cardiovascular Surgery*, **58,** 703 (1969)
96. Jaques, L. B. 'Heparin from different sources.' *Lancet*, **2,** 1262 (1972)
97. Jennings, E. R., Beland, A. J., Cope, J. A., Ellestad, M. H., Monroe, C. and Shadle, O. W. 'Citrate toxicity and the use of anticoagulant acid citrate dextrose blood for extracorporeal circulation.' *Surgery, Gynecology and Obstetrics*, **120,** 997 (1965)
98. Kaplan, J. A., Cannarella, C., Jones, E. L., Kutner, M. H., Hatcher, C. R. and Dunbar, R. W. 'Autologous blood transfusion during cardiac surgery. A re-evaluation of three methods.' *Journal of Thoracic and Cardiovascular Surgery*, **74,** 4 (1977)
99. Katz, S. E., Kornfeld, D. S., Harris, P. D. and Yeoh, C. B. 'Acute gastro-intestinal ulceration with open-heart surgery and aortic valve disease.' *Surgery*, **72,** 438 (1972)
100. Kayser, K. L. 'Blood-gas interface oxygenators versus membrane oxygenators.' *Annals of Thoracic Surgery*, **17,** 459 (1974)
101. Kessler, J. and Patterson, R. H., Jr. 'The production of microemboli by various blood oxygenators.' *Annals of Thoracic Surgery*, **9,** 221 (1970)
102. Kevy, S. V., Glickman, R. M., Bernhard, W. F., Diamond, L. K. and Gross, R. E. 'The pathogenesis and control of the haemorrhagic defect in open-heart surgery.' *Surgery, Gynecology and Obstetrics*, **126,** 313 (1966)
103. Kohlstaedt, K. G. and Page, I. H. 'The liberation of renin by perfusion of kidneys following reduction of pulse pressure.' *Journal of Experimental Medicine*, **72,** 201 (1940)
104. Kolobow, T., Zapol, W. M., Sigman, R. L. and Pierce, J. 'Partial cardiopulmonary bypass lasting up to seven days in alert lambs with membrane lung blood oxygenation.' *Journal of Thoracic and Cardiovascular Surgery*, **60,** 781 (1970)
105. Kornfeld, D. S., Heller, S. S., Frank, K. A., Edie, R. N. and Barsa, J. 'Delirium after coronary artery bypass surgery.' *Journal of Thoracic and Cardiovascular Surgery*, **76,** 93 (1978)
106. Krous, M. D., Mansfield, P. B. and Sauvage, L. R. 'Carotid artery hyperfusion during open-heart surgery.' *Journal of Thoracic and Cardiovascular Surgery*, **66,** 118 (1973)
107. Kusserow, B. K. and Larrow, R. 'Studies of leukocyte responses to prolonged blood pumping – effects upon phagocytic capability and total white cell count.' *Transactions of the American Society for Artificial Internal Organs*, **14,** 261 (1968)

108. Landé, A. J., Carlson, R. G., Patterson, R. H., Jr., Baxter, J. and Lillehei, C. W. 'Cardiac surgery with disposable membrane lungs.' *Transactions of the American Society for Artificial Internal Organs*, **18**, 532 (1972)
109. Landé, A. J., Edwards, L., Bloch, J. H., Carlson, R. G., Subramanian, V. A., Ascheim, R. S., Scheidt, S., Fillmore, S., Killip, T. and Lillehei, C. W. 'Clinical experience with emergency use of prolonged cardiopulmonary bypass with a membrane pump oxygenator.' *Annals of Thoracic Surgery*, **10**, 409 (1970)
110. Lawrence, G. H., McKay, H. A. and Sherensky, R. T. 'Effective measures in the prevention of intraoperative aeroembolus.' *Journal of Thoracic and Cardiovascular Surgery*, **62**, 731 (1971)
111. Lee, W. H., Jr., Brady, M. P., Rowe, J. M. and Miller, W. C., Jr. 'Effects of extracorporeal circulation upon behaviour, personality, and brain function: Part II, Haemodynamic, metabolic and psychometric correlations.' *Annals of Surgery*, **173**, 1013 (1970)
112. Lee, W. H., Jr., Krumhaar, D., Fonkalsrud, E. W., Schjeide, O. E. and Maloney, J. V. 'Denaturation of plasma proteins as a cause of morbidity and death after intracardiac operations.' *Surgery*, **50**, 29 (1961)
113. Lees, M. H., Herr, R. H., Hill, J. D., Morgan, C. L., Ochsner, A. J., Thomas, C. and Van Fleet, D. L. 'Distribution of systemic blood flow of the rhesus monkey during cardiopulmonary bypass.' *Journal of Thoracic and Cardiovascular Surgery*, **61**, 570 (1970)
114. Lemieuz, M., Tice, D. A., Reed, G. E. and Chauss, R. H. 'Chlorpromazine; adjunt to physiologic perfusion.' *Journal of Thoracic and Cardiovascular Surgery*, **53**, 425 (1967)
115. Lichti, E. L., Simmons, E. J., Jr. and Almond, C. A. 'Detection of microemboli during cardiopulmonary bypass.' *Surgery, Gynecology and Obstetrics*, **134**, 977 (1972)
116. Litwack, R. S., Gilson, A. J., Slonim, R., McCune, C. C., Kiem, I. and Gadboys, H. L. 'Alterations in blood volume during "normovolaemic" total body perfusion.' *Journal of Thoracic and Cardiovascular Surgery*, **42**, 477 (1961)
117. Litwack, R. S., Jurado, R. A., Lukban, S. B., Mitchell, B. A., Kahn, M., Berger, S., Estioka, M. R. and Aledort, L. 'Perfusion without donor blood.' *Journal of Thoracic and Cardiovascular Surgery*, **64**, 714 (1972)
118. Litwack, R. S., Slonim, R., Wisoff, B. G. and Gadboys, H. L. 'Homologous blood syndrome during extracorporeal circulation in man.' *New England Journal of Medicine*, **268**, 1377 (1963)
119. Madras, P. N., Morton, W. A. and Petschek, H. E. 'Dynamics of thrombus formation.' *Federation Proceedings*, **30**, 1665 (1971)
120. Mandelbaum, I. and Morgan, C. R. 'Pancreatic blood flow and its relationship to insulin secretion during extracorporeal circulation.' *Annals of Surgery*, **170**, 753 (1969)
121. Many, M., Giron, F., Birtwell, W. C., Deterling, R. A. and Soroff, H. S. 'Effects of depulsation of renal blood flow upon renal function and renin secretion.' *Surgery*, **66**, 242 (1969)
122. Maxwell, G. M., Rowe, C. G., Castillo, G., Shuster, B., White, D. H. and Crumpton, C. W. 'Haemodynamic effects of chlorpromazine: including studies of cardiac work and coronary blood flow.' *Anesthesiology*, **19**, 64 (1958)
123. McNamara, J. J., Boatright, D., Burran, E. L., Molot, M. D., Summers, E. and Stremple, J. F. 'Changes in some physical properties of stored blood.' *Annals of Surgery*, **174**, 58 (1970)
124. Mielke, C. H., Jr., de Leval, M., Hill, J. D., Macur, M. F. and Gerbode, F. 'Drug influence on platelet loss during extracorporeal circulation.' *Journal of Thoracic and Cardiovascular Surgery*, **290**, 144 (1973)

125. Moffitt, E. A, Tarhan, S., Goldsmith, R. S., Pluth, J. R. and McGoon, D. C. 'Patterns of total and ionized calcium and other electrolytes in plasma during and after cardiac surgery.' *Journal of Thoracic and Cardiovascular Surgery*, **65,** 751 (1973)
126. Moores, W. Y., Gago, O., Morris, J. D. and Peck, C. C. 'Serum and urinary amylase levels following pulsatile and continuous cardiopulmonary bypass.' *Journal of Thoracic and Cardiovascular Surgery*, **74,** 73 (1977)
127. Moran, J. M., Babka, R., Silberman, S., Rice, P. L., Pifarré, R., Sullivan, H. J. and Montoya, A. 'Immediate centrifugation of oxygenator contents after cardiopulmonary bypass.' *Journal of Thoracic and Cardiovascular Surgery*, **76,** 510 (1978)
128. Mukherjee, N. D., Beran, A. V., Hirai, J. *et al.* '*In vivo* determination of renal tissue oxygenation during pulsatile and non-pulsatile left heart bypass.' *Annals of Thoracic Surgery*, **15,** 345 (1973)
129. Mullin, P., Lee, S., Burd, S. *et al.* 'A new device for the rapid automated determination of the activated clotting time of whole blood.' *AmSECT Proceedings*, pp. 6–8 (1976)
130. Murphy, D. A., Norris, K. and Martin, M. 'The *in vitro* characteristics of a toroidal flow membrane oxygenator.' *Transactions of the American Society for Artificial Internal Organs*, **17,** 337 (1971)
131. Murphy, W., Trudell, L. A., Friedman, L. I., Kakvan, M., Richardson, P. P., Galletti, P. M. and Karlson, K. 'Laboratory and clinical experience with a microporous membrane oxygenator.' *Transactions of the American Society for Artificial Internal Organs*, **20,** 278 (1974)
132. Nakayama, K., Tamiya, T., Yamamoto, K., Izumi, T., Akimoto, S., Imori, T., Odaka, M. and Yasawa, C. 'High amplitude pulsatile pump in extracorporeal circulation with particular reference to haemodynamics.' *Surgery*, **65,** 798 (1963)
133. Norman, J. C., McDonald, H. P. and Sloan, H. 'The early and aggressive treatment of acute renal failure following cardiopulmonary bypass with continuous peritoneal dialysis.' *Surgery*, **56,** 240 (1964)
134. O'Connor, N. E., Sheh, J. M., Bartlett, R. H. and Gazzaniga, A. B. 'Changes in pulmonary extravascular water volume following mitral valve replacement.' *Journal of Thoracic and Cardiovascular Surgery*, **61,** 342 (1971)
135. Okies, J. E., Goodnight, S. H., Kitchford, B., Connell, R. S. and Starr, A. 'Effect of infusion of cardiotomy suction blood during extracorporeal circulation for coronary artery bypass surgery.' *Journal of Thoracic and Cardiovascular Surgery*, **74,** 440 (1977)
136. Pacifico, A. D., Digerness, S. and Kirklin, J. W. 'Acute alterations of bodyt composition after open intracardiac operations.' *Circulation*, **41,** 331 (1970)
137. Page, U. S., Bigelow, J. C., Carter, C. R. and Swank, R. L. 'Emboli (debris) produced by bubble oxygenators.' *Annals of Thoracic Surgery*, **18,** 164 (1974)
138. Panebianco, A. C., Scott, S. M., Dart, C. H., Takaro, T. and Echegaray, H. M. 'Acute pancreatitis following extracorporeal circulation.' *Annals of Thoracic Surgery*, **9,** 562 (1970)
139. Pappas, G., Winter, S., Kopriva, C. J. and Steele, P. P. 'Improvement of myocardial and other vital organ functions and metabolism with a simple method of pulsatile flow (IABP) during clinical cardiopulmonary bypass.' *Surgery*, **77,** 34 (1975)
140. Patterson, R. H., Jr. and Kessler, J. 'Microemboli during cardiopulmonary bypass detected by ultrasound.' *Surgery, Gynecology and Obstetrics*, **129,** 505 (1969)
141. Peirce, E. C., II. (Guest ed.) 'Clinical uses of membrane lungs.' *Mount Sinai Journal of Medicine*, **40,** 119 (1973)

142. Peirce, E. C., II. 'A comparison of the Landé–Edwards, the Peirce, and the General Electric–Peirce membrane lungs.' *Transactions of the American Society for Artificial Internal Organs*, **16,** 358 (1970)
143. Peirce, E. C., II. *Extracorporeal Circulation for Open-heart Surgery*. Springfield: Thomas (1969)
144. Peirce, E. C., II. 'Is the blood-gas interface of clinical importance?' *Annals of Thoracic Surgery*, **17,** 526 (1974)
145. Peirce, E. C. II, Corrigan, J. J., Kent, B. B., Cate, C. L., Johnson, R. L. and Dreves, A. E. 'Comparative trauma to blood in the disc oxygenator and membrane lung.' *Transactions of the American Society for Artificial Internal Organs*, **15,** 33 (1969)
146. Peskin, G. W., O'Brien, K. and Rabiner, S. F. 'Stroma-free haemoglobin solution: the 'ideal' blood substitute?' *Surgery*, **66,** 185 (1969)
147. Proctor, R. R. and Rapaport, S. I. 'The partial thromboplastin time with kaolin.' *American Journal of Clinical Pathology*, **36,** 212 (1961)
148. Rabelo, R. C., Oliveira, S. A., Tanaka, H., Weigl, D. R., Verginelli, G. and Zerbini, E. J. 'The influence of the nature of the prime on post-perfusion pulmonary changes.' *Journal of Thoracic and Cardiovascular Surgery*, **66,** 782 (1973)
149. Ratliff, N. B., Young, G., Jr., Hackel, D. B., Mikat, E. and Wilson, J. E. 'Pulmonary injury secondary to extracorporeal circulation. An ultrastructural study.' *Journal of Thoracic and Cardiovascular Surgery*, **65,** 425 (1972)
150. Reed, W. A. and Kittle, C. F. 'Observations on toxicity and use of antifoam.' *Archives of Surgery*, **78,** 220 (1959)
151. Relihan, M. and Kitwin, M. S. 'Effects of stroma-free haemoglobin solution on clearance rate and renal function.' *Surgery*, **71,** 395 (1972)
152. Replogle, R. L. 'Use of corticosteroids during cardiopulmonary bypass: possible lysosome stabilization.' *Circulation*, **33,** and **34** (**Suppl. I**), 86 (1966)
153. Replogle, R. L. and Gross, R. E. 'Renal function during extracorporeal circulation.' *Journal of Surgical Research*, **1,** 91 (1961)
154. Replogle, R. L., Levy, M., DeWall, R. A. and Lillehei, R. C. 'Catecholamine and serotonin response to cardiopulmonary bypass.' *Journal of Thoracic and Cardiovascular Surgery*, **44,** 638 (1962)
155. Rittenhouse, E. A., Hessel, E. A., Ito, C. S. and Merendino, K. A. 'Effect of dipyridamole on microaggregate formation in the pump oxygenator.' *Annals of Surgery*, **175,** 1 (1972)
156. Romero, E. G., Castillo-Olivares, J. L., O'Connor, F., Guardiola, J. and Aymerich, D. F. 'The importance of calcium and magnesium ions in serum and cerebrospinal fluid during cardiopulmonary bypass.' *Journal of Thoracic and Cardiovascular Surgery*, **66,** 668 (1973)
157. Rosenblum, R. and Heidenberg, W. J. 'Post pump syndrome variant of post transfusion hepatitis.' *Archives of Internal Medicine*, **122,** 204 (1968)
158. Rosendorf, L. L., Daicoff, G. and Baer, H. 'Sources of gram negative infection after open-heart surgery.' *Journal of Thoracic and Cardiovascular Surgery*, **67,** 195 (1974)
159. Roughton, F. J. W. 'Transport of oxygen and carbon dioxide'. In *Handbook of Physiology: Respiration I*. Ed. W. Fenn and H. Rahn, Ch. 31, p. 767. Rockville, Maryland: American Physiological Society (1965)
160. Rudy, L. W., Heymann, M. A. and Edmunds, L. H. 'Distribution of systemic blood flow during total cardiopulmonary bypass in rhesus monkeys.' *Surgical Forum*, **21,** 149 (1970)
161. Rudy, L. W., Heymann, M. A. and Edmunds, L. H. 'Distribution of systemic blood flow during cardiopulmonary bypass.' *Journal of Applied Physiology*, **34,** 194 (1970)

162. Sakerno, T. A., Lince, D. P., White, D. N., Lynn, R. B. and Charrette, E. J. P. 'Monitoring of electroencephalogram during open-heart surgery.' *Journal of Thoracic and Cardiovascular Surgery*, **76,** 97 (1978)
163. Sallam, I. A. 'Prophylactic antibiotics in open-heart surgery.' *Surgery Digest*, **8,** 7 (1973)
164. Salzman, E. W. 'Role of platelets in blood-surface interactions.' *Federation Proceedings*, **30,** 1503 (1971)
165. Sanderson, J. M., Wright, G. and Simms, F. W. 'Brain damage in dogs immediately following pulsatile and nonpulsatile blood flows in extracorporeal circulation.' *Thorax*, **27,** 275 (1972)
166. Sanderson, R. G., Ellison, J. H., Benson, J. A., Jr. and Starr, A. 'Jaundice following open-heart surgery.' *Annals of Surgery*, **165,** 217 (1966)
167. Schaff, H. V., Hauer, J. M., Bell, W. R., Gardner, T. J., Donahoo, J. S., Gott, V. L. and Brawley, R. K. 'Autotransfusion of shed mediastinal blood after cardiac surgery – a prospective study.' *Journal of Thoracic and Cardiovascular Surgery*, **75,** 632 (1978)
168. Scheinman, M. M., Sullivan, R. W., Hutchinson, J. C. and Hyatt, K. H. 'Clinical significance of changes in serum magnesium in patients undergoing cardiopulmonary bypass.' *Journal of Thoracic and Cardiovascular Surgery*, **61,** 135 (1971)
169. Selmonosky, C. A. 'Studies on urinary urea concentration after cardiopulmonary bypass: a sensitive index of altered renal haemodynamics.' *Annals of Surgery*, **172,** 226 (1969)
170. Sessler, A. D., Taswell, H. F., Moffitt, E. A. and Kirklin, J. W. 'Heparinized versus acid-citrate-dextrose blood for cardiopulmonary bypass.' *Mayo Clinic Proceedings*, **40,** 859 (1965)
171. Shah-Mirany, J., Najafi, H., Serry, C., Callaghan, R. and Yang, J. 'Pathophysiological alterations in perfused and nonperfused lungs during cardiopulmonary bypass.' *Annals of Thoracic Surgery*, **10,** 402 (1970)
172. Shepard, R. B. and Kirklin, J. W. 'Relation of pulsatile flow to oxygen consumption and other variables during cardiopulmonary bypass.' *Journal of Thoracic and Cardiovascular Surgery*, **58,** 694 (1969)
173. Silva, J., Jr., Hoeksema, H. and Fekety, F. R. 'Transient defects in phagocytic functions during cardiopulmonary bypass.' *Journal of Thoracic and Cardiovascular Surgery*, **67,** 175 (1974)
174. Spaeth, E. E., Roberts, G. W., Yadwadkar, S. R., Ng, P. K. and Jackson, C. M. 'The influence of fluid shear on the kinetics of blood coagulation reactions.' *Transactions of the American Society for Artificial Internal Organs*, **19,** 179 (1973)
175. Stanley, P., Bertranou, E., Forest, F. and Langevin, L. 'Toxicity of ethylene oxide sterilization of polyvinyl chloride in open-heart surgery.' *Journal of Thoracic and Cardiovascular Surgery*, **61,** 309 (1971)
176. Stein, J. H. and Perris, T. F. 'The physiology of renin.' *Archives of Internal Medicine*, **131,** 860 (1973)
177. Subramanian, V., Lowman, J. and Gans, H. 'Effect of extracorporeal circulation on reticuloendothelial function.' *Archives of Surgery*, **97,** 330 (1968)
178. Subramanian, V., McLeod, J. and Gans, H. 'Effect of extracorporeal circulation on reticuloendothelial function. I. Experimental evidence for impaired reticuloendothelial function following cardiopulmonary bypass in rats.' *Surgery*, **64,** 775 (1968)
179. Sveinsson, I. S. 'Postoperative psychosis after heart surgery.' *Journal of Thoracic and Cardiovascular Surgery*, **70,** 717 (1975)
180. Swan, H. 'Clinical hypothermia: a lady with a past and some promise for the future.' *Surgery*, **73,** 736 (1973)

181. Tan, C–K., Glisson, S. N., El–Etr, A. A. and Ramakrishnaiah, K. B. 'Levels of circulating norepinephrine and epinephrine before, during, and after cardiopulmonary bypass in man.' *Journal of Thoracic and Cardiovascular Surgery*, **71,** 928 (1976)
182. Tarhan, S. and Moffitt, E. A. 'Anaesthesia and supportive care during and after cardiac surgery.' *Annals of Thoracic Surgery*, **11,** 64 (1971)
183. Taylor, K. M., Wright, G. S., Reid, J. M., Bain, W. H., Caves, P. K., Walker, M. S. and Grant, J. K. 'Comparative studies of pulsatile and non-pulsatile flow during cardiopulmonary bypass II. The effects on adrenal secretion of cortisol.' *Journal of Thoracic and Cardiovascular Surgery*, **75,** 574 (1978)
184. Timmis, H. H., Hardy, J. D., Davis, D. J. and Raju, S. 'Intracranial pressure during cardiopulmonary bypass.' *Annals of Surgery*, **174,** 887 (1970)
185. Trinkle, J. K., Helton, N. E., Bryant, L. R. and Gridden, W. O. 'Pulsatile cardiopulmonary bypass: clinical evaluation.' *Surgery*, **68,** 1074 (1970)
186. Trinkle, J. K., Helton, N. E., Wood, R. E. and Bryant, L. R. 'Metabolic comparison of a new pulsatile pump and a roller pump for cardiopulmonary bypass.' *Journal of Thoracic and Cardiovascular Surgery*, **58,** 562 (1969)
187. Trudell, L. A., Friedman, L. I., Kakvan, M., Galletti, P. M. and Richardson, P. D. 'Evaluation of a disposable membrane oxygenator.' *Transactions of the American Society for Artificial Internal Organs*, **18,** 538 (1972)
188. Tufo, H. M., Ostfeld, A. M. and Shekelle, R. 'Central nervous system dysfunction following open-heart surgery.' *Journal of the American Medical Association*, **212,** 1333 (1970)
189. Turnier, E., Osborn, J. J., Gerbode, F. and Popper, R. W. 'Magnesium and open-heart surgery.' *Journal of Thoracic and Cardiovascular Surgery*, **64,** 694 (1972)
190. Varco, R. L. (Ed.) 'Conference on mechanical surface and gas layer effects on moving blood.' *Federation Proceedings*, **30,** 1475 (1971)
191. Vasko, K. A., Riley, A. M. and DeWall, R. A. 'Poloxalkol (pluronic F–68): a priming solution for cardiopulmonary bypass.' *Transactions of the American Society for Artificial Internal Organs*, **18,** 526 (1972)
192. Vroman, L., Adams, A. L. and Lings, M. 'Interactions among human blood proteins at interfaces.' *Federation Proceedings*, **30,** 1494 (1971)
193. Vroman, L. and Leonard, E. F. 'The behaviour of blood and its components at interfaces.' *Annals of the New York Academy of Science*, **283,** (1977)
194. Wallace, H. W., Mooz, E. D. and Blakemore, W. S. 'Amino acid response to open-heart surgery.' *Annals of Surgery*, **178,** 600 (1972)
195. Walsh, J. H., Purcell, R. H., Morrow, A. G., Chanock, R. M. and Schmidt, P. J. 'Post-transfusion hepatitis after open-heart operations.' *Journal of the American Medical Association*, **211,** 261 (1970)
196. Weedn, R. J., Coalson, J. J. and Greenfield, L. J. 'Effects of oxygen and ventilation on pulmonary mechanics and ultrastructure during cardiopulmonary bypass.' *American Journal of Surgery*, **120,** 584 (1970)
197. Wellons, H. A., Jr. and Nolan, S. P. 'Prevention of air embolism due to trapped air in filters used in extracorporeal circuits.' *Journal of Thoracic and Cardiovascular Surgery*, **65,** 476 (1973)
198. Wells, R. E., Bygdeman, M. S., Shahariar, A. A., Matloff, J. M. and Harken, D. E. 'Use of a polyol in the prevention of haemolysis due to an antifoam agent in pump oxygenators.' *Circulation*, **37,** 168 (1968)
199. Welsh, G. F., Dozois, R. R., Bartholemew, L. G., Brown, A. L. and Danielson, G. K. 'Gastrointestinal bleeding after open-heart surgery.' *Journal of Thoracic and Cardiovascular Surgery*, **65,** 738 (1973)
200. Wesoloski, S. A., Sauvage, L. R. and Pine, R. D. 'Extracorporeal circulation: the role of the pulse in maintenance of the systemic circulation during heart-lung bypass.' *Surgery*, **37,** 663 (1954)

201. Williams, K. R. and Blustein, R. 'Evaluation of a disposable bubble oxygenator.' *Journal of Thoracic and Cardiovascular Surgery*, **50,** 35 (1965)
202. Woods, J. E., Taswell, H. F., Kirklin, J. W. and Owen, C. A. 'The transfusion of platelet concentrates in patients undergoing heart surgery.' *Mayo Clinic Proceedings*, **42,** 318 (1967)
203. Witoszka, M. M., Tamura, H., Indeglia, R., Hopkins, R. W. and Simeone, F. A. 'Electroencephalographic changes and cerebral complications in open-heart surgery.' *Journal of Thoracic and Cardiovascular Surgery*, **66,** 855 (1973)
204. Zapol, W., Pontoppidan, H., McCullough, N., Schmidt, V., Bland, J. and Kitz, R. 'Clinical membrane lung support for acute respiratory insufficiency.' *Transactions of the American Society for Artificial Internal Organs*, **18,** 553 (1972)
205. Zapol, W. M. and Qvist, J. *Artificial Lungs for Acute Respiratory Failure*. New York: Academic Press (1976)

2

Extracorporeal Circulation Using the Rotating Disc Oxygenator

Earle B. Kay, David Mendelsohn and Hossein Naraghipour

via trita, via tuta

Introduction

The basic mechanism of the Kay–Cross rotating disc oxygenator[1,2] is a series of 60–120 siliconized Teflon-coated stainless steel discs, 0.4 mm in thickness and 12.2 cm in diameter, mounted 4.5 mm apart by means of siliconized stainless steel spacers on a rotating central shaft. The disc assembly is supported horizontally within a silicone-coated pyrex cylinder 13, 20, or 25 inches in length, depending upon the demands on the oxygenator being used. The diameter of the cylinder is 13.3 cm. The ends are gasketed by siliconized stainless steel plates with provisions for the necessary input and output connections (*Figure 2.1*). Fitting snugly in the bottom of the cylinder is a coiled Gebauer heat exchanger.

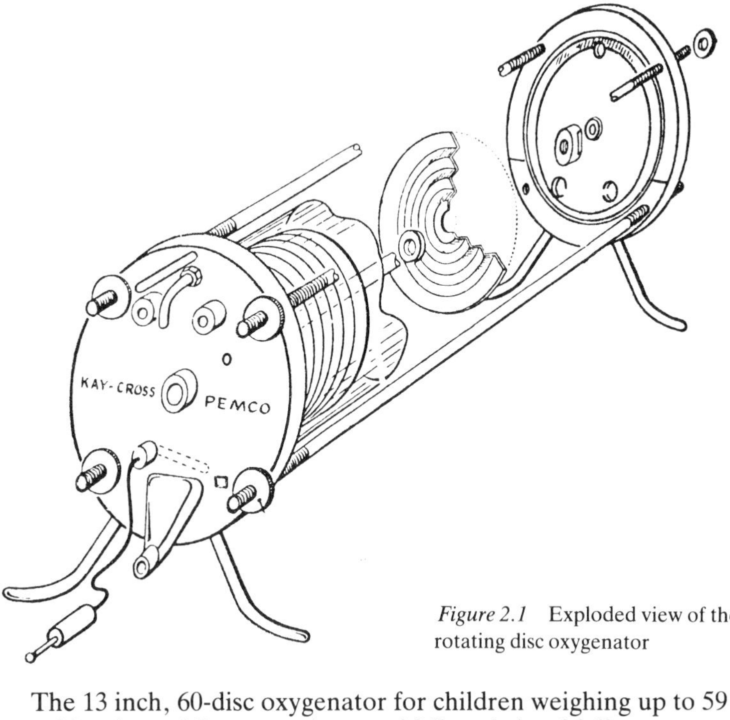

Figure 2.1 Exploded view of the Kay–Cross rotating disc oxygenator

The 13 inch, 60-disc oxygenator for children weighing up to 59 pounds is capable of providing a maximum of 3 litres/min of fully oxygenated blood. The 21 inch, 93-disc oxygenator for patients weighing between 60 and 159 pounds provides a maximum flow of 4.5 litres/min. The large 25 inch, 113-disc oxygenator provides a flow of 6 litres/min. The venous blood introduced at one end is filmed upon the uppermost two-thirds aspect of the discs as they rotate. As the chemical reaction between haemoglobin and oxygen and carbon dioxide is short, the rotation of the discs at 120 revolutions per minute (rev/min) allows the filming of blood to be changed sufficiently frequently to provide for new films to be constantly presented for brief exposures. If necessary, the rev/min can be increased to 140 without significant columning of blood, but this increases haemolysis in long pump runs. The effective oxygenating area at 120 rev/min for the intermediate oxygenator is 208 m^2. By rapid exposure of the blood film to oxygen a large minute area in a comparatively small apparatus can be achieved. Bubbles brought to the oxygenator from the cardiotomy suction are easily expelled during the filming process. This method of oxygenation is free from gaseous microembolism.

Directional blood flow occurs at the bottom of the oxygenator cylinder. As the discs rotate a film of blood is formed upon the discs. As the blood moves to the following discs, the successive filming increases oxygen saturation and carbon dioxide elimination.

Though the original flat discs are still used by some, we recommend the convoluted discs developed in 1958[3] because of their greater surface area and oxygenation capacity. The discs are stamped with a 90 degree impression in a concentric manner which increases the oxygenating surface area per disc by 38 per cent over the flat discs (*Figure 2.2*). The optimal size

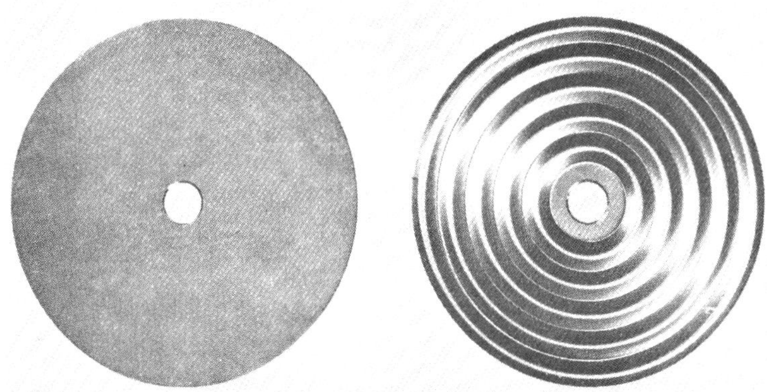

Figure 2.2 Flat and convoluted discs

oxygenator for the size of patient being perfused at physiological flows provides arterial saturations between 95 and 100 per cent and venous saturations between 70 and 74 per cent.

Oxygen is introduced into the cylinder through a metallic tube positioned in the upper part of the oxygenator. The metallic tube has numerous holes with the distal holes larger than the proximal ones so that the gas diffuses evenly inside the oxygenator. Five litres/min of oxygen is adequate to saturate the blood. The gaseous exchange within the disc oxygenator is governed by the same biochemical reactive and physical laws which govern such changes within the normal lungs. Several factors control gaseous exchange within the rotating disc oxygenator. They are the rotation speed of the discs, the flow rate of blood, the flow volume of gases into the oxygenator, the blood level and the temperature.

With 5 litres/min oxygen flow into the oxygenator and a disc rotation of 120 rev/min there is a tendency to produce a respiratory alkalosis due to wash-out of CO_2. This becomes clinically significant when the $P\text{CO}_2$ is below 25mmHg. This may increase cerebral vascular resistance and cerebral anoxia. Maintaining the $P\text{CO}_2$ at near normal level may indirectly prevent metabolic acidosis which may accompany respiratory alkalosis. As such, it is necessary to add 1 to 3 per cent carbon dioxide (10 ml/min) to the oxygenator to prevent hypocarbia.

Pumps

Though Sigmamotor pumps were used initially, laboratory studies on pump output, arterial line pressures, haemolysis and perfusion led to the use of modified DeBakey type roller pumps[2]. The pump consists of a system of two rollers diametrically positioned which compress the rubber latex pump chamber over a 200 degree arc with a circumferential distance of 11 inches (*Figure 2.3*). The distance of each of the rollers from the pumping track can

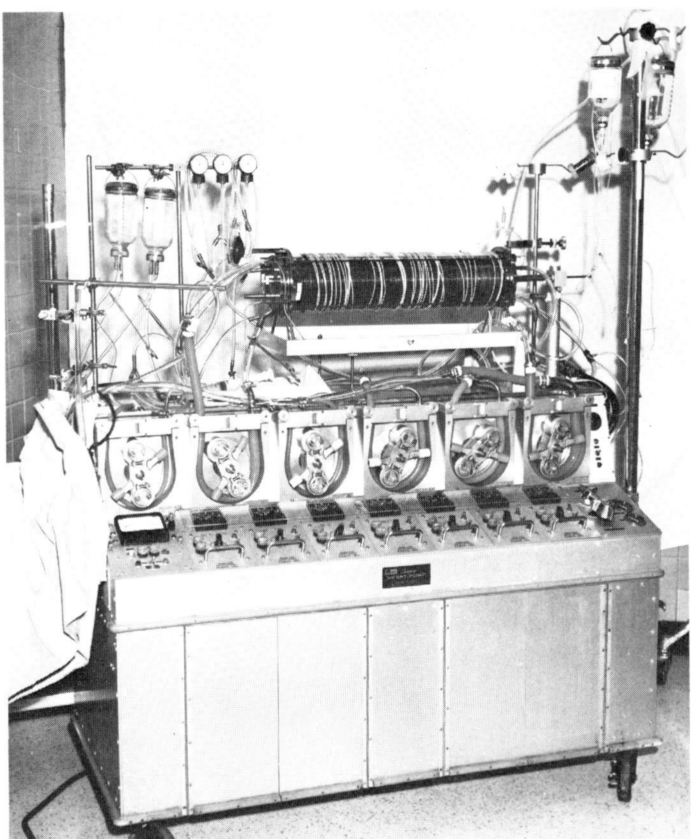

Figure 2.3 Kay–Cross disc oxygenator with DeBakey type roller pumps

be adjusted by a small screw which alters its centre of rotation in relation to the roller arc and thus its distance from the track. A rubber latex pump chamber can be varied in size for optimum stroke volume, corresponding to the size of the oxygenator.

A 3 foot length of ½ inch internal diameter tygon tubing connects the pump to the oxygenator. A 7 foot length of ⅜ inch internal diameter tygon tubing is connected to the arterial cannula. By tightly occluding the rollers the amount of blood destruction per passage through the pump is increased. By adjusting the rollers to be non-occlusive a large backflow through the pump decreases the stroke volume to the extent that rapid pump speeds are necessary to produce sufficient flow rates. With a non-occlusive setting the effect of the resistance in the perfused subject markedly changes the calibrated flow of the pump. With a compromise between these two settings to a just-non-occlusive setting, haemolysis is decreased and only a small back flow is permitted. The non-occlusive roller setting of the pump is calibrated against a simulated peripheral resistance as well as graded sizes of arterial cannulae. The roller pump output is so designed that it provides for a greater pulsatile flow output per revolution of the rollers than is obtained with a non-pulsatile flow. The arterial and venous pressures and the vascular resistance are lower during pulsatile bypass. The pulsatile flow by means of the roller pump apparently improves cellular oxygenation[5]. The arterial pH and P_{O_2} are consistently higher and the lactate–pyruvate ratio is lower. This is supported by the high venous P_{O_2} determinations in patients with pulsatile bypass. Pulsatile flow also results in less haemolysis, less defibrination and a smaller decline in platelet count and haematocrit.

Heat exchanger

The Gebauer heat exchanger employed with a disc oxygenator consists of a system of coils placed in the bottom of the oxygenator cylinder. This system consists of a series of ⅛ inch internal diameter stainless steel tubes semicircular moulded and connected in parallel, placed in the bottom of the oxygenator cylinder (*Figure 2.4*). Inflow and outflow conduits pass the end-plate of the disc oxygenator near the top and are then connected to a thermal regulatory unit.

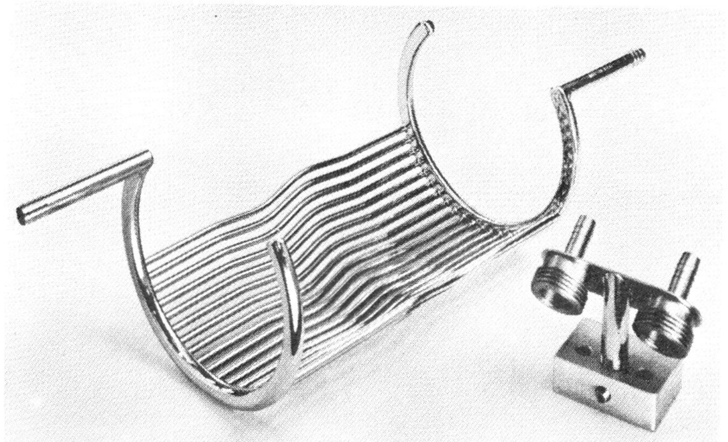

Figure 2.4 Gebauer heat exchanger

Coronary perfusion

If the aorta is to be clamped and opened for extended periods, coronary perfusion is employed. A variety of cannulae have been designed to be inserted into the coronary orifices. Some of these are metal with flexible ends to be held in place by hand, while others are flexible and are secured by ligature.

The blood for coronary perfusion comes directly from the arterial end-plate of the disc oxygenator through a ¼ inch internal diameter tygon tube. A roller pump is placed in each of the coronary lines for perfusion. A pressure reservoir and manometer are connected to each coronary line by a Y-shaped connector in order to measure both the resistance to the perfusion and the volume of flow being perfused. A small reservoir in the line provides a safety factor against resistance increases due to malposition of the cannulae. Usually 200 to 250 ml/min flow is perfused through each of the coronary lines at a mean pressure of 100 mmHg. In the event that one coronary cannula prevents operative exposure or if suitable flow is not being obtained, only one coronary artery is perfused, usually with a higher flow rate.

Arterial and venous lines and suction systems

A 3 foot length of ½ inch internal diameter tygon tubing is used to connect the arterial pump to the disc oxygenator and a 9 foot long, ⅜ inch internal diameter tygon tubing connects the pump to the arterial cannula in the ascending aorta. A 21 inch extension of the latex tubing extends beyond the pump in the arterial line which acts as a depulsator, so that arterial flow is just mildly pulsatile. The two vena-caval cannulae are connected to a single ⅜ inch internal diameter tygon tubing, 9 feet in length, by a Y-shaped connector. The latex tube is connected to the venous pump head. There is a 2 foot long, ½ inch internal diameter tygon tubing which connects the venous pump to the input end-plate of the disc oxygenator. Central venous pressure during a pump run is monitored using a 6 foot length of ¼ inch internal diameter tygon tubing connected to the catheter which is placed within the superior vena cava.

There are two field sumps which pass through a filter system and a cardiotomy reservoir. One of these is usually used to decompress the left ventricle. These are connected to the venous end-plate of the disc oxygenator. Filter systems are never used on the arterial line.

Priming and transfusion requirements

The priming volumes of the three sizes of oxygenators are: 1300, 3700 and 4500 ml. The depth of the priming solution within the cylinder should be approximately 4 cm. A 2 cm rise or fall in the level does not interfere with the oxygenating safety. The priming solution consists usually of 50 per cent blood and 50 per cent diluent. One-half the diluent is low molecular weight dextran to prevent intravascular haemoagglutination and the rest is Normosol. Blood is introduced into the oxygenator through a filter to remove any aggregates of fibrin, platelets or red blood cells.

The haematocrit at the onset ranges between 26 and 32 per cent and persists during the initial one-half of the pump run. The haematocrit is determined periodically. A higher flow rate is used with a lower haematocrit to provide adequate oxygenation. Mannitol is added within the first 30 minutes. The patient's temperature is maintained at around 30°C. This is usually obtained within five minutes. Ice slush is frequently employed initially in the pericardial sac for quick cardioplegia. Rewarming is usually instituted between 20 and 30 minutes prior to completion of the bypass. During this period of rewarming, 500 to 1500 ml of urinary output increases the haematocrit to a satisfactory level. The volume of blood used during the bypass varies between 1 and 4 units depending upon the size of the patient, the surgical technique and whether or not it is a primary or secondary operation.

Fresh blood is preferred and is collected a few hours before surgery in plastic bags which contain 15 mg of heparin per 500 ml of blood. Blood stored for 24–48 hours may also be used. If so, this is used for priming, and fresh blood is added later if necessary. Because of the low haemolysis, and satisfactory haematocrit at the completion of the operation, the blood in the oxygenator is collected in 500 ml plastic bags and used postoperatively. This is preferred to using additional units for it represents a good portion of the patient's own blood and minimizes the danger of hepatitis or postoperative pump syndrome. The average total blood usage during surgery in the last 100 patients operated upon was 2.5 litres. The average 24 hour thoracotomy drainage was 800 ml. The total blood usage during surgery and the first 24 hours postoperatively was 3.5 litres. In only 4 patients was it necessary to reoperate for haemostasis. This demonstrates that our present technique of perfusion is physiological and atraumatic to the blood and the clotting mechanism.

Total and partial perfusion

At the beginning and also at the end of the bypass only a portion of the total blood flow passes through the pump oxygenator. We believe that commencing and discontinuing the complete heart–lung bypass should be done gradually in order to allow ample time for cardiocirculatory adjustments to take place. At the beginning of heart-lung bypass a period of hypotension may initially occur which may be due to some blood cell incompatibility, allergic response or venous pooling. Another factor which contributes to hypotension is reduction of peripheral resistance by temporary dilatation of the arterioles. If stored blood is used, the high concentration of potassium and low pH may result in hypotension. With the pump running, the hypotension lasts usually only for a short period of time, following which the condition becomes stable.

Immediately after starting the perfusion the level of the blood in the oxygenator might fall from a reduction in the venous return. This may be due to sequestration of the blood in the dilated veins, particularly in the spanchnic area. The filling pressure of the right ventricle is reduced by drainage of the blood to the oxygenator. At the termination of the cardiac operation, while the heart is being supported, there is gradual reduction in pump flow, as myocardial contractility improves.

A transition from partial to total perfusion is achieved by occluding the venae cavae or by reducing the venous pressure through increased venous pump suction so that the venous blood is completely diverted from the right atrium to the extracorporeal apparatus. The venomotor reflex, which normally alters the cardiac output in response to the baroceptor signals, is greatly diminished. This may result in up to a 50 per cent fall in venous return during the initial part of total perfusion. Although not usually necessary, a small dose of norepinephrine can temporarily return the flow to a normal level.

In infants and children, flow rates of 80–120 ml/kg per min, are employed. Adolescents and adults are perfused with 45–50 ml/kg per min. Certain guidelines are followed in determining optimal flow rates. These include colour of conjunctivae, skin and tissue turgor, venous pressure, mean arterial pressure and urinary output. Constant urinary output is one of the best indices of adequate tissue perfusion and oxygenation. In older patients, in the presence of hypothermia vasoconstriction may lead to abnormally high mean arterial pressures. In such an event the pump output is not decreased, but instead the patient is partially rewarmed. With the onset of partial perfusion the venous pressure is maintained at 5–10 mm of water. As the perfusion flow augments and becomes stabilized, the rotation speed of the venous pump is gradually increased to reduce the venous pressure to between –3 and 0, thus diverting the blood from the heart to the oxygenator. Usually 3–4 minutes are necessary to reach full perfusion.

In left-side heart surgical procedures, and in patients requiring myocardial revascularization, the venae cavae are not occluded so that the negative venous pressure withdraws the coronary sinus blood to the oxygenator. This prevents engorgement of the pulmonary vascular bed and return to the left side of the heart and consequently minimizes the amount of left ventricular decompression. In patients with hypertrophied hearts, congested lungs and tissue fluid retention, requiring valve surgery, an increase in venous return is usually noted at the time of, or shortly after, the cardiotomy and decompression. This excess blood, which amounts to 300–800 ml, is collected in a reservoir in the sump system. This blood is later transfused back to the patient.

At the conclusion of the bypass the venous pressure is gradually returned to physiological levels. In the presence of advanced pulmonary vascular disease the venous pressure and right ventricular pressure are slightly elevated to overcome the pulmonary vascular resistance. In patients with valve surgery the left ventricular filling volume and pressure are regulated by monitoring the left atrial pressure postoperatively. The haemoglobin and haematocrit are readjusted if necessary. The calculated dose of protamine is given and careful haemostasis is made. Pacemaker wires are inserted routinely in all patients with mitral or multiple valve surgery, and in patients with coronary artery disease and conduction defects or arrhythmias. Drainage tubes are placed in the pericardium and in the anterior mediastinum. Pleural thoracotomy tubes are inserted if necessary. The above tubes are connected to closed thoracotomy drainage bottles without suction. A gastric tube is inserted to prevent gastric distension and aspiration of gastric fluid. The patient is weighed and a roentgenogram of the chest is obtained. Tracheobronchial aspiration is performed as required. Blood samples are drawn for blood gas analysis and chemical determinations. The necessary corrective steps are then taken if any abnormalities exist.

Patients are usually extubated in the operating room. Postoperatively humidified oxygen mixed with air is supplied by a hood for the first night, and through a nasal catheter afterwards. Intubation and mechanically controlled respiration is employed when indicated.

Clinical method of cardioplegia

We employ hypothermic cardiac arrest, maintaining the oesophageal temperature at 28–30°C. In cases in which ventricular fibrillation does not occur spontaneously, ice-slush saline is placed in the pericardial sac until fibrillation occurs. The coronary arteries are perfused by the systemic arterial perfusion with blood cooled to 28–30°C when the aorta is not clamped. In no instance do we clamp the aorta during bypass surgery for myocardial revascularization. If the aorta is clamped and opened for aortic valve surgery, the coronary arteries are perfused through two separate cannulae with cooled blood, and the heart usually remains at a standstill. At the completion of the operative technique, rewarming of the blood and myocardium is performed by slowly raising the temperature of the heat exchanger over a period of 10–15 minutes. The heart is allowed to fill with blood by discontinuing the intracardiac decompression, and the venous pressure is gradually increased by reducing the revolutions of the venous pump. Electric counter-shock is used to defibrillate the heart. Prior to electric defibrillation the apex of the left ventricle is elevated, and the site of the opening in the left ventricle is reopened to allow any retained air to escape. The aorta is clamped and a second small vent is made in the base of the aorta. Succinylcholine is given and the heart is shocked, unless spontaneous stystole has occurred. In the event of delay in establishing complete cardiocirculatory response, calcium is first employed. If after adequate calcium therapy, bradycardia exists, isoproterenol is administered. If a heart rate of 80–100 beats per minute is obtained and the blood pressure is adequate, no further medication is provided. Rarely are vasoconstrictor drugs used. The heart is allowed to pump against the clamped aorta, to free itself of any additional undetected residual air through the aortic vent. The aortic clamp can then be opened. Since this technique has been routinely employed during the past five years there have been no instances of cerebral air embolism.

A second period of total or partial heart-lung bypass may be employed in patients with poor ventricular function and low systemic blood pressure.

The pump units

We have three pump units available for clinical use in addition to those employed in the research laboratory. The first and simplest is a three-pump unit used in the cardiac intensive care unit for circulatory support of patients in congestive heart failure, patients in shock from an extensive myocardial infarction and patients with a low postoperative cardiac output. One pump is used for the arterial line, a second pump for the venous line and a third for suction if required. The appropriate oxygenators are used, but usually a smaller size is selected for partial support of the circulation and respiration. Consequently, considerably less priming volume is required. Usually a filter and reservoir system is not employed with a support pump unit. All cannulations are performed at the groin site. Partial support is maintained usually for less than 12 hours and frequently for 6 to 8 hours. No detrimental changes have been noted in the blood chemistry or clotting mechanism, and invariably these parameters were improved. This pump oxygenator system is always available on an emergency basis.

A four-pump unit is employed in patients for myocardial revascularization. This provides one pump for the venous return, one for the arterial output, a third for ventricular decompression and a fourth for general sump purposes. A six-pump unit is employed in patients requiring aortic or multiple valve surgery. In addition to the above-mentioned four pumps, two pumps are used for separate right and left coronary perfusion (*Figure 2.3*).

Ideal perfusion

The ideal perfusion is that which best replaces the action of the heart and lungs while these are excluded from the circulation. The best criterion for an ideal perfusion is the complete return to normal function of all the organs and systems after termination of the heart-lung bypass.

Some responsibilities of the perfusionist must be emphasized. The first is the immaculate cleansing of all reusable parts of the heart-lung machine. Every amount of old protein from previous uses must be removed and all surfaces must be satisfactorily resiliconized daily. Periodically the discs are completely stripped of the silicone build-up. After the oxygenator is assembled and the tubing connected, the entire unit is cleansed by immersing the venous inlet tube in a large container of saline. This is circulated through all the tubing and oxygenator and discharged from the arterial output. This eliminates any lint, residual detergent, and other debris. The perfusionist ensures that the heart-lung machine is safely reassembled and that all connections are secure. Before the perfusion is started, it is important to check the following: the delivery of humidified oxygen, as well as the proper concentration of CO_2, into the oxygenator, the heat exchanger temperature, the rotation of the discs and, finally, the patency of the arterial and venous lines. The operator of the machine must be able to communicate with the surgeon regarding any difficulties. The perfusion rate must be equal to the basic cardiac output. The mean arterial pressure, monitored by a catheter in the radial artery, must be maintained at

60–80 mmHg in order to provide sufficient pressure to all vascular beds. Venous pressures are kept at physiological levels at the onset and at the termination of the heart-lung bypass. During perfusion the venous pressure is maintained at a slightly negative level in order to prevent cerebral and hepatic damage.

Extremely high oxygenation during perfusion is avoided. The arterial oxygen saturation is usually maintained at 95–100 per cent. It is important to maintain the venous oxygen saturation near 70 per cent. In general, a mixed venous oxygen saturation of 60 per cent or lower means inadequate tissue perfusion. The mixed venous $P\text{CO}_2$ should be about 40 mmHg. Blood haemoglobin and haematocrit should be checked periodically. Very diluted blood must be avoided because it results in a lower oxygen content. The excretory function of the kidneys should remain within physiological limits. The number of blood cells should not decrease, and denaturation of plasma proteins should be minimized.

It is preferable to use the ascending aorta as the site of arterial cannulation. We use a pump for controlled venous return to the oxygenator. This has the advantage of maintaining the patient's blood volume more accurately and allows the operator to determine the amount of blood to be diverted from the heart. When the bypass is total the arterial pump should provide an output near normal for that particular patient. For an adult patient with valvular disease, the arterial perfusion flow is around 50 ml/kg per min. For children less than 10 years old, the arterial flow is 70–100 ml/kg per min. If metabolic acidosis develops following a prolonged heart-lung bypass, this means inadequate perfusion, and it must be appropriately treated. Special attention should be paid to the venous return and blood level in the oxygenator. If the venous pressure increases and the blood level in the oxygenator drops, the venae cavae cannulae are either kinked, are too small or are inserted too far into the venae cavae with their ends in the hepatic veins or innominate vessels. The position of the tapes around the venae cavae should be inspected. If the venous pressure is low, and at the same time the level in the oxygenator is falling, the patient is hypovolaemic due to blood loss. Less often, this may be due to a collection of blood in the reservoir from the open-heart decompression line or to venous pooling. The commonest cause of arterial hypotension is loss of circulating volume. The presence of aortic insufficiency or of a patent ductus arteriosus may also account for low blood pressure.

In the course of perfusion the sump suction needs careful watching. This may require rather precise adjustment because the greatest amount of damage to the blood takes place in the suction system. To minimize blood damage a very wide suction tip is used. The suction must be just enough to keep the field clear. Excessive suction of air with blood will greatly increase the haemolysis. When suction is not employed, the suction pump is turned off. Excessive air in a suction system is also a potential source of contamination from room air. The blood should be aspirated from the cardiac chambers before it enters the pericardial cavity. There will be an increase of haemolysis and loss of thromboplastin when the blood comes into contact with the pericardial or pleural cavities. The efficacy of the technique of extracorporeal perfusion as described above evidences itself in minimal postoperative cerebral, pulmonary and renal complications.

Analysis of last 100 operated patients

The efficacy of a pump oxygenating system is attested to by the results obtained with its use. The various parameters attained in the last 100 patients operated upon with the use of the Kay–Cross rotating disc oxygenator were purposely analysed for presentation in this chapter. *Table 2.1* lists the surgical techniques employed and the final haemolysis observed in these 100 patients.

Table 2.1

Procedure	*Total pts*	*Pump time* *<2h*	 *2–3h*	*Haemolysis* *<50%*	 *<75%*	 *<100%*	 *>100%*
		No.pts	No.pts	No.pts	No.pts	No.pts	No.pts
CAD 1	7	6	1	6	1	0	0
CAD 2	19	10	9	13	5	1	0
CAD 3	15	5	10	6	4	2	3
CAD + aneurysm							
1 "	4	2	2	4	0	0	0
2 "	2	1	1	1	1	0	0
3 "	4	1	3	1	1	1	1
Valves							
Single	25	5	20	8	8	4	5
Single + CAD 1	4	0	4	0	0	1	3
Single + CAD 2	4	0	4	1	0	0	3
Multiple	10	3	7	2	4	3	1
ASD	4	4	0	3	0	1	0
Tetralogy	1	0	1	1	0	0	0
VSD	1	1	0	1	0	0	0

Fifty-one patients had myocardial revascularization by aorta to coronary artery, saphenous vein bypass grafts, and 10 of these had in addition resection of ventricular aneurysms. There were no operative deaths, but 2 patients died during the postoperative period. Forty-three patients had heart valve replacement; 10 of them had double valve replacement and 8 had additional single or multiple saphenous vein bypass grafts for myocardial revascularization. There were no operative deaths, but 3 patients in this group died postoperatively. There were 6 congenital defects repaired with no operative mortality. The total operative mortality for this group of 100 patients was 5 per cent.

The capacity of the oxygenating system is attested to by the fact that 8 patients weighed between 195 and 235 pounds. The average perfusion time in these patients was 2 hours and 40 minutes. There was an average haemolysis of 116 milligrams of free haemoglobin per 100 ml. All of these 8 heavy patients had uncomplicated postoperative courses.

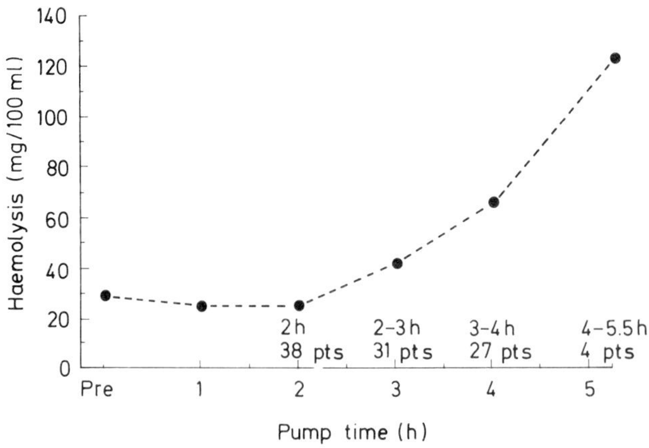

Figure 2.5 Relation of haemolysis to the perfusion time (pts = patients)

Figure 2.5 demonstrates the average perfusion time in relation to haemolysis. In this series of 100 patients operated upon, 4 who had heart-lung bypass for over 4 hours had haemolysis of more than 65 milligrams/100 ml. There was only an increase of 10 milligrams/100 ml at up to 3 hours of perfusion time. The average heart-lung bypass duration in the other 4 patients was 5.5 hours. The haemolysis in these 4 patients averaged 130 milligrams/100 ml. Haemolysis appears to be directly proportional to the duration of the bypass.

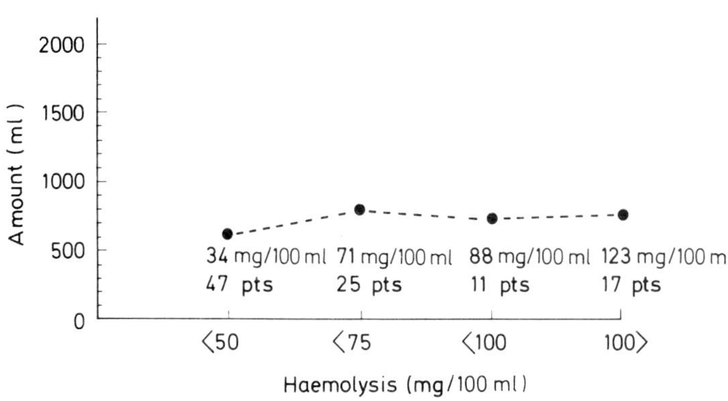

Figure 2.6 First 24 hours postoperative blood loss in relation to haemolysis

Figure 2.6 demonstrates graphically the postoperative blood loss in relation to the increase in haemolysis during heart-lung bypass. In the past, the degree of haemolysis has frequently been used as an index for blood trauma produced by the pump oxygenator system. It has been felt that destruction of the red blood cells would be similar to that of the other blood elements, such as platelets and fibrinogen, which are involved in the clotting mechanism. It was of interest to note that in this series of 100 patients, postoperative chest drainage remained fairly constant at 800 ml/patient regardless of the degree of haemolysis. However, it must be emphasized that the overall increase in haemolysis was relatively insignificant. This atraumatic action to the blood by the Kay–Cross rotating disc oxygenator is further reflected in the fact that only 4 patients required secondary postoperative haemostasis. In 3 of these patients definite bleeding sources were found.

Figure 2.7 demonstrates the average amount of blood used during and after heart-lung bypass in 100 patients. The oxygenator was primed with 2500 ml of blood and about 800 to 1100 ml diluent. In the course of the

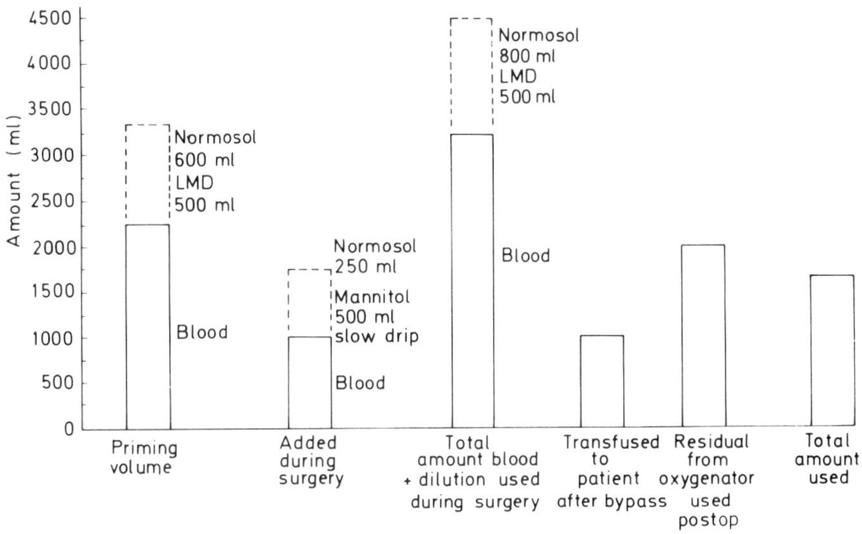

Figure 2.7 Graphic presentation of the amount of blood and diluent used for priming the oxygenator; the amount transfused to the patient after completion of heart-lung bypass and postoperatively; and total blood used (LMD = low molecular weight dextran)

perfusion, 1000 ml of blood, 500 ml of Mannitol Solution and 250 ml of Normosol Solution were added to the oxygenator. After completion of the heart-lung bypass, 1000 ml of blood from the oxygenator were reinfused through the arterial line into the patient to restore blood volume. The central venous pressure was usually increased to 12 cm of water. The residual blood in the oxygenator was then drained into plastic bags for use in the postoperative period.

Figure 2.8 and *2.9* are typical examples of the physiological response attained during and immediately after the heart-lung bypass procedure in patients with heart valve replacement and myocardial revascularization.

Other indices of the physiological efficacy of the perfusion or of the pump oxygenator system are the incidence and types of postoperative complications. In the group of 100 cardiac patients subjected to various operative procedures, many of whom sustained lengthy periods of heart-lung bypass, there was no incidence of renal complications nor was there any incidence of cerebral damage due to poor cerebral perfusion or air embolization. Four

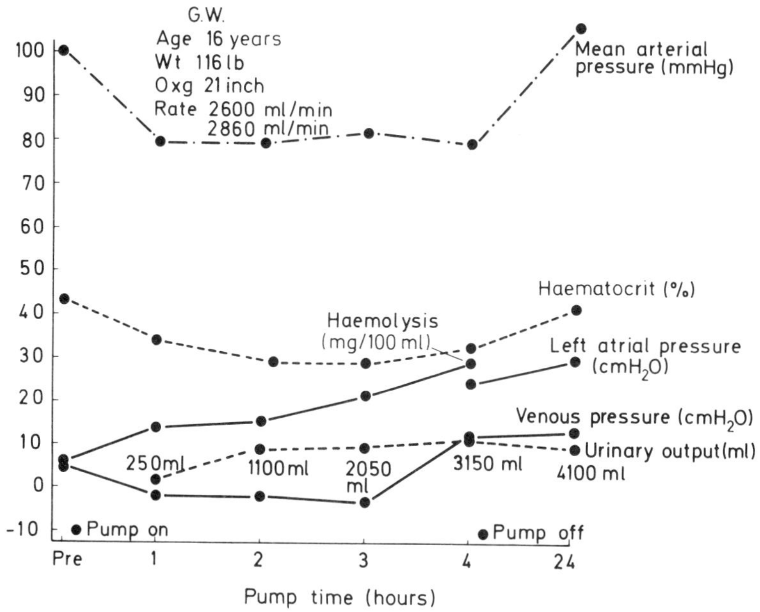

Figure 2.8 Evolution of arterial pressure, venous pressure, haemolysis, haematocrit, urinary output and left atrial pressure during perfusion in a patient undergoing aortic and mitral valve replacement and 24 hours after

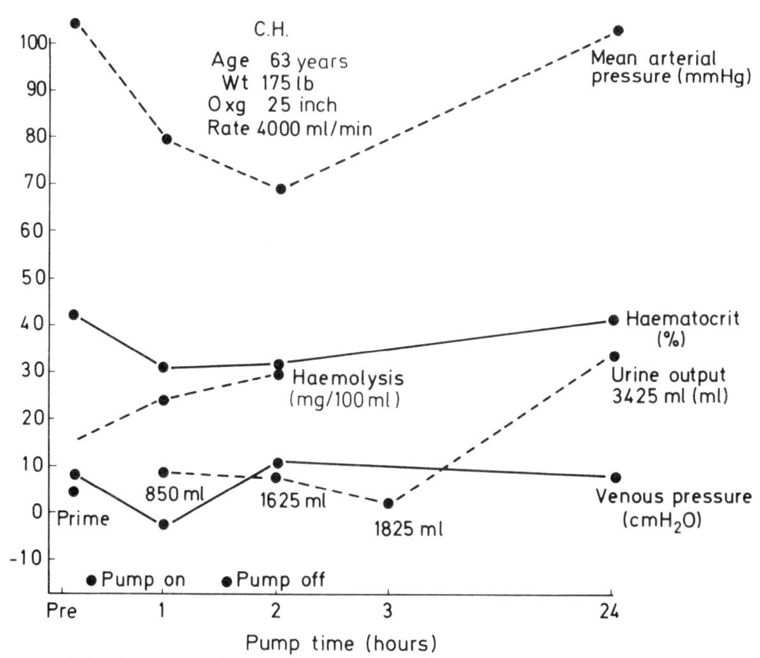

Figure 2.9 Evolution of arterial pressure, venous pressure, haemolysis, haematocrit and urinary output during perfusion in a patient undergoing surgery for coronary revascularization

patients developed transient mental depressive states 3 to 5 days postoperatively, which lasted 2 to 3 weeks. This occurred in the older age group of patients in whom cerebral arteriosclerosis was suspected.

Eight patients had postoperative gastrointestinal bleeding. Three of them had a previous history of peptic ulcer and 4 were on steroid therapy for bronchospasm. One of these patients required partial gastrectomy for control of the bleeding.

Two postoperative deaths after myocardial revascularization were the result of fulminating bronchopneumonia due to enterobacter species. Six other patients developed various degrees of pulmonary complications in the postoperative period. Three of them had focal atelectasis and 2 had lobar atelectasis which required bronchial aspiration. One patient had pulmonary embolization which was treated medically.

We have been satisfied with the performance of the rotating disc oxygenator in over 4000 extracorporeal perfusions since January 1956. Battling with time in order to provide a short perfusion to assure success has never concerned us. Our main concern has always been how well we can correct surgically the defect, rather than how fast we can get the patient off the operating table. Our objective has always been to provide every means possible in our view to increase the safety and effectiveness of the operative procedure. The safety and efficiency of the rotating disc oxygenator has allowed us to operate successfully up to 9 hours in complicated cases. Serial acid–base balance studies have verified our clinical experience in over 300 patients on whom such studies were performed.

We have considered on a number of occasions the advisability of changing to disposable oxygenating units. Such units work perfectly well in fairly short, uncomplicated cases. Perhaps the disc oxygenator is more of a machine than is necessary in such instances. However, we have always enjoyed that factor of additional safety provided by a disc oxygenator knowing that when 'things were getting tough' we had all the capacity we needed and the time necessary to allow us maximal accomplishment. Two of the objections to the disc oxygenator are the time and personnel necessary for maintenance, and the larger priming volume. The overall results with its use justify the time and personnel necessary for its operation. More strict attention to haemostasis and blood loss, and the use in the postoperative period of the blood left in the oxygenator at the end of the heart-lung bypass, have significantly reduced the requirements for blood.

Addendum

Since writing this paper, certain changes have been made in our program with the use of an oxygenator. We have recently employed a Bentley Q-200 Temptrol oxygenator which has been used particularly in patients with anticipated short runs and uncomplicated pathology. We still use the disc oxygenator for longer and more complicated perfusions. This includes the majority of patients having re-do operations where the anticipated blood loss from adhesions is greater.

By using the residual blood in the disc oxygenator postoperatively the total 24 hour blood usage has averaged 3.5 litres per patient with the use of the Bentley Q-200 as compared to 6.5 litres with the disc oxygenator. This program has resulted in a 24 hour haematocrit of 38.9 mg/100 ml in patients with the use of the Bentley, as compared to 37 mg/100 ml for those patients on the disc oxygenator.

References

1. Cross, F. S., Berne, R. M., Hirose, Y. and Kay, E. B. 'Description and evaluation of a rotating disc type reservoir oxygenator.' *Surgical Forum*, **7**, 274 (1956)
2. Head, R., Coenen, J.P., Angola, E., Nogueira, C., Mendelsohn, D. and Kay, E.B. 'Operation of the roller pump for extracorporeal circulation.' *Journal of Thoracic and Cardiovascular Surgery*, **39**, 210 (1960)
3. Kay, E. B., Gallajda, J., Lux, A. and Cross, F. S. 'The use of convoluted discs in the rotating disc oxygenator.' *Journal of Thoracic and Cardiovascular Surgery*, **36**, 268 (1958)
4. Kay, E. B., Zimmerman, H. A., Berne, R. M., Hirose, Y., Jones, R. D. and Cross, F. S. 'Certain clinical aspects in the use of the pump oxygenator.' *Journal of the American Medical Association*, **162**, 639 (1956)
5. Shepard, R. B. and Kirklin, J. W. 'Relation of pulsatile flow to oxygen consumption and other variables during cardiopulmonary bypass.' *Journal of Thoracic and Cardiovascular Surgery*, **58**, 694 (1969)

3

The Membrane Lung

M. L. Bramson, J. J. Osborn and Frank Gerbode

exitus acta probat

Introduction

The first clinical use of a membrane lung was reported in 1958 by Clowes[2]. Until then, extracorporeal gas exchange had been accomplished by devices using large direct blood-gas contact surfaces, such as bubble and filming.

The initial impetus to membrane lung development was an intuitive belief that since the human lung effects gas exchange by diffusion through the alveolar membrane, which avoids direct blood-gas contact, nature's way must be physiologically preferable and should be copied.

More objective evidence favouring membrane lungs, indicating reduced trauma to the blood and the patient (haemolysis, denaturation of plasma proteins, 'pump lung'), gradually became available[11, 12].

Another strong stimulus was the later discovery that clinically effective, closed-chest, partial perfusion with membrane oxygenation could be performed safely for days, rather than hours, and could be used successfully to treat some categories of patients in acute pulmonary insufficiency who otherwise could not be saved[6, 8].

It has also been clinically demonstrated[1] that a similar technique is capable of reversing the vicious circle of cardiogenic shock and gives reasonable hope of significantly lowering the present mortality rate of around 90 per cent.

The continuing energetic and widespread research and development in the field of membrane perfusion systems are a natural and welcome consequence of those experiences.

According to Drinker[3], the first practical membrane system in routine use in surgery was the Bramson Heart-Lung Machine, starting in 1965. Since then a number of other membrane lung designs, such as the General Electric–Peirce[13, 14], the Landé–Edwards, the Travenol and Kolobow, have also come into clinical use. Currently, however, only two, the Travenol and the Sci-Med (formerly the 'Kolobow') are being used extensively. They all have the important practical advantage of being fully disposable, which the Bramson lung is not.

Nevertheless, because of our extensive clinical experience with the latter, and also because it was the first in the field, it forms the subject of the detailed description of design and function presented in this chapter. It has in fact been used for over 500 open-heart operations and for treating more than 35 cases of acute pulmonary insufficiency by prolonged partial perfusions lasting from less than 1 day to more than 20 days (*see* Chapter 23).

Essential and/or desirable characteristics of systems for the total or partial perfusion of adults

Haemodynamic characteristics

For total perfusion of adults the flow rate obtainable (i.e. the maximum venous drainage by gravity) is usually 3–4.5 litres/min. However, a young patient weighing 90 kg may produce a venous outflow up to 6 litres/min. The system should therefore be capable of handling such a flow rate. The pressure gradient through the artificial lung should not (for practical reasons and to avoid excessive haemolysis) exceed 150 mmHg at maximum flow.

To permit meaningful performance comparisons between different artificial lungs, Galletti *et al.* have defined 'rated flow' as the perfusion flow at which an artificial lung is capable of raising the oxygen saturation of venous blood with an haematocrit of 40 per cent from 65 per cent to an arterial oxygen saturation of 95 per cent. 'Rated oxygen transfer' is that which occurs at rated blood flow, and at 65 per cent venous oxygen saturation. For total perfusion of adults, the rated flow needed has been found in practice to be at least 3.5 litres/min.

Gas exchange

The oxygen transfer capacity should be between 200 and 300 ml/min. At 6 litres/min blood flow this represents a 20–30 per cent step-up in oxygen saturation (assuming the haemoglobin is 12.4 g/100 ml). This transfer capacity varies with the blood flow rate and, inversely, with the venous oxygen saturation.

The carbon dioxide excretion rate, when using 100 per cent oxygen in the gas circuit, should be approximately equal to the rate of oxygen uptake.

Priming volume

The priming volume of the complete extracorporeal circuit should of course be as small as possible. Usually, 1500 ml is an attainable goal (this does not include any reserve held available in the priming reservoir to compensate for surgical or other fluid losses).

Minimum haemolysis and other blood damage

The amount of plasma-free haemoglobin (PFH) formed per hour depends upon the haemodynamics of the system. It cannot be measured when a patient is in circuit, since the amount eliminated by his kidneys is unknown. However, the level of PFH should not exceed 60–80 mg/100 ml during perfusion. Platelet loss and plasma protein denaturation depend upon the blood contact surfaces and on the streamline geometry.

Gas and particulate emboli

Complete and rapid elimination of gas bubbles from the extracorporeal circuit must be feasible during priming, and efficient bubble traps in the circuit must be capable of handling any bubbles entering accidentally during perfusion–for example, through a leaky venous cannulation. Any foam from coronary return suction must be eliminated by incorporating a defoaming system in the coronary suction return line.

Filters capable of removing particulate emboli should be inserted both in the coronary suction line and the arterial line to the patient. (Such emboli may consist of dust, fat, clumped platelets or debris from the surgical field.)

Constant extracorporeal volume

For ease of perfusion management, it is important (especially with membrane lungs in which the volume is not defined by a visible blood level) that the extracorporeal blood volume be essentially constant. Otherwise, when significant changes occur in the patient's arterial or venous pressure, the perfusionist will be in doubt whether volume changes in the artificial lung are responsible for the loss or gain in the patient's blood volume, or whether there are other causes (vasodilation or surgical losses, etc.). His correct reaction depends on that knowledge. Constant volume also simplifies automatic arterial pump control.

Integral heat exchange

Since the patient's temperature must be controllable by a heat exchange device, it is clearly preferable if this is achieved without additional equipment and/or blood contact surfaces. Integral heat exchange within the lung is therefore desirable.

Recirculation

Some artificial lungs cannot achieve adequate gas exchange by a single passage of blood through them. In such cases recirculation is adopted, which means that the flow rate through the lung is greater than the perfusion flow to the patient. There are, however, several disadvantages to such an arrangement. It increases the haemodynamic pressure drop through the lung, it usually necessitates more than one pump in the circuit, it increases the haemolysis and it complicates the automatic pump control.

Automatic pump control

The highest rate of venous flow obtainable by gravity from the patient determines the maximum perfusion rate. It is nearly always desirable to use that rate. But since it varies with the patient's condition and many other factors, close and constant attention to the 'manual' pump speed control is necessary. This can become an almost intolerable burden on the perfusionist, especially when the procedure lasts several days. By automating this control so that the pumping rate is always equal to the venous outflow rate, perfusion management is simplified, not only because continuous attention to the pump control is unnecessary, but also because minor or major changes in venous flow rate become instantly obvious by the automatic change in pump speed. Remedial action, if required, can then be taken without delay.

Disposability

It is clearly desirable that hospitals should save the skilled man-hours required after each use to disassemble and reassemble, test and sterilize non-disposable artificial lungs. Hence, subject to adequate performance, a disposable 'cartridge' which comes in a sterile package is a keenly desired solution which has already been attained by several lung developers[9, 10, 14].

Minimal thrombogenicity of blood contact surfaces

This quality is of great importance when membrane lungs are used for prolonged perfusions because it permits the use of low concentrations of heparin, which in turn reduces the danger of uncontrollable bleeding.

Membrane lung systems compared with direct blood-gas contact systems

Advantages

(1) The most important advantage is the low overall time-related trauma to the patient demonstrated by the feasibility of prolonged life support (up to 20 days). This can be regarded as indirect evidence of significantly lower morbidity, even after short perfusions.
(2) Specifically, the *in vitro* haemolysis rate (8.2 mg/100 ml per h) of the Bramson membrane lung was respectively 9.7 per cent, 8.4 per cent and 14.7 per cent of the rates measured in strictly comparable 6 hour tests with three conventional oxygenators (one filming and two bubbling)[15].
(3) A constant blood volume is attainable in an extracorporeal circuit which comprises a membrane lung. Good perfusion management is thereby facilitated.
(4) Constant blood volume also simplifies automatic pump control, which in turn insures utilization at all times of the maximum available venous flow rate from the patient.
(5) By the same token, changes in pump speed give instant and obvious warning of physiological or technical irregularities which may call for remedial action.
(6) Membrane lungs can be designed with integral heat exchange, thus avoiding additional blood contact surfaces and/or equipment for temperature control.
(7) Foam cannot form within the membrane lung (so long as blood pressure is not allowed to fall below atmospheric).
(8) The disposable membrane lung now being developed will almost certainly be cost-competitive with non-membrane lungs of equal capacity.

Disadvantages

If not totally disposable, the processing and testing of a membrane lung after each use is time-consuming and requires skilled personnel.

Rationale for the use of a membrane lung system

Now, after about 15 years of research and development, the rationale for the use of membrane lungs may be summarized.

For prolonged perfusions membrane lungs must be used because so far no other type of artificial lung has been clinically successful when circulatory support has been needed for several days.

For cardiac surgery – in which perfusions last 3 to 4 hours at the most – bubbling and filming oxygenators are being used routinely and successfully. Nevertheless, a reasonable inference of time-related blood damage (which after short perfusions does not prevent, but may delay or otherwise affect full recovery) can be drawn from the fact that patients have never survived non-membrane perfusions lasting days, rather than hours.

The question whether to use membrane lungs for cardiac surgery, then, becomes a matter of balancing this indirect evidence against such mundane factors as cost and convenience. If and when these latter factors become favourable to the membrane lung, a rationale for its universal use will no doubt be considered established.

Physics of gas exchange through membranes and liquids

When a liquid flows along a solid surface, a semistagnant boundary layer is formed in which the flow velocity varies from zero at the surface to that of the general flow at a small distance from the surface. That distance is the thickness of the 'boundary layer'.

When gas diffuses through a membrane into or out of blood it must also diffuse through the boundary layer, whose resistance is sometimes greater than that of the membrane.

Fick's law states, in effect, that the volume of gas diffusing through a layer of plasma in unit time is proportional to (1) the solubility of the gas in plasma; (2) the gas partial pressure difference (gradient) between the two sides of the layer; and (3) the area of the layer; and it is inversely proportional to the thickness of the layer. The layer must, therefore, be kept as thin as possible, which in practice can be achieved by providing gently turbulent flow, or 'mixing', through thin blood passages.

Gas diffusion through a membrane obeys the same law.

The Bramson membrane heart-lung machine

Figure 3.1 shows the system in actual clinical use for prolonged circulatory support.

Membranes

The membranes in the lung are made of silicone rubber* impregnated into an open-weave fibreglass, supporting fabric, 0.002 inch thick, with an overall thickness of 0.005 to 0.0055 inches.

Gas-to-gas diffusion tests of these membranes have indicated an oxygen transmission of approximately 150 ml/m^2 per minute per atmosphere and carbon dioxide transmission of 780 ml/m^2 per minute per atmosphere.

*Dow Corning

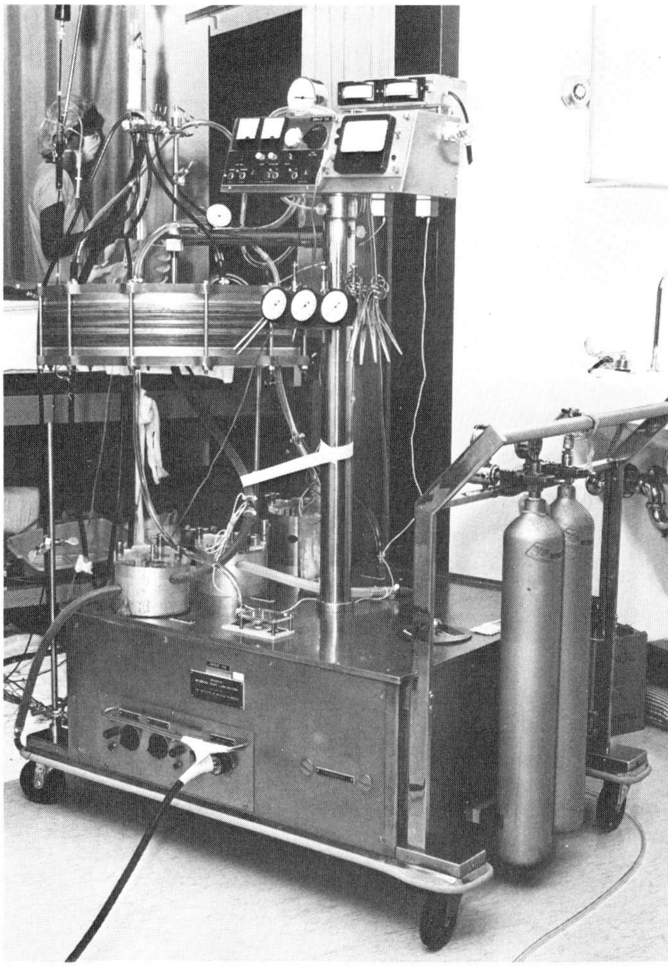

Figure 3.1 The Bramson membrane heart-lung machine. The 'drum' at the upper left is the membrane lung. (Photo taken in the CPU during prolonged extracorporeal circulation.)

The partial pressure gradients available in an artificial lung to which 100 per cent O_2 is supplied (in excess) are about 650 mmHg for oxygen and about 50 mmHg for CO_2 (since the $P\text{CO}_2$ of the blood should not exceed about 50 mmHg and cannot of course be less than zero on the gas side of the membrane).

This apparent 13 to 1 (partial pressure gradient) factor operating against the CO_2 transfer as compared with the O_2 transfer is eliminated in practice by two fortuitous facts: (1) since CO_2 is about 30 times more soluble in plasma than O_2, the resistance of the boundary layer to CO_2 diffusion is negligible; (2) the diffusion coefficient of the membrane for CO_2 is over 5 times better than for O_2. As a result the O_2 and CO_2 transfer rates are in practice approximately balanced in this lung.

Engineering design

Membrane lung design is a problem in fluid logistics (Galletti *et al.*[4])
The adult-size lung is a circular drum (*Figure 3.1*) containing 15 'sandwiches' or 'cells'. The stacking order of one cell is shown in *Figure 3.2*. The thickness of the blood screen (*Figure 3.3a*) defines the blood path between the two

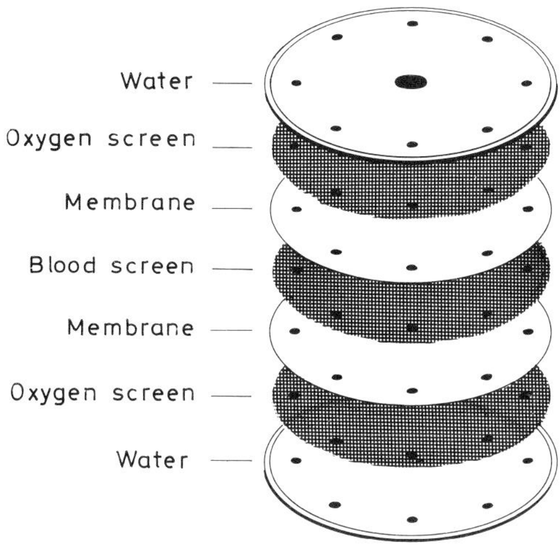

Figure 3.2 The stacking order of one of the 15 'cells' of the membrane lung

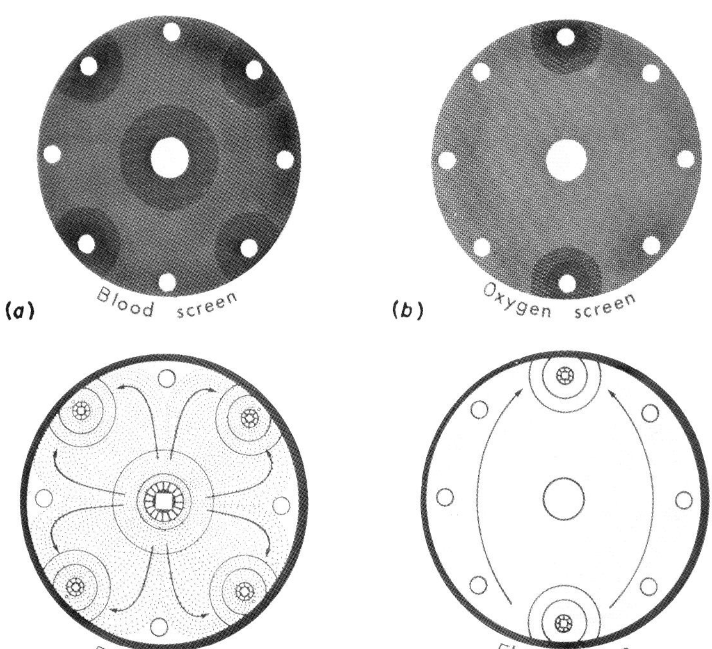

Figure 3.3 (*a*) Shows a blood screen and the blood flow pattern through each blood screen. (*b*) Shows an oxygen screen and the gas flow pattern through it

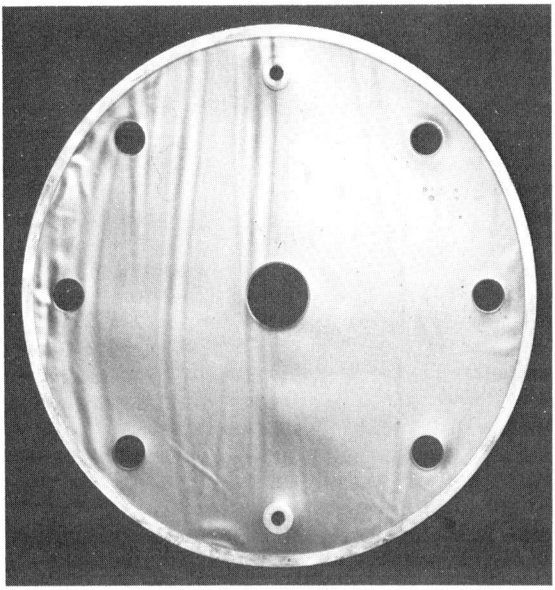

Figure 3.4 A water mattress. The central hole and six of the peripheral holes in the double plastic (PVC) disc are edge-welded. Distribution discs are located at the two remaining holes. When assembled the water manifold bolts (*Figure 3.3a*) pass through these holes

membranes which are pressed onto the screen by two pressurized water mattresses (*Figure 3.4*).

Two oxygen screens (*Figure 3.3b*) are inserted between the membranes and the mattresses, thus giving access of oxygen to each dry membrane surface. The oxygen screens also transmit mechanically the water mattress pressure to the membranes. These pressurized mattresses serve the following purposes: (1) by uniformly supporting the membranes they protect them against bulging and tearing stresses; (2) provided the water pressure is always set to exceed the blood pressure, they insure constant and minimum blood volume (as defined by the thickness of the blood screens) in the lung; (3) by preventing bulging of the membranes, they compel the blood flow to conform to the blood screen mesh, thus insuring the break-up of the plasma boundary layer by gentle turbulence; (4) by circulating the water and controlling its temperature, integral heat exchange is provided within the lung at no cost in additional equipment or blood contact surfaces.

Manifold systems

The lung is a 'drum' measuring 24 inches in diameter and 6 inches in overall thickness. It contains 15 blood cells (with a total effective membrane area of 6 square metres), 30 oxygen screens and 16 water mattresses. *Figure 3.5a* shows a stainless steel manifold bolt with one distributing ring. The bolt is tubular and externally of square cross-section. Eight such bolts provide gas inlet and outlet, water inlet and outlet and four blood outlets. The central blood inlet bolt is shown in *Figure 3.5b*. It is of larger diameter and also serves as the suspension point for the lung. Blood, gas or water flows through the spaces between the square bolts and the circular holes in the distributing rings and, in parallel, through all of the blood cells, all of the

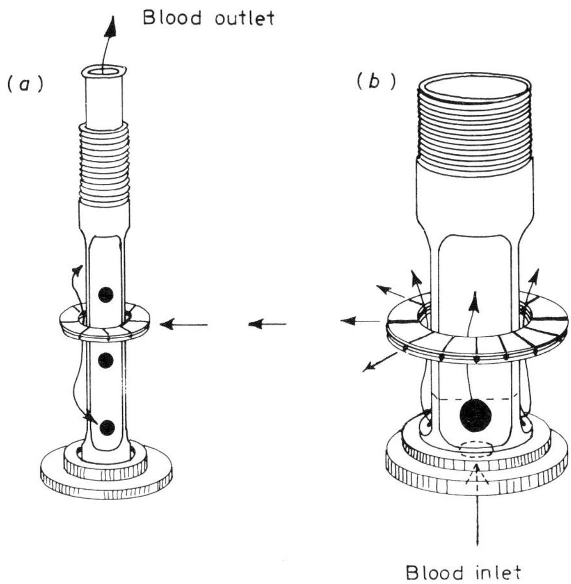

Figure 3.5 (*a*) Shows one of the eight peripheral manifold bolts. There are four 'blood out' bolts, two water bolts (one 'in' and one 'out') and two oxygen bolts (one 'in' and one 'out'). All these are identical. (*b*) Shows the central blood inlet manifold bolt with one of the 15 polyethylene distribution washers

oxygen screens and all of the water mattresses respectively. The distributing rings are injection mouldings, and one nut on each bolt tightens all joints along it.

Figure 3.3a and *3.3b* show the screens and flow patterns for blood and gas.

Circuit and controls for cardiac surgery

Blood circuit (*Figure 3.6*)

Venous blood from the patient enters a 'T' connector in the line between the priming reservoir and a slack plastic bladder or 'atrium', in which the blood level is automatically kept constant. At a lower corner of this bladder a small box is attached which contains a light bulb and a photoelectric cell on opposite sides of the bladder. When the blood level rises it gradually

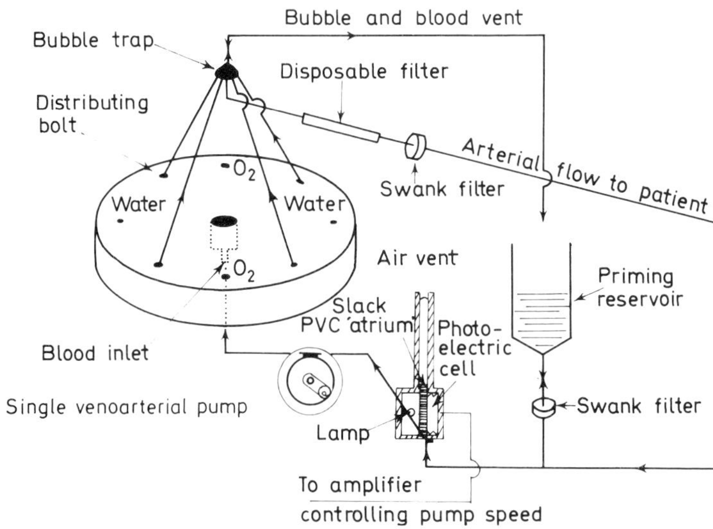

Figure 3.6 The extracorporeal blood circuit

obscures the light reaching the photoelectric cell. This produces a proportional signal which is amplified to control the speed of the arterial pump. (This is the only pump in the circuit and no recirculation is used.) From the 'atrial' bladder the blood passes through the pump into the central blood inlet of the lung, traversing all 15 cells radially in parallel. It emerges from the upper ends of the four blood outlet manifold bolts into four plastic tubes joined together in a disposable bubble trap. Here the stream changes direction and flows downward through a tubular and a 'Swank' filter forming part of the arterial line to the patient.

Two gauges show the lung inlet and outlet pressures and there is an alarm and circuit breaker (defeatable) which prevents a preset line pressure from being exceeded. When desired, such as during priming, the speed control can be switched from automatic to manual.

Oxygen circuit (*Figure 3.7*)

Oxygen enters the lung at one of the oxygen manifold bolts, passes through the 30 oxygen screens (*Figure 3.3b*) also in parallel, and emerges into the

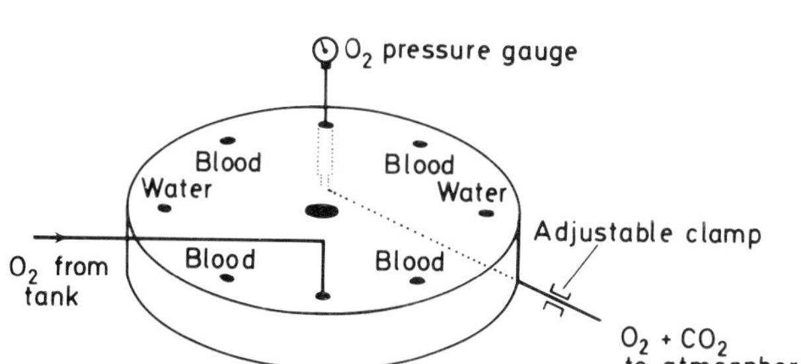

Figure 3.7 The oxygen circuit

atmosphere at the lower end of the diametrically opposite oxygen bolt. If it is desired to raise the arterial Po_2, oxygen pressure can be increased by a slight throttling of the gas outflow at this point. To keep the Pco_2 in the gas phase low, a large excess of gas flow (about 15 ℓ/min) is used. During total perfusions oxygen with 2 per cent or 4 per cent CO_2 has been found to ensure balanced gas exchange while preventing CO_2 elimination beyond physiologically desirable rates.

Water circuit (*Figure 3.8*)

Water from a tank pressurized from a standard compressed nitrogen bottle is circulated through the water mattresses by a small centrifugal pump and returned to the tank. The water temperature is controlled by means of a coil of copper tubing in the tank through which hot or cold water from the

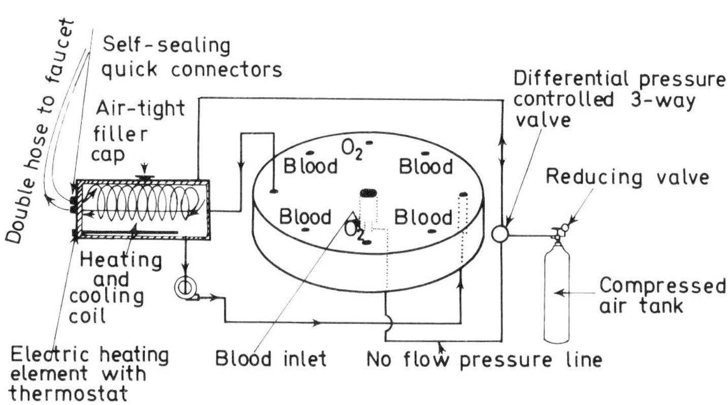

Figure 3.8 The water circuit

nearest faucet can be circulated. (A double rubber hose with self-sealing quick connectors is used for this purpose.) This provides quick cooling if called for, and rewarming. For slow warming a thermostatically controlled electric heater in the tank is used.

The gas pressure in the water tank is controlled by a specially developed three-way valve, which automatically maintains a constant excess over the blood inlet pressure in the lung. The differential is set at about 150 mmHg.

Cardiotomy suction return

The standard chassis comprises three suction roller pumps–one for ventricular venting and the other two for coronary return and general suction from the surgical field.

Modified circuitry for prolonged partial perfusion

The equipment used for prolonged circulatory support of patients in acute pulmonary insufficiency has been slightly modified in the light of experience.

Since heparin must be more closely controlled at lower levels than during short perfusions, it has been found essential to eliminate from the blood circuit all stagnant or semi-stagnant regions. Four such regions were found. Two capillary polyvinyl chloride tubes connecting blood entry and exit to the respective pressure gauges, as well as the gauges, were eliminated and substituted by electronic leads and instrumentation performing the same function.

One capillary polyvinyl chloride tube connecting blood entry with the differential pressure controller was also eliminated. In this case no other instrumentation is needed, since it has been found safe and satisfactory merely to set the water circuit pressurization at a fixed level of 600 mmHg. Lastly, a stagnant region was found in the corner of the 'atrial' bladder where the photoelectric control box was attached. This was redesigned and the stagnant region eliminated.

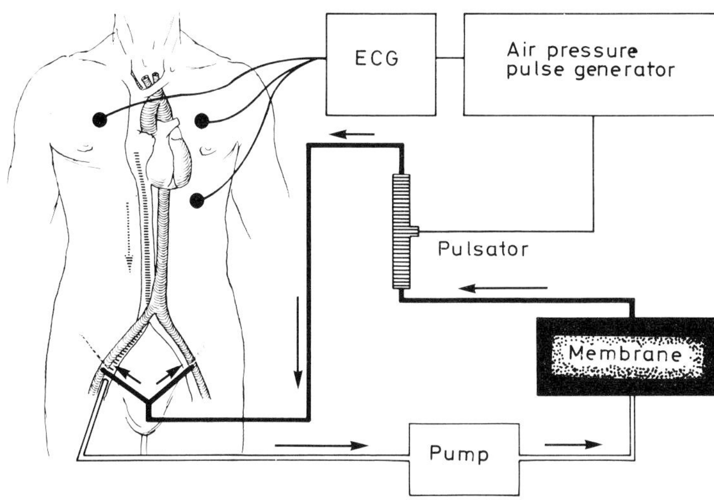

Figure 3.9 Circuit diagram and circulation for membrane lung perfusion combined with diastolic augmentation

Clinical performance of the Bramson heart-lung machine

We have reported elsewhere[13] on a series of 22 consecutive clinical perfusions using this equipment. The following is a quotation from that report: '. . . the longest perfusion lasted 730 minutes and the shortest lasted 28 minutes with an average duration of over two hours. Blood flow through the oxygenator ranged from 2 to 4 ℓ/min. Mean blood pressure during perfusion was 80 mmHg. The oxygenating capacity of the membrane lung was very satisfactory. The mean $P\text{O}_2$ of the arterialized blood was 157 mmHg. The mixed venous $P\text{O}_2$ ranged from 31 to 57 mmHg, with a mean of 39 mmHg during perfusion. Carbon dioxide elimination was also excellent. The mixed venous $P\text{CO}_2$ was never over 50 mmHg (mean 41.4). The mean $P\text{CO}_2$ gradient from the venous to the arterial side of the lung was 6.7 mmHg.

'Metabolic acidosis was never a problem during perfusion. About half of the cases showed a slight rise in the standard bicarbonate; the other half showed a slight fall. The mean change was – 0.2 mEq. The arterial pH had a range of 7.32 to 7.63, with a mean of 7.44.

'Urinary flow persisted normally during perfusion in all of the patients in whom it was measured and there was no evidence of postoperative renal damage due to perfusion.

'The mean platelet count at the end of perfusion was measured in 6 patients. In 4 of these patients serial platelet counts were carried out at 5 minute intervals. The mean count at the onset was 220 000/mm^3; the mean lowest count during perfusion was 91 000/mm^3, while the mean count at the end of perfusion was 125 000/mm^3. Thus, there was a tendency for the

Table 3.1 Characteristics of the Landé–Edwards, General Electric–Peirce, Kolobow and Bramson membrane lungs

	Landé–Edwards	*General Electric–Peirce*	*Kolobow*	*Bramson*
Membrane area (m^2)	3.0	3.0	3.5	6.0
Rated flow (ℓ/min)	1.5	1.35	3.5	4.25
Specific rated flow (ℓ/min per m^2)	0.5	0.45	1.0	0.71
Oxygen transfer at rated flow (ml/min)	84	78	150	230
Specific oxygen transfer at rated flow (ml/min per m^2)	28	26	43	38
Priming volume—lung only (ml)	500	600	350	1100
Specific priming volume—lung only (ml/m^2)	167	200	100	183
Plasma-free haemoglobin	Remains within control levels	10%/hour *in vitro* at 1 litre/min per m^2 flow	Remains within control levels	Remains within control levels
How is plasma boundary layer controlled	By recirculation	Cones moulded in membranes	Nylon mesh incorporated in membranes	Screens in blood path
Recirculation (%)	200	10	None	None
Constant blood volume	No	No	Yes	Yes
Heat exchange	None	None	External	Yes
Total disposability	Yes	Yes	Yes	No
No. of lungs needed for total perfusion of adults	2 or 3	2	1 or 2 smaller	1
Lung cost per perfusion	$400 or $600	$800	$200 to $350	$250

platelet count to rise during perfusion, a finding we had not observed with our disc oxygenator.

'Haemolysis in the lung was minimal. During *in vitro* recirculation of 2 litres of human blood at 3 litres/min against a pressure of 100 mmHg the rise in plasma haemoglobin was 10 mg/h. During clinical perfusions the amount of haemolysis appeared to be related to the amount of open-heart suction. The rise in plasma haemoglobin ranged from 12 mg/100ml per hour to over 40 mg/100ml per hour the higher value being reached when blood was sucked from the pleural space for re-use. It is not possible to measure the haemolysis produced by passage through the lung as separate from that produced by the pump and the arterial cannula, but assuming reasonable values for pump and cannula haemolysis, the amount due to circulation through the lung itself would be under 10 mg/100ml per hour of perfusion. The pressure gradient through the lung at a flow rate of 3 ℓ/min was 15 mmHg at a blood temperature of 32°C. It rose as the blood temperature dropped. At a flow rate of 2.6 ℓ/min and a blood temperature of 17°C the gradient across the lung was 45 mmHg.

'The heat exchanging capacity of the membrane lung was very large and as a practical matter was limited mainly by the flow and temperature of the water pumped through the spacing mattresses. The temperature of the arterial blood leaving the lung at normal flow rates came very close to reaching the temperature of the circulating water. Because the heat exchange capacity of the lung exceeded what seemed to us to be safe rates of induction of hypothermia or of rewarming, we did not explore how fast the patient could be cooled or rewarmed. Adults were easily cooled or rewarmed at a rate of 0.5°C per minute . . .'

Subsequent clinical experience (the series now exceeds 500 perfusions at this Centre) has shown essentially a similar performance of the system.

The performance and other characteristics of four types of membrane lungs are set forth in *Table 3.1*. The information has been obtained from published reports, mostly written by the respective designers. It was accumulated in 1976 and is of interest mainly to permit comparison of the various lung types.

Perfusion procedure for cardiac surgery – open-chest total body perfusion

Pre-priming

Before allowing any flow into the blood circuit the water circuit must be filled (using distilled or demineralized water) and pressurized (with nitrogen), setting the reducing value at 15 psi.

The blood circuit may now be filled with heparinized Ringer's lactate (or other preferred electrolyte solution) and flushed two or three times, using the procedure for debubbling as well as rinsing.

For these purposes the recirculating line is used, partially clamped to maintain the pressure around 100 mmHg. Once this pressure is established it should not be allowed to drop, so as not to prolong the debubbling procedure.

To eliminate any danger of air embolism or foaming, it is essential, both during pre-priming and priming, that the circuitry and the procedure be such as to make it impossible for the pressure in the blood space to fall below atmospheric. This can most simply be done by suspending the priming reservoir above the level of the lung.

Priming

When all air has been eliminated, the solution is slowly displaced by 1500 ml of fresh, heparinized donor blood. To increase the fluid reserve an additional 500 ml of heparinized solution is added to the priming reservoir. The surgical sash can now be filled by allowing repeated rapid flush-through from the control bladder via the pump, lung and surgical sash back to the priming reservoir, where any air from the sash is eliminated. At this point or earlier, slow warming can be started by switching on the immersion heater in the water circuit.

The arterial line is now clamped, and slow recirculation is started until perfusion is called for. It is good practice, while waiting, to switch the pump control to 'automatic', then controlling the pumping rate by adjusting a screw clamp on the gravity line from the priming reservoir to the control bladder.

Starting perfusion

Starting the perfusion is simply done by the following manoeuvres:

(1) The gravity line from the priming reservoir and the recirculating line are simultaneously clamped, thus stopping the pump and retaining the pressure in the circuit.
(2) All clamps on the arterial and venous lines, except the large venous screw clamp, are removed.
(3) The latter is slowly opened, thereby starting the perfusion.

When full perfusion is called for it is obtained by fully opening the venous screw clamp. The perfusion rate can be read directly from the pump speed indicator.

General perfusion management

Adding blood volume

If the patient's central venous or mean arterial pressure or both indicate hypovolaemia, volume may be added by allowing flow from the priming reservoir into the control bladder. This immediately speeds up the arterial pump and, since no 'pooling' can occur in the lung, the exact volume added is at once supplied to the patient.

Removing blood from the patient

If by accident or otherwise the patient is deemed to be hypervolaemic a measured amount of blood can be removed from the circuit by briefly opening the clamp on the recirculating line. It is convenient to have a calibrated volume scale on the priming reservoir.

Increasing the gas exchange capacity of the lung

In cases of exceptionally heavy metabolic oxygen demand, oxygen transfer may be increased by 20–30 per cent by the simple means of slightly throttling the O_2 outflow from the lung. When doing so, the oxygen pressure in the lung must not be allowed to exceed the lowest (i.e. outlet) pressure of the blood, so that even if a pinhole were present in a membrane no gas emboli could occur.

In general, raising the oxygen pressure to 200 mmHg should be safe.

Conversely, since routinely the gas mixture used is 4 per cent CO_2 in 96 per cent O_2, by merely switching to 100 per cent oxygen the $P\text{CO}_2$ gradient is increased by 30 mmHg, which will produce a more-than-adequate corresponding increase in the CO_2 transfer capacity.

Heparin dosage

In addition to the initial heparin dose, hourly maintenance of 1 mg of heparin per kg of body weight is given.

Going off perfusion

By slowly closing the venous screw clamp the arterial pump is slowed and stopped. The manual pump speed control should now be set to zero and the switch thereafter changed from 'automatic' to 'manual'. If at this point there is little or no reserve in the priming reservoir, 500 to 1000 ml of heparinized solution should be added, and the clamp between the reservoir and control bladder should be removed. If, as is frequent, transfusion is now required to normalize the patient's blood pressure, any needed proportion of the extracorporeal blood volume can now be delivered from the lung by operating the manual pump control.

Changes in technique for prolonged partial perfusion

Apart from the minor changes in instrumentation referred to above, and in the control of clotting time described in detail in Chapter 14, there are only the following slight changes in set-up and procedure for prolonged perfusion. Packed red cells, instead of whole blood, are used for priming. Since the patients are awake, even though mildly sedated, their metabolic rates and oxygen demand are substantially greater than those of anaesthetized patients undergoing open-heart surgery. The total systemic flow may in a large and young patient amount to 10 ℓ/min or more. Seventy-five per cent thereof, or approximately 7.5 ℓ/min, may easily be diverted through the artificial lung, which therefore may need a larger capacity. We therefore routinely use a 20-cell lung (instead of the standard 15-cell lung) in the emergency membrane heart-lung machine standing by for prolonged perfusions.

To eliminate any unnecessary thrombogenic contact surfaces, the Swank filter in the arterial line is omitted. However, the filter in the line from the priming reservoir is initially retained, so that all donor blood is filtered.

After a few hours of perfusion the priming reservoir and the Swank filter (which contain stagnant regions) are disconnected from the circuit. The distal end of the recirculating line is connected to the control bladder, and a flow of about 50 ml/min is allowed to prevent stagnation in that line.

The silastic tube of the arterial pump is generously lubricated every 24 hours.

Summary

The design and development of new membrane lungs, and the refining and perfecting of those which have reached the clinical stage, is continuing. Currently that work is mainly focused on combining advances in efficiency and patient safety with improvements in production methods and costs.

The main stimulus is the clearly established time-related trauma to the blood caused by non-membrane lungs. These have never permitted patient survival after 6 hours of perfusion; and although patients do survive such treatment for 2, 3 or 4 hours, it seems reasonable to deduce that they will have suffered some damage, most of which is now avoidable. Another stimulus to further development is the clinical confirmation of the feasibility of prolonged perfusions with membrane oxygenation as a life-saving procedure in some otherwise lethal cases of acute cardiopulmonary insufficiency.

Because of the authors' direct clinical experience with it, our original Bramson membrane lung was selected for detailed description and analysis of its performance, circuitry and perfusion protocols. It is the bases of our current and future development work. It is desirable, but difficult, to predict a definite trend in the present phase of membrane lung development. Some lungs are of the 'sandwich' type; others of the spiral coil, hollow fibre, oscillating or rotating disc types. Yet one trend is clear: the demand for total disposability.

To comply with that trend, while retaining, or improving, the functional characteristics of our said membrane lung, promising development work is proceeding and is estimated to reach the clinical stage in 1981.

Membrane lungs may thus be said to be in a technologically exciting phase, and the volume of new developments reinforces our belief that they hold the future for extracorporeal oxygenation.

References

1. Bramson, M. L., Hill, J. D., Osborn, J. J. and Gerbode, F. 'Partial veno-arterial perfusion with membrane oxygenation and diastolic augmentation.' *Transactions of the American Society for Artificial Internal Organs*, **15**, 412 (1969)
2. Clowes, G. H. A. Jr. and Neville, W. E. 'The membrane oxygenator.' In *Extracorporeal Circulation*, Ed. J. G. Allen. pp. 81–100. Springfield: Thomas (1958)

3. Drinker, A. 'Progress in oxygenator design.' *Anaesthesiology*, **37,** 245 (1972)
4. Galletti, P. M., Richardson, P. D., Snider, M. T. and Friedman, L. I. 'Standardized method for defining the overall gas transfer performance of artificial lungs.' *Transactions of the American Society for Artificial Internal Organs*, **18,** 359 (1972)
5. Gerbode, F., Osborn, J. J. and Bramson, M. L. 'Experiences in the development of a membrane heart-lung machine.' *American Journal of Surgery*, **114,** 16 (1967)
6. Hill, J. D., de Leval, M., Fallet, R. J., Bramson, M. L., Eberhart, R. C., Schulte, H. D., Osborne, J. J., Barber, R. and Gerbode, F. 'Acute respiratory insufficiency: treatment with prolonged extracorporeal oxygenation.' *Journal of Thoracic and Cardiovascular Surgery*, **64,** 551 (1972)
7. Hill, J. D., de Leval, M., Mielke, C. H., Jr., Bramson, M. L. and Gerbode, F. 'Clinical prolonged extracorporeal circulation for respiratory insufficiency: haematological effects.' *Transactions of the American Society for Artificial Internal Organs*, **18,** 546 (1972)
8. Hill, J. D., O'Brien, T. G., Murray, J. J., Dontigny, L., Bramson, M. L., Osborn, J. J. and Gerbode, F. 'Prolonged extracorporeal oxygenation for acute post-traumatic respiratory failure (shock lung syndrome). Use of the Bramson membrane lung.' *New England Journal of Medicine*, **286,** 629 (1972)
9. Kolobow, T. and Zapol, W. M. 'Partial and total extracorporeal respiratory gas exchange with the spiral membrane lung.' In *Mechanical Devices for Cardiopulmonary Assistance*, Vol. 6. *Advances in Cardiology*, pp. 112–132. Eds R. H. Bartlett, P. A. Drinker and P. M. Galletti. Basel: S. Karger (1971)
10. Landé, A. J., Edwards, L., Bloch, J. H., Carlson, R. G., Subramanian, V., Ascheim, R. S., Scheidt, S., Fillmore, S., Killip, T. and Lillehei, C. W. 'Prolonged cardiopulmonary support with a practical membrane oxygenator.' *Transactions of the American Society for Artificial Internal Organs*, **16,** 352 (1970)
11. Lee, W. H. Jr., Krumhaar, D., Derry, G., Sachs, D., Lawrence, S. H., Clowes, G. H. A. Jr. and Maloney, J. V. Jr. 'Comparison of the effects of membrane and non-membrane oxygenators on the biochemical and biophysical characteristics of blood.' *Surgical Forum*, **12,** 200 (1961)
12. Lee, W. H. Jr., Krumhaar, D., Fonkalsrud, E. W., Schjeide, D. A. and Maloney, J. V. Jr. 'Denaturation of plasma proteins as a cause of morbidity and death after intra-cardiac operations.' *Surgery*, **50,** 29 (1961)
13. Osborn, J. J., Bramson, M. L., Hill, J. D., Main, F. B., Kerth, W. J. and Gerbode, F. 'Clinical experience with a disposable membrane oxygenator.' *Bullétin de la Société Internationale de Chirurgie*, **25,** 346 (1966)
14. Peirce, E. Converse, II, Corrigan, J. J., Kent, B. B., Cate, C. L., Johnson, R. L. and Dreves, A. E. 'Comparative trauma to blood in the disc oxygenator and membrane lung.' *Transactions of the American Society for Artificial Internal Organs*, **15,** 33 (1969)
15. Ryon, D. M. and Mathewson, W. F. '*Development of the General Electric–Peirce Lung*.' Personal communication (1970)
16. Schulte, H. D. 'Hamolyse in der Herz-Lungen-Machine. Klinische Vergleichsstudien und experimentelle Untersuchungen unter Besonderer Berüchsichtigung der Bramson-Membranlunge.' p. 69. *Thesis submitted to the Medical Faculty of the University of Dusseldorf, July 1971* (1971)

4

Clinical Use of the Travenol TMO Membrane Oxygenator

Delos M. Cosgrove and Floyd D. Loop

audi alteram partem

Historical background

Since 1812 when Cesar LeGallois[35] first suggested replacing the heart by a pump which would provide a continuous supply of arterial blood the search has continued to perfect such a support system. Brown-Sequard[20] in the 1850s noted that blue blood could be aerated and altered to red blood by a whipping technique. In 1896, Ludwig and Schmidt[37] artificially oxygenated the blood by agitating it in a balloon during extracorporeal circulation. Many ingenious devices for oxygenation were devised to perfuse and maintain isolated organs during the ensuing years. A major turning point came with the introduction of heparin by McLean[40] in 1916, thus making it possible for experiments to progress from single organ perfusion to total body support. In 1937 Gibbon's[22] report of the successful use of cardiopulmonary bypass during a period of experimental total pulmonary artery occlusion provided a major impetus for oxygenator development. With a screen oxygenator, in 1953, he first used cardiopulmonary bypass successfully for closure of an atrial septal defect in an 18-year-old girl[21]. Subsequent to this, several varieties of oxygenators were devised and examined. Those which proved to be most efficient were screen oxygenators, the rotating disc device[7] and several varieties of bubble oxygenators[16]. These were later replaced by the disposable devices widely used today.

Major problems associated with the use of the cardiopulmonary bypass involved trauma to the blood causing destruction of erythrocytes and platelets, and embolization of gas and thrombi[17, 34]. This destruction was thought to produce vasoactive substances which resulted in damage to other organs[50]. These problems were caused by direct exposure of the blood to gas and served as a stimulus for development of membrane oxygenators[33].The observation of gas exchange through a synthetic membrane was made by Kolff[28] in 1944 when he observed the arterialization of blood as it passed through the cellophane chambers of the first artificial kidney. The first true oxygenator was described 11 years later by Kolff and associates[29] who used the device successfully in animal perfusions.

Encouraged by these investigations, Clowes and Neville[13] undertook a study of the membrane oxygenator, and in 1958 reported a series using their oxygenator for cardiac surgical procedures. After this demonstration that patients could be adequately supported with an oxygenator which eliminated the blood gas interface, several groups developed research programmes in this direction. Early membrane oxygenators suffered from poor oxygen transfer capability and, therefore, required large surface areas and large priming volumes making them cumbersome and unreliable. Efforts were directed at finding more suitable membranes, but the search progressed slowly. Teflon was shown to have 5 to 6 times greater oxygen exchange capacity and silicon rubber had a permeability for oxygen 40 times that of Teflon. Early attempts to produce a thin silicon rubber membrane were frought with difficulties because of the uneven quality and low mechanical strength.

Early in the history of membrane oxygenators, the idea occurred that small pores in the blood-gas barrier could minimize the resistance to gas diffusion of most plastic materials, while preserving physical separation of the blood and gas streams. The first prototypes utilized microporous polyethylene,[38] sintered nickel,[32] or hydrophobic polymers of cellulose acetate[6]. It was soon recognized that a pore size less than 10 microns and preferably about one micron would be necessary to prevent blood or plasma from passing through the membrane. Initial concern for blood leakage into the gas phase, and microbubble embolization in the opposite direction when the pressure of the oxygen was permitted to exceed that of the blood, did much to dampen the initial interest in the microporous membrane concept. In 1969, two separate membrane formulations were suggested to circumvent these problems. Dantowitz *et al.*[14] described a gas exchange device in which the surface of a microporous matrix of Teflon and carbon was coated with a thin, continuous silicone polymer film, and Lautier *et al.*[31] achieved a similar result with a sheet of synthetic paper made impermeable by impregnation with a polysiloxane. These reports established the feasibility of large scale, continuous blood oxygenation through microporous materials. The oxygen transfer coefficients achieved compared most favourably with those of other membrane oxygenator configurations. The CO_2 transfer capability was much higher than that of standard membrane lungs, and approached the performance of bubble oxygenators. The continuous skin of silicone on the microporous substrate was soon found unnecessary. The problem of blood or plasma oozing through the membrane was resolved by directing appropriate attention to the distribution as well as to the median value of pore size. The fear of damage to the blood associated with direct exposure of blood to the gaseous atmosphere proved unfounded, as was the concern for microbubble release in the bloodstream.

During this period, Eiseman *et al.*[18] combined the advantages of Teflon and a microporous membrane (Gortex). This joined the strength and heat seal ability of Teflon with the excellent gas transfer capability of a microporous membrane. The surface of a microporous membrane is a hybrid. Most of the surface is direct gas interface and the remainder is inert hydrophobic polymer. Under normal perfusion pressure, plasma does not ultrafilter through the microscopic pores because the surface tension of the fluid film is greater than the transmural hydrostatic pressure. It has been postulated that the fluid film contains a cell-free protein monolayer which does not interchange freely with proteins in the flow path. Consequently, the surface exposed to flowing blood is similar to the protein adsorbed surface characteristic of a solid membrane. This being the case, the haematological effects of prolonged blood exposure to microporous membranes should resemble those seen with solid membrane devices more than direct gas interface systems.

The initial laboratory work by Bartlett *et al.*[5] comparing the Teflon membrane with a silicon rubber membrane demonstrated excellent membrane characteristics and confirmed the adequacy of gas transfer and the benign interaction with formed elements of the blood. In 1974, Karlson *et al.*[27] reported using this membrane for cardiac surgical perfusions. The first commercially available membrane was made of expanded fibrillated tetrafluorethylene with pore size between 3 and 5 microns in diameter. This membrane demonstrated occasional problems with 'lung oedema' and the design was modified. Currently, the Travenol TMO membrane is manufactured from polypropylene and has a pore size of 1–2 microns. Lung oedema is no longer reported. In its present form this oxygenator has become widely used and there are numerous publications describing its clinical application. Data comparing its clinical performance with that of bubble oxygenators are becoming available.

Oxygenator design

The basic configuration of the oxygenator is an accordion-pleated design. This results in a flat rectangular oxygenator with 30 blood phase envelopes alternating with 30 gas envelopes (*Figure 4.1*). The membrane material is a sheet of microporous polypropylene reinforced with a mesh of polyvinyl

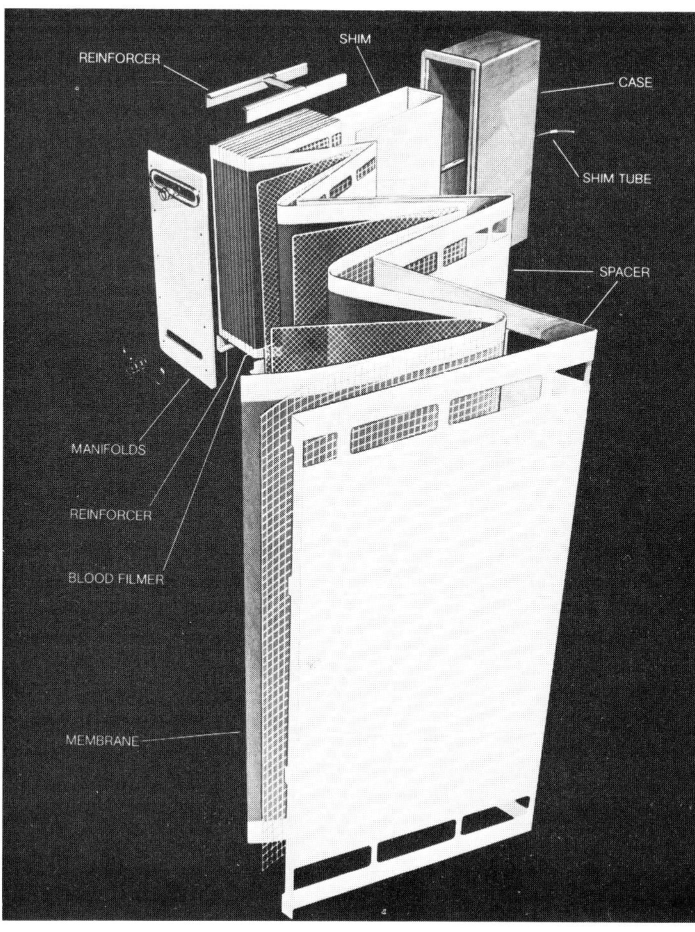

Figure 4.1 Schematic demonstration of the accordion-pleated design of the membrane and the shim which regulate the blood space thickness. The entire membrane configuration is contained in the case and is disposable

chloride-coated fibreglass. The pore size is 1–2 microns. A fine nylon screen separates the membrane surfaces in the blood phase and a thin stiff paperboard sheet separates the folds in the gas phase. The membrane surface is 2.25 m^2, but the actual exchange area is less, due to the masking effect of the various supporting screens used in the blood and gas phases. A flat rectangular polyvinyl chloride 'shim' bag is inserted in the middle of the back of the membrane. It serves to compress the blood layers and may be inflated to any desired pressure through a tube connecting it to the outside pressure source, thus decreasing the thickness of the blood-phase envelopes and increasing oxygen transfer. The stack of membranes is enclosed in a rigid rectangular box, 27.5 × 15 × 7.15 cm. The long narrow side (27.5 × 7.15 cm) facing the blood spaces contains blood inlet and outlet ports. The opposite side facing the gas phase contains gas inlet and outlet ports and egress for the shim access tube. The oxygenator fits into a steel frame on its pump console. Gas phase pressure is automatically eliminated by a vent through a water column. The oxygenator is operated with about 10 per cent blood recirculation to eliminate the possibility of gas pressure ever exceeding the blood pressure.

Pump assembly

This oxygenator was designed to be used with a set of flexible, polyvinyl chloride reservoir bags, one venous and one arterial. The venous reservoir has connections for cardiotomy suction return, for vena-caval drainage, and for delivering blood to the oxygenator. A ¼ inch internal diameter × 18 inch length recirculation tube provides a connection between the venous and arterial reservoirs. The arterial reservoir has connections for one tube from the exit port of the oxygenator, one for a tube going to the patient, and the third one for a tube connected to a coronary perfusion unit. The oxygenator carriage was designed to hold the software components described above, i.e. the oxygenator, the reservoir bags, and the miniprime heat exchanger. The oxygenator fits tightly into a rigid metal box on the carriage which keeps the oxygenator from distending during use. The box encloses the oxygenator on all six sides. The side of the box that faces the gas phase side of the oxygenator has three functions: first, it provides connections for a shim pressure regulator, for a safety gas pressure blow-off device, and for oxygen input; second, it has a heater which thermostatically regulates the temperature of the gas entering the oxygenator to 40°C; and third, it forms a tight seal between the oxygen supply and the input oxygen port on the oxygenator. An adjustable rack for the reservoir set is mounted on a pole fastened to the top of the box. Appropriately spaced water connections for a Miniprime heat exchanger are beside the box. This oxygenator carriage can be used with any pump console having appropriately placed pumpheads with their respective speed controls (*Figure 4.2*).

Sarns has manufactured a special five-position, modular pump base with two blood suction pumpheads, a water temperature regulator, and two

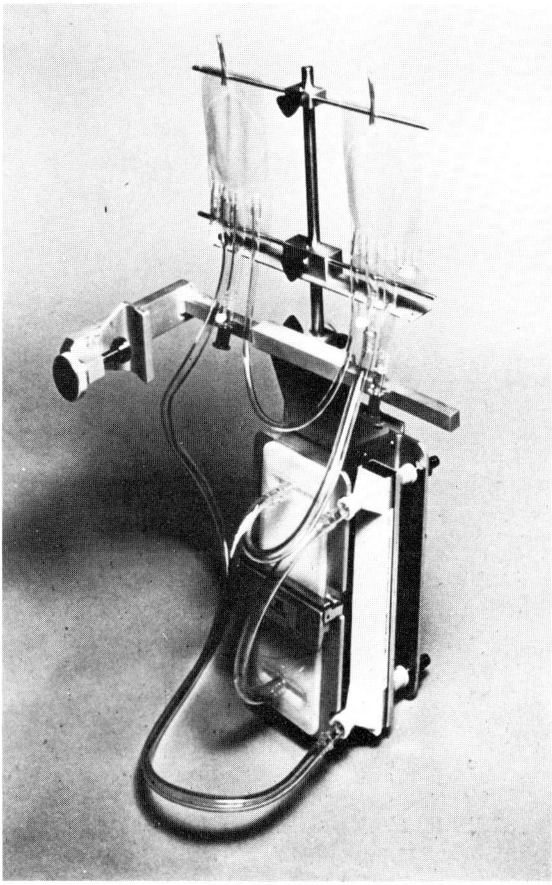

Figure 4.2 The oxygenator carriage and its venous and arterial reservoirs prior to attachment to the back of the pump console

oxygenator pumpheads. The speed control of the two oxygenator pumpheads is linked to one electrical control allowing the speed to be offset between them. This means that one pumphead (the 'master' pump) pumps a higher volume than the other (the 'slave' pump) during perfusion. This link can also be made by a geared mechanical device which straddles the speed controls of any two pumpheads not having the electrical linkage. This mechanical device is available from the oxygenator manufacturer. A control panel provided with the Sarns modular pump has four devices: first and second are a shim pressure regulator and an oxygen valve driven by a single oxygen line from a wall outlet; third is a gauge that shows the temperature of the oxygen entering the oxygenator; and fourth is an audible alarm activated by excessively low oxygen flow to the oxygenator (*Figure 4.3*).

A Cobe cardiotomy reservoir with an integrated Swank 20 micron filter allows filtration of all fluids entering the pump or being returned to the

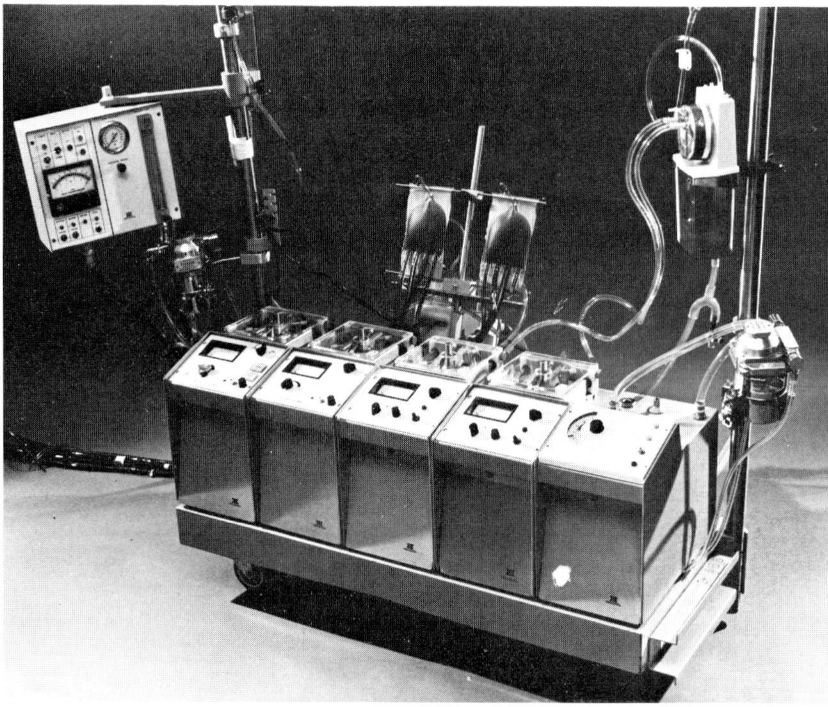

Figure 4.3 The entire pump oxygenator assembly and its control appearing as it is used clinically

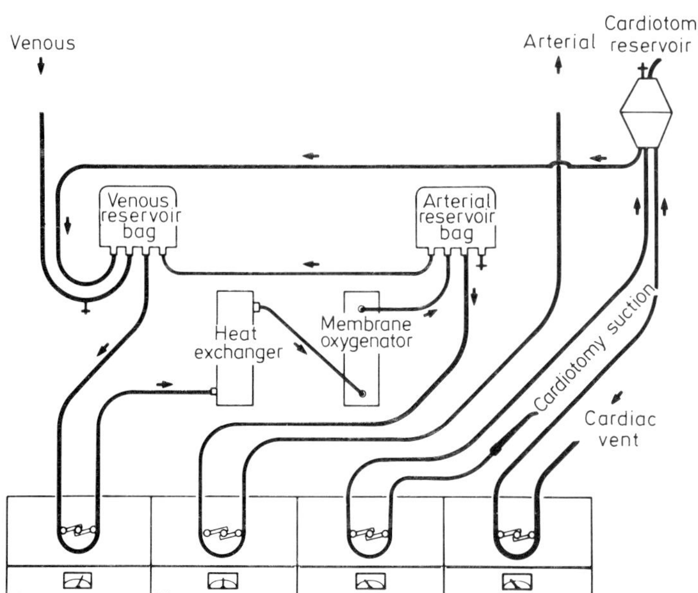

Figure 4.4 Schematic representation of the circuitry of the pump oxygenator assembly

oxygenator via the left-sided vent or the cardiotomy sucker. Travenol Miniprime hypothermia disposable heat exchangers are used and connected to the integrated thermal unit if euthermia is to be employed or to the Sarns heater cooler unit if hypothermia is required. The circuitry for the entire assembly is shown schematically in *Figure 4.4*.

Pump prime

The priming volume of the oxygenators is 450 ml and 2000 ml for the entire bypass circuitry. Blood is not used as a priming agent. The pump is primed with 2000 ml of a 2.5 per cent dextrose balanced electrolyte solution (*Table 4.1*). This solution is appropriately buffered with sodium bicarbonate to a pH of 7.46. Five thousand units of heparin are added to the prime initially and 2500 supplementary units are given for each additional litre of electrolyte solution used during bypass. The entire process of setting up the pump, priming and debubbling it takes an experienced perfusionist approximately 20 minutes.

Table 4.1 Electrolyte solution used for oxygenator priming. Prepared in 2.5 per cent dextrose in water

Sodium	102 mmol/ℓ
Potassium	5 mmol/ℓ
Calcium	5 mmol/ℓ
Magnesium	2 mmol/ℓ
Chloride	107 mmol/ℓ
Phosphate	2 mmol/ℓ
Gluconate	5 mmol/ℓ

Heparinization

Immediately before initiating cannulation of the heart, 3 mg/kg of heparin is administered intravenously and an additional dose of 1.5 mg/kg is given one hour after the initial dose. This is repeated every hour. After termination of bypass and removal of the cannulae, protamine sulphate is administered. The dosage is determined by the use of activated clotting times, or 1.5 mg of protamine is given for each mg of heparin administered either intravenously or via the pump during the entire operation.

Perfusion technique

During cardiopulmonary bypass both perfusion pressure and flow rate are regulated. The flow at euthermia is 2 ℓ/min per m^2 of body surface area and is gradually and progressively reduced as systemic hypothermia is induced.

While maintaining satisfactory flow rates the mean blood pressure is maintained between 60 and 90 mmHg. This is often manipulated at the surgeon's request either by intravenous administration of nitroglycerine, sodium nitroprusside for vasodilation or by neosyneperine for vasoconstriction.

Monitoring during bypass

Fifteen minutes after the initiation of bypass, arterial and venous blood samples are obtained for blood gases, pH, serum potassium and haematocrit determinations. Unless abnormalities are found, these laboratory tests are repeated every 30 minutes. Oxygenation is adjusted by increasing or decreasing the 'shim' pressure while the CO_2 is determined by the rate of oxygen flow 'washing' through the oxygenator. Metabolic acidosis is treated by administering sodium bicarbonate. It is seldom necessary to add potassium during bypass because of the large potassium load administered with the cardioplegic solution. Similarly, blood is very seldom added during bypass despite haematocrit levels in the low twenties during perfusion.

Blood salvage

At the completion of bypass the patient is vasodilated with intravenous nitroglycerine. As much of the oxygenator content as possible is returned to the patient via the arterial line consistent with satisfactory right and left ventricular filling pressures. After the cannulae have been removed and the patient is in a stable condition, the remainder of the pump oxygenator contents are salvaged by collecting it into blood bags for later transfusion. It is always possible to obtain at least 500 ml from the pump circuitry by careful drainage, and it is frequently possible to salvage as much as 1000–1500 ml. The pump contents are not centrifuged to obtain packed cells because this wastes plasma and some formed elements of the blood.

Clinical results

Since Gibbon's pioneering efforts, many oxygenators have been developed and marketed which indicates a lack of complete satisfaction with any particular oxygenator. Major problems resulting from bubble oxygenators include trauma to the formed elements of the blood and microembolization of oxygen and platelets. The nature of the destruction of formed elements and denaturation of proteins has been well documented and shown to be secondary to the blood-gas interface[33] while microemboli formation has been shown to be greater in bubble oxygenators[10]. The rationale for the use of membrane oxygenators is thus established, and its efficacy in eliminating these two main problems has been demonstrated by prolonged clinical perfusion[4, 26, 44, 51]. To achieve clinical acceptance for routine cardiac surgery, the membrane oxygenator must be practical and reliable, economically comparable to current oxygenators and superior to existing methods in clinical practice.

The Travenol TMO membrane oxygenator has now been used in approximately 4000 clinical cases at the Cleveland Clinic during the past two years. It has been extremely reliable and practical to assemble and operate with respect to set-up time, priming volume, and efficiency of gas exchange. Initially, it was used only for cases expected to have a long perfusion duration such as reoperations, combined valve surgery and revascularization, or revascularization with more than three grafts. Its ability has been proven in those difficult situations, and it is now used in virtually all cases. The cost of the unit has decreased and is at present only slightly more expensive than most commercially available bubble oxygenators.

The question of superiority of this type of oxygenator as compared to the traditional bubble oxygenator is more difficult to evaluate, but data are gradually accumulating on this subject from numerous centres including our own. The most important areas where differences have been examined are (1) trauma to formed elements of the blood; (2) pulmonary function; and (3) neurologic function.

Damage to red cells is most commonly assessed by serum haemoglobin levels and many comparisons have demonstrated a lower serum haemoglobin level with membrane perfusions[2, 11, 12, 43]. It is well recognized that contact of blood with the pericardial surface is the most important source of haemolysis[40, 45] and, therefore, the serum haemoglobin level probably represents an inaccurate determinant of red blood cell trauma produced by the oxygenator. Lactate dehydrogenase resulting from red cell damage may represent a better measure of red cell trauma. The levels were higher in patients perfused with bubble oxygenators than in those with the membrane oxygenators[2]. The ultimate determinant of red cell destruction or sublethal damage may be evidenced by the need for red cell replacement. A significant reduction in blood utilization has been reported by several authors[9, 12, 39], and in our series it was noted in patients with perfusions longer than two hours. The incidence of reoperation for bleeding has decreased in all major series and no comparison of these two oxygenator types has demonstrated any significant difference, although postoperative chest tube drainage has been reported to be less[36].

It is well known that the number and function of circulating platelets is greatly reduced with the onset of cardiopulmonary bypass and that these parameters do not begin to return to normal until the first postoperative day[15]. It has been further demonstrated that in longterm perfusions the platelet number will decrease to zero when a bubble oxygenator is used but will reach equilibrium with platelet production when membrane oxygenation is employed[19]. Clinically, several authors[2, 23, 39] have reported higher platelet counts with the Travenol TMO membrane oxygenator in comparative series, but this was most dramatically demonstrated in perfusions lasting more than two hours. Platelet function has not been frequently investigated, but Kvarstein *et al.*[30], Solis *et al.*[47] and Wright *et al.*[49] have demonstrated improved platelet adhesiveness postoperatively in patients perfused with membrane oxygenators.

To evaluate critically the clinical function of bubble and membrane oxygenators on formed elements of the blood, a randomized prospective study of 80 direct myocardial revascularization patients, 40 using the Travenol TMO membrane oxygenator as previously described, and 40 using

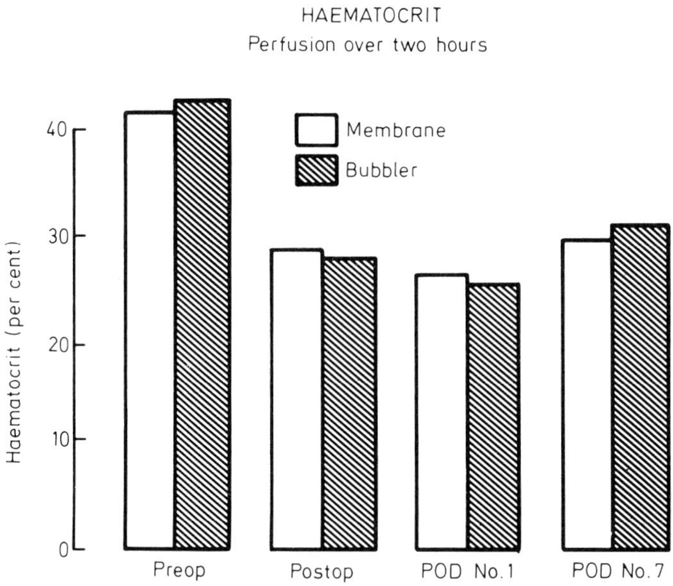

Figure 4.5 The haematocrit values preoperatively, immediately following the operation, and on the first and seventh postoperative days, do not show any statistically significant differences between the groups investigated

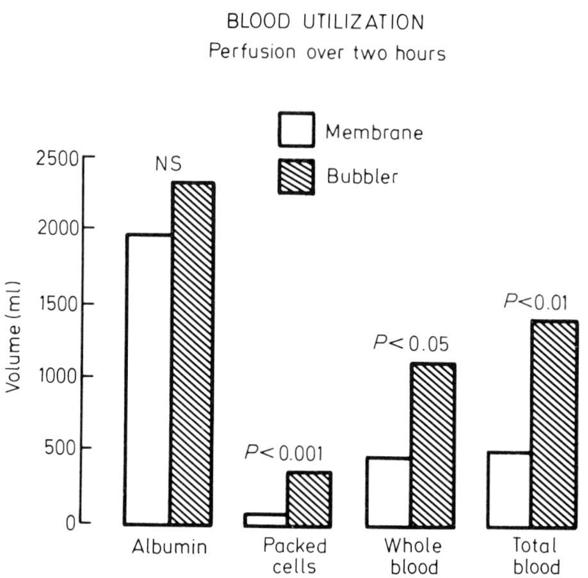

Figure 4.6 The blood requirements were statistically significantly higher for the bubble oxygenator group in order to maintain similar levels of haematocrit

the Travenol Variflo bubble oxygenator, was undertaken. No statistically significant differences could be demonstrated in the haematological parameters. Similarly, the amount of chest tube drainage, blood and colloid requirements, and incidence of re-exploration for bleeding were not statistically significantly different. Considering that a short perfusion might not stress the systems adequately to demonstrate potential differences, a subset of 20 patients, 10 in each group, having perfusions longer than two hours were compared using the same criteria. A favourable trend in all haematological parameters was noted for the membrane oxygenator, but this only achieved statistical significance as far as blood replacement was concerned. In this subgroup the haematocrit levels preoperatively, immediately postoperatively, and on the first and seventh postoperative days were similar (*Figure 4.5*). The blood required to maintain these haematocrit levels differed markedly. A statistically significant greater amount of packed cells, whole blood and total blood was transfused to patients in the bubble oxygenator group (*Figure 4.6*). The higher, although not statistically significant, serum lactic dehydrogenase, bilirubin, and serum haemoglobin values suggest greater blood trauma from the bubble oxygenator. Similarly, a smaller leucocyte response, higher platelet count, and less postoperative chest tube drainage suggest less trauma to blood during oxygenation (*Table 4.2*). Our data and the accumulated consensus from other authors reporting on the membrane oxygenator indicate that this form of oxygenation is less

Table 4.2 Data from patients with perfusion durations longer than 2 hours (mean values)

Clinical and laboratory data	*Membrane oxygenator (10 patients)*	*Bubble oxygenator (10 patients)*	*P-Value*
Perfusion duration (min)	124	133	NS
Haematocrit postop	28.7	27.9	NS
Serum haemoglobin	58	65	NS
LDH, first postop day	246	307	NS
Bilirubin, first postop day	1.7	2.0	NS
Platelets postop	152 800	139 400	NS
Platelets, first postop day	156 500	127 100	NS
White blood cells, first postop day	7 370	8 270	NS
Chest tube drainage	620	891	NS
Packed cells infused	50	325	<.01
Whole blood infused	450	1 100	<.05
Total blood given	5 000	1 425	<.01

traumatic to red blood cells, platelets, and probably results in less blood utilization.

Pulmonary dysfunction following cardiopulmonary bypass has been reported and its pathological changes have been well described[3, 45]. The bubble oxygenator is incriminated in causing denaturation of proteins leading to pulmonary vasculitis with capillary leakage of plasma[42] and increased pulmonary vascular resistance due to the release of histamine and serotonin[50]. Hill and his colleagues[25] reported endothelial swelling in the lungs of puppies that were perfused with a bubble oxygenator but this did not appear in those animals perfused with a membrane artificial lung. These changes were associated with increased pulmonary vascular resistance. This finding was confirmed clinically by Byrick and Noble[9] who compared membrane oxygenators with bubble oxygenators and found a much greater increase in pulmonary vascular resistance and accumulation of lung water in patients perfused with a bubble oxygenator. No investigators have reported any comparative data demonstrating the superiority of one method or another in terms of postoperative blood gases. In our series there was no appreciable difference in gases between groups or in a subset of patients having the longest perfusion. Thus it appears that membrane oxygenators have a lower incidence of pulmonary dysfunction, although this is not evidenced by blood gas determinations.

Neurological dysfunction following cardiac surgery is a well recognized problem[8, 48] and the pathological findings in the brains of patients dying after cardiac surgery have been well documented[1]. Particulate matter was present, and this led to the investigation of the amount of particulate matter produced by an oxygenator. Carlson *et al.*[10] reported that a Bentley oxygenator produced 18 000 particles per minute as opposed to only 1500 for the Landé–Edwards membrane oxygenator by Solis *et al.*[47]. These counts were reduced by a factor of ten when a Pall filter was placed in the arterial line, but the membrane oxygenator was still superior. It was hoped that this would translate into improved neurological function postoperatively, but recently Hessel *et al.*[23] compared the mental and neurological functions of patients by objective criteria and were unable to demonstrate any significant advantages.

The Travenol TMO membrane oxygenator is a reliable, efficient, practical, and economically attractive device. Its advantages over bubble oxygenators appear to be a reduction in trauma to formed elements of the blood and a decrease in microemboli. This appears to have clinical significance in reducing blood utilization and in decreasing pulmonary dysfunction after bypass. These and other potential advantages would probably be most apparent in perfusions lasting longer than two hours. More work remains to be done for the clinical evaluation of this oxygenator which appears to offer significant potential advantages.

References

1. Aguilar, M. J., Gerbode, F. and Hill, J. D. 'Neuropathologic complications of cardiac surgery.' *Journal of Thoracic and Cardiovascular Surgery*, **61**, 676 (1971)
2. Alon, L., Turina, M. and Gattiker, R. 'Membrane and bubble oxygenator; A clinical comparison in patients undergoing aortocoronary bypass procedures.' *Herz*, **4**, 56 (1979)
3. Awad, J. A., Lemieux, J. M., and Lou, W. 'Pulmonary complications following perfusion of the lungs.' *Journal of Thoracic and Cardiovascular Surgery*, **51**, 767 (1966)

4. Awad, J. A., Matte, J. and Brassard, A. 'Prolonged extracorporeal respiration with a membrane gas exchanger.' *Journal of Thoracic and Cardiovascular Surgery*, **66,** 40 (1973)
5. Bartlett, R. H., Fong, S. W., Woldanski, C., Hung, E., Styler, D. and MacArthur, C. 'Haematologic responses to prolonged extracorporeal circulation (ECC) with microporous membrane devices.' *Transactions of the American Society for Artificial Internal Organs*, **21,** 250 (1975)
6. Berman, H. J., Fallon, K., Halkett, J. A. E. and Schwartz, J. 'Elimination of CO_2 from blood through hydrophobic millipore and teflon membranes.' *Federation Proceedings*, **23,** 496 (1964)
7. Björk, V. O. 'Brain perfusions in dogs with artificially oxygenated blood.' *Acta Chirurgica Scandinavica (Suppl. 137)*, **96,** 1 (1948)
8. Branthwaite, M. A. 'Neurological damage related to open-heart surgery. A clinical survey.' *Thorax*, **27,** 748 (1972)
9. Byrick, R. J. and Noble, W. H. 'Postperfusion lung syndrome. Comparison of Travenol bubble and membrane oxygenators.' *Journal of Thoracic and Cardiovascular Surgery*, **76,** 685 (1978)
10. Carlson, J. G., Larde, A. J., Twichell, J., Baxter, J. and Lillehei, C. W. 'Prolonged cardiopulmonary support with disposable membrane oxygenator.' *New York State Journal of Medicine*, **72,** 2513 (1972)
11. Chopra, P. S., Dufek, J. H., Kroncke, G. M., Dacumos, G. C., Celesia, G. G., Troner, S. P., Marshall, J. R., Jefferson, J. W., Loring, L. L. and Kahn, D. R. 'Clinical comparison of the General Electric–Peirce membrane lung and bubble oxygenator for prolonged cardiopulmonary bypass.' *Surgery*, **74,** 874 (1973)
12. Clark, R. E., Beauchamp, R. A., Magrath, R. A., Brooks, J. D., Ferguson, T. B. and Weldon, C. S. 'A comparison of bubble and membrane oxygenators in short and long perfusion.' Presented at the American Association of Thoracic Surgeons. Boston (1979)
13. Clowes, G. H. A. Jr. and Neville, W. E. 'The membrane oxygenator.' In *Extracorporeal Circulation*. Ed. J. G. Allen. Springfield: Charles C. Thomas (1958)
14. Dantowitz, P., Borsanyi, A. S., Deibert, M. C., Snider, M. T., Scherler, M., Lipsky, M. H. and Galletti, P. M. 'A blood oxygenator with preformed membrane-lined, capillary channels.' *Transactions of the American Society for Artificial Internal Organs*, **15,** 138 (1969)
15. DeLeval, M. R., Hill, J. D., Mielke, C. H., Jr., Macur, M. F. and Gerbode, F. 'Blood platelets and extracorporeal circulation.' *Journal of Thoracic and Cardiovascular Surgery*, **69,** 144 (1975)
16. DeWall, R. H., Grage, T. B., McFee, A. S. and Chiechi, M. A. 'Theme and variations on blood oxygenators: I. bubble oxygenators.' *Surgery*, **50,** 931 (1961)
17. Dobell, A. R. C., Mitri, M., Galva, R., Sarkozy, E. and Murphy, D. R. 'Biologic evaluation of blood after prolonged recirculation through film and membrane oxygenators.' *Annals of Surgery*, **161,** 617 (1965)
18. Eiseman, B., Birnbaum, D., Leonard, R. and Martinez, E. J. 'A new gas permeable membrane for blood oxygenators.' *Surgery, Gynecology and Obstetrics*, **135,** 732 (1972)
19. Fong, S. W., Burns, N. E., Williams, G., Waldanski, C., Gazzaniga, A. B. and Bartlett, R. H. 'Changes in coagulation and platelet function during prolonged extracorporeal circulation in sheep and man.' *Transactions of the American Society for Artificial Internal Organs*, **20,** 239 (1974)
20. Galletti, P. M. and Brecher, G. A. *Heart-lung Bypass*. New York: Grune and Stratton (1962)
21. Gibbon, J. H., Jr. 'The application of a mechanical heart and lung apparatus to cardiac surgery.' *Minnesota Medicine*, **37,** 171 (1974)

22. Gibbon, J. H., Jr. 'Artificial maintenance of the circulation during experimental occlusion of the pulmonary artery.' *Archives of Surgery*, **34,** 1105 (1937)
23. Hessel, E. A., Johnson, D. D., Ivey, T. D., Dillard, D. H. and Miller, D. W., Jr. 'Membrane versus bubble oxygenator for open-heart surgery: A prospective randomized study.' (*Abstr.*) *American Journal of Cardiology*, **43,** 425 (1979)
24. Hewitt, R. L. and Creech, O., Jr. 'Special communication: History of the pump oxygenator.' *Archives of Surgery*, **93,** 680 (1966)
25. Hill, D. G., deLanerolle, P., Aguilar, M. J. and Hall, J. D. 'The pulmonary pathophysiology of membrane and bubble oxygenators,' *Transactions of the American Society for Artificial Internal Organs*, **21,** 165 (1975)
26. Hill, J. D., deLeval, M. R., Fallat, R. J., Bramson, M. L., Eberhart, R. C., Schulte, H. D., Osborn, J. J., Barber, R. and Gerbode, F. 'Acute respiratory insufficiency: Treatment with prolonged extracorporeal oxygenation.' *Journal of Thoracic and Cardiovascular Surgery*, **64,** 551 (1972)
27. Karlson, K. E., Murphy, W. R., Kakvan, R., Anthony, P., Cooper, G. N., Jr., Richardson, P. D. and Galletti, P. M. 'Total cardiopulmonary bypass with a new microporous teflon membrane oxygenator.' *Surgery*, **76,** 935 (1974)
28. Kolff, W. J. and Berk, H. T. J. 'Artificial kidney: A dialyser with a great area.' *Acta Medica Scandinavica*, **117,** 121 (1944)
29. Kolff, W. J., Effler, D. B., Groves, L. K., Peereboom, G. and Moraca, P. P. 'Disposable membrane oxygenator (heart-lung machine) and its use in experimental surgery.' *Cleveland Clinic Quarterly*, **23,** 69 (1956)
30. Kvarstein, B., Vasage, S. T., Tjonneland, S., Cappelan, C., Jr. and Aune, H. 'The adhesiveness of blood platelets before during and after cardiopulmonary bypass.' *Scandinavian Journal of Thoracic and Cardiovascular Surgery*, **11,** 57 (1977)
31. Lautier, A., Rey, P., Bizot, J., Faure, A., Sausse, A. and Laurent, D. 'Comparison of gaseous transfer through synthetic membranes for oxygenators.' *Transactions of the American Society for Artificial Internal Organs*, **15,** 144 (1969)
32. Lawn, L. and McCance, R. A. 'Artificial placentae: a progress report.' *Acta Paediatrica Scandinavica*, **53,** 317 (1964)
33. Lee, W. H., Jr. and Hairston, P. 'Structural effects on blood proteins at the gas-blood interface.' *Federation Proceedings*, **30,** 1615 (1971)
34. Lee, W. H., Krumhaar, D., Fonkalstrud, E. W., Schjeide, O. A. and Maloney, J. V., Jr. 'Denaturation of plasma proteins as a cause of morbidity and death after intracardiac operations.' *Surgery*, **60,** 29 (1961)
35. LeGallois, C. J. J. *Experiments on the principle of life, and particularly on the principle of the motions of the heart, and on the seat of this principle*. Translated by N. C. and J. G. Nancrede. Philadelphia: M. Thomas (1813)
36. Liddicoat, J. E., Bekassy, S. M., Beall, A. C., Glaeser, D. H. and DeBakey, M. E. 'Membrane versus bubble oxygenator: clinical comparison.' *Annals of Surgery*, **181,** 747 (1975)
37. Ludwig, C. and Schmidt, A. 'Das Verhalten der Gase, Welche mit dem Blut durch die reizbaren Saugethiermuskelz stromen.' *Arbeiten auf der Physiologischen Anstalt zu Leipzig*, **3,** 1 (1869)
38. McCaughan, J. S., Weeder, R. R., Schuder, J. C. and Blakemore, W. S. 'Evaluation of new nonwettable microporous membranes with high permeability coefficients for possible use in a membrane oxygenator.' *Journal of Thoracic and Cardiovascular Surgery*, **40,** 574 (1969)
39. McKenzie, F. N., Heimbecker, R. O., Barnicoat, K. T. N., Robert, A., Gergeley, N. F., Del Maestro, R. and Wall, W. 'Bloodless open-heart surgery with atraumatic extracorporeal circulation.' *Canadian Medical Association Journal*, **112,** 1073 (1975)

40. McLean, J. 'The discovery of heparin.' *Circulation*, **19,** 75 (1959)
41. Morris, K. N., Kinross, F. M. and Stirling, G. R. 'Haemolysis of blood in the pericardium: The major source of plasma haemoglobin during total body perfusion.' *Journal of Thoracic and Cardiovascular Surgery*, **49,** 250 (1965)
42. Neville, W., Kontaxis, A., Gavin, T. and Clowes, G. H. A., Jr. 'Postperfusion pulmonary vasculitis. Its relationship to blood trauma.' *Archives of Surgery*, **86,** 126 (1963)
43. Niguidula, F. N., Romano, A., Eldredge, W. J. and Lemole, G. M. 'Clinical experience with membrane oxygenators on infants and children: Comparison with bubble oxygenator on 154 consecutive patients.' (*Abstr.*). *American Journal of Cardiology*, **39,** 261 (1977)
44. Pyle, R. B., Helton, W. C., Johnson, F. W., Hornung, J. R., Hunt, C. E., Trumball, H. R., Lindsay, W. G. and Nicoloff, D. M. 'Clinical use of the membrane oxygenator.' *Archives of Surgery*, **110,** 966 (1975)
45. Ratliff, N. B., Young, W. G., Jr., Hackel, D. B., Mikat, E. and Wilson, J. W. 'Pulmonary injury secondary to extracorporeal circultion. An ultrastructural study.' *Journal of Thoracic and Cardiovascular Surgery*, **65,** 425 (1973)
46. Siderys, H., Herod, G. T., Halbrook, H., Pittman, J. N., Rubush, J. L., Kasebaker, V. and Berry, G. R., Jr. 'A comparison of membrane and bubble oxygenation as used in cardiopulmonary bypass in patients: The importance of pericardial blood as a source of haemolysis.' *Journal of Thoracic and Cardiovascular Surgery*, **69,** 708 (1975)
47. Solis, R. T., Kennedy, P. S., Beall, A. C., Noon, G. P. and DeBakey, M. E. 'Cardiopulmonary bypass: Microembolization and platelet aggregation.' *Circulation*, **52,** 103 (1975)
48. Tufo, H. M., Ostfeld, A. M. and Shekelle, R. 'Central nervous system dysfunction following open heart surgery.' *Journal of the American Medical Association*, **212,** 1333 (1970)
49. Wright, J. S., Fisk, G. C., Torda, T. A., Stacey, R. B., Hicks, R. G. 'Some advantages of the membrane oxygenator for open heart surgery.' *Journal of Thoracic and Cardiovascular Surgery*, **69,** 884 (1975)
50. Yong, N. K., Eiseman, B., Spencer, F. C., and Rossi, N. 'Increased pulmonary vascular resistance following prolonged pump oxygenation.' *Journal of Thoracic and Cardiovascular Surgery*, **49,** 580 (1965)
51. Zapol, W., Pontoppidan, H., McCullough, N., Schmidt, V., Bland, J. and Kitz, R. 'Clinical membrane lung support for acute respiratory insufficiency.' *Transactions of the American Society for Artificial Internal Organs*, **18,** 553 (1972)

5

The Polystan (Rygg–Kyvsgaard) System for Extracorporeal Oxygenation and Circulation

Inge H. Rygg and Colin G. Green

gratia gratiam parit

Introduction

The increased interest in extracorporeal circulation in the early 1950s led to experimental work within this field at Rigshospitalet, the University Hospital of Copenhagen, concerning both venovenous cooling and cardiopulmonary bypass.

Early studies in extracorporeal circulation resulted in the first clinical open-heart operation with cardiopulmonary bypass at Rigshospitalet in June 1956. In the autumn of the same year the first publications appeared concerning the Polystan (Rygg–Kyvsgaard) disposable bubble oxygenators[10,11].

During the years 1956 and 1957, a rather intensive study resulted in several improvements of the earlier designed oxygenators. Reports on these design changes were given at the European Society of Cardiovascular Surgery in Torino in June 1957 and at the First Work Conference on Extracorporeal Circulation in Chicago in September, 1957[5,6,12]. Since then the principal design of the oxygenators has been virtually unchanged.

The design principles of the heart-lung machine

The basic concept from the start of the experimental work was to develop a combined oxygenating and pumping system with the oxygenator and tubing circuitry to be disposable items. The experience gained with the early types of pump-oxygenators resulted in a design based upon gravity drainage of the venous blood directly into the oxygenator and a coronary suction system based upon the same principle. Changes in blood volume in the oxygenator were monitored by the use of a simple mechanical weighing system that constantly displayed the weight of the oxygenator. A single roller pump – the only one required – returned the blood from the oxygenator to the patient.

This rather simple set-up has been used since 1956. Weighing the oxygenator and its contents is a particular advantage at the start and end of the perfusion, as any degree of partial perfusion can easily be obtained and maintained by setting the pump speed at the desired level and controlling the venous inflow by means of a variable venous line clamp whilst observing the weight of the oxygenator. The use of this mechanism also enables extracorporeal/intracorporeal blood volume changes to be easily controlled and recorded.

The Rygg–Kyvsgaard Mark IV heart-lung machine is shown in *Figure 5.1*. The entire machine is manufactured from stainless steel. Its lower portion contains the arterial pump, the drive-motor and gear box and a vacuum pump for the suction system. The oxygenator is suspended within the stainless steel frame and is attached to a weighing mechanism which displays the weight of the oxygenator on a scale readable from the top of the machine. On the upper left- and right-hand corners of the machine are located two control handles – one for regulation of the arterial pump speed and one for regulation of a venous clamp that enables the venous line to be

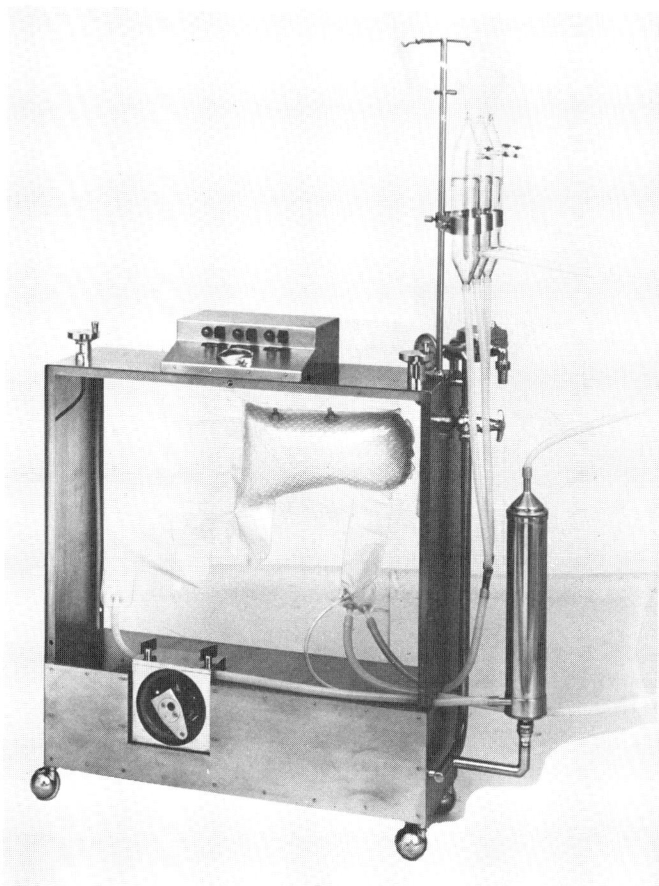

Figure 5.1 The Rygg–Kyvsgaard Mark IV heart-lung machine. (Reproduced from Rygg[7] by courtesy of FADL Publishing House, Copenhagen)

gradually occluded or released. On the right-hand side of the machine is a vertical pole which supports the three suction chambers that are an integral part of the suction system. A reusable annular-type heat exchanger is mounted on the right-hand side of the machine. *Figure 5.2* shows the latest type of the heart-lung machine, which is built as a modular system. In this machine the single-roller pump has been replaced by a double-roller pump

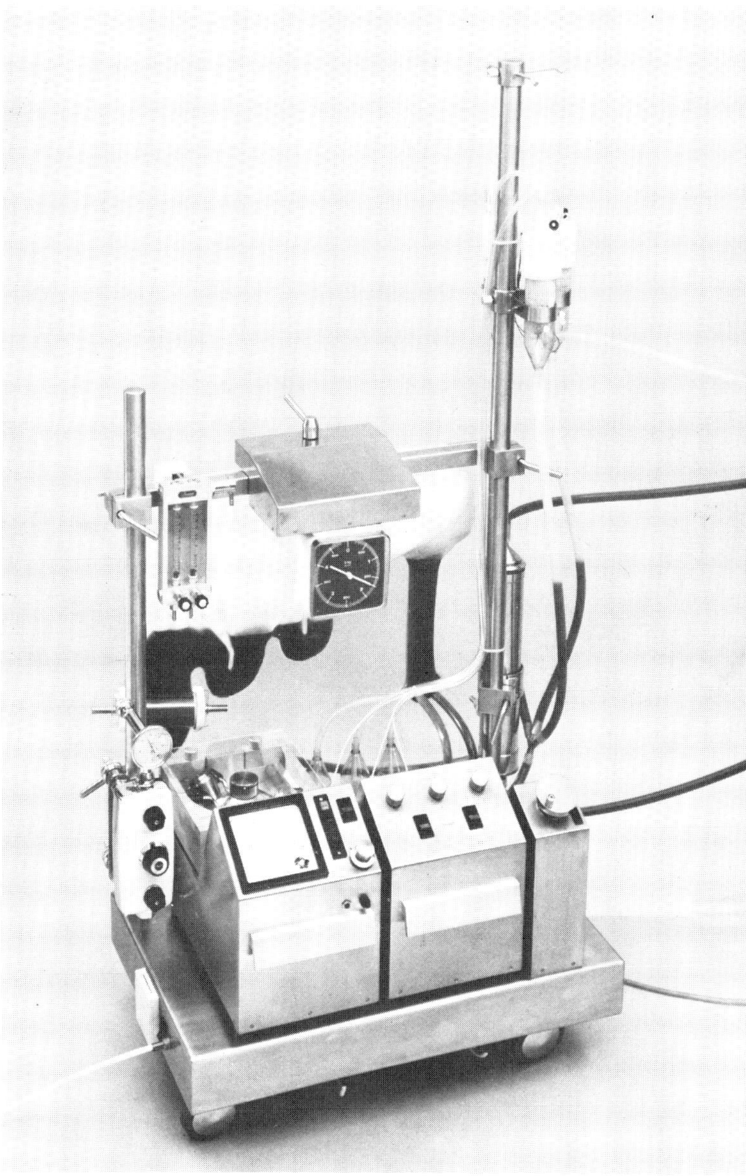

Figure 5.2 The new modular heart-lung machine

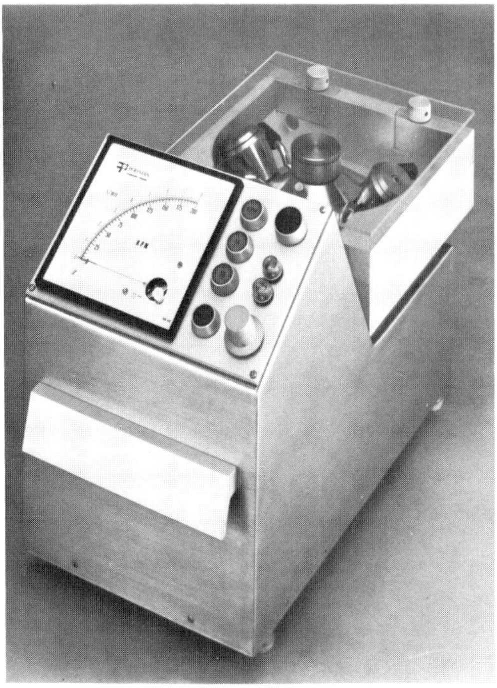

Figure 5.3 Polystan modular pump with Verticlude pump head

module of a new type (*Figure 5.3*). In conventional double-roller pumps the occlusiveness of the pump tubing is adjusted by moving the rollers independently or simultaneously in a radial direction. By contrast, the new 'Verticlude' pump head (*Figure 5.4*) relies on a vertical movement of the complete roller assembly, thereby ensuring that both rollers will identically occlude the pump tubing at all times. By use of recalibration buttons the direct read-out flow scale can be used with various tubing diameters.

Next to the pump module is the suction module containing the vacuum sources and controls for the vacuum suction system. The disposable chambers for the system are mounted on the right-hand side accessory pole. The venous clamp is mounted on the console base next to the suction module.

The oxygenator

Experiments with the early types of Polystan (Rygg–Kyvsgaard) oxygenators showed that filtration of the blood was necessary, due to the presence of air microbubbles in the blood after defoaming. Therefore, certain precautions had to be taken in order to avoid the reformation of bubbles after the filtration. New bubbles were found to be formed where the blood was allowed to flow in a high velocity stream against an underlying surface. A

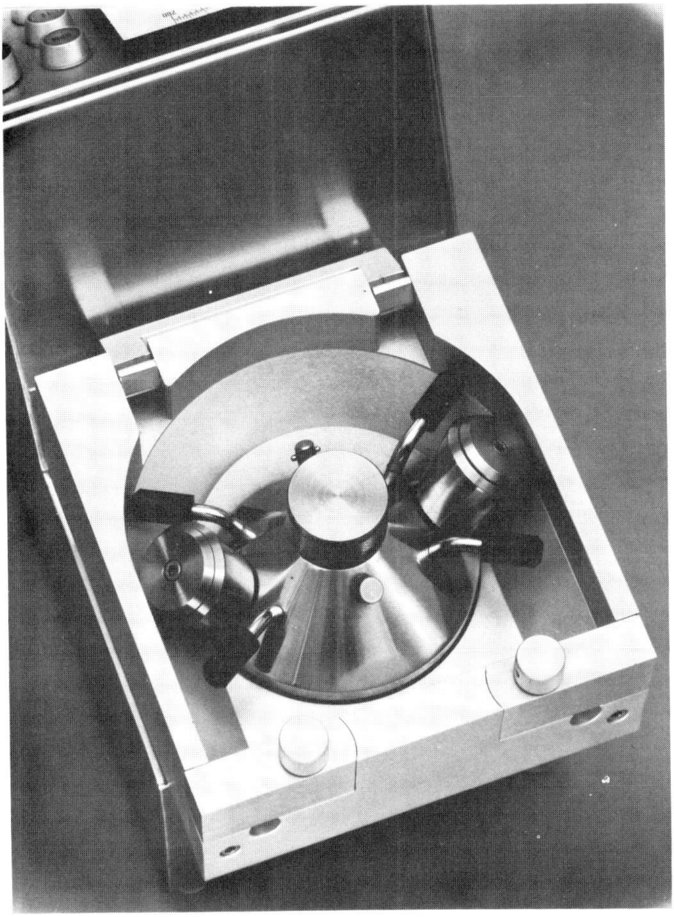

Figure 5.4 Verticlude pump head

free fall of the blood had to be avoided. A sufficiently smooth flow pattern was obtained by an almost horizontal direction of the flow and a priming volume that secured large cross-sectional areas of the blood in the arterial reservoir after defoaming and filtration. The incorporation of a U-shaped trap after the defoaming section proved to be advantageous both as a bubble trap and as a natural site for filtration of the blood. Based upon these observations, a design for disposable bubble oxygenators, suitable for gravity drainage of the venous blood directly into the oxygenator, was developed at the beginning of 1957.

Three conventional types and three Venotherm oxygenators incorporating an integral heat exchanger are now available (*Table 5.1*). The principal design is still used and is shown in *Figures 5.1, 5.2, 5.5* and *5.6*. Blood from the vena cavae and from the suction system enters the oxygenator through two inlets at the bottom of the oxygenating column where a mixture of O_2 and CO_2 is supplied through an oxygen dispenser. At the top of the column, the blood passes through a defoaming chamber filled with polypropylene

Table 5.1 Polystan (Rygg–Kyvsgaard) oxygenators. Flow rates, minimum priming volumes and maximum volume capacity

Oxygenator type	*Maximum blood flow rate (ml/min)*	*Minimum priming volume (ml)*	*Maximum volume capacity (ml)*
Venotherm with heat exchanger			
VT–7000 High Prime Adult	7000	1600	4900
VT–5000 Low Prime Adult/Paediatric	7000	1200	2900
VT–2000 Infant	2000	600	1500
Oxygenator without heat exchanger			
RK–7000 High Prime Adult	7000	1700	4900
RK–5000 Low Prime Adult/Paediatric	7000	1300	2900
RK–2000 Infant	2000	650	1500

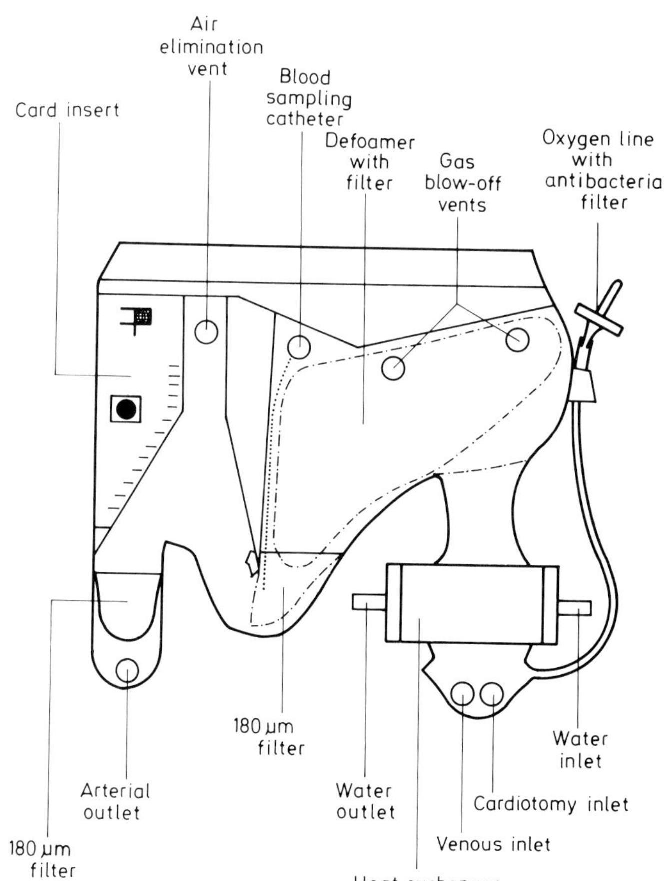

Figure 5.5 Schematic drawing of the Polystan (Rygg–Kyvsgaard) Venotherm oxygenator

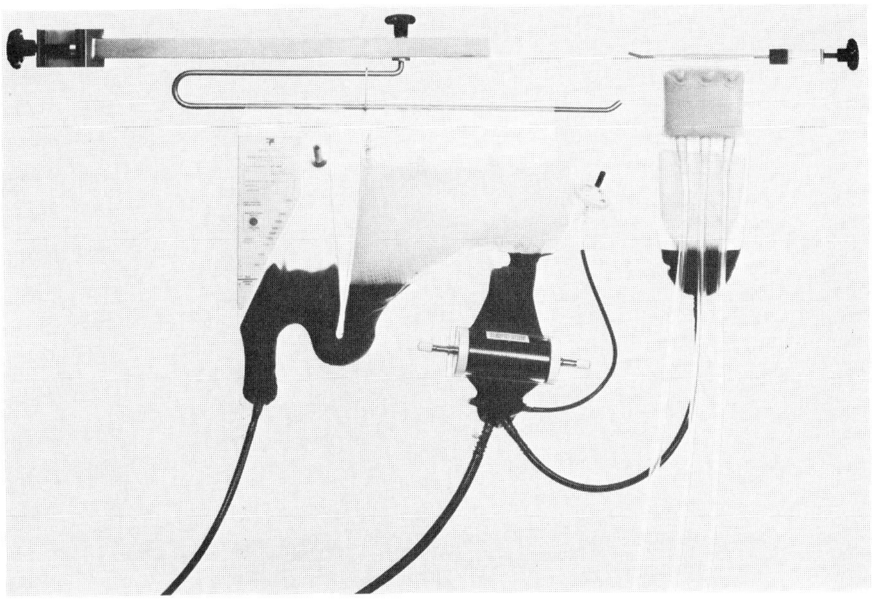

Figure 5.6 Polystan (Rygg–Kyvsgaard) Venotherm oxygenator with cardiotomy blood reservoir attached

fibres coated with antifoam material. After defoaming, the blood passes through a filter that surrounds the entire defoamer and passes through one U-shaped trap, containing a fine-meshed filter, as it enters the arterial reservoir. The blood leaves the arterial reservoir after passing through one or more fine-meshed filters.

All air in the last section of the arterial reservoir is removed before commencing perfusion. If the oxygenator should accidentally be emptied, this section collapses and closes off the arterial outlet, thus functioning as a safety valve, making it impossible to inadvertently pump air into the arterial line.

In designing the oxygenators due attention has been paid to permit the storage of blood in the oxygenator from patients in whom large volume changes may occur. The arterial reservoir can, therefore, not only be primed with a relatively low volume of fluid, but can also store a relatively large volume of perfusate if necessary.

Figure 5.5 and *5.6* show the Venotherm oxygenator in which the disposable heat exchanger is incorporated in the oxygenating column. The heat exchanger consists of a corrugated stainless steel cylinder with a surface area of 1005 cm^2. The heat exchanger is incorporated in the oxygenating column immediately above the two venous inlets and the oxygen dispenser. Without increasing the venous inflow resistance significantly, the heat exchanger in this position is extremely efficient. This is due to the effect of increased 'stirring' of blood across its surface. The presence of the heat exchanger in this position has also contributed to a higher oxygenating efficiency. There are two reasons for this. Firstly, the ascent of the bubbles from the oxygen dispenser to the top of the oxygenating column has been slowed down, and consequently the contact time between bubbles and venous blood has been increased. Secondly, the vertical corrugations in the heat exchanger have the effect of distributing the bubbles more evenly across the complete width of the oxygenating column.

The present range of oxygenator types is listed in *Table 5.1* together with their recommended maximum blood flow rates, minimum priming volumes and maximum volume capacities.

The cardiotomy suction system

The suction system for handling the intracardiac blood that should be returned to the oxygenator is based upon the gravity drainage principle in which blood is aspirated into one or more suction chambers by means of a negative pressure and then flows by gravity from each chamber to an inlet at the bottom of the oxygenating column.

For each suction line used, a suction chamber is positioned at the level of the patient's heart and serves the purpose of continuously re-establishing the gravity drainage when air is aspirated along the sucker line. Defoaming is facilitated by the negative pressure and takes place inside each chamber which is coated with antifoam material or provided with antifoam-coated plastic fibres which also serve as gross filters. The negative pressure required for the correct function of each chamber corresponds to the pull of gravity exerted by a column of blood with an effective height equal to the difference in the level between the blood surface in the oxygenator and the patient's heart. As this negative pressure is limited, the capacity of the system is dependent upon the diameter, or, more correctly, on the flow resistance of the tubes and sucker tips used. The suction system is seen in the photographs of the heart-lung machine in *Figures 5.1* and *5.2* and is diagrammatically illustrated in *Figure 5.7*.

Three suction lines, each provided with a suction chamber, are used during the perfusion. The blood outlet lines from each chamber are joined together by means of a four-way connector just before the venous inlet connector at the bottom of the oxygenating column of the oxygenator. It is essential for the function of the suction system that the four-way connector is placed well below the blood level in the oxygenator.

In the Mark IV model of the heart-lung machine the negative pressure is created by a common vacuum pump placed in the lower portion of the apparatus. The common line from this pump is connected to a stainless steel tube mounted on the right upper corner of the oxygenator frame which also serves as a holder for the three disposable suction chambers. The tubes distributing the negative pressure to the chambers are provided with a constriction of such a dimension that the maintenance of negative pressure in any of the chambers is secured, even when air is sucked through one or more of the suction lines. The negative pressure in each individual chamber is adjusted by a side-arm inlet on each vacuum applicator cover.

In the new modular heart-lung machine system the vacuum module contains two vacuum pumps, and the negative pressure in each individual chamber is adjusted by vacuum controls on the front panel of the module.

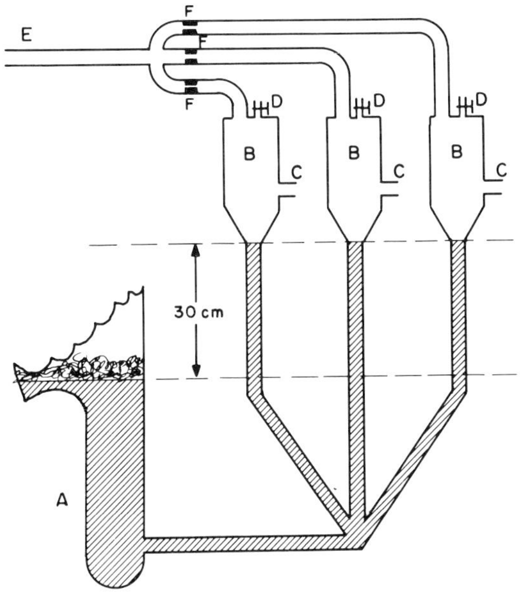

Figure 5.7 Vacuum suction system. A = oxygenator; B = disposable suction chamber; C = suction line; D = air inlet with adjustable clamp; E = vacuum supply line; F = constriction

Adjustment of the negative pressure takes place after the oxygenator and extracorporeal tubing have been primed and while the priming volume is still recirculating. The inlets to each chamber are clamped, and the negative pressure is increased sufficiently to raise the column of blood in the outlet tube of each chamber from the level of blood in the oxygenator to the outlet of the chamber. The vacuum suction module contains the electronic circuitry for the automatic level-sensing electrodes which are placed on each suction chamber. When the blood level reaches the upper electrode contact, air is automatically introduced into the vacuum supply line to that particular chamber, thereby allowing the chamber to drain to the oxygenator. When the level reaches the lower electrode contact, strong suction is re-established. With this system the level of the negative pressure is adjusted by means of the control knobs on the vacuum suction module.

Table 5.2 The capacity of a single gravity suction line

Tubing and suction tips	*Blood transport (ml/min)*
Silicone tube only, 10 mm*, 100 cm long	2900
Silicone tube with 8 mm* caval cannula tip	2200
Silicone tube with 6 mm* caval cannula tip	1800
Silicone tube with 5.2 mm* caval cannula tip	1500
Silicone tube with 3.7 mm* caval cannula tip	600

*internal diameter

The capacity of a single suction line is shown in *Table 5.2*. Suction lines with a 10 mm internal diameter are used for carrying the blood from the heart to the suction chambers. It is important that these suction lines be placed straight and horizontal in order to avoid traps of blood and air. The outlet lines from each chamber all have a 12 mm internal diameter. The degree of haemolysis caused by this gravity suction system in an experimental set-up is shown in *Table 5.3*. The damaging effect is considerably

Table 5.3 Increase in plasma haemoglobin after 100 passages of the same sample of blood through the pump and the gravity suction line (1 μmol/ℓ = 1.61 mg/100ml)

Size of sucker	*Numer of expts.*	*Haemolysis (μmol/ℓ)*
5.2 mm sucker, no admixture of air	2	20 (17–22)
8 mm caval cannula, admixture of air	2	64 (40–87)

increased by the mixing of air and blood ('audible suction') as in other systems.

This kind of cardiotomy suction has been used since 1957 to our entire satisfaction. The three suction lines are used for left ventricular venting, for aspiration with a cardiotomy sucker, and as an extra sucker for rapid removal of larger amounts of blood or drainage of a left-superior vena cava.

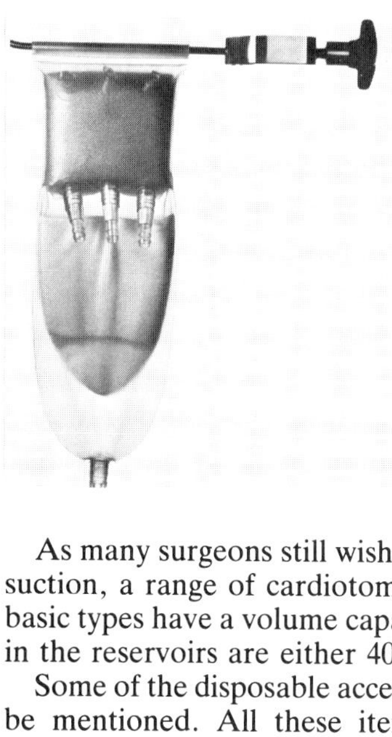

Figure 5.8 Polystan cardiotomy reservoir

As many surgeons still wish to use roller pumps for handling cardiotomy suction, a range of cardiotomy reservoirs are available (*Figure 5.8*). The basic types have a volume capacity of either 1000 or 2000 ml, and the filters in the reservoirs are either 40 microns or 120 microns.

Some of the disposable accessories used in open-heart surgery will briefly be mentioned. All these items as well as the oxygenators, heart-lung machine and cardiotomy reservoirs have been designed in co-operation with, and manufactured by, Polystan A/S*.

Venous catheters

These specially shaped caval catheters shown in *Figure 5.9* have been used since 1957. The catheters are made from polyvinyl chloride and have either a straight or bent tip. The basket-shaped tip is tapered, and a ring is placed on the bent catheters at the point of passage through the atrial wall. This ring is used as a convenient site for atrial attachment by snaring of the pursestring

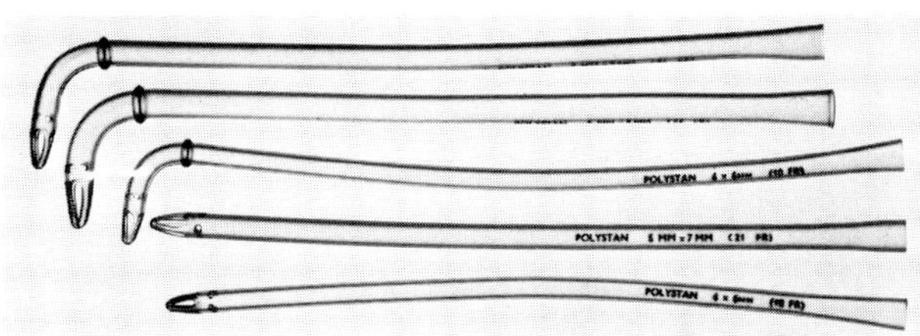

Figure 5.9 Straight and bent venous catheters also suitable for ventricular decompression and suction tips

suture. The bent catheter occupies only a small space in the right atrium, and this type of catheter is particularly useful in the Mustard procedure for transposition of the great vessels. The catheters are easy to introduce and are also suitable for apical or transatrial venting of the left ventricle. The straight catheters are suitable as cardiotomy suction tips and for left ventricular venting as well as for caval drainage.

Coronary perfusion cannulae

Cannulae for coronary perfusion are thin-wall plastic tubes with either a self-inflating balloon, a cone or a ring-shaped tip. The shape of the balloon cannula is shown in *Figure 5.10a*. The part of the cannula which is surrounded by the balloon is hardened. The interior of the balloon communicates with the lumen of the cannula through a hole. This construction ensures expansion of the balloon against the coronary arterial wall during the perfusion. The balloons are made of latex and are able to withstand an internal pressure of about 200 mmHg before being enlarged beyond their original size.

*Polystan A/S, Generatorvej 41, DK-2730 Herlev, Denmark

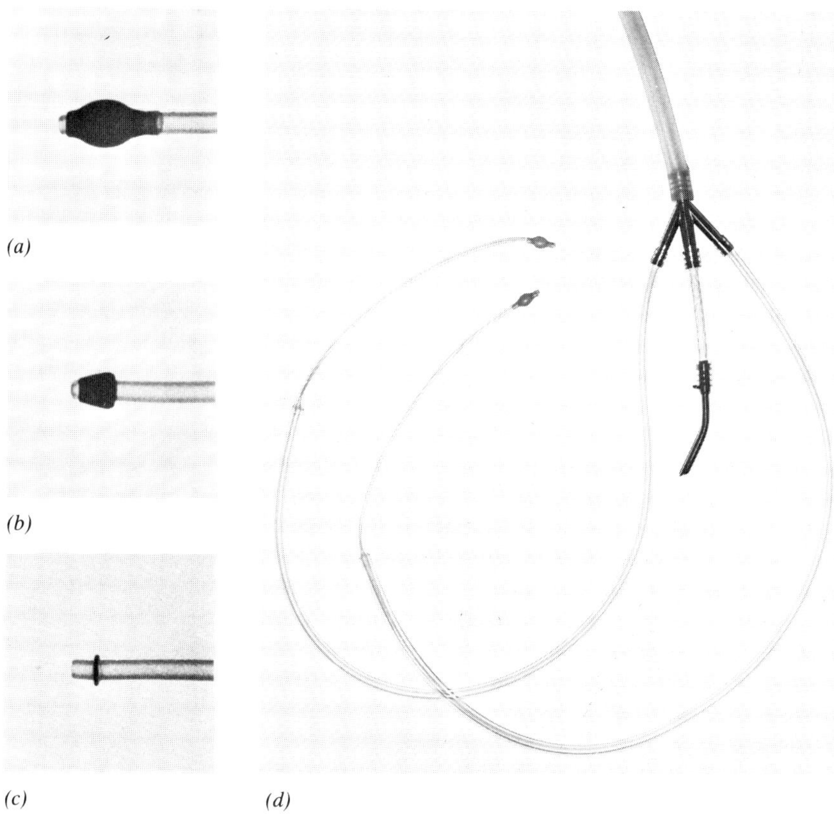

Figure 5.10 (*a*) Tip of balloon-type coronary perfusion cannula. (*b*) Tip of cone-type coronary perfusion cannula. (*c*) Tip of ring-type coronary perfusion cannula. (*d*) The arterial line showing the arterial cannula and the coronary perfusion cannulae

In order to avoid obstruction of the anterior descending coronary artery, in cases of its early branching from the main left stem, a cannula with a conical tip is used (*Figure 5.10b*). Cannulae with ring-tips (*Figure 5.10c*) are used for cannulation of small right coronary arteries. All cannulae are available with either straight or bent tips.

As shown in *Figure 5.10d* the coronary perfusion lines are taken from the arterial line. This method has worked very satisfactorily in our hands. At the present time coronary perfusion is not used in our clinic as it has been replaced by cold cardioplegia by means of the Brettschneider solution.

Connectors

All tubing circuits require that connectors be used in several places to join pieces of tubing to one another. A range of disposable polycarbonate connectors are available in various sizes and configurations (*Figure 5.11*).

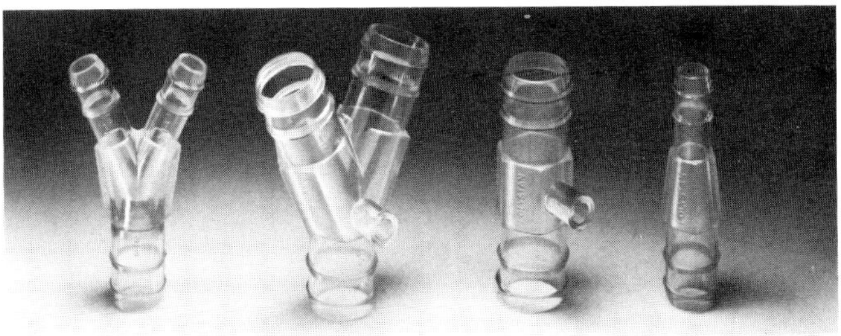

Figure 5.11 Disposable tubing connectors

Assembly of the heart-lung machine

The following is the procedure used for assembling the heart-lung machine in our department.

The tubing from the oxygenator, through the arterial pump and to the patient has the same diameter as the tubing which carries the venous blood from the patient to the oxygenator. When using the smallest oxygenator type for perfusion of newborns we use an 8 mm arteriovenous loop. Tubing with a 10 mm internal diameter in the arteriovenous loop is used for all other cases except for perfusions where flow rates above 4 litres per minute are anticipated. In these situations the tubing from the oxygenator and through the pump head has a 12 mm diameter and is reduced to a 10 mm diameter for the arterial line, whilst the venous line has an internal diameter of 12 mm.

Assembly of the machine is carried out in the following order. On a sterile, draped table the oxygenator is attached to the suction chambers by assembling the three chamber outlet lines to the special four-way connector. Fitted to this connector is a short length of tubing into which is inserted a micropore filter*. By way of another short tubing length the filter is then attached to one of the two inlets at the bottom of the oxygenating column. The arterial pump tubing segment is attached to the outlet of the arterial reservoir. A steel rod for mounting the oxygenator in the heart-lung machine is passed through the channel along the upper edge of the oxygenator. The oxygenator with the above mentioned tubing assemblies is then placed on the console. A short length of tubing connects the oxygen filter to the gas flowmeter outlet. The pump tubing is placed in the arterial pump and the vacuum chambers are mounted in their special bracket on the right-hand accessory pole. After this initial assembly the machine is transported to the operating theatre where the water lines are attached to the water mixing valve and heat exchanger. The gas supply lines are attached to the gas flowmeter and the electrical power to the heart-lung machine is turned on. The last part of the assembly consists of attaching the arterial end of the arteriovenous loop to the arterial pump outlet tubing. The

*Bentley PF 427

venous end of the arteriovenous loop is passed through the venous clamp and fitted to the venous inlet connector at the bottom of the oxygenating column. Finally the open-heart suction lines are connected to the inlets of the disposable suction chambers. Before priming the oxygenator and circuitry the gas supply to the oxygenator is started at a flow of 100–200 cc/min. The gas contains a mixture of 95 per cent O_2 and 5 per cent CO_2. When blood or part-blood prime is being used, the introduction of gas to the oxygenator maintains the patency of the pores in the oxygen dispenser. The vents at the top of the defoaming section must always be opened before the gas supply is turned on. The total minimum priming volumes (for oxygenator and the arteriovenous loop) are a few hundred ml greater than the minimum priming volumes indicated in *Table 5.1*.

When the total priming volume has been introduced into the oxygenator, the pump is started and the prime is recirculated through the arteriovenous loop so that it is filled and all air is removed. During recirculation of the prime the air in the last arterial reservoir section of the oxygenator is removed through the air elimination vent at the top of the 'chimney' in the arterial reservoir. This procedure ensures that the last reservoir section of the oxygenator, should it be inadvertently emptied of fluid during the perfusion, will collapse, and the arterial outlet connector will be sealed, thereby preventing the introduction of air into the arterial line during the perfusion.

When recirculating the prime, the heat exchanger is supplied with water at a temperature around 35°C in order to bring the prime up to this temperature.

During the recirculation the negative pressure is also adjusted in the suction chambers as previously described, and the occlusion of the arterial pump is checked once again.

Finally, the arterial pump is adjusted to its lowest rate and then stopped, and the venous line is clamped by closing the venous clamp. The arteriovenous loop can now be divided on the operating table and connected to the arterial cannula and venous catheters. The weight of the oxygenator is recorded.

Priming solutions

During the recent two years our policy has been to avoid the use of blood or albumin before and during the perfusion in all patients except in infants and small children. Accordingly the priming volume consists of pure Ringer's solution for all adults and children over 15 to 20 kg in weight. This usually reduces the haematocrit to between 20 and 25 per cent and occasionally even below this level. The haematocrit tends to increase slightly during the perfusion. With this degree of dilution the blood pressure during the perfusion is usually low, in the range of 30–60 mmHg. This arterial pressure is accepted as adequate, and the administration of drugs for the elevation of pressure is avoided. After termination of heart-lung bypass the perfusate is reinfused to all patients except infants and small children. At this stage vasodilation with chlorpromazine is normally induced in adults.

The VT-5000 Venotherm oxygenator is used for all patients above 20 kg, with the exception of big patients with large heart volumes and big patients subjected to coronary artery bypass graft procedures. In these two categories we use the VT-7000 Venotherm oxygenator. In patients weighing between 20 kg and 50 kg the arteriovenous lines are 10 mm internal diameter as is also the arterial pump segment. In patients above 50 kg in weight the arterial line is 10 mm, the venous line is 12 mm and the pump segment is also 12 mm internal diameter. The standard prime for the total extracorporeal circuit when the VT-5000 Venotherm oxygenator is being used with a 10 mm arterial and a 12 mm venous line consists of 1700–2000 ml lactated Ringer's solution, 50 ml of 50 mg/100ml glucose, 1 g ascorbic acid, 200 mg Pluronic F-68, 40 mmol sodium bicarbonate and 8500–10 000 iu heparin. The standard prime for the VT-5000 Venotherm oxygenator with 10 mm lines consists of 1500 ml lactated Ringer's solution, 50 ml of 50 mg/100ml glucose, 1 g ascorbic acid, 200 mg Pluronic F-68, 30 mmol sodium bicarbonate and 7500 iu of heparin. When the VT-7000 is used, the total priming volume is 2300–2500 ml. Pluronic and ascorbic acid are used to reduce platelet aggregation.

Operating the heart-lung machine during perfusion

Before commencing the perfusion the oxygen and carbon dioxide supply to the oxygenator is adjusted, and the water supply to the heat exchanger is set to a minimum of 35°C. Perfusion is commenced by starting the arterial pump at its slowest speed. At the same time the venous clamp is opened enough to maintain a constant weight of the oxygenator. The rate of the arterial pump is slowly increased, while the gravity drainage is increased by gradually opening the venous clamp. Monitoring the weight of the oxygenator ensures that a balanced venous blood inflow and arterial outflow may be maintained. This balanced increase in the arterial output is maintained until the calculated pump flow rate has been obtained.

In most of the patients the venous clamp is fully released so that free venous drainage is obtained, usually resulting in a drop of the central venous pressure to zero. In cases where partial cardiopulmonary support of the circulation is still desired, the venous clamp is maintained to keep a certain venous pressure or a certain weight of the oxygenator.

The arterial pump flow rate for total cardiopulmonary bypass at euthermic levels corresponds to a minimum of 2.4 ℓ/min per m^2. During hypothermia at around 30°C the rate is decreased to 2.0 ℓ/min per m^2 and in paediatric cardiac surgery, with hypothermia around 25°C or below, the rate is often decreased to 0.8 ℓ/min per m^2.

In order to obtain rapid cooling in cases where deep hypothermia is required, the pump flow rate is maintained at around 2.4 ℓ/min per m^2 throughout the cooling period. This same blood flow rate is always used during rewarming.

In periods with circulatory arrest the extracorporeal blood volume may be recirculated at around 100 ml/min through a shunt connecting the arterial and venous lines at the operating table.

The arterial pump flow is recorded at various stages of the perfusion. At our institution the mean systemic arterial and venous pressures and the oesophageal and rectal temperatures are recorded continuously during the perfusion.

During perfusions combined with hypothermia, cooling is commenced when a stable heart-lung bypass has been reached. The temperature of the water supply to the heat exchanger during the cooling period is lowered to approximately 14°C. After this period the temperature of the water is adjusted to maintain the body temperature required by the surgeon – for adults usually between 28°C and 30°C. Rewarming takes place slowly and care is exercised to avoid temperature differentials of more than 12°C between the water supplied to the heat exchanger and the patient's oesophageal temperature.

Blood from the oxygenator may be returned to the patient as long as there is sufficient volume in the arterial reservoir to ensure a safe blood level in the oxygenator. In many cases extra volume must be added to the extracorporeal circuit during the perfusion. In the great majority of cases the extra volume consists only of additional lactated Ringer's solution while blood is very seldom used. The amount of fluid added is always recorded, and by reading the weight of the oxygenator at the end of the perfusion the total volume which has been administered to the patient can be easily determined.

The perfusion is terminated by slowly occluding the venous line with the venous clamp and at the same time reducing the output of the arterial pump, under the control of the oxygenator weight. At the end of the perfusion it is often necessary to give blood from the oxygenator to the patient under the control of the central venous and left atrial pressures.

Chlorpromazine is given to the patients for vasodilatation and in most adult patients the oxygenator blood volume is returned to the patient before decannulation. After the termination of heart-lung bypass the gas flow to the oxygenator is reduced to about 100/200 cc/min (95 per cent O_2 and 5 per cent CO_2) and the heart-lung machine is kept ready until the arterial and venous cannulae have been removed.

Gas flow rate

The gas flow rate used in modern bubble oxygenators, including the present Polystan series, has been reduced in recent years. This has been done in order to minimize the traumatic effect of bubbling and defoaming, which has been the main cause of haemolysis during perfusion. The gas flow/blood flow ratios are now at physiological levels, but still so high that admixture of CO_2 in the oxygen is usually necessary. The high oxygenating capacity of the oxygenators makes constant regulation of the gas flow rate necessary in order to avoid excessively high oxygen tensions, especially during hypothermic perfusions. Usually the gas flow rate is related to the blood flow rate, which is kept more or less constant at 2.0 to 2.4 ℓ/min per m^2 in the majority of cases. However, in paediatric cardiac surgery combined with deep hypothermia, the blood flow rate is often much reduced, and unless this reduction is fixed, a correlation between gas flow and blood flow rates may be difficult. Nevertheless, the gas flow/blood flow ratio is helpful as a guideline for the regulation of gas supply.

At our institution the gas supply has been regulated by a servocontrol unit in which the continuously measured P_{O_2} is the variable parameter which is regulated to a value around 100 mmHg with ranges between 80 and 120 mmHg. Even though these values may be regarded as higher than

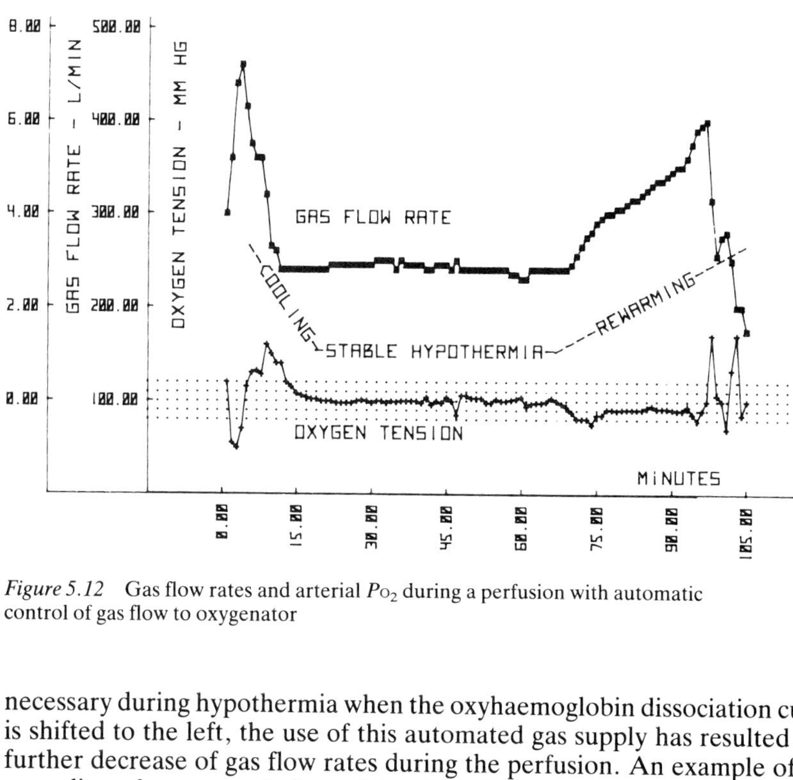

Figure 5.12 Gas flow rates and arterial P_{O_2} during a perfusion with automatic control of gas flow to oxygenator

necessary during hypothermia when the oxyhaemoglobin dissociation curve is shifted to the left, the use of this automated gas supply has resulted in a further decrease of gas flow rates during the perfusion. An example of the recordings from a perfusion with a blood flow rate of 5000 ml/min and oesophageal temperature of 30°C during hypothermia is shown in *Figure 5.12*. From the data obtained, the guidelines for a stepwise manual regulation of the gas flow rate is shown in *Table 5.4*. The values during deep hypothermia are the results from perfusions of infants and children and are also valid for perfusions with reduced blood flow rates down to 0.8 ℓ/min per m^2 (1/3 of normal). Such low gas flow rates require the use of very accurate gas flowmeters capable of measuring flows to below 100 cc/min.

The gas flow rate during priming and recirculation prior to perfusion or during periods of circulatory arrest is the lowest necessary to prevent fluid from entering into the oxygen dispenser. This amounts to 100 cc/min for the infant sizes and to 200 cc/min for the larger sizes of oxygenators.

Table 5.4 Gas to blood flow ratios $\frac{GF}{BF}$ and CO_2 percentages at different periods of perfusion

Period	$\frac{GF}{BF}$	CO_2 *percentage*
Start of perfusion	1.5	3
Cooling	1.0	5
Stable hypothermia at 30°C	0.6	5
Stable hypothermia at 25°C	0.4	5
Stable hypothermia at 20°C	0.3	5
Rewarming	0.8–1.0	3
End of perfusion with partial cardiopulmonary support	0.5	3

The percentage of CO_2 in the oxygen is 5 per cent during priming and recirculation and during cooling and stable hypothermia. During perfusions at 'euthermic' levels (34–37°C) and during rewarming 3 per cent CO_2 is used. It should be noted that the gas supply can only be reduced to the minimum necessary for adequate CO_2 removal.

Filtration

As previously described, all Polystan (Rygg–Kyvsgaard) bubble oxygenators are provided with arterial reservoir filters. A further filtration takes place in the defoaming fibres and also in a woven filter surrounding these fibres.

Up to 1961 the filters consisted of a roll of nylon fibres or compressed polyurethane sponges in the descending limbs of the two U-shaped traps. These filters proved to be very effective in removing small bubbles. An additional filter was placed in the arterial line between the pump and the patient. It contained a fine-mesh stainless steel screen. In this last filter, deposition of fibrin was constantly found, and it was thought to be the cause of cerebral and/or renal embolism. In an early series of animal experiments embolic lesions were found in 50 per cent of the animals with this filter as compared to 10 per cent without. No arterial line filter has since been used, except in a small series of clinical perfusions for investigational purposes. Further experiments led to the incorporation in the oxygenator of the present filters woven from monofilament thread instead of the fibre or sponge filters. Gross deposits are avoided by filters in this position, where the blood passes at a steady and low velocity flow and under low pressure. A recent study has confirmed the influence of the flow and pressure pattern on filtration. In a pump circuit with recirculation of the same sample of freshly drawn, human heparinized blood, a filter was exposed to a steady gravity flow under low pressure or to pulsatile flow under pressure created by a roller pump. Commercially available Dacron-wool, Polyester-urethane or woven filters with pore sizes down to 25 microns were tested. With the filter in the venous line (gravity flow) no haemolysis was found. The number of platelets and leucocytes decreased in the blood, and they were practically all removed by Dacron-wool filtration. Placed distal to the pump all the filters increased the haemolysis to almost double that of the control pump circuit, without a filter. Platelets and white cells decreased very rapidly, and Dacron-wool filtration was again the most damaging procedure. Microscopic examination revealed a higher degree of fibrin deposition in the filters which were placed distal to the pump. This increase in haemolysis found in recirculation experiments does not necessarily have any relation to the findings during clinical perfusion.

An examination of the different filters in the oxygenator revealed many kinds of particles, as shown in *Table 5.5*. During these clinical perfusions the

Table 5.5 Particles found by microscopic examination of the four filters of the Rygg–Kyvsgaard thermo-oxygenator following clinical perfusions

Defoaming filter	*First trap filter*	*Second trap filter*	*Last filter*
Fibrin	Small fibrin threads Minor clots	Platelets and white cells	Platelets and white cells
Blood clots	Platelets and white cells		
Platelets and white cells	Heart muscle cells		
Heart muscle cells	Minor calcific particles Cholesterol crystals		
Endothelial cells			
Fragments of calcified tissue			
Cholesterol crystals			
Fibroblasts			
Cancer cells			

filter usually situated in the cardiotomy suction line was placed between the oxygenator and the pump.

The first filtration takes place in the filter surrounding the defoaming fibres, where most of the deposits were found. Single clots, cells and threads of fibrin were found in the first trap filter, whereas the last two filters contained only platelets and leucocytes, isolated or as aggregates. Interestingly, cancer cells, believed to originate from a bronchial carcinoma, were found in one of the filters. No signs of growth have been detected in the patient so far.

In a series of perfusions with the commercially available filter described by Patterson and Twichell[4], placed proximal as well as distal to the pump, equal amounts of cellular deposits were found in the filters. From the microscopic picture it was concluded that the deposits of platelets and white cells in the filters seemed to be related to the length of the perfusion. Fibrin deposition was somewhat more pronounced in the filter placed distal to the pump.

In our opinion there is ample evidence that filters inserted in the arterial line are traumatic to the blood and may cause the release of fibrin and other particulate matter as a result of the pressure and flow variations existing in this position. Filters should preferably be placed in sections of the extracorporeal circuit where such pressure variations do not exist and through which the linear velocity of the blood is low. Consequently, apart from the filters in the oxygenator, we only use one filter in the cardiotomy suction line.

Acid–base balance

The acid–base balance of the patients is altered somewhat at the beginning of the perfusion by the difference in buffer capacity between the priming fluid and the blood of the patient. Changes in pH and base excess (BE) are usually towards the acid side. The changes are, however, dependent on the

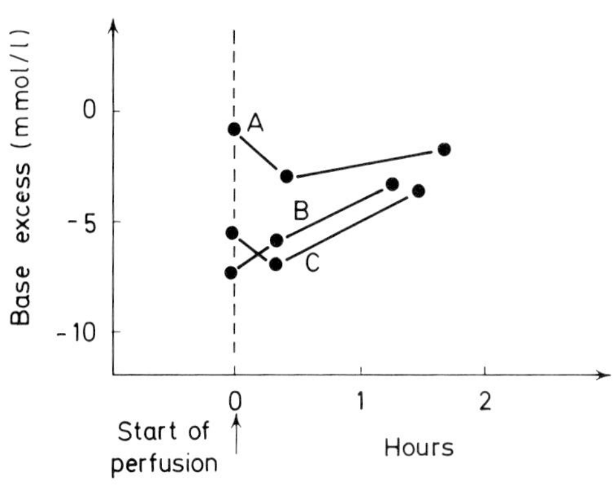

Figure 5.13 Changes in base excess during extracorporeal circulation. Group A comprises 20 patients in whom the preperfusion sample had a value higher than −5. Eight patients in group B had initial values lower than −5. Sodium bicarbonate was not given to the patients of groups A and B. In group C, comprising 6 patients, the initial values were −3.8 to −6.7. These patients were treated with sodium bicarbonate (90 mmol for adults, and correspondingly lower doses for children)

acid–base situation of the patient before the onset of perfusion. Patients with severely impaired circulation often have an accumulation of metabolic acid equivalents to such a degree that their balance improves by the mixing and dilution with the priming fluid.

During perfusions with relatively high blood flow rates and adequate oxygenation, increases of the BE or the standard bicarbonate are often seen. Even during perfusions combined with moderate or deep hypothermia, accumulation of acid metabolites does not occur. The tendency towards spontaneous correction of the acidosis following circulatory arrest during profound hypothermia was previously described by Rygg, Borgeskov and Arnfred[8].

It has been our practice to correct the acid–base disturbances often seen in patients with a poor circulatory condition before the start of perfusion. However, from *Figure 5.13* it can be seen that such a correction is hardly necessary, as the improvement of the circulation produced by an adequate perfusion generally enables the patient to eliminate the existing acid metabolites.

Haemolysis

Haemodilution and reduced gas flow rates have reduced the trauma to the blood to such an extent that no correlation exists between the duration of perfusion and haemolysis in many clinical cases. This relates to perfusions at haematocrits around 20 to 25 per cent and without heavy open-heart suction. It means that haemolysis under such conditions is so low that the production of plasma haemoglobin has decreased to the level of its elimination rate by the organism. The importance of haemodilution and reduction of gas flow rates in order to reduce haemolysis caused by bubble oxygenation is shown in *Figure 5.14*. The figure illustrates the correlation between the haemolysis and the gas flow rate at a pump speed of 2 or 4 ℓ/min. Experimentally, the increase in plasma haemoglobin was recorded after 100 passages of the same sample of blood through the oxygenator. Freshly drawn heparinized human blood was used and the recirculation performed at room temperature. A mixture of oxygen and carbon dioxide (95 per cent O_2 and 5 per cent CO_2) was used in the oxygenator in order to keep the pH within normal ranges. The gas was not humidified and the blood was not filtered before use. From the values in *Figure 5.14* the haemolysis caused by the action of the pump alone should be subtracted. This amounts to a maximum of 13 μmol/ℓ (21 mg/100ml) at a pump speed of 4 ℓ/min. It follows that haemolysis can be reduced by haemodilution.

These experimental observations confirm the clinical findings in a group of patients with tetralogy of Fallot in which the rate of haemolysis was dependent on the haemoglobin concentration of the perfusate[9].

The damaging effect of bubble oxygenation on the red blood cells has been expressed as the haemolysis found per 100 litres of gas delivered to the oxygenator. Apart from a similar dependence on the concentration or red cells expressed by the haemoglobin concentration, no significant difference in the haemolysis caused by 100 litres of gas was found whether it was supplied at 2, 4, 5 or 6 ℓ/min. This observation suggests that it is the energy required in the formation and the breakdown of a certain amount of bubbles or foam which is the determining factor. The defoaming process seems to be most traumatic, rendering the amount of foam which is allowed to be formed during oxygenation of special importance.

Compared to the oxygenating process, the pumping of the blood, even against pressure, causes but little haemolysis as already mentioned. The

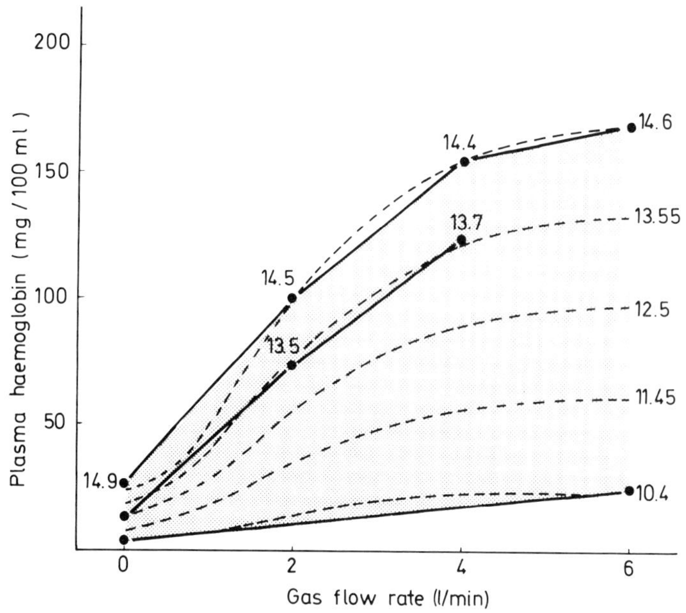

Figure 5.14 Increase in plasma haemoglobin after 100 passages of the same sample of blood through the pump and oxygenator, in relation to the gas flow rate for different haemoglobin concentrations, indicated by the numbers on the different lines. The continuous lines are observations, the dotted lines are estimates at a linear proportionality between haemoglobin concentration and haemolysis. 1 mg haemoglobin/100 ml equals 0.62 mmol/l (Reproduced from Rygg[7] by courtesy of FADL Publishing House, Copenhagen)

intracardiac suction may, however, be rather traumatic if a mixture of air and blood is transported as in 'audible aspiration'.

A previous study[15] revealed the trauma inflicted upon the blood by the intracardiac suckers. In 12 patients who were previously operated upon (mitral valve disease) and in whom the open-heart suckers were continuously used, the mean hourly rate of haemolysis was 25 μmol/ℓ as compared to only 14 μmol/ℓ in 21 patients with isolated aortic valve disease in whom open-heart suction was scarcely used. The degree of haemodilution was comparable, and the difference was statistically significant (1 μmol/ℓ = 1.61 mg/100ml). It may be stressed that haemodilution to a degree that causes a considerable reduction of haemolysis is necessary during open-heart surgery merely to obtain acceptable conditions for intracardiac suction and avoidance of homologous blood administration. The many beneficial effects of haemodilution are described elsewhere in this book as is also the 'homologous blood syndrome'. The improved quality of perfusion obtained through recent years has made it possible to perform routine perfusions of 3 to 5 hours' duration.

Damage to blood constituents other than red blood cells

During perfusion with the Polystan (Rygg–Kyvsgaard) oxygenator the number of circulating platelets diminished by about 50 per cent[8, 15]. Similar figures have been reported by other investigations[13]. *Figure 5.15* shows that platelet counts were identical in the postoperative period whether haemodilution was used or not. From this figure, it can also be seen that in the 5

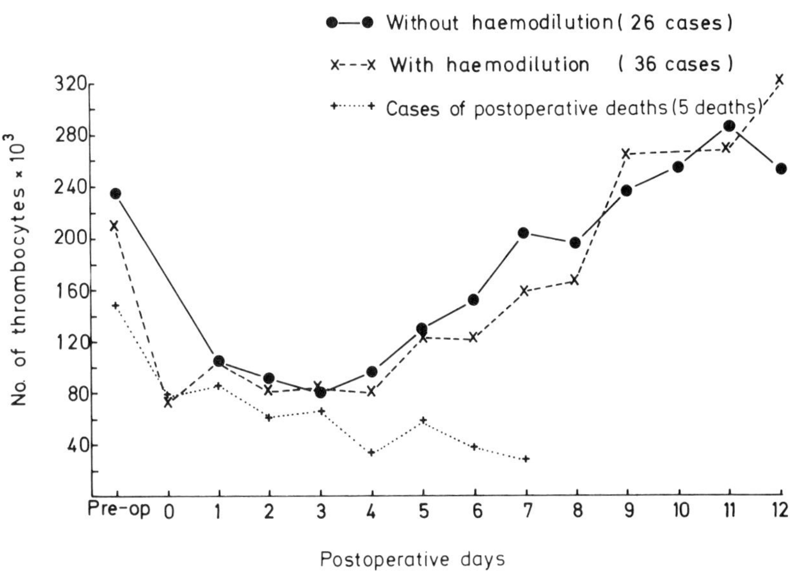

Figure 5.15 Platelet counts before and after extracorporeal circulation with the Polystan (Rygg–Kyvsgaard) oxygenator

fatal cases the platelet counts were low before as well as after heart-lung bypass. All these 5 patients died from low cardiac output, and the low platelet counts are probably a reflection of their poor circulatory status before and after bypass leading to intravascular coagulopathy and perhaps a decreased production of thrombocytes. *Figure 5.10d* also shows that after the ninth postoperative day the average platelet count exceeds the preoperative value. This phenomenon is also encountered following general surgical procedures[14].

In a previous investigation it was stated that coagulation was not impaired following extracorporeal circulation with the Rygg–Kyvsgaard thermo-oxygenator[15]. Fibrinogen depletion has not occurred (*Figure 5.16*) and no changes in coagulation parameters have been found immediately following bypass, except those attributable to the haemodilution or to inadequate dosage of protamine suphate. Furthermore, electrophoretic studies revealed that the relative concentrations of most plasma proteins were practically unaffected by extracorporeal circulation. Apart from a very

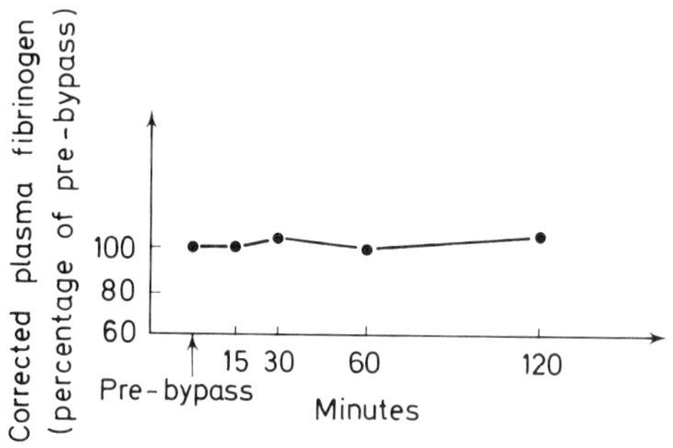

Figure 5.16 Relative concentrations of plasma fibrinogen, corrected for the haemodilution, during 14 clinical perfusions. (Reproduced from Valentin *et al.*[15] by courtesy of *Scandinavian Journal of Thoracic and Cardiovascular Surgery*)

small decrease in the albumin fraction, a pronounced fall in haptoglobin was seen due to the linking of haptoglobin to free haemoglobin. Other globulin fractions showed a small increase.

Final considerations

Bubble oxygenation is, at the moment, the most widely used principle for heart-lung bypass during open-heart surgery. Bubble oxygenation is only slightly more traumatic than membrane oxygenation, the benefits of which only become significant after several hours of perfusion[1, 2, 3]. The direct contact between blood and oxygen is not thought to be more deleterious to blood than its contact with other non-endothelial surfaces, provided the oxygen is properly humidified and mixed with CO_2. The trauma of bubble oxygenation seems mainly to be related to the strong forces involved in the formation and breakdown of foam. By improving the methods for distribution of the bubbles in the blood and the methods for reducing foam formation, it is believed that the bubble diffusion principle for artificial oxygenation will become even less traumatic in the years to come.

Summary

The construction of the Polystan (Rygg–Kyvsgaard) system for extracorporeal circulation and oxygenation and the underlying principles are reported. The current techniques for extracorporeal circulation employed at the department of Thoracic Surgery, Rigshospitalet, Copenhagen, are described. The extent of damage to blood constituents is surveyed.

It is concluded that the number and severity of complications attributable to the perfusion *per se* is acceptable and that bubble oxygenation will have a place in the clinical practice of tomorrow.

References

1. Alon, L., Turina, M. and Gattiker, R. 'Membrane and bubble oxygenators. A clinical comparison in patients undergoing aortocoronary bypass procedures.' *Herz*, **4,** 56 (1979)
2. Fleming, J. S., Bentall, H. H., Sapsford, R. N. and Melrose, D. G. 'Comparison between bubble and membrane oxygenators: preliminary report of a clinical trial.' *In press*, (1979)
3. Gullestad, S. and Skagseth, E. 'A comparative clinical study between the Travenol Teflon membrane oxygenator and the Polystan (Rygg–Kyvsgaard) bubble oxygenator.' Presented at the Scandinavian Association of Thoracic and Cardiovascular Surgery, 8 September 1976, Trondheim, Norway (1976)
4. Patterson, R. H., Jr. and Twichell, J. B. 'Disposable filter for microemboli.' *Journal of the American Medical Association*, **215**, 76 (1971)
5. Rygg, I. H. 'Discussion on oxygenators'. In *Extracorporeal Circulation*. Ed. J. G. Allen, p. 108. Springfield: Thomas (1958)
6. Rygg, I. H. 'Discussion on pumps.' In *Extracorporeal Circulation*. Ed. J. G. Allen, p. 39. Springfield: Thomas (1958)
7. Rygg, I. H. *Studies in Extracorporeal Circulation*. Copenhagen: FADL (1973)
8. Rygg, I. H., Borgeskov, S. and Arnfred, I. 'A case of prolonged deep hypothermia during cardiopulmonary bypass.' *Scandinavian Journal of Thoracic and Cardiovascular Surgery*, **3,** 197 (1969)
9. Rygg, I. H., Borgeskov, S., de la Mata, R. C., Frederiksen, T. and Rosen, J. 'An evaluation of the perfusion and surgical technique related to extracorporeal circulation in an early series of open-heart operations of tetralogy of Fallot.' *Danish Medical Bulletin*, **18** (Suppl. 2), 101 (1971)
10. Rygg, I. H., Engell, H. C. and Kyvsgaard, E. 'A heart-lung machine with disposable polyethylene oxygenator system.' *Danish Medical Bulletin*, **3,** 200 (1956)
11. Rygg, I. H. and Kyvsgaard, E. 'A disposable polyethylene oxygenator system applied in a heart-lung machine.' *Acta Chirurgica Scandinavica*, **112,** 433 (1956)
12. Rygg, I. H. and Kyvsgaard, E. 'Further development of the heart-lung machine with Rygg–Kyvsgaard plastic bag oxygenator.' *Minerva Chirurgica*, **8,** 1402 (1958)
13. Salzman, E. W. 'Blood platelets and extracorporeal circulation.' *Transfusion*, **2,** 274 (1963)
14. Storm, O. 'Post-operative thrombozytosen.' In *Thrombozytäre Gerinnungsstorungen*. Ed. L. Zuckschwerdt and J. A. Theiss, p. 221. Stuttgart: F. K. Schattauer-Verlag (1967)
15. Valentin, N., Nielsen, V. G., Bersteen, O. and Rygg, I. H. 'The Rygg–Kyvsgaard thermo-oxygenator. A clinical trial.' *Scandinavian Journal of Thoracic and Cardiovascular Surgery*, **18,** 176 (1974)

6

Clinical Use of the Shiley Oxygenating System

Michele F. Roesler, Anand P. Tandon and
Marian I. Ionescu

a fonte puro pura deuit aqua

Introduction

During the last few years considerable progress in the development of new types of oxygenators has been achieved. The evolution of oxygenator design is dramatically illustrated by comparison between, for example, a Melrose or Kay–Cross and a modern disposable oxygenator with its incorporated heat exchanger (*Figure 6.1*). Currently available models must offer high standards of reliability, gas exchange performance and heat exchange efficiency with minimal trauma to blood constituents. Furthermore, compactness, ease of assembly and reasonable cost are important factors to be taken into account.

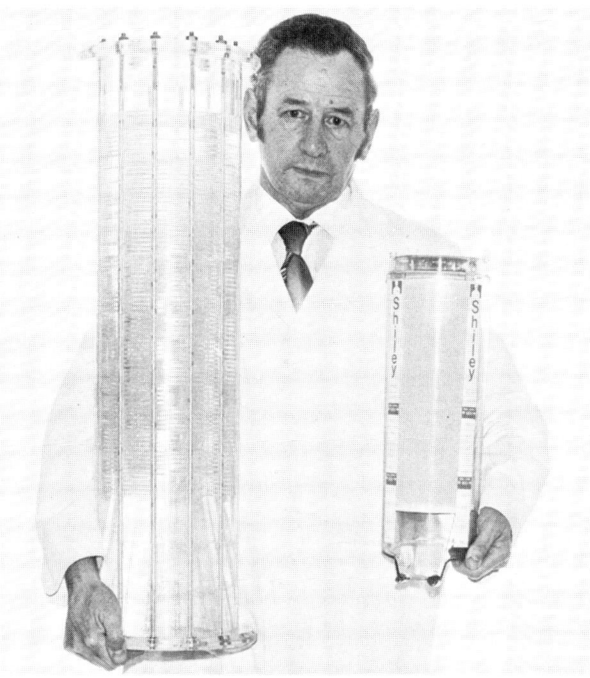

Figure 6.1 Twenty years apart. Comparison of the size of the Melrose and the Shiley oxygenator

There is a great deal of debate about the choice between membrane and bubble oxygenators. Laboratory and clinical data indicate that membrane oxygenators have certain attractions[7, 20, 33, 35]. In particular, they appear to be less traumatic to blood constituents during long perfusions[7–34], while offering the theoretical and practical advantage of independent control of arterial oxygen and carbon dioxide saturation. However, bulk, cost and difficulty of assembly limit their widespread clinical use for routine cardiac surgical operations. For these reasons we believe that the present generation of bubble oxygenators has a substantial place in modern cardiac surgery. This chapter considers the clinical use of the Shiley bubble oxygenating systems.

Description of apparatus

The oxygenator

The model S-100-A Shiley oxygenator has the same general configuration as the previous S-100 model. It has a compact body composed of two cylinders (*Figure 6.2*). The gas inlet (1) is connected to the base of the smaller cylinder

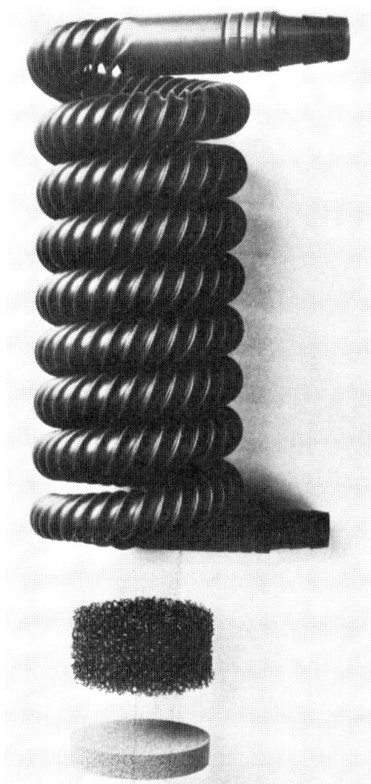

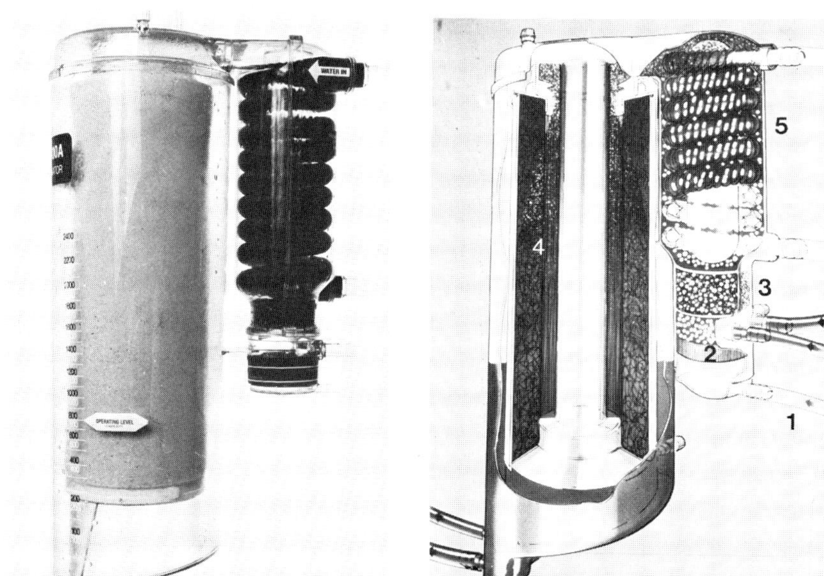

Figure 6.2 The Shiley S-100-A oxygenator-heat exchanger. 1 = gas inlet; 2 = gas disperser; 3 = porous sponge; 4 = reticulated polyurethane sponge; 5 = anodized aluminium coil. *Left*: photograph. *Right*: schematic view. *Top*: components contained in the oxygenating column

and the gas dispersed through the blood by a gas sparger (2) made from epoxy-bonded glass beads*. The blood and gas mixture then passes through an open-cell porous sponge (3) whose pore size (10 pores/in^2) and thickness have been chosen to optimize the exchange of oxygen and carbon dioxide. The sponge induces laminar mixing. Defoaming takes place in a reticulated polyurethane sponge (4) coated with Dow Corning† antifoam A compound. A nylon tricot cloth surrounding the defoaming sponge provides the final filtration of the blood entering the arterial reservoir.

The heat exchanger

The heat exchanger is an integral part of the oxygenator (*Figure 6.2*). It is composed of a helically coiled and axially twisted aluminium tube which is either polyurethane coated (S-100) or anodized (S-100-A) according to the model. This is placed above the open-cell porous sponge in the venous reservoir. The grooves between the helical fins are designed to provide an increased surface area for thermal transfer during the cooling and rewarming of blood required for hypothermic perfusions. Moreover they continue the laminar mixing process. The inlet and outlet of the water and blood in the heat exchanger are disposed in such a way that the water flows from the top to the bottom while the blood flows in the opposite direction. This creates a counter-current mechanism. As the coil of the heat exchanger is moulded in one piece there are no seals or welds in locations which could lead to a water to blood leak. Shiley has produced two models of oxygenator, the S-100 and S-100-A. They differ in the quality of the heat exchanger tubing. In the S-100-A model it is made of anodized aluminium which replaced the polyurethane-coated aluminium tubing of the previous S-100 model. This modification was introduced by the manufacturer in order to further improve the efficiency of the heat exchanger.

The cardiotomy reservoir

The Shiley cardiotomy reservoir (*Figure 6.3*) consists of a clear polycarbonate cylinder (total capacity 2400 ml). Blood is returned to the top of the cylinder via three inlets, two for intracardiac suction and one for the left heart vent. Blood passes through an inner, cylindrically shaped, reticulated polyurethane sponge coated with Dow Corning antifoam A compound and covered with a nylon tricot cloth. The defoamed blood passes through the cloth into the outer reservoir from where it is gravity-drained into the oxygenator via an outlet at the base of the cylinder. There are three priming points at the top of the unit. The reservoir can efficiently handle blood at flow rates of up to 5 ℓ/min. The manufacturers recommend that the pressure in the reservoir should be monitored and kept below 200 mmHg.

As the Shiley cardiotomy reservoir does not incorporate a micropore filter, a blood filter is interposed in-line between the cardiotomy reservoir and the oxygenator (*Figure 6.3*).

*Tegraglass, 3M Corporation, Minneapolis, Minnesota, USA
†Dow Corning Corporation, Midland, Michigan, USA

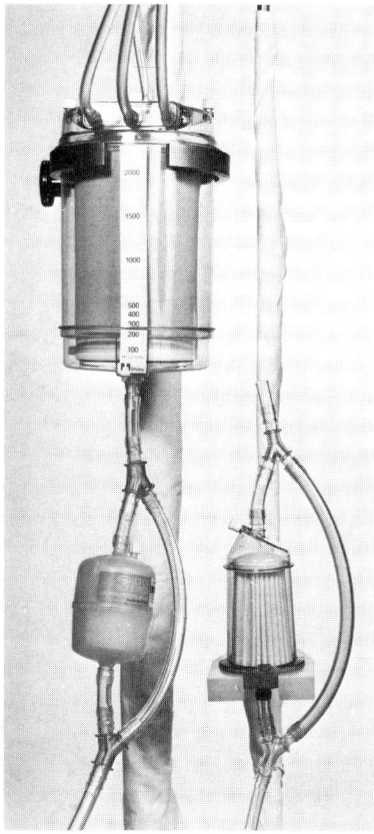

Figure 6.3 The Shiley cardiotomy reservoir with two types of blood filters (Pall Ultipore on the left and Johnson and Johnson Intercept on the right)

The circuit

At the Leeds General Infirmary the Shiley disposable oxygenator is used in conjunction with a Pemco pump console unit*, Shiley cardiotomy reservoir†, Shiley tygon tubing† and either Pall Ultipore** or Intercept†† blood filters. The total priming volume of the entire extracorporeal circuit is 1600–1800 ml. This comprises 800 ml for the oxygenator, 100 ml for the filter and cardiotomy reservoir and 900 ml for the connecting tubing. The prime consists of an isotonic dextrose-saline solution containing potassium, calcium, magnesium, chloride, gluconate and phosphate (*Table 6.1*). Variable volumes of bicarbonate and 50 per cent dextrose are added during heart-lung bypass as required by the clinical situation. Three grams of potassium chloride per m^2 surface area are added slowly into the circuit early after commencing the heart-lung bypass.

*Pemco Inc., Cleveland, Ohio, USA.
†Shiley Laboratories Inc., Irvine, California, USA.
**Pall Miomedical Ltd., Portsmouth, UK.
††Johnson and Johnson Co., New Brunswick, New Jersey, USA.

Table 6.1 Priming solution for the heart-lung machine

Components	*mmol/ℓ*
Sodium	101.2
Potassium	5.0
Chloride	105.8
Calcium	2.5
Magnesium	0.8
Gluconate	2.5
Phosphate	1.2
Dextrose	25.0 g
Freshly distilled water	1.0 ℓ

Description of the perfusion procedure

For virtually all open-heart surgical procedures a median sternotomy approach and cannulation of the ascending aorta and both venae cavae is used. Cannulation of the femoral or external iliac artery is reserved for aortic aneurysms and for the third reoperations on the aortic valve.

While preparation is being made for cannulation, the scrub nurse passes the arterial and venous line ends to the perfusionist operating the pump. The lines are connected to the heart-lung machine, primed, cut and secured to the drapes. Tapes are passed around the aorta and both venae cavae. Two concentric pursestrings are placed just proximal to the innominate artery on the convex surface of the ascending aorta. The pursestring for the superior vena cava cannula is placed at the base of the right auricular appendage at a distance from the right coronary artery. The pursestring for the inferior vena cava cannula is placed in the right atrial wall just above the insertion of the inferior vena cava. Cardioplegic, hypothermic arrest is routinely used and in the absence of aortic incompetence a small pursestring is placed 2 cm proximal to the aortic cannulation site, again on the convex aspect of the ascending aorta. All the pursestrings are passed through tourniquets. Intracardiac pressures are routinely recorded prior to cannulation. A loading dose of heparin (3 mg/kg body weight) is injected by the surgeon directly into the right atrium. While gentle traction is applied caudally to the aorta using the umbilical tape, a partially-occluding Satinsky clamp is placed tangentially around the aortic pursestrings. A small incision is made and probed with the tip of an arterial clamp to ensure that the lumen has been reached. A clamped USCI* cannula of adequate size with right-angle tip but without lateral holes is inserted through the incision, both pursestrings are snared, the cannula connected to the primed arterial line and the clamp

*United States Catheter and Instrument International Inc., Massachusetts, USA.

removed. A heavy silk ligature is tied around the tourniquets and cannula. The cannula is also secured by a suture to the skin and drapes at the level of the upper end of the incision.

The right auricular appendage is excluded with a Satinsky clamp, and incised and the muscular bands completely divided with scissors. The tricuspid valve and atrial septum are explored by direct digital palpation. A Portex* venous cannula is inserted and advanced just proximal to the junction of the superior vena cava with the innominate vein. The pursestring is snared and a ligature tied around the tourniquet and the cannula. The latter is joined to the venous line via one limb of a 'Y' connector. At this stage partial bypass is gradually instituted.

While the assistant applies gentle traction on the pursestring near to the inferior vena cava, a Bland Sutton forceps is placed at the opposite corner of the oval-shaped pursestring. An incision is made in the right atrial wall through which the second venous cannula is inserted and advanced into the inferior vena cava. The cannula is connected to the other limb of the 'Y' connector of the venous line and the pursestring snared. Total heart-lung bypass is established by snaring the vena caval tourniquets. Cooling is started and the aorta cross-clamped when the desired temperature is reached. The heart is decompressed in order to avoid left ventricular distension. The aortic root is opened for operations on the aortic valve, the

Table 6.2 Blood flow rates of perfusion according to body temperature

Temperature (°C)	*Blood flow (ℓ/min per m^2 BSA*)*
36.5	2.5–2.3
29	2.0–1.8
26	1.8–1.6

*BSA = body surface area

left atrium is incised for mitral valve procedures, or a vent tube is inserted through a stab wound into the apex of the left ventricle for coronary bypass procedures. At the beginning of perfusion a flow of 2.4 ℓ/min per m^2 of body surface area is used and this is progressively reduced as the temperature is lowered to accommodate increasing vascular resistance (*Table 6.2*). Superior vena cava and arterial pressures are continuously monitored. The urine output is measured and the following parameters recorded at 15 minute intervals: arterial and venous blood gases and acid–base balance, haemoglobin, haematocrit and platelet count. Oesophageal, rectal, skin (dorsum of the foot) and heat exchanger water temperatures are continually monitored. The blood volume in the oxygenator is monitored and maintained above a minimum safe level according to the arterial blood flow. The blood from the open-heart suckers is normally returned to the oxygenator unless debris or fat droplets are seen in large amounts. If the volume of blood in the

*Portex Ltd., Hythe, Kent, UK.

oxygenator is insufficient it is supplemented using blood, plasma or crystalloid solution according to the haematocrit. At present the myocardium is protected using total body hypothermia, cold cardioplegia and topical hypothermia. For short procedures such as closure of secundum type atrial septal defect or straight-forward mitral valve replacement the body temperature is lowered to 26–28°C, while for complex cases such as multiple valve replacement, combined procedures, repair of tetralogy of Fallot or reoperations, a central temperature of 20–26°C is preferred. A lower temperature is also used in cases of predominant aortic stenosis with heavy calcification where, though the operating time may not be unduly long, the myocardium is hypertrophied and does not tolerate ischaemia and hypoxia. Systemic cooling is supplemented by topical hypothermia induced with intermittent bathing of the heart with saline solution at 4°C. This saline solution is not returned to the oxygenator. For cardioplegia an electrolyte solution containing 16 mmol of potassium, 16 mmol of magnesium, 49 mmol of chloride and 273 mg of procaine per litre at 4°C is used. In cases in which the aorta is not open the solution is infused under pressure into the aortic root by a cannula inserted through the small aortic pursestring. For cases where the aorta is open the solution is infused directly into the left and right coronary arteries via coronary cannulae intermittently held in the ostia. Usually 200–300 ml of cardioplegic solution are infused initially for each square meter of body surface area and half this amount infused every 30–45 minutes during the aortic cross-clamp duration. The temperature of the ventricular septum is recorded and maintained below 20°C. Coronary perfusion is no longer in use at our institution. Attention to monitoring of the septal temperature seems particularly important where a valvular lesion coexists with a coronary narrowing requiring grafting as the potential for ischaemia is greater in this situation. This is also true of many reoperations where complete dissection of the heart from the pericardium is not safe and therefore topical hypothermia is ineffective. It is important to try to avoid long periods of ventricular fibrillation which seem to produce metabolic and ultrastructural myocardial disturbances[1, 15, 16, 26].

Towards the end of the procedure and before rewarming, venting of the left ventricle is instituted when this has not been previously necessary. In patients subjected to aortic valve replacement or in those with direct myocardial revascularization the vent is placed at the beginning of the procedure either through the right superior pulmonary vein and across the mitral valve or through the apex of the left ventricle. For venting through the superior pulmonary vein a Ferguson* cannula is employed. Due to its J-shaped tip it is guided more easily through the mitral valve towards the apex of the left ventricle. This shape is best maintained by stiffening the tube in cold saline. For an apical vent and for a vent through a mitral prosthesis a size 22 F cannula is used. If a vent is to be passed through the mitral valve towards the left ventricular apex an additional hole is cut in the cannula at about 10 cm from its tip in order to vent the left atrium simultaneously. This is also useful in removing air before discontinuation of the heart-lung bypass.

Towards the end of the operative procedure, rewarming is commenced. There are now data available relating the patient's body surface area to the

*'Argyle' Ferguson vena caval catheter, Sherwood Medical Industries Inc., St. Louis, Missouri, USA

time required for a Shiley heat exchanger to rewarm through a given temperature range (*see below*). Knowing the approximate duration of the final steps of the procedure, one is better able to decide when rewarming should commence – for instance following aortic valve replacement, rewarming is started as the aortotomy incision is being closed. No attempt is made to discontinue the heart-lung bypass until the oesophageal temperature has reached 36.5–37°C and acceptable blood gas and serum potassium values have been established.

A crucial step before discontinuing perfusion is the meticulous expulsion of air from the left cardiac chambers. This *must* be achieved before the heart starts ejecting. For mitral procedures the vent tube placed across the mitral valve prosthesis will keep the valve incompetent so that air in the ventricle can be expelled into the atrium. Before the left atrial suture line is completely closed, the anaesthetist inflates the lungs, draining blood and trapped air from the pulmonary veins into the left atrium. The left atrial suture line is held open by artery forceps while saline is infused into the atrium until it overflows and no more air bubbles are seen emerging. The left atrial suture line is then finally closed. This manoeuvre is helped by simultaneously and temporarily releasing the tourniquet from around the superior vena cava and allowing blood to enter the right and left side of the heart. The left ventricular vent is maintained on gravity drainage in order to prevent distension of the left ventricle. When the heart is full of blood the superior vena cava is snared again to prevent ejection of blood in the aorta. The heart is gently dislocated and a large-bore needle attached to a syringe is used to aspirate residual air from the apex of the left ventricle and from the roof of the left atrium. At this stage the aorta is unclamped but ejection prevented by temporarily increasing the perfusion flow to 3 ℓ/min per m^2. The coronary cannula previously used for the infusion of the cardioplegic solution into the aortic root is now connected to an open-heart suction line thus removing any air which may escape into the aorta. Both venae cavae are unsnared and on most occasions the heart will spontaneously resume contraction and left ventricular ejection will progressively increase as the perfusion flow is gradually reduced. If ventricular fibrillation is present the heart is electrically defibrillated and as soon as the first ejection occurs gentle pressure is applied with fingers to the anterior aspect of the ascending aorta to direct possible air towards the venting coronary cannula. Perfusion flow is gradually reduced allowing the heart to take over the circulation. After aortic valve replacement the procedure is similar. A vent through the mitral valve is already in position, the transverse aortotomy is closed from either end leaving a central gap sufficient to allow expulsion of air when the left heart is filled and starts ejecting. A vent needle is inserted into the convex aspect of the ascending aorta and the aortic incision gap finally closed with a mattress suture on Teflon pledgets. During coronary artery bypass graft surgery the risk of air embolism is considerably smaller as the left heart chambers are not opened. Exerting gentle suction, by gravity drainage on the vent tube placed in the apex of the left ventricle, appears to be, however, a precautionary method for such operations. When surgical procedures on the tricuspid valve are performed the heart is allowed to beat but it is decompressed by a vent tube.

Discontinuing the extracorporeal circulation

Once air is expelled from the heart and cardiac action is established, the left ventricular vent can be safely withdrawn into the atrium. The vent tube is used initially to monitor the left atrial pressure and soon it is removed and replaced by a percutaneous radiopaque 16 E-Z Cath* which is used to monitor the left atrial pressure in all cases both in the operating theatre and in the Intensive Care Unit. The E-Z catheter is inserted into the left atrium through the skin and through the thickness of the left atrial suture line. A mattress suture with large Teflon pledgets is tied around the catheter. With this technique significant bleeding following later removal of the catheter has not been encountered. (Only one reoperation for bleeding from the catheter site has been performed in more than 1500 patients.)

After discontinuing the heart-lung bypass, one venous line (from the superior vena cava) is clamped and removed. If the heart is able to maintain adequate systemic arterial pressure the contents of the oxygenator are gradually returned to the patient through the arterial cannula. The left atrial pressure is closely monitored and kept initially around its preoperative value. If the heart is unable to maintain an adequate circulation the cardiopulmonary bypass is promptly reinstituted, using high flow perfusion while blood gases, acid–base balance and potassium levels are reassessed. Arrhythmias may be a problem at this stage and these might respond to electrical pacing or to pharmacological treatment though they may resolve spontaneously. With this policy of early reinstitution of supportive perfusion very rarely one is forced into using inotropic drugs or balloon pumping for discontinuing bypass. While this is inevitably associated with the drawback of increased average perfusion time, the use of inotropic support has its own disadvantages in terms of increased myocardial oxygen demand at this critical time. Once the cardiovascular dynamics are stable the air vent needle from the aorta and the second venous cannula are removed and the oxygenator emptied while protamine sulphate is being injected. This must be given slowly to avoid rapid peripheral vasodilation producing a sudden fall in systemic arterial pressure. The aortic cannula is removed and haemostasis secured. Temporary atrial and ventricular epicardial pacemaker wires are inserted in every case as this has proved a valuable asset in the early postoperative management of many patients.

Materials and methods

Performance of the oxygenator and heat exchanger were assessed first in the laboratory and later during routine clinical use.

The oxygenator

Three each of the S-100 and S-100-A oxygenators were tested *in vitro*. Fresh bovine blood diluted with normal saline (Hb 11.9 g/100 ml, at a temperature

*Deseret Pharmaceutical Co. Inc., Sandy, Utah, USA

Table 6.3 Open-heart operations performed with the use of the S-100 and S-100-A Shiley disposable oxygenators

Surgical procedure	*Number of patients* *S-100*		*S-100-A*	
Aortic valve replacement		45		14
with: MVR	*6*			
Replacement of ascending aorta	*2*		*2*	
SVBG	*7*		*2*	
Mitral valve replacement		75		14
with: Tricuspid annuloplasty	*6*		*2*	
SVBG	*6*		*5*	
Repair of coronary to LA fistula	*1*			
Repair of ASD	*2*			
Mitral and aortic valve replacement		35		8
with: SVBG	*2*			
Tricuspid annuloplasty	*6*		*1*	
Closure of PDA			*1*	
Mitral and tricuspid valve replacement		5		2
Mitral, aortic and tricuspid valve replacement		5		
LV aneurysmectomy		15		
with: SVGB	*8*			
SVGB		33		6
Resection of HOCM		1		
Repair of ASD		9		
with: Anomalous pulmonary venous drainage	*3*			
Pulmonary infundibulectomy	*1*			
Repair of Fallot's tetralogy		2		1
TOTAL		225		45

MVR = mitral valve repair; SVBG = saphenous vein bypass graft; LA = left atrium; ASD = atrial septal defect; PDA = patent ductus arteriosus; HOCM = hypertrophic obstructive cardiomyopathy

of 37°C) was passed through the oxygenator at regulated rates of 2 to 6 ℓ/min. A gas mixture containing 97 per cent oxygen and 3 per cent carbon dioxide (premixed in a cylinder) was passed simultaneously through the gas inlet at the same flow rate, maintaining a gas flow/blood flow ratio of 1/1. The $P\text{O}_2$ and $P\text{CO}_2$ of the blood entering and leaving the oxygenator were measured and oxygen and carbon dioxide transfer rates in cc/min were calculated.

Clinical experience with the Shiley S-100 and S-100-A oxygenators at the Leeds General Infirmary currently refers to 360 patients (225 with S-100 and

135 with S-100-A). Data on the first 271 consecutive patients are reviewed, 225 were perfused with the Shiley S-100 and 46 with the S-100-A model. The surgical operations performed on these patients are outlined in *Table 6.3*.

During bypass the gas mixture used for all patients was 97 per cent oxygen and 3 per cent carbon dioxide, available in premixed cylinders, anaesthesia being maintained with 0.5 per cent Halothane. The gas mixture was maintained constant irrespective of the temperature. The gas flow was adjusted to maintain optimum PO_2 and PCO_2. For each patient the age, body surface area, total bypass time and postoperative blood loss at 6 and 24 hours were recorded. During each perfusion, blood flow and gas flow rates were recorded every 15 minutes and a mean gas flow/blood flow ratio calaculated. The following parameters were measured before perfusion, every 15 minutes during heart-lung bypass and after bypass: arterial PO_2, PCO_2, pH, non-respiratory pH, haemoglobin, haematocrit and platelet count. The blood gas and acid–base measurements were made using a Corning Model 165 pH blood gas analyser* and the values were corrected for temperature. The haematological data were obtained with a Coulter counter†. The free plasma haemoglobin was measured every 10 minutes during heart-lung bypass using the Cyanmethaemoglobin method and an SP 500 ultraviolet Spectrophotometer**[9].

The heat exchanger

In the laboratory three S-100 and three S-100-A oxygenators were tested. A schematic diagram of the heat exchanger test circuit is shown in *Figure 6.4*. Water was obtained direct from the mains and flow measurements were made with a calibrated flowmeter†† (11.6 ℓ/min). The water temperature was controlled by a heated water bath. Bovine blood (haematocrit 31 per cent) was circulated using a calibrated roller pump. The temperature of the blood entering the heat exchanger was maintained by an in-line cooler also connected to the mains water supply. Thermocouples were used to monitor the temperature of the water entering (T_{WI}) and leaving (T_{WO}) and of the blood entering (T_{BI}) and leaving (T_{BO}) the heat exchanger. Several measurements were made at each blood flow. These allowed the calculation of a performance factor[22] by substituting in the formula:

$$\text{Performance factor} = \frac{T_{BO} - T_{BI}}{T_{WI} - T_{BI}}$$

Such performance factors were obtained for each oxygenator tested at blood flow rates of 2 to 6 ℓ/min.

In the operating theatre an estimate of heat exchanger efficiency was obtained in 74 patients perfused with the S-100 and 46 patients perfused with

*Corning Scientific Instruments, Medfield, Massachusetts, USA
†Coulter Electronics Ltd., Harpenden, Hertfordshire, UK
**Unicam Ltd., Cambridge, UK
††G.E.C., Elliott Process Instruments Ltd., Rotameter Works, Croydon, UK

the S-100-A oxygenator. The time required for cooling to and rewarming from the minimum temperature recorded with an oesophageal Thermistore* was measured. The majority of patients were cooled to 29°C. Of the 46 patients perfused with the S-100-A, a group of 15 who underwent complex operations or multiple valve replacements were electively cooled to 26°C. Under operating conditions the temperature of the water entering the heat exchanger was regulated by a Thermocirculator†. The water flow provided by this unit was measured with a flow meter and was found to be consistently

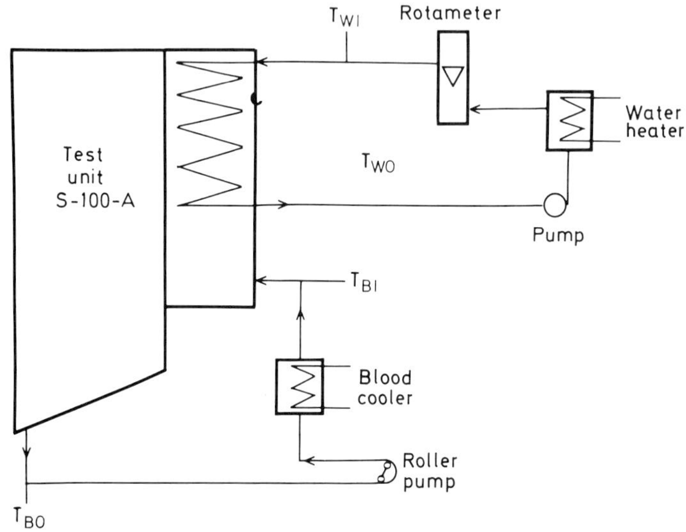

Figure 6.4 Schematic diagram of the experimental circuit for testing the heat exchanger. The temperatures in the circuit are measured by thermocouples. T_{WI} = water entering the heat exchanger; T_{WO} = water leaving the heat exchanger; T_{BI} = blood entering the oxygenator; T_{BO} = blood leaving the oxygenator. (Reproduced from Roesler, Bull and Ionescu[30] by courtesy of *The Journal of Cardiovascular Surgery*)

around 8 ℓ/min. During cooling the temperature of the water in the thermocirculator was held at least 10° lower than the minimum oesophageal temperature planned for that perfusion. During rewarming the temperature of the water in the heat exchanger never exceeded 42°C and the pressure was not allowed to rise above 250 mmHg.

In a further 46 patients perfused with the Shiley S-100-A model, measurements were obtained similar to those used to calculate the performance factor in the laboratory circuit. The temperature of the water passing in and out of the heat exchanger and the blood circulating in and out of the oxygenator were monitored using in-line Thermocouples** (*Figure*

*Yellow Springs Instrument Co., Yellow Springs, Ohio, USA
†Churchill Instrument Co. Ltd., Perivale, Middlesex, UK
**Elektro Laboratoriet, Ellab, A/S, Copenhagen, Denmark

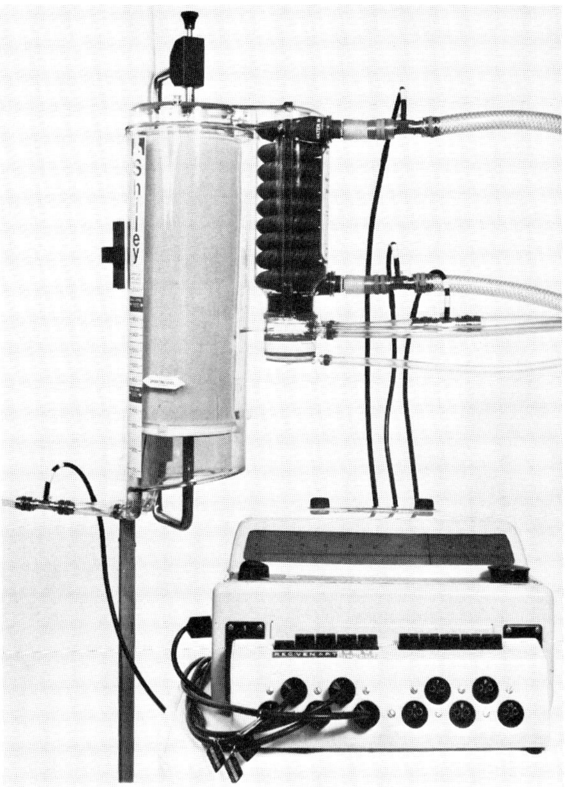

Figure 6.5 The position of the thermocouples for monitoring the temperature of the water and the blood at the entrance to, and exit from, the heat exchanger and the oxygenator, respectively

6.5). The oesophageal thermistore and the in-line thermocouples were calibrated against the same standards. No attempt was made to systematically vary the blood flow during perfusion. Measurements taken thus allowed calculation only of a mean '*in vivo*' performance factor using the same equation as above.

Results

The oxygenator

The findings of the *in vitro* studies of the gas exchange capability of the Shiley oxygenator are summarized in *Table 6.4*. At a blood and gas flow rate of 3 ℓ/min the oxygen transfer rate was 188 cc/min with a carbon dioxide transfer rate of 102 cc/min.

The clinical data from 271 patients perfused with the Shiley S-100 and S-100-A oxygenators are summarized in *Table 6.5* and the laboratory data in *Table 6.6*. The mean gas flow/blood flow ratio when using the Shiley S-100

Table 6.4 *In vitro* gas transfer for the Shiley S-100 and S-100-A bubble oxygenators at a gas flow to blood flow ratio of 1:1

Blood flow rate ℓ/min	*O_2 transfer rate cc/min*	*CO_2 transfer rate cc/min*
2	128	70
3	188	102
4	248	171
5	291	201
6	367	267

oxygenator was 0.87 (range 0.6–1.7) while with the Shiley S-100-A oxygenator it was 1.08 (range 0.4–1.2). For the Shiley S-100 model the mean arterial PO_2 ± standard error (SE) during perfusion was 192 ± 5.0 mmHg, the PCO_2 was 44 ± 0.4 mmHg and the pH 7.36 ± 0.003 while for the Shiley S-100-A model the figures were: PO_2 215 ± 6.8 mmHg, PCO_2 39 ± 0.8 mmHg and pH 7.39 ± 0.07. No difference was therefore demonstrated between the

Table 6.5 Clinical data from 225 patients perfused with the S-100 and from 46 patients perfused with the S-100-A Shiley disposable oxygenators

	S-100		*S-100-A*	
	Mean	*Range*	*Mean*	*Range*
Patient's BSA	1.69	1.29–2.3	1.72	1.38–2.4
Patient's age	48	15–69	49	15–64
Blood flow rate (ℓ/min)	3.9	2.8–5.5	3.8	3.1–5.3
Gas flow rate (ℓ/min)*	3.5	2.0–6.7	4.1	3.2–5.3
Gas flow/blood flow ratio	0.87	0.6–1.7	1.08	0.4–1.2
Bypass time (minutes)	96	27–285	110	42–194
Pump priming volume (ml)	1700		1700	
Postoperative blood loss (ml/m^2)				
at 6 hours	130		119	
at 24 hours	292		270	

BSA = body surface area
*Mixture containing a fixed proportion of 97 per cent O_2 and 3 per cent CO_2

performance of the S-100 and S-100-A models as far as gas transport was concerned.

The fall in platelet count was acceptable at around 30 per cent of the initial count. Free plasma haemoglobin per 60 minutes of heart-lung bypass was 26.2 ± 1.7 mg/100 ml for the Shiley S-100 and 21.5 ± 1.5 mg/100 ml for the S-100-A model. The postoperative blood loss was low[17] and only two patients from the entire series were reoperated upon for surgical bleeding.

The heat exchanger

Figure 6.6 shows the relationship between the performance factor and the blood flow for the two oxygenators tested in the laboratory circuit. The S-100-A with its anodized aluminium coil was superior to the S-100 model with polyurethane coated aluminium tubing. For example, at a blood flow rate of 4 ℓ/min the performance factor of the S-100-A was 0.50 ± 0.014 while for the S-100 it was 0.35 ± 0.017.

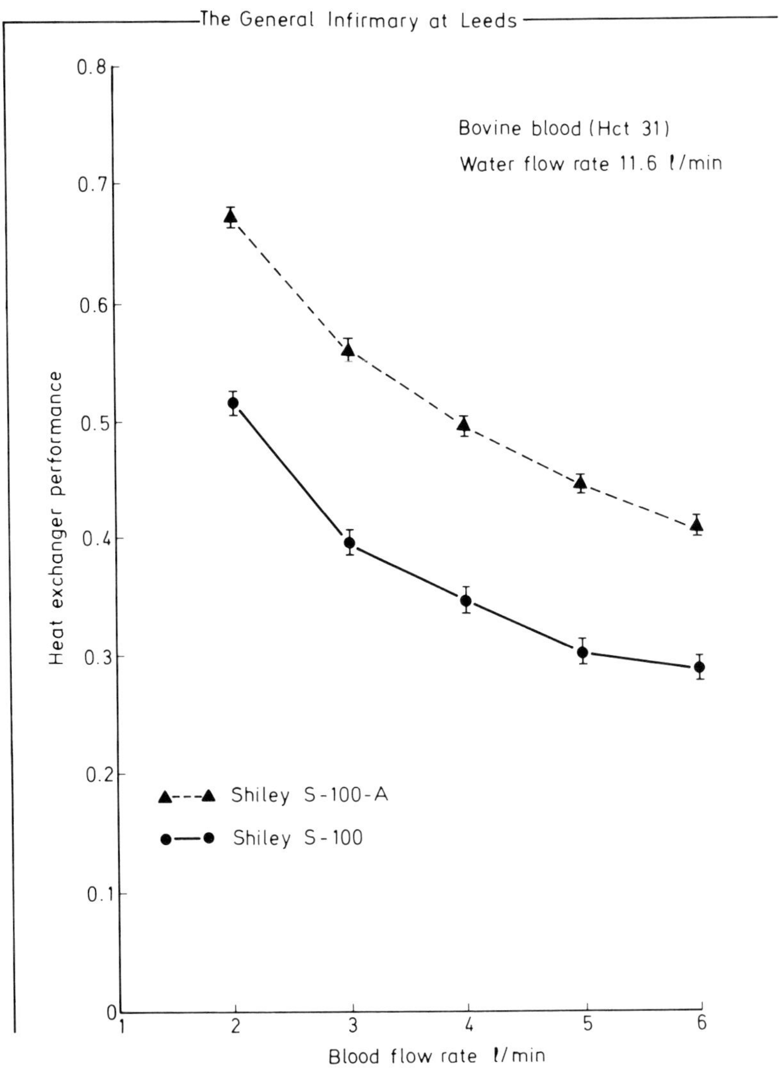

Figure 6.6 Graphic presentation of the relationship between heat exchanger performance factor and blood flow for the Shiley S-100 and S-100-A oxygenators. (Reproduced from Roesler, Bull and Ionescu[30] by courtesy of *The Journal of Cardiovascular Surgery*)

Table 6.6 Laboratory data from 225 patients perfused with the S-100 and 46 patients perfused with the S-100-A Shiley disposable oxygenators

	Shiley S-100 oxygenator						*Shiley S-100-A oxygenator*					
	Before bypass		*During bypass*		*After bypass*		*Before bypass*		*During bypass*		*After bypass*	
Laboratory parameters	*Mean*	*Standard error*	*Mean*	*Standard error*	*Mean*	*Standard error*	*Mean*	*Standard error*	*Mean*	*Standard error*	*Mean*	*Standard error*
P_{O_2} (mmHg)	150	±3.4	192	±5	150	±2.9	165	±8	215	±6.8	146	±4.2
P_{CO_2} (mmHg)	38	±0.5	44	±0.4	35	±0.2	38	±0.8	39	±0.8	34	±0.5
pH	7.36	±0.006	7.36	±0.003	7.36	±0.003	7.4	±0.2	7.39	±0.07	7.44	±0.01
Non-respiratory pH[18, 19]	7.38	±0.004	7.43	±0.003	7.40	±0.003	7.4	±0.01	7.39	±0.01	7.40	±0.01
Haematocrit (%)	39.4	±0.38	23.5	±0.29	31.3	±0.22	40	±0.71	23	±0.53	39	±0.35
Haemoglobin (g/d1)	13.8	±0.14	7.6	±0.09	12.7	±0.06	13.7	±0.3	8.1	±0.18	12.8	±0.12
Platelets ($\times 10^9/\ell$)	216	±4.1	100	±3.1	129	±2.3	201	±8.5	122	±2.54	141	±5.84
Free plasma haemoglobin (mg/100 ml per 60 min of bypass)			26.2	±1.7					21.5	±1.5		

Table 6.7 Performance of the heat exchanger incorporated in the Shiley disposable oxygenator

Number of patients			*Cooling time (min) from 36.5° to 29.6°C (range 26–30°C)*						*Rewarming time (min) from 29.6° (range 26–30°C) to 37°C*					
			Mean		*Range*		*Minutes per 1°C*		*Mean*		*Range*		*Minutes per 1°C*	
S-100	*S-100-A*	*Body surface area (m²)*	*S-100*	*S-100-A*	*S-100*	*S-100-A*	*S-100*	*S-100-A*	*S-100*	*S-100-A*	*S-100*	*S-100-A*	*S-100*	*S-100-A*
43	9	1.3 to 1.6	7	6.6	3–16	3–11	1.0	0.9	24	13	11–36	9–14	3.4	1.7
113	23	1.6 to 1.8	9.1	6.7	4–30	3–12	1.5	0.9	26	15	20–43	8–22	3.7	1.9
69	14	greater than 1.8	13.0	7.0	4–45	3–14	1.9	1.0	34	19	15–52	11–25	4.5	2.3

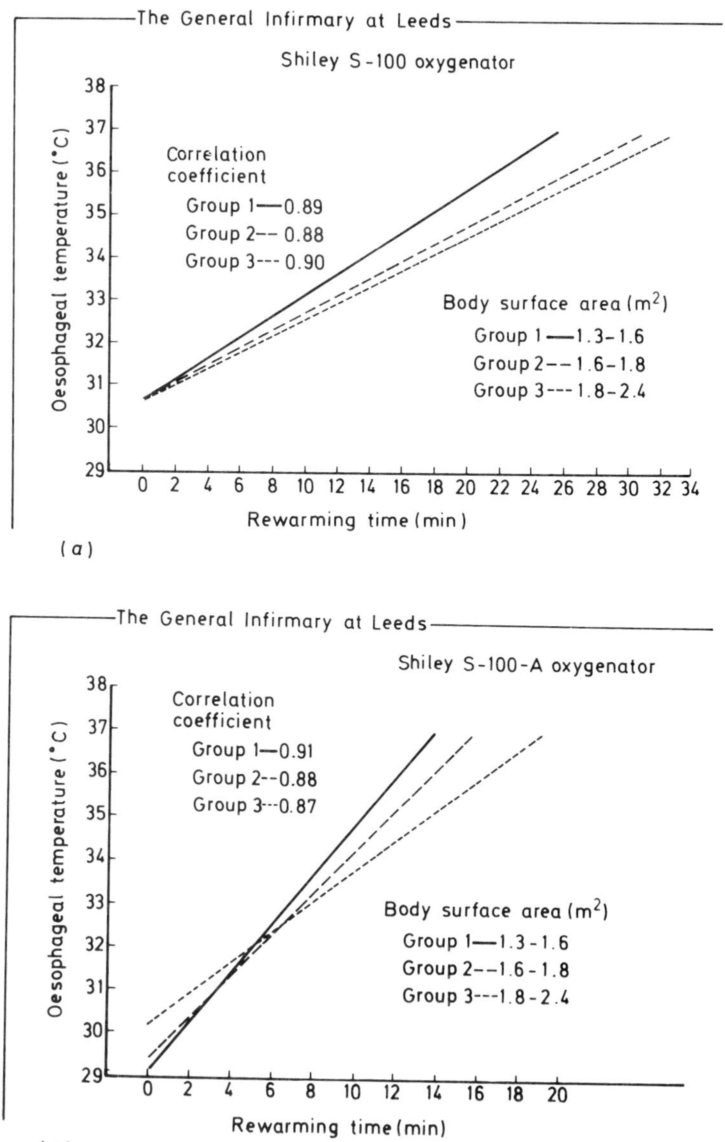

Figure 6.7 Rewarming times for (*a*) the Shiley S-100 and (*b*) the Shiley S-100-A oxygenators according to patient body surface area

Table 6.7 and *Figure 6.7* show the mean cooling and rewarming times from the temperatures of 36.5°C to 29.6°C and from 29.6°C to 37°C for the groups of patients perfused with the two oxygenator models. The results were subdivided according to the patient's body surface area. In practice, the time required for cooling and rewarming through this range for a patient of average build (1.6 – 1.8 m^2 body surface area BSA) was 9.1 and 26

Table 6.8 Performance of the heat exchanger incorporated in the Shiley S-100-A oxygenator. (Data from 15 patients)

Body surface area		*Cooling time (min) from 36.5° to 26°C*			*Rewarming time (min) from 26° to 37°C*		
Mean	*Range*	*Mean*	*Range*	*Minutes per 1°C*	*Mean*	*Range*	*Minutes per 1°C*
1.76	1.28–1.92	12.4	5–21	0.8	23	17–38	2.2

minutes for the S-100 model and 6.7 and 15 minutes, respectively, for the S-100-A model. In the group of 15 patients cooled to 26°C (mean BSA 1.76 m^2) the mean cooling and rewarming times were 12.4 and 23 minutes respectively (*Table 6.8*). All these data refer to a water flow rate through the heat exchanger of 8 ℓ/min.

Discussion

The oxygenator

The gas flow/blood flow ratios for both oxygenators could be maintained around 1. General studies have demonstrated that excessive gas flow and uncontrolled entry of oxygen into a column of blood creates turbulence, haemolysis and persistent gas microemboli[3, 21]. These may be responsible for a sequence of detrimental metabolic events[2, 6, 23, 34]. The Shiley oxygenator, however, is capable of efficient gas exchange at low gas flows relative to blood flows. This may be attributable to two factors concerned with the design of the oxygenator. Firstly, the gas passes through a diffuser which delivers bubbles of small diameter to the blood. In a bubble oxygenator the oxygen transfer efficiency is related to the size of the bubbles[13]. Secondly, after the gas and blood have passed through the porous sponge where most of the gas exchange occurs, they enter the rest of the oxygenating chamber where prolonged contact of blood with gas bubbles is probably enhanced by the helical shape and the presence of the fins of the heat exchanger coil. The duration of the contact of the gas bubble with the blood seems to be important in producing efficient gas transfer.

However, occasionally, unnecessarily high P_{O_2} values were encountered during perfusion suggesting that an even lower gas flow may have been sufficient. On the other hand, during rewarming P_{CO_2} tended to rise so that relatively high gas flow rates were required during this stage. It should be mentioned, however, that this increase in P_{CO_2} during rewarming was the consequence of using a gas mixture with a fixed proportion of 97 per cent oxygen and 3 per cent carbon dioxide. This implies that lower average gas flow/blood flow ratios could have been achieved if facilities for varying the concentrations of the gases in the mixture were available. More recently, separate cylinders of oxygen and carbon dioxide with finely calibrated gas flow meters have been used to generate a variable gas mixture for the oxygenator. Under these circumstances the gas flow/blood flow ratios averaged 0.8 (range 0.58–1).

Another important factor in assessing the safety of an oxygenator is the amount of trauma inflicted to blood constituents, particularly platelets and red cells. Platelet numbers were measured before, during and after perfusion and the degree of haemolysis estimated as the mean free plasma haemoglobin per 60 minutes of perfusion. These measures, however, represent a simplified view of the situation. Recent studies[12] indicate, for instance, that platelets are taken up in the spleen and liver during perfusion so that a decrease in platelet count does not necessarily reflect damage induced by the oxygenator. Red cell trauma might be better evaluated by a study using labelled red cells so that a formal estimate of their half-life as affected by perfusion could be obtained. A second possibility would be the measurement of the total free haemoglobin excreted through the kidney in, for instance, 24 hours from the start of perfusion. Preliminary studies were made in 30 patients using this method but the high urinary output consequent upon non-haemic prime diluted the free haemoglobin present so that its final concentration was usually below that required by the sensitivity of the assay method. For practical purposes the simple tests used provide sufficient data to allow comparison with other oxygenators.

The heat exchanger

There are two different approaches to the evaluation of a heat exchanger. Measurements of times required for cooling and rewarming a patient can be made. These are directly useful to the operating surgeon who must decide the stage of the procedure at which cooling and rewarming should start. However, cooling and rewarming times will depend on the type of patient. Therefore a measurement independent of the individual variables should be available.

Most of the heat exchangers employed in cardiac surgery consist basically of two conduits, one carrying blood and one carrying water with an interface between them. The temperature changes as the blood passes through the apparatus and is related to the temperature gradient across the blood-water interface. As this gradient will vary along the interface, its measurement must be made, in practice, at an arbitrary point. The temperature of water and blood at the inlet and outlet of the heat exchanger can be measured. The temperature change of the blood will be given by the temperature of the blood out minus the temperature of the blood in ($T_{BO} - T_{BI}$) and the initial temperature gradient across the blood-water interface will be given by the temperature of the water in minus the temperature of the blood in ($T_{WI} - T_{BI}$), from where the formula for the performance factor

$$= \frac{T_{BO} - T_{BI}}{T_{WI} - T_{BI}}$$

The performance factor defined in this way gives an assessment of the heat exchanger efficiency. Ideal heat exchange would be expressed as a performance factor of 1.0. The performance factor of a given heat exchanger varies with blood and water flow rates but it should be constant under constant conditions of use, thus providing a valuable means for comparison of various heat exchangers. However, as Bethune, Gill and Wheeldon[8] point out, variations in water flow may play a significant part in determining the performance of a heat exchanger. It would be desirable to establish the optimal water flow rate for a given heat exchanger.

The heat exchanger of the S-100-A model is efficient with cooling and rewarming times 30 to 50 per cent shorter than those of the previous S-100 model. In the absence of other modifications this improvement is due to the introduction of anodized aluminium tubing which is thinner and has a better thermal conductivity than polyurethane-coated aluminium. Both models incorporate a counter-current mechanism for water and blood flow. Accidental inversion of the water inlet and outlet connections giving concurrent water and blood flow reduces the heat exchanger performance up to 30 per cent[28]. An efficient heat exchanger is mandatory in modern cardiac surgery. For example, in the presence of uncontrolled bleeding, urgent reinstitution of bypass, rapid cooling and reduction of blood flow may allow retrieval of a life-threatening situation.

The cardiotomy reservoir

A cardiotomy reservoir serves two main functions; it acts as a defoamer and filter and also as a blood storage reservoir for the blood recovered by open-heat suckers and ventricular vent devices. This blood contains large proportions of air and debris. Air and fat microemboli, calcium and aggregates from the stored blood are detrimental to the brain and other organs[1, 10]. Most cardiotomy reservoirs contain a defoaming substance and filters to remove these emboli. However, they do not completely clear the blood of bubbles. This limitation is inherent in the design of many cardiotomy reservoirs. Any turbulence or frothing generated within the reservoir produces more microemboli and may prevent a proportion of blood from coming into contact with the defoaming substance. These problems have been thoroughly investigated by Pearson, Watson and Waterhouse[27] who suggested that improvements in the design and mode of use of cardiotomy reservoirs may reduce the number of gaseous microemboli in the effluent blood.

As the Shiley cardiotomy reservoir does not incorporate a filter a separate blood filter is interposed between the cardiotomy reservoir and oxygenator in our perfusion circuit. Recent studies have suggested that the filter placed in this position enhances bubble extraction better than if it is placed in the arterial line.

Modern micropore filters are of three kinds; depth filters, screen filters and combination filters. Blood passing through a depth filter comes into contact with a large surface area of foreign material which traps microaggregates by adhesion. Filtration through a screen-type filter is purely mechanical, microaggregates being trapped by sieving through a mesh of known pore size. Combination filters have been successfully used in extracorporeal circulation since 1970. However, reduction in platelet numbers following filtration has been consistently reported[4, 11]. Until recently a screen filter (Pall Ultipore) was used in our circuit. Filtration was effected by a mesh screen, pore size 40 μm. The passage of blood through this filter does not result in significant removal of platelets or alteration of other plasma constituents[5]. However, Litwin and Hurley[24] suggest that a filter pore size of 20 μm is optimal as this effectively removes 98 per cent of potentially harmful microaggregates. At present a combination-type filter (Johnson and Johnson Intercept) is used at our institution. Blood passed through an outer cloth screen (170 μm), a Dacron wool depth filter and finally a screen of nylon mesh (pore size 20 μm). This unit produces a significant reduction in the number of microaggregates in all size ranges[25].

Micropore filters are used in our unit not only in an extracorporeal circuit but also when large volumes of stored blood are transfused in order to prevent infusion of microaggregates which seem to play an important part in the pathophysiology of post-traumatic pulmonary insufficiency[29].

Conclusion

At the Leeds General Infirmary[30, 31] experience with the Shiley S-100 and S-100-A disposable oxygenators broadly confirms the preliminary studies of other groups [14, 32]. In particular, oxygenation of the blood and removal of carbon dioxide are adequate at low gas flow/blood flow ratios. Furthermore, the heat exchanger performance, particularly with the newer S-100-A model, is very satisfactory. No complications attributable to the oxygenator were encountered in a large series of patients subjected to open-heart surgery.

References

1. Aberg, T. 'Effect of open-heart surgery on intellectual function.' *Scandinavian Journal of Thoracic and Cardiovascular Surgery*, (Suppl.) p. 15 (1974)
2. Aberg, T. and Kihlgren, M. 'Cerebral protection during open-heart surgery.' *Thorax*, **32,** 525 (1977)
3. Anderson, M. N. and Kuahiba, K. 'Blood trauma produced by blood oxygenators: a comparative study of five different units.' *Journal of Thoracic and Cardiovascular Surgery*, **57,** 238 (1969)
4. Barrett, J., Dhurandhar, H. N., Miller, E. and Litwin, M. S. 'A comparison *in vivo* of Dacron wool (Swank) and Polyester mesh (Pall) micropore blood transfusion filters in the prevention of pulmonary microembolism associated with massive transfusion.' *Annals of Surgery*, **182,** 690 (1975)
5. Barrett, J., Miller, E. and Litwin, M. S. 'Filtration characteristics of Polyester mesh (Pall) micropore blood transfusion filter.' *Archives of Surgery*, **111,** 56 (1976)
6. Bartlett, R. H. and Gazzaniga, A. B. 'Physiology and pathophysiology of extracorporeal circulation.' In *Current Techniques in Extracorporeal Circulation*. Eds M. I. Ionescu and G. H. Wooler, pp. 1–44. London: Butterworths (1976)
7. Beall, A. C., Jr., Solis, R. T., Kakvan, M., Morris, G. C., Jr., Noon, G. P. and de Bakey, M. E. 'Clinical experience with the Teflon disposable membrane oxygenator.' *Annals of Thoracic Surgery*, **21,** 144 (1976)

8. Bethune, D. W., Gill, R. D. and Wheeldon, D. R. 'Performance of heat exchangers in whole body perfusion circuits.' *Thorax*, **30,** 569 (1975)
9. Blakney, G. B. and Dinwodie, A. J. 'A spectrophotometric scanning technique for the rapid determination of plasma haemoglobin.' *Clinical Biochemistry*, **8,** 96 (1975)
10. Branthwaite, M. A. 'Prevention of neurological damage during open-heart surgery.' *Thorax,* **30,** 258 (1975)
11. Buley, R. and Lumley, J. 'Some observations on blood microfilters.' *Annals of the Royal College of Surgeons of England*, **57,** 262 (1975)
12. de Leval, M., Hill, J. D., Mielke, H., Bramson, M. L., Smith, C. and Gerbode, F. 'Platelets kinetics during extracorporeal circulation.' *Transactions of the American Society for Artificial Internal Organs*, **18,** 355 (1972)
13. Hammond, G. L. and Bowley, W. W. 'Bubble mechanics and oxygen transfer.' *Journal of Thoracic and Cardiovascular Surgery*, **71,** 422 (1976)
14. Hartley, M. B. and Relley, W. B. 'A comparative study of two disposable oxygenators.' *AmSECT Proceedings, 15th International Conference*, **5,** 63 (1977)
15. Hottenrot, C. E., Maloney, J. V. and Buckberg, G. D. 'Studies of the effects of ventricular fibrillation on the adequacy of regional myocardial flow.' *Journal of Thoracic and Cardiovascular Surgery*, **68,** 615 (1974)
16. Hottenrot, C. E., Towers, B., Kurkji, H., Maloney, J. V. and Buckberg, G. D. 'The hazard of ventricular fibrillation in hypertrophied ventricles during cardiopulmonary bypass.' *Journal of Thoracic and Cardiovascular Surgery*, **66,** 742 (1973)
17. Ionescu, M. I., Tandon, A. P., Roesler, M. F. and Mary, D. A. S. 'Blood loss following extracorporeal circulation for heart valve surgery.' In *Techniques of Extracorporeal Circulation*, 2nd Edn. Ed. M. I. Ionescu, p. 345. London: Butterworths (1981)
18. Kappagoda, C. T., Deverall, P. B., Stoker, J. B., Panday, J. and Linden, R. J. 'Postoperative alkalaemia.' *Journal of Thoracic and Cardiovascular Surgery*, **66,** 305 (1973)
19. Kappagoda, C. T., Linden, R. J. and Snow, H. M. 'An approach to the problems of acid base balance.' *Clinical Science*, **39,** 169 (1970)
20. Karlson, K. E., Murphy, W. R., Kakvan, M., Antony, P., Cooper, G. M., Jr., Richardson, P. D. and Galletti, P. M. 'Total cardiopulmonary bypass with a new microporous Teflon membrane oxygenator.' *Surgery*, **76,** 935 (1974)
21. Kessler, J. and Patterson, R. H., Jr. 'The production of microemboli by various blood oxygenators.' *Annals of Thoracic Surgery*, **9,** 221 (1970)
22. Kreith, F., *Principles of Heat Transfer*, 2nd Edn. p. 497. Scranton: International Textbook Company (1968)
23. *Lancet*. Editorial. 'Brain damage after open heart surgery.' *Lancet*, **2,** 399 (1975)
24. Litwin, M. S. and Hurley, J. J. 'The filtration of blood'. In *Surgery Annual*, **10,** Ed. L. M. Nyhus. New York: Appleton-Century-Crofts (1978)
25. Marshall, B. E., Wurzel, H. A., Neufel, G. R. and Klinberg, P. L. 'Effects of intersept micropore filtration of blood on microaggregates and other constituents.' *Anaesthesiology*, **44,** 525 (1976)
26. Najafi, H., Henson, D., Dye, W. S., Javid, H., Hunter, J. A., Callagan, R., Eisenstein, R. and Julian, O. C. 'Left ventricular haemorrhagic necrosis.' *Annals of Thoracic Surgery*, **7,** 550 (1969)
27. Pearson, D. T., Watson, B. G. and Waterhouse, P. S. 'An ultrasonic analysis of the comparative efficiency of various cardiotomy reservoirs and micropore blood filters.' *Thorax*, **33,** 352 (1978)
28. Reed, C. C. and Clark, D. K. *Cardiopulmonary Perfusion*. Houston: Texas Medical Press, Inc. (1975)

29. Reul, G. J., Greenberg, S. D., Lefrak, E. A., McCollum, B. W., Beall, A. C., Jr. and Jordan, G. O. 'Prevention of post-traumatic pulmonary insufficiency.' *Archives of Surgery*, **106,** 386 (1973)
30. Roesler, M. F., Bull, C. and Ionescu, M. I. 'Clinical and laboratory evaluation of the Shiley S-100-A oxygenator heat exchanger.' *Journal of Cardiovascular Surgery*, **21,** 271 (1980)
31. Roesler, M. F., Bull, C. and Ionescu, M. I. 'Clinical experience with the Shiley S-100 disposable blood oxygenator.' *Journal of Extracorporeal Technology*, **10,** 180 (1978)
32. Sabatelli, P. 'Clinical experience with 100 Shiley S-100 oxygenators.' *AmSECT Proceedings*, **9,** 145 (1977)
33. Siderys, H., Herod, G. T., Halbrook, H., Pittman, J. N., Rubush, J., Kasebaker, V. and Berry, G. R. 'A comparison of membrane and bubble oxygenators as used in cardiopulmonary bypass in patients.' *Journal of Thoracic and Cardiovascular Surgery*, **69,** 708 (1975)
34. Solis, R. T., Kennedy, P. S., Beall, A. C., Jr., Noon, G. P. and DeBakey, M. E. 'Cardiopulmonary bypass – microembolization and platelets aggregation.' *Circulation*, **52,** 103 (1975)
35. Subramanian, V. A. and Berger, R. L. 'Comparative evaluation of a new disposable rotating membrane oxygenator with bubble oxygenator.' *Annals of Thoracic Surgery*, **21,** 48 (1976)

7

Cardiotomy Reservoirs and Blood Filters

Derek T. Pearson

finem respice

Introduction

Several investigators have described the deleterious effects resulting from the functional replacement of the heart and lungs by a pump oxygenator during open-heart surgery[1, 2, 3, 14, 15, 16]. The brain would appear to be particularly susceptible to damage in this context. Many reports indicate the wide variety of disturbances in cerebral function ranging from mild delirium and psychosis to overt focal and diffuse neurological deficits[14, 39, 70] which can nullify the benefits of open-heart surgery.

As well as disturbances produced by systemic arterial hypotension[13, 32, 70], reduction in cerebral blood flow[12] and non-pulsatile perfusion flow[54, 72], the incidence of neurological dysfunction is increased if the patient is over 50-years-old and the duration of heart-lung bypass exceeds 120 minutes[32, 70].

The significance of microemboli in the production of an alteration in cerebral physiology is well documented[4, 36, 50, 62]. Emboli of fat[19, 24], calcium[8], antifoam[20], denatured proteins[38] and aggregated blood elements[48] have been implicated in the causation of the widespread organ dysfunction which may follow open-heart surgery. Gaseous microemboli originating from the heart, pulmonary veins and pump oxygenator system can also cause alterations in myocardial and cerebral physiology during cardiac surgery[25, 27, 28, 37, 64]. *Table 7.1* summarizes the more important

Table 7.1 Cerebral dysfunction during open-heart surgery. Aetiological factors

A. Haemodynamic		
Age of patient		
Duration of heat-lung bypass		
Systemic arterial pressure during heart-lung bypass		
Cerebral blood flow during heart-lung bypass		
Pulsatile versus non-pulsatile flow		
B. Embolic		
Gaseous microemboli from	(i)	heart and pulmonary veins
	(ii)	pump oxygenator
Foreign material from	(i)	oxygenator (cotton fibres, silicone, plastic chips)
	(ii)	pump (spallation of pump tubing)
	(iii)	operative equipment (talcum powder, thread, dust, cloth particles)
Red cell, platelet and leucocyte aggregates		
Fibrin		
Calcium and arteriosclerotic debris		
Denatured proteins		
Fat globules		

aetiological factors involved in the production of neurological dysfunction following open-heart surgery.

Improvement in pump oxygenator design, perfusion techniques and management of haemodynamic parameters during cardiopulmonary bypass can reduce the number of microemboli entering the systemic arterial circulation and may result in a reduction in morbidity and mortality following open-heart surgery[15, 27, 34, 57].

Gaseous microemboli occurring during open-heart surgery

Gaseous microemboli originating from the pump oxygenator system during cardiopulmonary bypass have been described by Selman, McAlpine and Ratan[55] who used a transparent chamber in the arterial line and with the aid of magnification were able to detect these microemboli. Following a preliminary report by Austen and Howry in 1965[7] describing the use of ultrasound to detect bubbles and particulate matter, many other workers have used this technique[27, 40, 50, 63] to define the various sources of gaseous microemboli and relate events during perfusion to their production. The use

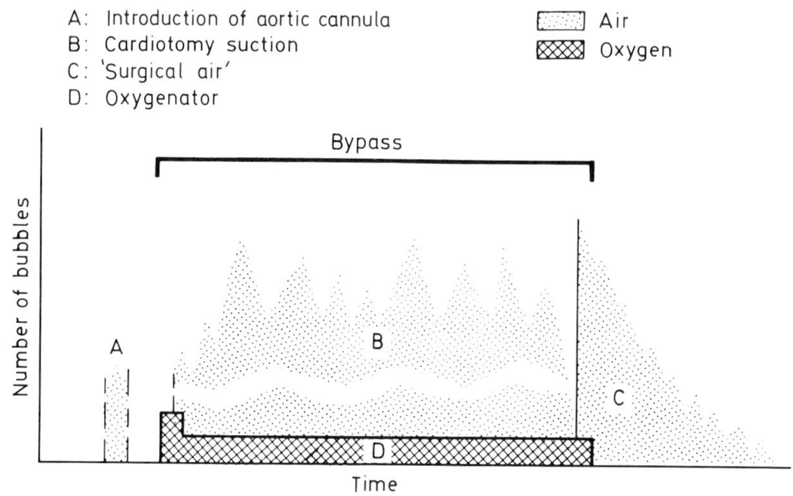

Figure 7.1 Schematic diagram indicating the source and type of gaseous microemboli entering the systemic arterial circulation during open-heart surgery

of an ultrasonic transducer placed over the carotid artery during open-heart surgery[27] has shown that gaseous microemboli were released into the systemic arterial circulation following recognizable surgical manoeuvres and from the pump oxygenator. The number of gaseous microemboli related to various events during the operation is shown schematically in *Figure 7.1*.

Cannulation of the heart

Cannulation of the ascending aorta may admit gaseous microemboli into the systemic circulation as may insertion of the caval cannulae through the right atrial wall in the presence of an intracardiac septal defect even when there is a left-to-right shunt.

Gaseous microemboli from the oxygenator

It is well recognized that the oxygenator is a potent source of gaseous microemboli[27, 40]. Before institution of cardiopulmonary bypass the pump oxygenator system is primed with fluid which is recirculated through a 'ductus loop'. Bethune[10] has suggested that when the priming fluid is incorporated within the patient at the start of heart-lung bypass, the pressure difference between free and dissolved gases in the circulating blood will favour the growth of any gaseous microemboli originating from the prime, particularly if nitrous oxide is utilized as an inhalational anaesthetic up to the time perfusion begins. Nitrous oxide, being a highly soluble gas, will tend to come out of solution in the blood and cause an enlargement of the gaseous microemboli of air and oxygen introduced from the oxygenator until equilibrium is reached between the nitrous oxide remaining in solution in the blood and that in the bubbles. Injected microemboli will thus increase in size. To prevent this complication it has been recommended that the bypass circuit should be flushed with carbon dioxide, which is a highly soluble gas, before priming with warmed fluids. Recirculation of the priming fluid should take place without introduction of gas into the oxygenator. Nitrous oxide should be discontinued ten minutes prior to the institution of perfusion thus allowing most of the nitrous oxide to be eliminated via the lungs. The number of gaseous microemboli originating from the oxygenator is usually high at the beginning of perfusion, decreasing rapidly with time[21], but the numbers could be reduced by applying the techniques described above.

Improvements in the design of bubble oxygenators leading to a reduction in oxygen flow/blood flow ratios has diminished the number of gaseous microemboli remaining in the blood following oxygenation and defoaming[58]. However, the number of gaseous microemboli originating from several different types of oxygenator have produced confusing results[35, 55, 58, 61], presumably due to the differences in monitoring techniques. Although it is recognized that the techniques currently available do not quantify the precise number of microemboli, they do, however, provide an accurate sample[40, 50]. Consequently it is difficult to compare studies originating from different cardiac surgical centres. Factors which increase the number of gaseous microemboli originating from bubble oxygenators[27, 40] include:

(1) A high oxygen flow to blood flow ratio.
(2) A low level of blood in the oxygenator.
(3) Agitation of the oxygenator during perfusion.
(4) Splashing within the oxygenator.
(5) Addition of cold fluids to the oxygenator.

The production of gaseous microemboli by disc oxygenators has been described by Gallaher and Pearson in 1973[27]. Increasing the rate of disc rotation and maintaining a high level of blood in the oxygenator are factors which increase the number of gaseous microemboli in the perfusion fluid. The close spacing of the discs in the oxygenator was also related to the production of gaseous microemboli. The membrane oxygenator, having no blood to gas interface or defoamer, is claimed to produce less gaseous microemboli than bubble oxygenators[34, 61]. If gaseous microemboli are introduced into the oxygenator from the cardiotomy suction system, by entrainment of air at the venous cannulae or by infusion of cold fluids, these emboli will pass into the arterial line of the heart-lung machine.

Numerous gaseous microemboli are well tolerated by the majority of patients. Respiratory and neurological dysfunction are rarely found in the spectrum of complications following open-heart surgery, yet when present they can be related both to the length of perfusion and to the patient's age[40]. Nevertheless, the conduct of the perfusion, the choice of an oxygenator, as well as the knowledge and control of the factors which may cause gaseous microemboli production can influence the outcome of the surgical procedure.

Heat exchanger

It has been demonstrated *in vitro* and inferred that also during clinical perfusions a significant increase in the number of gaseous microemboli may be caused by a temperature gradient of more than 10°C between the water inflow to the heat exchanger and the circulating blood during the rewarming phase of perfusion[21]. It is, therefore, important to maintain as low a temperature gradient as possible, commensurate with the rate of rise of the patient's temperature. Too rapid cooling of the blood using a heat exchanger has been identified as a cause of cerebral damage in children[11] though this cannot be attributed to gaseous microemboli.

Blood pumps

It has been demonstrated by Bass and Longmore[9] that negative pressures which develop behind each pump roller are potentially capable of inducing microbubble formation by the phenomenon of cavitation.

Cardiotomy suction

During cardiopulmonary bypass, the venous blood is drained into the pump oxygenator, arterialized, and returned to the systemic arterial circulation. Since both venae cavae can be cannulated separately through the right atrium, it is possible to withdraw the entire systemic venous blood, by gravity, into the oxygenator even when the right side of the heart is opened, provided that tourniquets are applied around the caval cannulae. In operations on the left side of the heart a single cannula placed in the right atrium for venous drainage will suffice. In this situation, as well as when both venae cavae are cannulated but not occluded by tourniquets, the venous blood returning directly to the right heart cavities (including that from the coronary sinus, the anterior coronary veins and Thebesian vessels) will be included in the venous drainage to the oxygenator.

If no cardiotomy suction is performed, any blood entering the right atrium which does not drain via the venous cannulae fills the right ventricle, is ejected into the pulmonary vascular bed and returns to the left heart to be pumped into the aorta. However, if the heart is arrested and no ejection is possible, acute cardiac dilatation and flooding of the pulmonary circulation with pulmonary oedema will occur. Total cardiopulmonary bypass and a dry operative field require the removal of coronary sinus blood by suction through the right atrial or ventricular cardiotomy or by vents placed in the left atrium or left ventricle. The bronchial venous blood returning to the left atrium creates similar problems. When the heart is arrested and there are no cardiac septal defects to allow the blood to drain into the right heart, pulmonary and cardiac damage will occur if venting of this blood does not take place.

Under normal circulatory conditions coronary and bronchial blood flow amount to approximately 10 per cent of the cardiac output. The collateral circulation through the lungs may be increased in cardiac disease and some 20 to 50 per cent of the output from the pump oxygenator may pass through systemic to pulmonary anastomoses in patients with cyanotic congenital heart disease. This situation is similar to that created by the presence of either a patent ductus arteriosus or the surgically-produced systemic-to-pulmonary-artery shunts when, during cardiopulmonary bypass, the heart and lungs are flooded with blood at systemic arterial pressure.

A patent ductus arteriosus or an artificially-produced anastomosis must be ligated or clamped during perfusion, and a left-sided superior vena cava clamped or preferably drained by a separate cannula. Any distension of the left ventricle due to aortic incompetence can be prevented by cross-clamping the aorta or by decompressing the left ventricle with a vent tube.

The intracardiac blood from collateral anastomoses often cannot be reduced during euthermic clinical perfusions. Under such circumstances the total amount of blood returning to the heart (coronary sinus and bronchial flow) exceeds 10 per cent of the cardiac output.

It is essential that any cardiotomy drainage system should be capable of coping with large volumes of blood aspirated from the cardiac chambers. Furthermore, it is necessary to compensate for the blood diverted via cardiotomy suction with a comparable increase in output from the pump oxygenator. Myocardial contractility must be sufficiently well preserved to ensure that the heart does not distend prior to the institution of cardiotomy suction and left ventricular decompression or following their withdrawal.

When gravity systemic venous drainage is inadequate or when there is a need for a considerable aspiration of blood from the open heart, this blood will necessarily be mixed with air. An efficient and safe cardiotomy suction system should, therefore, have the following capabilities[42]:

(1) Large storage capacity.
(2) Minimal degree of suction to avoid blood trauma.
(3) Minimal admixture of air.
(4) Reliable defoaming capacity.

It is now considered that a wide variety of microemboli can be returned to the oxygenating system and therefore the incorporation of a filter in the cardiotomy reservoir is advantageous[52, 63].

Several authors have identified cardiotomy suction as a potent source of particulate[21,61] and gaseous microemboli[27, 40, 52, 63]. Various cardiotomy reservoirs have been designed to incorporate filters and defoaming chambers in an attempt to remove these microemboli. The bubbles created by suction are qualitatively different from those generated in the oxygenator as they consist mainly of nitrogen, a relatively insoluble gas. The admission to a bubble oxygenator of a volume of blood, collected over a short period of time from a cardiotomy reservoir, results, after a certain time delay (sufficient to allow the blood to traverse the oxygenator), in an increase in

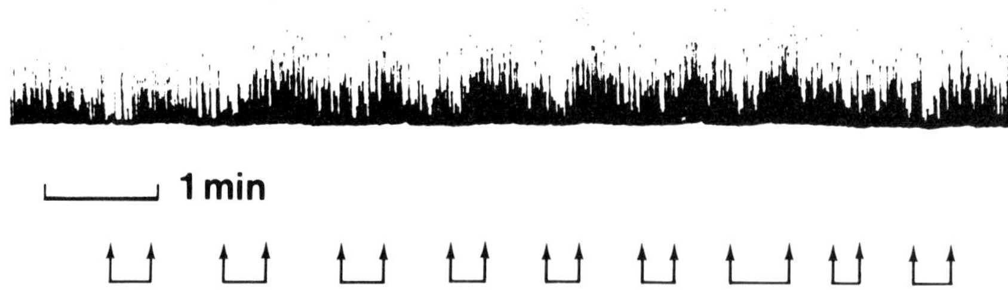

Figure 7.2 Phasic changes in ultrasonic echoes attributable to gaseous microemboli detected in the arterial line from the oxygenator following intermittent admission of cardiotomy suction blood from the cardiotomy reservoir

the number of gaseous microemboli detected in the arterial line (*Figure 7.2*). The persistence of these microemboli, after passage through both the defoamer in the cardiotomy reservoir and in the oxygenator, indicates their stability.

Recent work at our institution[52] has enabled a comparison to be made of the efficiency of various commercially-available cardiotomy reservoirs and micropore blood filters used to remove gaseous microemboli from the coronary suction blood, and to define perfusion techniques which influence the performance of the reservoirs and minimize the gaseous microemboli load to the patient. These will be described later in the chapter.

Surgical air

Cross-clamping of the aorta is used during open-heart surgery in the presence of aortic incompetence of a degree which hinders technically the replacement of the mitral valve. It may also be used to provide maximal visibility and relaxation of the heart during intracardiac repair of various abnormalities. Cross-clamping of the aorta is an absolute prerequisite for surgical operations on the aortic valve. Aortic clamping may be associated with the infusion of cardioplegic solution either directly into the coronary arteries or into the aortic root. Air can collect between the aortic clamp and the aortic valve, and even when the root of the aorta is vented either through the aortic suture line or by aspiration using a wide-bore needle, gaseous microemboli may enter the systemic arterial circulation when the cross-clamp is removed.

Following cardiotomy for the repair of a septal defect or during exposure of the left-side heart valves, cardiac ejection is prevented until the heart is filled with blood, air pockets are displaced and bubbles trapped in muscular traveculae are finally removed. Many techniques have been described to avoid the potential hazards of systemic air embolism during open-heart surgery. The use of a drain attached to suction, inserted through a stab wound in the apex of the left ventricle[41], may be combined with induced ventricular fibrillation[47, 56], flooding of the operative field with carbon dioxide[18, 46] and aspiration of the pulmonary veins and cardiac chambers with a needle[69], all in an attempt to reduce air embolism. Vents can be placed into the left side of the heart via the right superior pulmonary vein and air removed from the aorta using a wide-bore needle either draining freely in the pericardial sac or attached to controlled suction. None of these techniques has completely eliminated the incidence of air embolism[27] and further studies are needed to assess the relevance of surgical air in the development of postoperative cerebral complications.

Using intracardiac cinephotography[69] it has been demonstrated that air retained by gravity and trapped by anatomical intracardiac structures is nearly all removed by the commonly-used aortic and ventricular vents, but several small bubbles remain firmly attached to the endocardial surface. This may explain the findings[27] that gaseous microemboli can be detected on occasions for periods of up to one hour in the carotid artery after resumption of effective cardiac action following the end of cardiopulmonary bypass. Some of these emboli may originate in the pulmonary veins[49] and it is important that pulmonary veins are cleared of air when the left side of the heart has been opened.

Particulate microemboli occurring during open-heart surgery

There have been extensive investigations of the effects of mechanical pumping and artificial oxygenation on blood constituents. Haemolysis, thrombocytopenia, hypofibrinogenaemia and aggregation of red blood cells with denaturation of plasma proteins are related to the blood-surface and blood-gas interactions in the pump oxygenator circuit. Mechanical trauma induced by the compression effects of the pumps on the blood is potentiated by turbulence induced at connections, during oxygenation and following cardiotomy suction. It is also recognized that during cardiopulmonary bypass considerable quantities of foreign material are released into the pump oxygenator and operative field and may eventually be injected into the patient via the arterial cannula.

Particulate contamination from pump oxygenators

The degree of particulate contamination from seven commercially available types of bubble oxygenator in common use has been evaluated. The recirculation of the priming solution through a filter with a pore size of 5 microns has resulted in the removal of large quantities of particulate matter mainly consisting of fibres but also plastic chips and unidentifiable material. By adopting a washing and micropore filtration technique during the preparation of the pump oxygenator, Reed and his colleagues[53] have reported a significant reduction in the incidence of neurological complications following open-heart surgery.

An additional source of particulate emboli has been identified in relation to spallation of plastic tubing particles into the lumen of the conduits of the pump oxygenator by the erosive and fatiguing action of the rollers in the pump head[31]. The number and size of the particles generated by this means varies according to the type and batch of the tubing used, and the degree of occlusion and speed of the roller pumps.

Extracorporeal oxygenation for open-heart surgery involves the use of an antifoaming agent in the bubble oxygenator and cardiotomy reservoir to remove bubbles from the blood following oxygenation or cardiotomy suction. The substance in general use is a silicone, dimethyl polysiloxane[20]. Recent work[71] has confirmed the extensive literature concerning the release of droplets of silicone into the blood from the oxygenator during open-heart surgery, and described the presence of silicone in the brain and kidneys of patients who did not survive the operative procedure.

Oxygen utilized in cardiopulmonary bypass comes into intimate contact with the blood during bubble oxygenation. This gas contains viable bacterial contaminants[43] which can be removed by a gas line filter with a pore size of 0.2 microns.

Donor blood

It is well established that donor blood contains particulate microemboli[44, 73]. Debris accumulates in the blood in an amount and at a rate dependent upon duration of storage and type of anticoagulant used[67]. Such debris consists of intact and fragmented red cells, leucocyte and platelet aggregates, fibrin and denatured proteins. These microemboli are not removed by the standard filter supplied with blood-administration sets and are known to cause blockage of the pulmonary capillary bed as described during massive intravenous transfusion of blood to patients treated for shock[32, 45]. Donor blood added to the priming fluid or infused during cardiopulmonary bypass is not filtered in the lungs but enters the systemic arterial circulation directly, and there is good evidence that the particulate emboli in the donor blood can affect cerebral function[51].

Pump oxygenator

The oxygenator can induce the formation of leucocyte and platelet aggregates[5, 22, 23] due to the presence of blood-surface and blood-gas interfaces and the admixture of donor and patient blood[6, 26]. The number of platelet aggregates is reduced by the use of membrane oxygenation[23, 65]. Other factors which cause platelet and leucocyte aggregates within the pump oxygenator system include contact of the blood with foreign surfaces[68], systemic arterial hypotension[66], and the release of substances from haemolysed red cells which promote aggregation[4, 38]. Blood trauma can lead to denaturation of plasma proteins[38] with an increase in circulating lipids[19] and this in turn augments the microemboli load to the patient.

Cardiotomy suction

A large part of the red cell destruction which occurs during cardiopulmonary bypass is the result of mechanical trauma and turbulence induced by cardiotomy suction and it is well documented that aspiration of blood from the pericardium and intracardiac chambers causes microaggregation of the formed blood elements[48, 60]. Blood returning to the cardiotomy reservoir may also contain fibrin, calcium from calcified heart valves, talcum powder, dust, particles of thread and cloth and even hair[2].

Extracorporeal micropore blood filters

There are two basic types of filter, a screen filter composed of Dacron or nylon mesh where filtration depends upon the pore size of the mesh, and depth filters, composed of polyurethane foam, nylon, glass wool or Dacron wool. In this second type filtration depends upon adsorption of particulate matter.

Filters have been used during cardiopulmonary bypass in the following locations:

(1) Between the cardiotomy reservoir and the oxygenator. A filter in this position would need to extract foreign material aspirated from the heart and pericardium, remove a large quantity of aggregates and gaseous microemboli generated by coronary suction and should also have a low resistance to flow to enable the filtered blood to pass under gravity into the oxygenator.

(2) In the arterial line between the pump and the patient. This filter needs to be easily primed, made bubble-free and made to function at blood flow rates up to 6 ℓ/min without producing haemolysis. The pressure gradient across the filter should always be monitored during perfusion and a bypass line included in the circuit to circumvent the filter if it becomes occluded.

(3) In the venous line between the patient and the oxygenator. Filters in this location require characteristics similar to arterial line filter.

(4) In the transfusion line to a peripheral vein of the patient to filter stored blood or blood from the oxygenator transfused at the end of the heart-lung bypass.

    Transfusion filters should have a high filtering capacity, be of low priming volume and have a low resistance to blood flow.

The effectiveness of micropore arterial line filtration using continuous microembolic monitoring by ultrasound has been performed by Loop and his colleagues[40]. All the commercially available filters tested decreased the number of microemboli passing to the patient in the arterial line. It was found that a 20 micron woven mesh nylon filter, as well as a Dacron wool filter has, in this respect, a filtration efficiency greater than 90 per cent. The authors could not detect any alteration in leucocytes, platelets and plasma haemoglobin values beyond the limits normally encountered during perfusion without filtration. None of the filters tested showed an unacceptably high pressure gradient during cardiopulmonary bypass.

Using electronic particle size analysis, Solis and his colleagues[63] have demonstrated that none of the six commercially available cardiotomy reservoirs that were tested was effective in removing a significant number of microemboli smaller than 32 microns in the blood presented to them. There was considerable variation in the ability of the reservoirs to filter particles larger than 32 microns. To improve the filtration efficiency of the reservoirs, four in-line blood filters were installed beyond the reservoirs. The results indicated that all the filters removed a significant volume of microemboli greater than 32 microns but that the filters varied in their ability to remove microemboli below 32 microns. The Dacron wool and woven filters were the most effective in the removal of particles in the large and small size range.

Concern has been expressed that micropore blood filtration could remove or damage useful blood elements. An ideal filter should be capable of elimination of aggregates of damaged or non-functional cells, leaving normally-functioning platelets, red cells and leucocytes to pass through the filter medium. Skagseth and his associates[59] have not observed increases in postoperative bleeding in patients treated with micropore filters in the pump oxygenator circuit. A review of the literature suggests that these devices should be an integral part of the extracorporeal circuit[29]. Although it would be expected that the use of both cardiotomy and arterial line filters would provide more complete filtration of microemboli, it has been shown that arterial line filtration is not enhanced by the presence of filters in the cardiotomy circuit[40]. However, extra protection against microemboli entering the systemic arterial circulation can be obtained by the addition of a cardiotomy filter in those operations involving increased open-heart suction such as valve replacement, intracardiac correction of complex congenital heart disease and aortic aneurysmectomy.

During the last few years extracorporeal blood filtration has gained importance and is increasing in popularity. The use of micropore filtration can reduce the gaseous and particulate microembolic load to the patient during open-heart surgery and has now been reported to produce a significant decrease in patient morbidity and mortality[1, 14, 40, 48], particularly in patients over 65 years of age[55]. However, it is worthy of note that not all investigators are convinced of the need for arterial line filtration during cardiopulmonary bypass. Some surgeons still rely only on the filtration provided by the material surrounding the defoamer in bubble oxygenators. Heimbecker, Robert and McKenzie[30] have demonstrated that an arterial line micropore filter can be a grave source of platelet and fibrin destruction due to excessive turbulence and high frequency vibration of the filter mesh induced by the high blood velocity through the filter. This phenomenon did not occur when the filter was placed below the cardiotomy reservoir and subject to a lower blood flow rate. The authors conclude that whilst the filter in the arterial line is beneficial during recirculation of the priming fluid of the oxygenator it should be removed prior to cardiopulmonary bypass. In the patients investigated there was an improvement in platelet counts and a reduction in postoperative chest drainage when an arterial line filter was not used and it was presumed that this was due to the elimination of a degree of consumptive coagulopathy. Neurological changes did not occur in the absence of an arterial line filter. Much of the published work on arterial line filtration does not include details of the monitoring of heparin therapy. Many of the established protocols for heparin and protamine administration during extracorporeal circulation are inadequate and it has been considered that if the possibility of disseminated intravascular coagulation is to be confidently excluded then an adequate programme of monitoring heparin therapy and its protamine neutralization is essential. It is well documented that there is a threefold variation in sensitivity to heparin in patients who have open-heart surgery and that the variability of the heparin decay rate can show a range of from less than 1 hour to 4 hours[17].

The analysis of the comparative efficiency of various cardiotomy reservoirs and blood filters in the removal of gaseous microemboli

Reference has already been made to the need during open-heart surgery to aspirate large volumes of blood from the cardiac chambers, both during the surgical procedure and prior to the termination of cardiopulmonary bypass when the heart is vented, in order to remove the 'surgical' air. This blood contains large quantities of nitrogen microemboli as well as cellular aggregates and particulate matter. It has been demonstrated that commercially available cardiotomy reservoirs do not completely remove all the bubbles from the blood presented to them and that when the cardiotomy suction blood is returned to the oxygenator, the number of gaseous microemboli passing along the arterial line is increased[27, 40]. An *in vitro* analysis of the efficiency of various cardiotomy reservoirs and filters has been performed[52].

Method

An *in vitro* cardiopulmonary bypass circuit was constructed as shown in *Figure 7.3*. The main circuit consisted of a polycarbonate disc oxygenator with the arterial and venous connections joined by a loop of ⅜ inch diameter polyvinyl chloride tubing. The circuit was primed with heparinized acid-citrate-dextrose blood, which was then circulated at a constant flow rate of 2.5 ℓ/min by a double arm, non-pulsatile, roller pump (pump A). The temperature of the blood was maintained at 37°C by a heat exchanger. The detector head of the TM8 Microbubble Activity Monitor* was applied to the external surface of the circuit tubing. A continuous narrow beam of ultrasound was propagated by the transducer into the blood passing through the tubing, and as gaseous microemboli passed this beam the receiving transducer picked up modifications in the signal, which were processed by an electronic unit. The bubble counts were presented by a digital display in the size range selected on the sensitivity control. This detector position in the arterial line was used to compare the efficiency in removing microbubbles of the micropore filter in the cardiotomy return line and the micropore filter in the arterial line.

The blood was circulated without rotation of the discs in the oxygenator until the main circuit was free of gaseous microemboli. Blood was then pumped at 0.5 ℓ/min from the main circuit to the base of an open-ended jar by pump B. At the same time blood and air were aspirated from the jar by pump C, whose flow rate could be adjusted to vary the proportion of blood and air. This mixture simulating cardiotomy suction was discharged into the cardiotomy reservoir under investigation.

When a suitable volume of blood had collected in the cardiotomy reservoir it was returned to the main circuit either directly or through a

*Technique Laboratories, 1 High Street, Hartley Wintney, Hampshire, RG27 8PE, UK

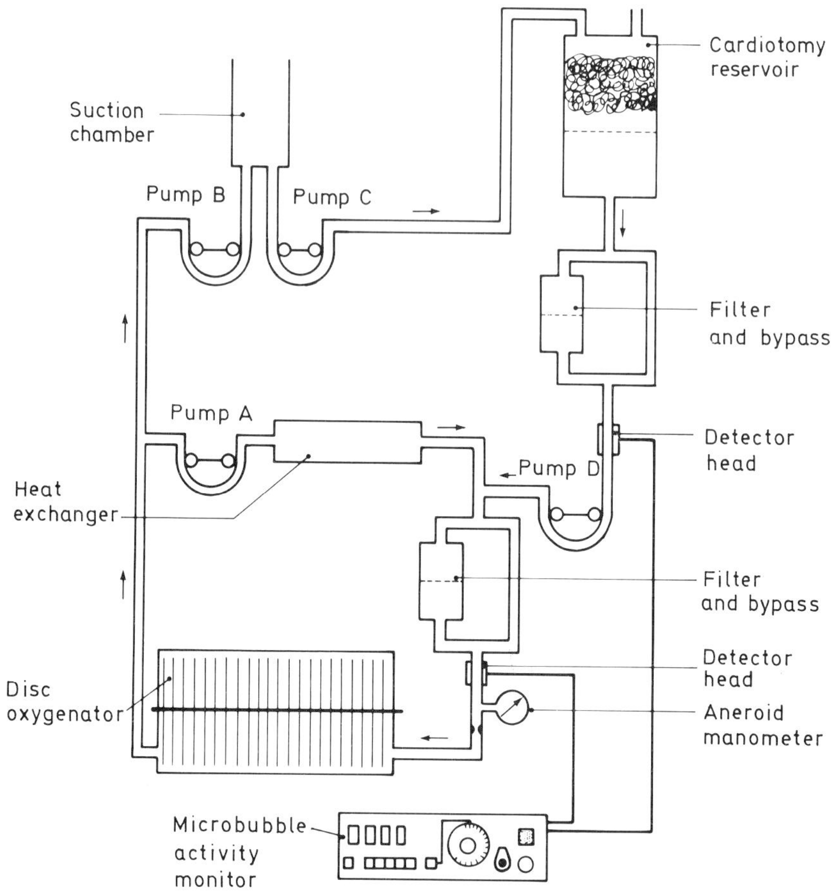

Figure 7.3 Schematic diagram of *in vitro* cardiopulmonary bypass circuit. (Reproduced from Pearson, Watson and Waterhouse[52] by courtesy of the Editor of *Thorax*)

micropore filter at 0.5 ℓ/min by pump D immediately or after a variable delay. The microbubble detector head was applied to the tubing distal to the cardiotomy reservoir, micropore filter, and bypass to assess the number and size of gaseous microemboli remaining in the blood.

Our first experiments showed that with a given cardiotomy reservoir the number of gaseous microemboli varied by less than 5 per cent in successive experiments when the effluent from the reservoir was monitored. This consistency enabled us to compare the efficiency of microbubble removal of different types of cardiotomy reservoirs and to measure the further improvement produced by microfiltration, either immediately below the reservoir or in the main circuit. Each experiment was repeated three times, and the main circuit was allowed to become bubble-free between each experiment.

Cardiotomy reservoirs and micropore filters tested

The following cardiotomy reservoirs and microfilters were investigated.

A. Polystan HL 282 DF cardiotomy reservoir.*
B. Polystan HL 280 DF cardiotomy reservoir.*
C. Polystan 40 cardiotomy reservoir.*
D. Bentley Q220 disposable expanded volume cardiotomy reservoir.†
E. Bentley Q120 disposable cardiotomy reservoir.†
F. Bentley Q220F disposable expanded volume cardiotomy reservoir with filter.†
G. Travenol 2-litres cardiotomy blood reservoir 5MO 391.‡
H. Travenol rigid cardiotomy reservoir 5MO 305.‡
I. Cobe cardiotomy reservoir 42–301.§
J. Cobe cardiotomy reservoir with Swank filter 42–300.§
K. Harvey disposable cardiotomy reservoir model H500.**
L. Bromlus cardiotomy suction filter and defoamer.††
M. Intersept arterial extracorporeal blood filter.‡‡
N. Intersept cardiotomy extracorporeal blood filter.‡‡
O. Pall Ultipor blood filter.§§

Results

Using a Polystan HL 282 DF cardiotomy reservoir, sequential experiments were carried out after collection of blood in the reservoir. This blood was pumped without micropore filtration past the detector head immediately after collection or after it had remained in the reservoir for varying periods of time. *Figure 7.4* shows the decline in the numbers of gaseous microemboli greater than 10 microns in diameter remaining in the blood as related to increasing storage time.

The relative speeds of pumps B and C determine the blood volume/gas volume ratio of the simulated cardiotomy suction blood. The effluent from a Polystan HL 282 DF cardiotomy reservoir showed an increasing number of gaseous microemboli as the proportion of air in the blood injected into the reservoir increased (*Figure 7.5*).

Using a blood volume/gas volume ratio of 1 to 2.7 in the simulated cardiotomy suction blood, an equal volume was successively injected into each of 12 commercially available cardiotomy reservoirs. The effluent was immediately pumped past the detector head without micropore filtration or after passage through an Ultipor filter. The results showed a wide variation in the ability of the reservoirs to remove gaseous microemboli, but, in all

*Albert Browne Ltd., Chancery House, Abbey Gate, Leicester LE4 0AA, UK
†Bentley Laboratories Ltd., 267 Cranbrook Road, Ilford, Essex, UK
‡Travenol Laboratories, Caxton Way, Thetford, Norfolk IP24 3SE, UK
§Cimid Ltd., Barnfield Road, Park Farm Industrial Estate, Folkestone, Kent, CT19 5EX, UK
**GU Manufacturing Co. Ltd., Plympton Street, London NW8 8AB, UK
††Avon Medicals Ltd., 1649 Pershore Road, Birmingham B30 3DR, UK
‡‡Johnson and Johnson Ltd., 260 Bath Road, Slough, Berks., SL1 4EA, UK
§§Pall Biomedical Ltd., Walton Road, Portsmouth PO6 1TD, UK

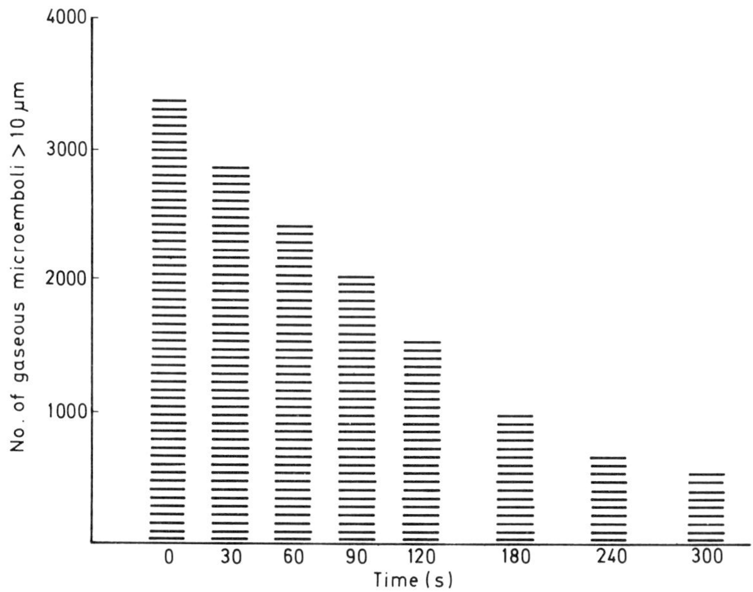

Figure 7.4 Number of gaseous microemboli smaller than 10 μm remaining in the effluent from a Polystan HL 282 DF cardiotomy reservoir as related to the duration of storage time. (Reproduced from Pearson, Watson and Waterhouse[52] by courtesy of the Editor of *Thorax*)

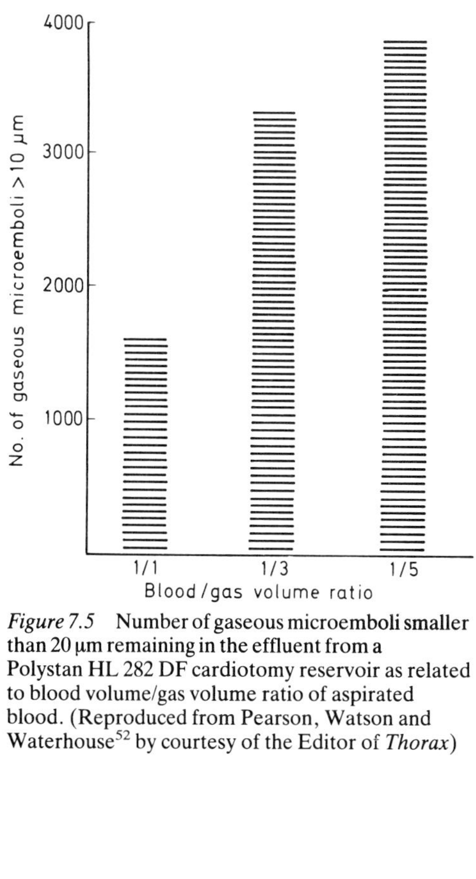

Figure 7.5 Number of gaseous microemboli smaller than 20 μm remaining in the effluent from a Polystan HL 282 DF cardiotomy reservoir as related to blood volume/gas volume ratio of aspirated blood. (Reproduced from Pearson, Watson and Waterhouse[52] by courtesy of the Editor of *Thorax*)

cases, performance was improved by using a micropore filter below the reservoir (*Figure 7.6*).

When a micropore filter and a bypass line were inserted into the main circuit the effluent from the cardiotomy reservoir could be discharged directly into this circuit with the detector head applied to the tubing distal to the filter (*Figure 7.3*). In this way the ability of a micropore filter to retain gaseous microemboli when sited in the simulated arterial line could be compared with its efficiency when sited below the cardiotomy reservoir. As

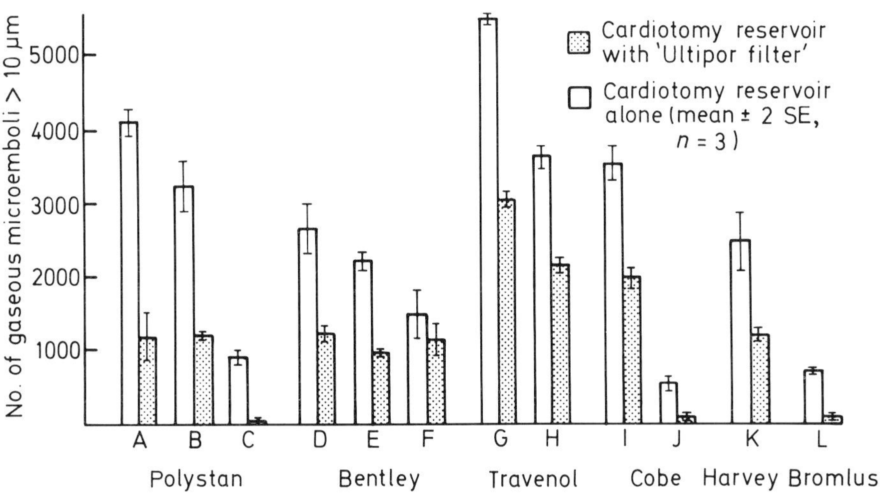

Figure 7.6 Comparative numbers of gaseous microemboli smaller than 10 µm remaining in the effluent from various cardiotomy reservoirs with and without filtration by a 40 µm Ultipor filter. (Reproduced from Pearson, Watson and Waterhouse[52] by courtesy of the Editor of *Thorax*)

the priming volume of the main circuit exceeded 3 litres, and the flow rate of pump A was maintained at 2.5 ℓ/min, no gaseous microemboli were counted twice, provided the duration of the counting did not exceed one minute. An aneroid manometer was placed in the main circuit and the line pressure distal to the filter was adjusted to 13.4 kPa (100 mmHg) by means of a screw clamp. The results (*Figure 7.7*) showed that the numbers of gaseous microemboli were reduced by a micropore filter inserted in the arterial line, but a much greater reduction was achieved by inserting the filter below the cardiotomy reservoir. A greater overall reduction in the number of gaseous microemboli was obtained when the 40 micron pore size Ultipor filter was replaced by the 20 micron pore size arterial line and cardiotomy Intersept filters.

The insertion of the 20 micron Intersept filter and the 40 micron Ultipor filter in parallel in the main circuit allowed direct comparisons of their efficiency by subjecting them alternately to a standard load of gaseous microemboli from the effluent of a cardiotomy reservoir. In addition, the size profile of the bubbles that passed through could be compared. The results confirmed the greater efficiency of the 20 micron filter. Most gaseous

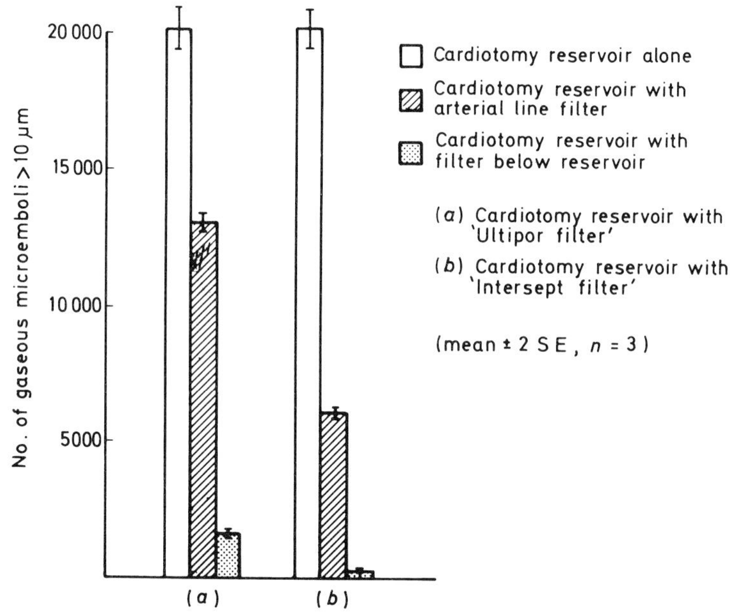

Figure 7.7 Comparison of efficiency of micropore filters sited below the cardiotomy reservoir and in a simulated arterial line. (Reproduced from Pearson, Watson and Waterhouse[52] by courtesy of the Editor of *Thorax*)

microemboli passing through this filter were in the 10–20 micron range, while the majority passing through the 40 micron filter were in the 10–30 micron range.

Discussion

The wide variation in the ability of various commercially available cardiotomy reservoirs and blood filters to remove bubbles from aspirated blood and produce an effluent relatively free from gaseous microemboli has been demonstrated *in vitro*.

The design of a reservoir can affect its performance. Some of those tested induced turbulence and frothing before admitting blood to the defoamer and also allowed a proportion of the blood to pass through the reservoir without coming into contact with the defoaming substance. Other reservoirs, having defoamed the blood, allowed it to splash into the storage part of the reservoir. All these factors increase the number of gaseous microemboli in the effluent.

A cardiotomy reservoir with improved filtration characteristics[63] needs to be developed, since, in the reservoirs tested, those that incorporated a 40 micron nylon mesh or Dacron wool filter performed the best. The three Polystan reservoirs were essentially similar in overall design but show a progressive improvement in efficiency as the pore size of the filter in the storage part of the reservoir is reduced from 180 through 120 to 40 microns.

The Bentley Q220F reservoir, incorporating a 27 micron filter, did not perform as well as expected. Not only did this unit suffer from splashing of the defoamed blood but it induced turbulence at the blood inlet ports.

An analysis of the design features of the reservoirs, assessed by correlation of their *in vitro* performance with the overall configuration of the reservoir, type of defoamer, and pore size of the incorporated filter material, suggests that optimal efficiency can be achieved by direct injection of aspirated blood into the defoaming substance and filtration by either Dacron wool or 40 micron nylon mesh. The defoamed and filtered blood should not be allowed to fall freely into the storage part of the reservoir.

Alterations in perfusion technique will influence the performance of the cardiotomy reservoirs. If the blood is stored in the reservoir for as long as possible within the confines of an adequate level in the oxygenator, not only will maintenance of a higher level reduce splashing of the defoamed blood but gaseous microemboli will have more time to dissipate. The greater the proportion of air mixed with blood in the aspirate from the open heart and pericardium, the more difficult it is for the cardiotomy reservoirs to remove gaseous microemboli completely. The speed of the suction pumps should be monitored continuously to allow as low an admixture of air with the blood as is compatible with the surgical technique.

Filtration of blood after passage through the cardiotomy reservoir reduces further the numbers of gaseous microemboli. The size and number of gaseous microemboli remaining in circulation is related to the pore size of the micropore filter used. However, microfiltration is only a partial solution to a problem best solved by avoiding factors responsible for the formation of microemboli and by choosing the most efficient cardiotomy reservoir. A simulated arterial line micropore filter is not as effective in removing gaseous microemboli as the same type of filter sited below the cardiotomy reservoir. During clinical perfusion, defoamed blood is returned to the oxygenator at a low flow rate by gravity, but when the filter is placed in the arterial line it is subjected to a much higher velocity and greater flow of blood. During the experiments the arterial line filter released gaseous microemboli into the main circuit when it was trapped. Considerable care was needed during priming of the filter to ensure that no gas was trapped in the filter medium.

Summary

Cerebral dysfunction has been reported to occur frequently following cardiac surgery especially in those operations involving the use of cardiopulmonary bypass. Although the use of a pump oxygenator for open-heart surgery has allowed significant advances to take place in this field, most of the commonly used oxygenators and pumps alter the blood in a manner which is detrimental to the perfused tissues.

The use of donor blood and the presence of a gas-blood interface in the oxygenator induce aggregation of the formed elements of the blood and generate gaseous microemboli. The surgeon is presented with the problem of aspiration of blood from the open heart and emptying the heart of air at the end of the intracardiac operation, both of which are potential hazards to the patient.

The use of micropore filters to remove debris from the oxygenator prior to cardiopulmonary bypass and to prevent the admission of gaseous and particulate emboli to the patient is gaining in popularity, though there still exists some doubt as to whether these filters damage the formed blood elements. There is no doubt that the advent of oxygenators which do not generate microemboli, the choice of atraumatic blood pumps, efficient cardiotomy reservoirs and the avoidance of the use of donor blood will eliminate many of the sources of microemboli. A high quality cardiopulmonary bypass so provided will make a significant contribution to the reduction in mortality and morbidity associated with open-heart surgery.

It is important that, during the choice of equipment from various manufacturers, consideration should be given to the efficiency of the cardiotomy reservoir and blood filters used. Considerable development has taken place in the field of artificial oxygenation but in the author's opinion this has not been paralleled by progress in cardiotomy design even though this device is an integral part of the pump oxygenator system for many open-heart surgical procedures. At our institution the ability of twelve commercially available cardiotomy reservoirs to remove bubbles from aspirated blood has been investigated by means of a simulated cardiopulmonary bypass circuit and an ultrasonic microbubble detector. The performance of these devices varied considerably. The number of gaseous microemboli remaining after passage of blood through the cardiotomy reservoir was reduced by: (a) holding the blood in the reservoir; (b) reducing the volume of air mixed with the aspirated blood; and (c) using a reservoir that did not induce turbulence and that contained integral micropore filtration material. Further micropore filtration of the blood after passage through the cardiotomy reservoir was beneficial in removing more gaseous microemboli. This work has been confirmed for particulate microemboli by other workers in the field, demonstrating the need for the development of a cardiotomy reservoir with improved filtration characteristics.

It is important that during cardiopulmonary bypass consideration is given to haemodynamic factors which influence the outcome of the operation, particularly when the patient's preoperative status is poor. Furthermore, it must be finally stated that the success of cardiopulmonary bypass is as dependent upon the equipment used as it is upon the perfusionist who operates the equipment.

References

1. Aberg, T. 'Effect of open-heart surgery on intellectual function.' *Scandinavian Journal of Thoracic and Cardiovascular Surgery*, (*Suppl.*) **15**, (1974)
2. Aberg, T. and Kihlgren, M. 'Cerebral protection during open-heart surgery.' *Thorax*, **32**, 525 (1977)
3. Aguilar, M. J., Gerbode, F. and Hill, J. D. 'Neuropathological complications of cardiac surgery.' *Journal of Thoracic and Cardiovascular Surgery*, **61**, 676 (1971)

4. Allardyce, D. B., Yoshida, S. H. and Ashmore, P. G. 'The importance of microembolism in the pathogenesis of organ dysfunction caused by prolonged use of the pump oxygenator.' *Journal of Thoracic and Cardiovascular Surgery*, **52,** 706 (1966)
5. Ashmore, P., Svitek, V. and Ambrose, P. 'The incidence and effects of particulate aggregation and microembolism in pump oxygenator systems.' *Journal of Thoracic and Cardiovascular Surgery*, **55,** 691 (1968)
6. Ashmore, P., Swank, R., Gallery, R., Ambrose, P. and Pritchard, K. H. 'Effect of Dacron wool filtration on the microembolic phenomenon in extracorporeal circulation.' *Journal of Thoracic and Cardiovascular Surgery*, **63,** 240 (1972)
7. Austen, W. G. and Howry, D. H. 'Ultrasound as a method to detect bubbles of particulate matter in the arterial line during cardiopulmonary bypass.' *Journal of Surgical Research*, **5,** 283 (1965)
8. Baglio, C. M. and Hunter, W. C. 'Calcific arterial embolisation accompanying commisurotomy.' *Journal of Thoracic Surgery*, **37,** 490 (1959)
9. Bass, R. M. and Longmore, D. B. 'Cerebral damage during open-heart surgery.' *Nature*, (*Lond*), **222,** 30 (1969)
10. Bethune, D. W. 'Organ damage after open-heart surgery.' (Letter). *Lancet*, **2,** 1410 (1976)
11. Björk, V. O. and Hultquist, G. 'Brain damage in children after deep hypothermia for open-heart surgery.' *Thorax*, **15,** 284 (1960)
12. Branthwaite, M. A. 'Cerebral blood flow and metabolism during open-heart surgery.' *Thorax*, **29,** 633 (1974)
13. Branthwaite, M. A. 'Detection of neurological damage during open-heart surgery.' *Thorax*, **28,** 464 (1973)
14. Branthwaite, M. A. 'Neurological damage related to open-heart surgery.' *Thorax*, **27,** 748 (1972)
15. Branthwaite, M. A. 'Prevention of neurological damage during open-heart surgery.' *Thorax*, **30,** 258 (1975)
16. Brennan, R. W., Patterson, R. H. and Kessler, J. 'Cerebral blood flow and metabolism during cardiopulmonary bypass.' *Neurology*, **23,** 665 (1971)
17. Bull, B. S., Korpman, R. A., Huse, W. M. and Briggs, B. D. 'Heparin therapy during extracorporeal circulation. 1. Problems inherent in existing heparin protocols.' *Journal of Thoracic and Cardiovascular Surgery*, **69,** 674 (1975)
18. Burbank, A., Ferguson, T. B. and Burford, T. H. 'Carbon dioxide flooding of the chest in open-heart surgery.' *Journal of Thoracic and Cardiovascular Surgery*, **50,** 691 (1965)
19. Caguin, F. and Carter, M. G. 'Fat embolisation with cardiotomy with use of cardiopulmonary bypass.' *Journal of Thoracic and Cardiovascular Surgery*, **46,** 665 (1963)
20. Cassie, A. B., Riddell, A. G. and Yates, P. O. 'Hazard of antifoam emboli from a bubble oxygenator.' *Thorax*, **15,** 22 (1960)
21. Clark, R. E., Dietz, D. R. and Miller, J. G. 'Continuous detection of microemboli during cardiopulmonary bypass in animals and man.' *Circulation*, **54,** 74 (1976)
22. Dutton, R. C. and Edmunds, L. H., Jr. 'Measurement of emboli in extracorporeal perfusion systems.' *Journal of Thoracic and Cardiovascular Surgery*, **65,** 523 (1973)
23. Dutton, R. C., Edmunds, L. H., Jr., Hutchinson, J. C. and Roe, B. B. 'Platelet aggregate emboli produced in patients during cardiopulmonary bypass with membrane and bubble oxygenators and blood filters.' *Journal of Thoracic and Cardiovascular Surgery*, **67,** 258 (1974)
24. Evans, E. A. and Wellington, J. S. 'Emboli associated with cardiopulmonary bypass.' *Journal of Thoracic and Cardiovascular Surgery*, **48,** 323 (1964)

25. Fishman, N. H., Carlsson, E. and Roe, B. B. 'The importance of the pulmonary veins in systemic air embolism following open-heart surgery.' *Surgery*, **66,** 655 (1969)
26. Gadboys, H. L., Slonim, R. and Litwak, R. S. 'Homologous blood syndrome: 1. Pulmonary observations on its relationship to clinical cardiopulmonary bypass.' *Annals of Surgery*, **156,** 793 (1962)
27. Gallagher, E. G. and Pearson, D. T. 'Ultrasonic identification of sources of gaseous microemboli during open-heart surgery.' *Thorax*, **28,** 295 (1973)
28. Groves, L. K. and Effler, D. B. 'A needle-vent safeguard against systemic air embolism in open heart surgery.' *Journal of Thoracic and Cardiovascular Surgery*, **47,** 349 (1964)
29. Guidoin, R., Laperche, Y., Martin, L., Awad, J. and Winchester, J. 'Disposable filters for microaggregate removal from extracorporeal circulation.' *Journal of Thoracic and Cardiovascular Surgery*, **72,** 502 (1976)
30. Heimbecker, R., Robert, A. and McKenzie, F. N. 'The extracorporeal pump filter—Saint or Sinner?' *Annals of Thoracic Surgery*, **21,** 55 (1976)
31. Hubbard, L. C., Kletschka, H. D., Olsen, D. A., Rafferty, E. H., Clausen, E. W. and Robinson, A. R. 'Spallation using roller pumps and its clinical implications.' *Proceedings of the American Society of Extracorporeal Technicians*, **27,** (1975)
32. Javid, H., Tufo, H. M., Najafi, H., Dye, W. S., Hunter, J. A. and Julian, O. C. 'Neurological abnormalities following open-heart surgery.' *Journal of Thoracic and Cardiovascular Surgery*, **58,** 502 (1969)
33. Jenevein, E. and Weiss, D. 'Platelet microemboli associated with massive blood transfusions.' *American Journal of Pathology*, **45,** 313 (1964)
34. Karlson, K. E., Murphy, W. R., Kakvan, M., Anthony, P., Cooper, G. N., Richardson, P. D. and Galletti, P. M. 'Total cardiopulmonary bypass with a new microporous Teflon membrane oxygenator.' *Surgery*, **76,** 935 (1974)
35. Kessler, J. and Patterson, R. H., Jr. 'The production of microemboli by various blood oxygenators.' *Annals of Thoracic Surgery*, **9,** 221 (1970)
36. *Lancet*. (Editorial). 'Brain damage after open-heart surgery.' *Lancet*, **2,** 399 (1975)
37. Lawrence, G. H., McKay, H. A. and Sherensky, R. T. 'Effective measures in the prevention of intraoperative aeroembolus.' *Journal of Thoracic and Cardiovascular Surgery*, **62,** 731 (1971)
38. Lee, W. H., Krumhaar, D., Fonkalsrud, E. W., Schjeide, O. A. and Maloney, J. V. 'Denaturation of plasma proteins as a cause of morbidity and death after intracardiac operations.' *Surgery*, **50,** 29 (1961)
39. Lee, W. H., Jr., Brady, M. P., Rowe, J. M. and Miller, W. C., Jr. 'Effects of extracorporeal circulation upon behaviour, personality and brain function. 2. Haemodynamic metabolic and psychometric correlations.' *Annals of Surgery*, **173,** 1013 (1971)
40. Loop, F. D., Szabo, J., Rowlinson, R. D. and Urbanek, K. 'Events related to microembolism during extracorporeal perfusion in man. Effectiveness of in-line filtration recorded by ultrasound.' *Annals of Thoracic Surgery*, **21,** 412 (1976)
41. Miller, B. J., Gibbon, J. H., Greco, V. F., Cohn, C. H. and Allbritten, F. F. 'The use of a vent for the left ventricle as a means of avoiding air embolism to the systemic circulation during open cardiotomy with the maintenance of the cardiorespiratory function of animals by a pump oxygenator.' *Surgical Forum*, **4,** 29 (1963)
42. Miller, D. R. and Allbritten, F. F. 'Coronary suction as a source of air embolism: an experimental study using the Kay–Cross oxygenator.' *Annals of Surgery*, **151,** 75 (1960)

43. Mortensen, J. D., Smith, S. M. and Hill, G. 'Bacterial contamination of oxygen used in cardiopulmonary bypass.' *Journal of Thoracic and Cardiovascular Surgery*, **41,** 675 (1961)
44. Moseley, R. V. and Doty, D. B. 'Changes in the filtration characteristics of stored blood.' *Annals of Surgery*, **121,** 329 (1970)
45. Moseley, R. V. and Doty, D. B. 'Death associated with multiple pulmonary emboli soon after battle injury.' *Annals of Surgery*, **171,** 336 (1970)
46. Nichols, H. T., Morse, D. P. and Hirose, T. 'Coronary and other air embolisation occurring during open cardiac surgery.' *Surgery*, **43,** 236 (1958)
47. Nicks, R. 'Air embolism in cardiac surgery: incidence and prophylaxis.' *Australian and New Zealand Journal of Surgery*, **38,** 328 (1969)
48. Osborn, J. J., Swank, R. L., Hill, J. D., Aguilar, M. J. and Gerbode, F. 'Clinical use of a Dacron wool filter during perfusion for open-heart surgery.' *Journal of Thoracic and Cardiovascular Surgery*, **60,** 575 (1970)
49. Padula, R. T., Eisenstat, T. E., Bronstein, M. H. and Camishion, R. C. 'Intracardiac air following cardiotomy; location, causative factors, and a method for removal.' *Journal of Thoracic and Cardiovascular Surgery*, **62,** 736 (1971)
50. Patterson, R. H. and Kessler, J. 'Microemboli during cardiopulmonary bypass detected by ultrasound.' *Surgery, Gynecology and Obstetrics*, **129,** 505 (1969)
51. Patterson, R. H., Jr., Wasser, J. S. and Porro, R. S. 'The effect of various filters on microembolic cerebrovascular blockade following cardiopulmonary bypass.' *Annals of Thoracic Surgery*, **17,** 464 (1974)
52. Pearson, D. T., Watson, B. G. and Waterhouse, P. S. 'An ultrasonic analysis of the comparative efficiency of various cardiotomy reservoirs and micropore blood filters.' *Thorax*, **33,** 352 (1978)
53. Reed, C. C., Romagnoli, A., Taylor, D. E. and Clark, D. K. 'Particulate matter in bubble oxygenators.' *Journal of Thoracic and Cardiovascular Surgery*, **68,** 971 (1974)
54. Sanderson, J. M., Wright, G. and Sims, F. W. 'Brain damage in dogs immediately following pulsatile and non-pulsatile blood flows in extracorporeal circulation.' *Thorax*, **27,** 275 (1972)
55. Selman, M. W., McAlpine, W. A. and Ratan, R. D. 'The effectiveness of various heart-lung machines in the elimination of microbubbles from the circulation.' *Journal of Thoracic and Cardiovascular Surgery*, **53,** 613 (1967)
56. Senning, A. 'Ventricular fibrillation during extracorporeal circulation used as a method to prevent air embolism and to facilitate intracardiac operations.' *Acta Chirurgica Scandinavica*, (*Suppl.*), p. 171 (1952)
57. Siderys, H., Herod, G. T., Halbrook, H., Pittman, J. N., Rubush, J., Kasebaker, V. and Berry, G. R. 'A comparison of membrane and bubble oxygenation as used in cardiopulmonary bypass in patients.' *Journal of Thoracic and Cardiovascular Surgery*, **69,** 708 (1975)
58. Simmons, E., MaGuire, C., Lichti, E., Helvey, W. and Almond, C. 'A comparison of the microparticles produced when two disposable-bag oxygenators and a disc oxygenator are used for cardiopulmonary bypass.' *Journal of Thoracic and Cardiovascular Surgery*, **63,** 613 (1972)
59. Skagseth, E., Frøysaker, T. and Refsum, S. B. 'Disposable filter for microemboli in cardiopulmonary bypass.' *Journal of Cardiovascular Surgery*, **15,** 318 (1974)
60. Solis, R. T. 'Blood filtration during cardiopulmonary bypass.' *Journal of Extracorporeal Technology*, **6,** 64 (1974)
61. Solis, R. T., Kennedy, P. S., Beall, A. C., Jr., Noon, G. P. and DeBakey, M. E. 'Cardiopulmonary bypass. Microembolisation and platelet aggregation.' *Circulation*, **52,** 103 (1975)

62. Solis, R. T., Noon, G. P., Beall, A. C. and DeBakey, M. E. 'Particulate microembolism during cardiac operation.' *Annals of Thoracic Surgery*, **17,** 332 (1974)
63. Solis, R. T., Scott, M. A., Kennedy, P. S. and Wilson, R. K. 'Filtration of cardiotomy reservoir blood.' *Journal of Extracorporeal Technology*, **8,** 69 (1976)
64. Starr, A. 'The mechanism and prevention of air embolism during correction of congenital cleft mitral valve.' *Journal of Thoracic and Cardiovascular Surgery*, **39,** 808 (1960)
65. Subramanian, V. A. and Berger, R. L. 'Comparative evaluation of a new disposable Rotating Membrane Oxygenator with bubble oxygenator.' *Annals of Thoracic Surgery*, **21**, 48 (1976)
66. Swank, R. L. 'Adhesiveness of platelets and leucocytes during acute exsanguination.' *American Journal of Physiology*, **202,** 261 (1961)
67. Swank, R. L. 'Alteration of blood on storage: measurement of adhesiveness of 'aging' platelets and leucocytes and their removal by filtration.' *New England Journal of Medicine*, **265,** 728 (1961)
68. Swank, R. L., Connell, R. S. and Webb, M. C. 'Platelet-leucocyte emboli; origins, effects and treatment.' *Journal of Extracorporeal Technology*, **5,** 23 (1973)
69. Taber, R. E., Maraan, B. M. and Tomatis, L. 'Prevention of air embolism during open-heart surgery. A study of the role of trapped air in the left ventricle.' *Surgery*, **68,** 685 (1970)
70. Tufo, M., Ostfeld, A. M. and Shekelle, R. 'Central nervous system dysfunction following open-heart surgery.' *Journal of the American Medical Association*, **212,** 1333 (1970)
71. Valentin, N. and Vilhelmsen, R. 'Blood and tissue silicone in extracorporeal circulation.' *Journal of Cardiovascular Surgery*, **17,** 20 (1976)
72. Wright, G. and Sanderson, J. M. 'Brain damage and mortality in dogs following pulsatile and non-pulsatile blood flows in extracorporeal circulation.' *Thorax*, **27,** 738 (1972)
73. Wright, G. and Sanderson, J. M. 'Cellular aggregation and destruction during blood circulation and oxygenation.' *Thorax*, **31,** 405 (1976)

8

The Use of Haemodilution and a Non-Haemic Prime for Cardiopulmonary Bypass

Richard N. Edie, Susan M. Haubert and James R. Malm

quae fuerunt vitia mores sunt

History

Blood prime

During the early days of cardiopulmonary bypass, it was accepted that fresh heparinized homologous blood should be used as the priming solution for the oxygenator. Soon there arose certain unforeseen problems associated both with the nature of the priming solution and the type of oxygenators. Since the performance of extracorporeal circulation acted, in effect, as an exchange transfusion between the patient and the priming solution, the relationship between the nature and amount of priming solution and the patient's blood volume became important. Obviously, if the priming solution was small, the exchange, no matter what the constitution of the priming solution, would be less deleterious than one with a large volume. The recent development of the satisfactory small prime bubble oxygenators has simplified perfusion fluid requirements and has been discussed at length in Chapter 6. This chapter then will be concerned primarily with the priming solutions.

The demand for and the use of fresh homologous blood led to immediate difficulties. The initial procurement of fresh blood put a great strain on blood banks and placed limitations on open-heart surgery especially for those who had rare blood types. The sequel of serum hepatitis was an all too frequent late complication related to the use of blood. Most important, however, there appeared certain intraoperative problems which occurred during cardiopulmonary bypass when a blood prime was used. It had been shown previously in experimental animals that soon after the commencement of perfusion with homologous blood there appeared a fall in both arterial pressure and systemic venous return. This event was associated with a decrease in circulating blood volume and a pooling of blood in the splanchnic circulation with subsequent hepatic congestion and portal hypertension[19]. This shock-like state created a severe metabolic acidosis and was accompanied by thrombocytopenia, leucopenia and red cell sequestration. Finally, coagulation abnormalities, pulmonary congestion, renal failure and cerebral insufficiency ensued. At first, attention was focused on the liver as the inciting organ until Ankeney and Murthy[1] excluded the liver from the circulation and found the above changes still occurred. In addition, this clinical picture did not appear when perfusates other than blood were used. It remained for Gadboys, Slonim and Litwak[24] to show that it was an incompatibility of the pooled homologous blood elements that was responsible for the above results. They postulated that this incompatibility reaction occurred not only between donor and recipient blood but also between the individual pooled donor blood elements. They termed this combination of sequelae the 'homologous blood syndrome' and through this work, clearly defined the areas where investigations into alternate priming solutions were necessary.

Alternative primes

Initially, it was felt that blood electively drawn and preserved with an anticoagulant solution could be used to obviate the procurement problems of fresh blood. Beginning in 1958, EDGLUGATE-Mg solution[57] was used as a preservative without significant problems but its commercial preparation was discontinued in 1961 because of potential nephrotoxicity. Foote, Trede and Maloney[22] then demonstrated that blood stored in an acid-citrate-dextrose (ACD) solution was acceptable for extracorporeal circulation and that the addition of calcium and heparin to the blood before bypass did not create any untoward effects. Though this preservative made the blood quite acidotic, it was felt initially that the natural buffers of the body could correct this base deficit. Buffering solutions such as tromethamine (THAM) soon were added to the ACD blood[34]. These buffers not only effectively neutralized the fixed acid of the priming solution but also helped to prevent further metabolic acidosis which occurred naturally during cardiopulmonary bypass. Despite this progress the previously mentioned problems with the use of blood continued: thus, further alternative priming solutions were sought.

It had been long known that physiologists had successfully perfused isolated organs in experimental animals with balanced electrolyte solutions. In 1959 Panico and Neptune[47, 40] designed a pump oxygenator in which the majority of the prime was normal saline. In this oxygenator, the saline prime layered on top of the patient's blood and thus reduced the quantity of blood necessary for perfusion. This development ushered in the concept of haemodilution and promoted experimental and clinical work in many centres[27, 61, 62]. In 1961 Cooley, Beall and Alexander[9] reported the successful clinical use of dextrose 5 mg/100ml in water as a prime for partial cardiopulmonary bypass in patients undergoing emergency pulmonary embolectomy. In addition, their experience using dextrose 5 mg/100ml in water as the complete prime in a bubble oxygenator for normothermic total cardiopulmonary bypass in 100 patients undergoing open-heart surgery further emphasized the efficacy of haemodilution[10].

Components and principles of haemodilution

Priming solutions

Acid-citrate-dextrose blood (alone and with diluents)

Soon after the report by Foote, Trede and Maloney[22], ACD blood was initiated widely as the sole priming solution. Buffers like THAM were added by some groups and alleviated the metabolic acidosis caused both by the priming fluid and by bypass itself. Interestingly, Malm *et al.*[34] found negligible metabolic acidosis in a group of patients using ACD blood plus THAM as opposed to those patients with heparinized blood both with and without THAM. Since at that time the majority of the oxygenators in use demanded a large volume prime, it was impossible for a total non-haemic prime to deliver a solution of adequate oxygen-carrying capacity to the patient. Thus, a number of investigators utilized numerous blood–electrolyte mixtures as a method of partial haemodilution. In an extensive study, Litwak *et al.*[30] employed ACD blood in various amounts along with 5 mg/100ml dextrose/Ringer's albumin prime with and without THAM. The beneficial results were immediately apparent. The overall biochemical abnormalities were minimal. Also, the urine output, both during and following bypass, increased in direct proportion to the amount of haemodilution and the buffer capacity of the prime. In addition there were less pulmonary and coagulation complications with these various mixtures of partial haemodilution. Sessler *et al.*[56] found similar results with haemodiluted perfusates as compared with undiluted heparinized blood.

Low molecular weight dextran (LMWD)

It had been known that dextran was an excellent plasma expander and that LMWD prevented sludging of red blood cells during shock-like states. Because of this effect on the microcirculation, studies were performed using LMWD as a perfusate. Long *et al.*[31] from Minnesota, used LMWD both alone and in various combinations with electrolyte solutions and found that urine output increased and haemolysis decreased. Also, coagulation abnormalities were not present unless the dosage of LMWD exceeded 20 ml/kg of body weight. In addition, the serum electrolytes and acid–base balance were not markedly altered. Using similar haemodiluted primes which included LMWD, Hepps *et al.*[28] found a marked reduction in adverse pulmonary changes but observed that the postoperative bleeding increased following the use of LMWD even though coagulation profiles were normal. Improvement in the above parameters was interpreted as representing adequate tissue perfusion during bypass. Whether the results were due to the nature of the perfusate or the expanded circulating plasma volume remained to be determined.

Dextrose 5 mg/100 ml in water

In order to confirm that some of the beneficial effects of LMWD were due to its haemodilution, dextrose 5 mg/100 ml in water was tried as a perfusate. The initial success by Cooley, Beall and Grondin[10] prompted others (Paton and Rosenkrantz)[48] to try this prime. Both groups utilized a bubble oxygenator, with either the DeWall–Lillehei or the disposable Travenol* bag, and kept haemodilution at a minimum (below 20 ml/kg of body weight). Both groups independently noted the excellent intraoperative and postoperative diuresis as the initial evidence of satisfactory tissue perfusion during cardiopulmonary bypass. As Cooley, Beall and Grondin[10] stated: 'After operation the patients usually demonstrate a prompt recovery of normal cerebral, pulmonary and renal function. Patients tended to be mentally alert immediately after operation and seldom had mental confusion or restlessness. Small, cutaneous petechiae, possibly the result of aggregations of cells, capillary sludging or platelet thrombi, were absent. Pulmonary congestion was not a complication.'

It was noted, however, that dextrose 5 mg/100ml in water, being a hypotonic perfusate, left the intravascular space during bypass in various amounts. As a result, in order to keep satisfactory flow rates and perfusion pressures, additional perfusate fluid had to be added during bypass. Also, it was necessary at the end of the bypass to reinfuse the majority of the perfusate in order to regain a normal blood volume. The combination of these factors led to an increase of the extracellular volume and a mild dilutional hyponatraemia which lasted anywhere from 7 to 10 days

*Travenol Labs. Inc., Los Angeles, California, USA

postoperatively. The effect of the above changes was mild, and the dilutional problem was easily treated with either fluid restriction and or diuretics. Furthermore, the hypotonicity of this prime was felt to be the cause of an increased haemolysis as measured by the plasma haemoglobin[48]. These disadvantages, however, were offset by the above-mentioned beneficial effects.

It was thus recognized that dextrose 5 mg/100ml in water could be satisfactorily used as a complete prime for either short perfusion and/or small volume primes or as an adjunct to other solutions when large volume primes were necessary or a longer bypass was anticipated.

Balanced crystalloid solutions

It soon became apparent, mainly through the independent experimental and clinical work by Roe and Neville and their associates, that crystalloid solutions of balanced electrolyte composition could satisfactorily perform as complete primes for oxygenators utilizing either small-or large-volume primes. Roe *et al.*[53] theorized that the major alteration of blood elements appeared at the gas-fluid interface and caused fluid transudation and intravascular agglutination with the resulting well-known clinical manifestations. The lowering of the blood viscosity with exchange fluids of composition similar to that which was present in the serum appears to have beneficial effects to the entire system. Roe used a small prime of a balanced electrolyte solution plus LMWD with a disposable Travenol bubble oxygenator. He lowered the patient's haematocrit to 25 per cent which, in effect, diluted the cellular and protein blood content by approximately 50 per cent. When additional fluid was needed during bypass, ACD blood was used if the haematocrit was less than 20 per cent and more electrolyte solution if the haematocrit was above this level. The most striking finding in these patients was the remarkable absence of metabolic acidosis, again interpreted as an index of adequate tissue perfusion. Any mild acidosis that did occur was easily resolved by the administration of small doses of sodium bicarbonate. In addition, the serum electrolyte pattern was remarkably stable, and postoperatively there were minimal renal and pulmonary problems. Finally, the trauma to the red blood cells as measured by free plasma haemoglobin was markedly reduced.

Neville *et al.*[42, 43], on the other hand, used buffered Ringer's lactate as the complete prime for the large-volume disc oxygenator. Again, similar results were obtained with the prevention of significant metabolic acidosis during and after perfusion associated with a striking increase in urinary output in the early postoperative period.

Adjuvant solutions

Certain other solutions were tried, not as a total non-haemic prime, but as adjuvants to other solutions. Mannitol had long been used as an osmotic diuretic in situations where haemolysis and/or diminished renal function was expected. In cases of prolonged cardiopulmonary bypass, mannitol was added to the perfusion fluid in order to forestall the detrimental effects of haemoglobinuria. Porter *et al.*[52] found that mannitol added to the perfusate decreased haemolysis and also the incidence of renal failure. They reasoned that during bypass there was an intraluminal renal deposition of haemoglobin pigments and that mannitol, by creating an osmotic diuresis, increased tubular flow. They also found that mannitol increased renal blood flow during periods of hypotension by decreasing renal vascular resistance.

Albumin and/or fresh-frozen plasma had a brief trial as a perfusate, as these solutions had physiological viscosity and osmolality and were readily available. The early clinical results with the use of albumin were good[21], but the expense of albumin and the high risk of hepatitis, primarily with the pooled fresh-frozen plasma, prohibited their wide utilization.

More recently, experimental work has been done utilizing the non-ionic detergent, Pluronic F68[59], a synthetic copolymer which is both hydrophobic and hydrophilic. Early investigation has shown that this substance may be useful, both as an entire, or adjuvant, priming solution. Its advantages, especially during long perfusions were its non-toxic effects, excellent oxygen and carbon dioxide carrying capacity, metabolic inertness, positive inotropic effect on the heart, and lastly, its prevention of haemolysis, fat embolization and protein denaturation. Further work with this substance is forthcoming.

Metabolic changes

Renal

With haemodilution, the absence of peripheral vasoconstriction and cyanosis, along with the excellent urinary output, were the initial observations of adequate tissue perfusion. This improvement in renal function led to immediate investigation. Mielke *et al.*[36] found pathological renal tubular cell changes in dogs subjected to extracorporeal circulation, with low urinary flow rates. These changes were abolished when higher urinary flow rates were produced during bypass by an osmotic diuresis. Neville *et al.*[41, 46] in clinical situations reported higher urinary outputs of lower osmolality during and after bypass coincident with the diminution of haematuria and felt that these results were secondary to the osmotic effects of the priming solutions. Das, Eraklis and Jones[14] found that a haemodiluted prime, made hyperosmolar by additional dextrose promoted an even greater initial diuresis in the first 6 hours postoperatively but then led to a state of relative dehydration unless adequate fluid replacement was given. Neville, Thomason and Hirsch[46] further reasoned that the improvement in renal function with haemodilution was due not only to the osmotic effect of the priming solution but also to the absolute blood volume dilution with subsequent increase in extracellular fluid volume. He felt that the buffered lactated Ringer's solution used in his studies potentiated urinary excretion by providing adequate renal perfusion by increased renal blood flow. In addition, he found that the lack of haematuria was directly related to the relatively hydrated state of the kidneys during the period of haemodilution. As a result of effective haemodilution, the absolute deposition of haemoglobin pigment in the kidneys during bypass was decreased and subsequent haematuria, oliguria and anuria avoided.

Many studies confirm the fact that there was a minimal change in sodium and chloride excretion but a marked increase in potassium loss[14, 16, 17].

Many explanations were given for the kaluresis and secondary hypokalaemia. First, the composition of the non-haemic prime necessitated the delivery of a large solute load with a high content of sodium to the distal tubules. As a result, potassium was exchanged for sodium at this level and thus excreted. Other factors such as renal tubular damage secondary to extracorporeal circulation, aldosterone effect secondary to surgical stress, and the cellular shifts of potassium in response to acid–base balance, were proposed as additional explanations for both the hypokalaemia and kaluresis. This finding had marked clinical significance as the level of serum potassium was closely correlated with cardiac arrhythmias and digitalis toxicity.

Pulmonary

Since pulmonary complications after cardiopulmonary bypass occurred frequently with blood primes, the effect of haemodilution on postoperative pulmonary function was quite important. With blood primes, congestion and pulmonary oedema were common, and it was believed that this clinical picture was due to a diffusion defect across the alveolar-capillary membrane. Gardner, Finley and Tooley[25] noted a significant reduction in pulmonary surfactant activity following cardiopulmonary bypass with whole blood primes both in dogs and humans. These studies showed increased surface tension and decreased compliance, coupled with pathological microscopic changes, presumed to be seondary to the loss of surfactant. This clinical and pathological picture was quite similar to that seen in hyaline membrane disease of the newborn. Camishon *et al.*[6] compared the effects of 50 per cent haemodilution and whole blood prime in dogs and found minimal changes in pulmonary compliance in the haemodilution group and marked changes in those receiving whole blood. Of the latter group, all animals died within eight hours. Neville *et al.*[44] observed increased polymorphonuclear cells along the intima of pulmonary blood vessels after bypass and related this to the use of homologous blood, the type of oxygenator and the duration of perfusion. They believed that this intravascular sequestration of polymorphonuclear cells added to the diffusion barrier, which was seen histopathologically by thickened alveolar walls, rounded, fluid-filled alveoli, haemorrhage and atelectasis. Heppe *et al.*[28] found in experimental animals that 50 per cent haemodilution with low molecular weight dextran resulted in distinctly less alveolar structural and functional change, with a marked reduction in protein-containing fluid in the alveoli. In addition, the minimal surface tension rose less in those dogs undergoing haemodilution perfusion for one hour than those with whole blood. Heppe *et al.* then applied this haemodilution principle to patients with a marked reduction in the postperfusion pulmonary complications. Thus, it was postulated that haemodilution gave a more effective perfusion to the alveoli during cardiopulmonary bypass, especially via the bronchial arteries. This theory was supported by the work of Finley *et al.*[20], who occluded one pulmonary artery in the dog, and showed that inadequate perfusion of the alveoli resulted in a loss or inactivation of surfactant, with resultant atelectasis. On the other hand, Mandelbaum, Giamonna and Schumacher[35] showed evidence of the possibility of a circulating surfactant inhibitor which could be responsible for the reduction or loss of pulmonary surfactant. They postulated that it might be due to the dilution of the inhibitor alone that haemodilution prevented pulmonary functional and structural changes.

Acid–base balance
When excessive haemodilution (greater than 100 ml/kg of body weight) was used, severe hypoxic acidosis resulted soon after the start of cardiopulmonary bypass. It was quickly discovered that the acidosis was directly proportional to the degree of haemodilution. Neville[41] found that, with haemodilution between 70 and 100 ml/kg body weight, acidosis could be partially corrected with sodium bicarbonate. It was not, however, until haemodilution was limited to between 50 and 70 ml/kg of body weight that the experimental animals survived. At this level of haemodilution, the oxygen-carrying capacity of the perfusate was not reduced to the extent that correction with buffering solutions was impossible. Neville further found that with Ringer's lactate solution as the prime, less acidosis occurred, and he related this to the ability of the lactate in the solution to compensate partially for the hypoxic acidosis itself.

In similar studies, Neville then compared the buffering ability of THAM and sodium bicarbonate during haemodilution and concluded that survival could be attained if the animals were kept well oxygenated and if acid–base changes were corrected during perfusion. There was no significant difference between the two buffering solutions. Cruz and Callaghan[11], in evaluating large and small non-blood primes, clearly showed that acidosis manifested by an excess lactate and glucose blood level was directly proportionate to the degree of haemodilution. The acidosis, it was felt, was the beginning of a vicious cycle which stimulated excess catecholamine secretion and, secondaily, hyperglycaemia. Malm *et al.*[33] found, during perfusion with a normal acid–base equilibrium, the absence of a significant rise in catecholamines as measured by plasma, epinephrine and norepinephrine levels. This fact was important because the rise in catecholamines further accentuated metabolic acidosis by increasing peripheral resistance and, subsequently, tissue hypoxia.

The above studies are in agreement with those of other investigators[30, 38, 42, 43, 53], who showed that with large volumes of haemodilution the addition of buffer base was mandatory. Also, buffering was recommended when small primes were used or longer perfusions anticipated. The overall conclusion, however, was that haemodilution or non-haemic primes could safely be used without severe or significant metabolic disturbances and that acid–base balance could be maintained with the use of buffering solutions.

Haematological alterations
Intra- and postoperative haemorrhage continue to be an important factor in open-heart surgery. The haematological alterations have been related to the duration of perfusion, the type of oxygenator, trauma to the blood elements by the open-heart suction system and, finally, to the use of the anticoagulant, heparin. Phillips, Malm and Deterling[51] using a DeWall bubble oxygenator, found that factor II (prothrombin), factor V (proaccelerin) and factor III (thromboplastin) generation were decreased during heparinization but reversed with protamine administration. The most important factor which caused severe bleeding was hypofibrinogenaemia due to a consump-

tive coagulopathy. This process began during perfusion and continued postoperatively. This result suggests that the activation of the fibrinolytic system was initiated by tissue extracts and trauma to the blood, and was one of the factors responsible for postoperative haemorrhage. Perkins[49] studied the effects of both different oxygenators and different perfusates. Electrolyte solutions caused a decrease in factor I, increased the fibrinolysis rate. The difference was the greatest at the end of bypass but progressively decreased afterwards.

With improved tissue perfusion by the use of non-haemic prime, coagulopathies and postoperative haemorrhage have been markedly decreased as reported by Neville[41] and Litwak *et al.*[30]. Neville noted increased postoperative bleeding only when the patients had either (fibrinogen), factor II (prothrombin) and factor V (proaccelerin) and previous transfusions or perfusions and then only when the preoperative coagulation profile was abnormal.

No definitive studies have proven that haemodilution itself has improved blood coagulation. The results, as mentioned above, indicated that haemodilution should be recognized, along with progress in oxygenators, open-heart suction systems and operative techniques, as a factor in the overall improvement in haematological alterations after heart-lung bypass.

Fluid balance and electrolyte distribution

Not all the effects of haemodilution or non-haemic primes are entirely beneficial, especially as far as fluid balance and electrolyte distribution are concerned. It was discovered early in the use of haemodilution that, usually, during bypass additional perfusate had to be used. Then at the completion of bypass it was necessary to reinfuse the patient with a large portion of the diluted perfusate in order to restore normal cardiovascular haemodynamics. This fluid load could be given to the patient safely with careful monitoring of central venous pressure and other functional parameters.

Numerous studies clearly demonstrated a consistent increase in the extracellular fluid compartment during and after haemodilution[3, 7, 8, 15, 26, 46]. Neville, Thomason and Hirsch[46] reported that, in addition to an expansion of the extracellular fluid, total body water and blood volume were increased. Of the latter, there was a significant increase in plasma volume associated with an actual decrease in the red blood cell mass. Cleland *et al.*[7] verified the increase in extracellular fluid, mainly the interstitial component, but showed that there was no increase in total body water as there was an actual decrease in both plasma volume and red blood cell mass. This work correlated well with that of DeBoer[15] and Cohn, Angell and Shumway[8]. The latter two groups then, in addition, compared fluid balance in patients with and without congestive heart failure and found a greater increase in the extracellular fluid volume in the failure group. This latter finding probably was related to neurohumoral factors causing further retention of salt and water.

These observers found that in the early postoperative period the excess extracellular and interstitial fluid re-entered the intravascular compartment and re-expanded the blood volume. This fluid shift occurred mainly during the first four postoperative days, when sodium excretion was at its lowest point[8]. Clearly, the knowledge of this fluid redistribution was important, for the re-entry of excess fluid into the intravascular space could promote congestive heart failure. As a result, fluid restriction and/or the judicious use of diuretics during this time was necessary.

The exact reasons for the above fluid shifts during and after haemodilution perfusion were unclear. It had been known that similar fluid alterations occur after major surgery with leakage of fluid out of the vascular compartment into the extracellular or interstitial space. Whether these changes are due to the stress of surgery, damage to cells and capillaries, or red cell sequestration has still not been totally explained. Das, Eraklis and Gross[13] and Beattie *et al.*[3] related the fluid shifts to the osmolarity and oncosity of the plasma. A minimal increase in tissue water and cation content was found following iso-osmolar perfusions, while a significant rise of intracellular water and cations followed the use of a hyperosmolar prime[13]. The expanded extracellular fluid volume associated with a reduced intravascular volume was directly related to a reduction in the serum oncotic pressure[3]. It was only after the first postoperative week that the fluid compartments were restored to preoperative levels coincident with a return of serum oncosity to normal. Whether the haemodiluted perfusate caused these fluid shifts purely by dilution or by directly injuring the cells themselves remains to be elucidated.

Haemodilution perfusion is also followed by changes in electrolyte distribution. The majority of studies indicated relatively minor changes in both intravascular and extravascular sodium and chloride concentrations[8, 14, 15, 46]. For the most part, the urinary excretion of both sodium and chloride was not altered significantly, though recently Cohn, Angell and Shumway[8] reported a marked decrease in urinary sodium during the first four postoperative days. Most important, however, was the finding of a consistent hypokalaemia and kaluresis after the use of haemodilution well documented by Das[14], Eraklis and Gross[13] in a study of 500 patients perfused with lactated Ringer's solution prime. Dieter, Neville and Pifarré[16, 17] showed that the changes in serum and urinary potassium were significantly accentuated by the preoperative use of diuretics and recommended prophylactic administration of potassium during the pre- and intraoperative period.

In addition, other observations regarding electrolytes and body metabolites have been published, but their clinical significance remains to be clearly defined. Dieter, Neville and Pifarré[17] reported a definite decrease in the serum content of carbon dioxide, calcium, phosphorus, magnesium and zinc. Das *et al.*[12, 14] found that calcium metabolism was fairly stable during haemodilution perfusion and related the changes in serum ionic calcium to the use of citrated blood. Dieter, Neville and Pifarré[17] correlated the fall in serum zinc with a rise in lactic acid dehydrogenase, a pattern seen also after myocardial infarctions. The fact that the concentration of zinc was high in both cardiac muscle and certain enzymes as lactic acid dehydrogenase, plus the similarity of the findings after haemodilution perfusion and myocardial infarction, left certain unanswered questions. Finally, work by Malm, Debbes and Nahas[32] and Moffitt *et al.*[38] has suggested that the perfusion medium has an effect on certain metabolites such as glucose, fatty acids and lactate, and may significantly alter metabolic pathways within the body.

Current clinical application of haemodilution and non-haemic primes

History

The progressive use of haemodilution has been reflected in the changing nature of the techniques used in the Thoracic Surgical Service of the Presbyterian Hospital in the City of New York. Until 1967, the disc oxygenator primed completely with buffered ACD blood was used. Beginning early that year, the Temptrol disposable bubble oxygenator* was introduced on a part-time basis, and by the middle of 1968 was in full-time use. Partial haemodilution was introduced at this time, with the prime consisting of an almost equal part of buffered ACD blood and balanced electrolyte solution. In March, 1971, the total non-haemic prime was introduced, and since then over 2000 open-heart operations have been performed using the subsequently described perfusion techniques.

Three different disposable oxygenators are used depending both on the size of the patient and the calculated flow. These oxygenators are the following:

(1) The Spiroflo BOS-10* adult oxygenator for flows of 2.8 ℓ/min and above.
(2) The Q-110 Temptrol* paediatric oxygenator for flows of 1.2 to 2.8 ℓ/min.
(3) The H-400† model infant oxygenator for flows up to 1.1 ℓ/min.

The Q-220F* model cardiotomy reservoir is used for open-heart suction. Incorporated in this device is a compressed foam rubber filter; thus a separate in-line suction filter is not necessary. With the exception of any medications, all blood and fluids used for the original or additional primes pass through this reservoir and filter.

Adult group

All adult patients are perfused with a flow calculated at 2.3 ℓ/min per m^2 and for this the BOS-10 model oxygenator is used for flows of 2.8 ℓ/min and above. All adult patients receive a total non-haemic prime, save for those patients with severe anaemia, marked congestive heart failure with anasarca or chronic infection.

The total non-haemic priming volume is 1700 ml dextrose 5 mg/100ml and lactated Ringer's solution and 300 ml of 25 per cent normal serum albumin (50 g/1000 ml of non-haemic priming fluid).

If a haemodiluted prime is used in the instances mentioned above the total priming solution is 1780 ml of which 500 ml is CPD (citrated phosphate dextrose) blood and approximately 1280 ml of other fluids. The latter is composed of 500 ml lactated Ringer's solution, 500 ml dextrose 5mg/100ml

*Bentley Laboratories, Santa Ana, California, USA
†William Harvey Research Corporation, Santa Ana, California, USA

and lactated Ringer's solution, 65 ml CPD solution in the blood, 200 ml (50 g) of 25 per cent normal serum albumin, 6 ml calcium chloride (600 mg), 8 ml sodium bicarbonate (8 mmol) and 2 ml sodium heparin (20 mg).

Careful monitoring of the blood balance and haematocrit is carried out throughout the bypass procedure. The haematocrit is checked at the start of bypass and at half-hourly intervals thereafter. If the calculated flow and a satisfactory perfusion pressure are maintained, no extra fluid is added to the perfusate. If either the flow or the pressure fall, and additional fluid is necessary, lactated Ringer's solution is added if the haematocrit is greater than 25 per cent; otherside CPD blood is used. The amount added is that which is necessary to refill the oxygenator reservoir to the minimal level while the calculated flow rate and perfusion pressure are maintained. For each additional 500 ml of CPD blood the following medications are also added: 2 ml sodium heparin (20 mg), 6 ml calcium chloride (600 mg) and 8 ml sodium bicarbonate (8 mmol).

Paediatric group

Paediatric patients are classified as those over 8 months of age or heavier than 5 kg weight and for them the flow is calculated at 2.3 ℓ/min per m^2. The Q-110 model oxygenator is used for calculated flows of 1.1 to 2.8 ℓ/min.

A total non-haemic prime is used for children over 20 kg weight or in instances of significant polycythaemia in smaller patients. The non-haemic prime for this oxygenator is 1200 ml which consists of 500 ml lactated Ringer's solution, 500 ml dextrose 5 mg/100ml and lactated Ringer's solution and 200 ml (50 g) of 25 per cent normal serum albumin. If a haemodiluted prime is used again the total volume is 1230 ml of which 500 ml is CPD blood. The remaining prime consists of 300 ml lactated Ringer's solution, 300 ml dextrose 5 mg/100ml and lactated Ringer's solution, 65 ml CPD solution in the blood, 2 ml sodium heparin (20 mg) and 200 ml (50 g) 25 per cent of normal serum albumin. Again, for each additional 500 ml of CPD blood used, heparin, sodium bicarbonate and calcium chloride are added.

Infant group

Infants are classified from newborn to 6 months of age or 5 kg in weight. For these patients the H-400 model oxygenator is used for flow rates up to 1.1 ℓ/min. At this age and size the flows are calculated at 210 ml/kg of body weight up to 6 weeks of age and at 200 ml/kg of body weight from 6 weeks to 6 months of age rather than on surface area basis. In the majority of infants the haemodiluted prime is used rather than a total non-haemic one. The priming volume is 747 ml and consists of 500 ml of CPD blood, 175 ml of dextrose 2.5 mg/100ml in half-strength normal saline, 65 ml CPD solution in the blood, 8 ml sodium bicarbonate (8 mmol), 6 ml calcium chloride (600 mg) 2 ml sodium heparin (20 mg), 50 ml (12.5 g) of 25 per cent normal serum albumin. If a non-haemic prime is used, such as in those cases of severe polycythaemia, the total priming volume is 650 ml of which 300 ml is lactated Ringer's solution, 300 ml dextrose 5 mg/100 ml and lactated

Ringer's solution and 50 ml (12.5 g) of 25 per cent normal serum albumin. Again, similar monitoring procedures are carried out, and replacement fluid is usually CPD blood. For each increment of blood used, proportionate amounts of sodium bicarbonate, sodium heparin, and calcium chloride are also added.

General perfusion technique

Total body heparinization is achieved prior to the start of bypass. After a baseline activated clotting time (ACT) determination, a dosage of 1 to 2 mg/kg of heparin is administered. Allowing 5 minutes for intravascular mixing a second ACT sample is obtained. ACTs are calculated using the Hemochron 800 blood coagulation timer*. This data is entered into a Texas Instrument TI-59 programmable calculator with a PC-100A thermal printer†. The calculator properly programmed then calculates future heparin dosage, based on the heparin-dose response curve, to maintain an ACT of between 480 to 600 seconds. At the termination of bypass the required protamine dosage is also calculated using the programmable calculator. During bypass, ACTs are checked every 30 minutes and 5 minutes after every heparin dose.

Cardiopulmonary bypass is instituted by arterial perfusion through the ascending aorta, if possible, or through one of the external iliac arteries. Large-bore venous catheters are placed in the superior and inferior venae cavae for venous drainage. The arterial pump is started slowly to allow mixing of the patient's blood with the priming fluid, while simultaneously the clamps are removed from the venous lines. The arterial flow is gradually increased until the calculated flow is reached, along with a satisfactory perfusion pressure. Thereafter the main perfusion pressure is maintained at approximately 50–80 mmHg and the central venous pressure below 10 mmHg. At the same time the accompanying oxygen flow delivered to the oxygenator is increased according to blood flow and temperature and the requirements of the oxygenator. A mixture of 98 per cent oxygen and 2 per cent carbon dioxide is used. Anaesthesia is maintained during bypass with such drugs as Morphine Sulfate, Valium and Curare given directly into the oxygenator. Halothane may also be used.

The patient's temperature is controlled by a heat exchanger incorporated in the Temptrol oxygenator and usually is lowered to 24°C for most adult patients.

The acid–base balance is checked at the beginning of bypass and any base deficit is corrected by sodium bicarbonate. The amount is calculated from the base deficit multiplied by the weight of the patient in kilograms. The arterial blood gases are checked again in one-half hour after the initial correction and any additional correction is then carried out. Urinary output is carefully monitored and for any significant haematuria or anuria, mannitol is added in amounts of 200 mg/kg of body weight if deemed necessary.

*International Technidyne, Metuchen, New Jersey, USA
†Texas Instrument, Lubbock, Texas, USA

Myocardial preservation is obtained with the use of cardioplegic solution at 4°C. The solution consists of 1000 ml Normosol-R, 30 mmol potassium chloride, 50 mmol sodium bicarbonate, and 25 g of 25 per cent normal serum albumin. The cardioplegic solution is injected by syringe either directly into the coronary ostia or into the root of the aorta. The dosage of cardioplegic solution is 30 ml/kg of body weight, an amount which renders a flaccid, non-fibrillating heart. The dosage is repeated approximately every 30 minutes. The solution has a pH of 7.5, an osmolality of 380 mmol, and a specific gravity of 1.017. The majority of this solution is discarded and not returned to the heart-lung machine.

At the completion of cardiopulmonary bypass, the blood balance is roughly calculated from the amount of perfusate used, the fluid loss in the operating field and the urinary output. By observing the cardiac action and output, arterial, central venous, and left atrial pressure, as much of the perfusion fluid as possible is transfused back into the patient. When the operating surgeon judges that the patient's blood balance has been restored, protamine sulphate is administered and decannulation is carried out.

Results

At the Columbia-Presbyterian Hospital, a non-haemic prime for extracorporeal circulation has been used recently in all patients over 20 kilograms in body weight. The data presented here are from an analysis over a 6 year period of the first 50 consecutive patients undergoing perfusion by this technique.

There was a striking decrease in the total amount of blood used for open-heart surgery. The previous average blood utilization for all open-heart surgery at our institution was 6500 ml. In contrast, an average of 750 ml of whole CPD preserved blood was used during bypass for all cases, and a total of 3200 ml of whole blood was used during an average adult hospitalization. This has resulted in a decrease in the incidence of hepatitis among the adult population. The use of the infant and paediatric disposable oxygenator reduced the initial blood prime to 500 ml and an average of 1200 ml of blood was used during the entire hospitalization of these patients.

Urinary flow during bypass varied between 20 and 100 ml/hour, with very few patients demonstrating haematuria. Urinary output ranged from 40 to 100 ml/hour during the first 12 hours postoperatively, a figure which was augmented easily with diuretics if clinically necessary. Metabolic acidosis was absent during bypass, as the pH ranged between 7.35 and 7.45 with the base excess being +5 or less. Any variations were easily corrected with sodium bicarbonate.

Coagulation parameters were studied during bypass and found within the normal range save for a consistent fall in the fibrinogen level to 125–185 mg/100ml. This value was presumed to be due to the haemodilution, as immediately postoperatively it returned to the normal range. Prothrombin times were always within 3 seconds of the control values and the Lee–White clotting times were not greater than 12 minutes. During bypass, the haematocrit averaged 31 per cent after the perfusate was supplemented by either blood or crystalloid solution. Immediately after bypass, following reinfusion of the perfusate, the haematocrit averaged 38 per cent. During the first 12 postoperative hours, the haematocrit was maintained above 30 per cent with the infusion of an average of 700 ml of blood per adult patient. During this same interval, the chest drainage averaged 500 ml of blood. Two patients required reoperation for persistent postoperative bleeding, and over the past two years the overall reoperation rate has been 5 per cent whereas previously it had been 10 per cent. This improvement obviously was due to many combined factors in addition to the use of the non-haemic prime.

Serum electrolytes and blood urea nitrogen were normal during bypass. The blood sugar was consistently elevated to the 400–600 mg/100 ml range, due to the dextrose content of the perfusate. Serum total protein, albumin and calcium were reduced proportional to the amount of haemodilution. Postoperatively, the serum electrolytes were again within the normal limits, including the serum potassium which averaged 3.5 mmol/ℓ (normal range for our laboratory 3.2–4.6 mmol/ℓ). Serum total protein and calcium returned to the normal range. The blood sugar initially remained elevated in the 200–400 mg/100ml range, but gradually returned to normal during the first 8 postoperative hours.

The disadvantages of the use of non-haemic prime have been few. The maintenance of calculated flows and perfusion pressures during bypass required additional perfusate in almost all cases. As a result, the patients returned to the recovery room with an expanded extracellular fluid volume and the adult patients weighed, on the average, between 4 and 6 pounds above their preoperative weight. It was clear, however, that the cardiovascular system could tolerate this excess fluid load and, with the use of fluid restriction and/or diuretics, the patients returned to their preoperative weights by the end of the first postoperative week.

Summary

The progress in extracorporeal circulation techniques over the past two decades has been remarkable. In many centres where blood is readily available, fresh blood is still used as perfusate. In the majority of cardiac centres, however, some form of haemodilution is used today, much to the relief of the suppliers of blood.

In discussing the development and the results of haemodilution, it is impossible to attribute all the progress in extracorporeal circulation to haemodilution alone as there have been many other factors, such as the improvement in equipment and operative technique, which have been equally important. In addition, the fact that numerous investigators used different combinations of haemodiluted solutions, along with a variety of oxygenators, led to difficulty in comparing results. Despite the above, certain definite statements can be made. A haemodiluted or a non-haemic priming solution have proved to be satisfactory and effective perfusates for cardiopulmonary bypass within the boundaries described above. The advantages of haemodilution as recorded by adequate tissue perfusion, diminution of pulmonary, renal, haematological and acid–base disturbances, far outweigh the disadvantages. With careful attention to details, the problems associated with haemodilution perfusion, such as the development of hypokalaemia, can be anticipated and adequately treated. Finally, modifications in haemodilution perfusates and perfusion techniques, such as have occurred at Presbyterian Hospital, can be expected to continue until the majority of the still unknown questions are answered.

References

1. Ankeney, J. S. and Murthy, S. K. 'A study of peripheral (IVC and SVC) and central (spanchnic) venous flow rates during extracorporeal bypass.' *Journal of Thoracic and Cardiovascular Surgery*, **44,** 589 (1962)
2. Baue, A. E., Nusbaum, M., Anstadt, G. and Blakemore, W. S. 'The pattern of lymphatic flow during extracorporeal circulation.' *Journal of Thoracic and Cardiovascular Surgery*, **50,** 648 (1965)
3. Beattie, H. W., Evans, G., Garnett, E. S. and Webber, C. E. 'Sustained hypovolaemia and extracellular fluid volume expansion following cardiopulmonary bypass.' *Surgery*, **71,** 891 (1972)
4. Bigelow, J. C., Dobbs, J. L. and Fogdahl, R. P. 'Acid-citrate dextrose vs. heparinized whole blood prime.' *Archives of Surgery, Chicago*, **96,** 65 (1968)
5. Blakemore, W. S. 'Diluents for priming in cardiopulmonary bypass.' *Surgery*, **62,** 981 (1967)
6. Camishon, R. C., Fraimow, W., Kelsey, D. M., Tokunaga, K., Davies, A. L., Joshi, P., Cathcart, R. T. and Pierucci, L. 'Effect of partial and total cardiopulmonary bypass with whole blood in haemodilution priming on pulmonary surfactant activity.' *Journal of Surgical Research*, **8,** 1 (1968)
7. Cleland, J., Pluth, H. R., Tauxe, W. N. and Kirklin, J. W. 'Blood volume and body fluid compartment changes soon after closed and open intracardiac surgery.' *Journal of Thoracic and Cardiovascular Surgery*, **52,** 698 (1966)
8. Cohn, L. H., Angell, W.W. and Shumway, N. E. 'Body fluid shifts after cardiopulmonary bypass.' *Journal of Thoracic and Cardiovascular Surgery*, **62,** 423 (1971)
9. Cooley, D. A., Beall, A. C., Jr. and Alexander, J. K. 'Acute massive pulmonary embolism: successful surgical treatment using temporary cardiopulmonary bypass.' *Journal of the American Medical Association*, **177,** 283 (1961)
10. Cooley, D. A., Beall, A. C., Jr. and Grondin, P. 'Open-heart operations with disposable oxygenators, 5% dextrose prime and normothermia.' *Surgery*, **52,** 713 (1962)
11. Cruz, A. B., Jr. and Callaghan, J. C. 'Haemodilution in extracorporeal circulation: large or small non-blood prime.' *Journal of Thoracic and Cardiovascular Surgery*, **52,** 690 (1966)
12. Das, J. B., Eraklis, A. J., Adams, J. G. and Gross, R. E. 'Changes in serum ionic calcium during cardiopulmonary bypass with haemodilution.' *Journal of Thoracic and Cardiovascular Surgery*, **62,** 449 (1971)
13. Das, J. B., Eraklis, A. J. and Gross, R. E. 'Water and cation content of red blood cells and muscle tissue before and after cardiopulmonary bypass.' *Journal of Thoracic and Cardiovascular Surgery*, **57,** 824 (1969)
14. Das, J. B., Eraklis, A. J. and Jones, J. E. 'Water and solute excretion following cardiopulmonary bypass with haemodilution.' *Journal of Thoracic and Cardiovascular Surgery*, **58,** 789 (1969)

15. DeBoer, A. 'Body fluid compartment change following large volume haemodilution.' *Archives of Surgery, Chicago*, **98**, 602 (1969)
16. Dieter, R. A., Neville, W. E. and Pifarré, R. 'Hypokalaemia following haemodilution cardiopulmonary bypass.' *Annals of Surgery*, **171**, 17 (1970)
17. Dieter, R. A., Neville, W. E. and Pifarré, R. 'Serum electrolyte changes after cardiopulmonary bypass with Ringer's lactate solution used for haemodilution.' *Journal of Thoracic and Cardiovascular Surgery*, **59**, 168 (1970)
18. Dieter, R. A., Neville, W. E., Pifarré, R. and Jasuja, M. 'Preoperative coagulation profiles and posthaemodilution cardiopulmonary bypass haemorrhage.' *American Journal of Surgery*, **121**, 689 (1971)
19. Dow, J. W. 'The shock state in heart-lung bypass in dogs.' *Transactions of the American Society for Artificial Internal Organs*, **5**, 240 (1959)
20. Finley, T. N., Swenson, E. Q., Clements, J., Gardner, R. E., Wright, R. R. and Severinghaus, J. W. 'Changes in mechanical properties, appearance of surface activity of extracts of one lung following occlusion of its pulmonary artery in the dog.' (Abstr.) *Physiologist*, **3**, 56 (1960)
21. Fisk, G. C. and Steedman, D. M. 'Haemodilution in clinical extracorporeal circulation: some effects on serum albumin.' *Australian and New Zealand Journal of Surgery*, **37**, 153 (1967)
22. Foote, A. V., Trede, M. and Maloney, J. V., Jr. 'An experimental and clinical study of the use of acid-citrate-dextrose (ACD) blood for extracorporeal circulation.' *Journal of Thoracic and Cardiovascular Surgery*, **42**, 93 (1961)
23. Gadboys, H. T., Litwak, R. S., Wallace, H. W., Kahn, M., Kochwa, S. and Buerger, W. 'Experimental large volume haemodilution with plasma.' *Journal of Thoracic and Cardiovascular Surgery*, **52**, 112 (1966)
24. Gadboys, H. T., Slonim, R. and Litwak, R. S. 'Homologous blood syndrome. 1. Preliminary observations on its relationship to clinical cardiopulmonary bypass.' *Annals of Surgery*, **156**, 793 (1962)
25. Gardner, R. W., Finley, T. N. and Tooley, W. H. 'The effects of cardiopulmonary bypass on surface of lung extracts.' *Bulletin de la Société Internationale de Chirurgie*, **21**, 542 (1962)
26. Gollub, S., Schechter, D. C., Schaefer, C., Svigals, R. and Bailey, C. P. 'Absolute haemodilution cardiopulmonary bypass: free water distribution and protein mobilization in body compartments.' *American Heart Journal*, **78**, 626 (1969)
27. Greer, A. E., Carey, J. M. and Zuhdi, N. 'Haemodilution principle of hypothermic perfusion: a concept obviating blood priming.' *Journal of Thoracic and Cardiovascular Surgery*, **43**, 640 (1962)
28. Hepps, S. A., Roe, B. R., Wright, R. R. and Gardner, R. E. 'Amelioration of the pulmonary postperfusion syndrome with haemodilution and low molecular weight dextran.' *Surgery*, **54**, 232 (1963)
29. Hirsch, D. M., Hadidian, C. and Neville, W. E. 'Oxygen consumption during cardiopulmonary bypass with large volume haemodilution.' *Journal of Thoracic and Cardiovascular Surgery*, **56**, 197 (1968)
30. Litwak, R. S., Gadboys, H. L., Kahn, M. and Wisoff, B. G. 'High flow total body perfusion utilizing diluted perfusate in a large prime system.' *Journal of Thoracic and Cardiovascular Surgery*, **49**, 74 (1965)
31. Long, D. M., Todd, C. B., Indeglia, R. A., Varco, R. L. and Lillehei, C. W. 'Clinical use of dextran-40 in extracorporeal circulation. A summary of 5 years' experience.' *Transfusion*, **6**, 401 (1966)
32. Malm, J. R., Debbas, E. and Nahas, G. G. 'Modified oxygenator performance fluid for cardiac surgery.' In *Body Fluid Replacement in the Surgical Patient*. Eds Charles L. Fox, Jr. and G. G. Nahas. p. 78. New York: Grune and Stratton (1970)

33. Malm, J. R., Manger, W. M., Sullivan, S. F., Pappas, E. M. and Nahas, G. G. 'The effect of acidosis on sympatho-adrenal stimulation.' *Journal of the American Medical Association*, **197,** 121 (1966)
34. Malm, J. R., Sullivan, S. F., Patterson, R. W., Bowman, F. O., Jr. and Nahas, G. G. 'The use of ACD blood titrated with THAM in extracorporeal circulation.' *Transactions of the American Society for Artificial Internal Organs*, **9,** 216 (1963)
35. Mandelbaum, I., Giamonna, S. T. and Schumacher, H. B. 'Extracorporeal circulation, pulmonary compliance and pulmonary surfactant.' *Journal of Thoracic and Cardiovascular Surgery*, **48,** 881 (1964)
36. Mielke, J. E., Hunt, J. C., Maher, F. T. and Kirklin, J. W. 'Renal performance during clinical cardiopulmonary bypass with and without haemodilution.' *Journal of Thoracic and Cardiovascular Surgery*, **51,** 229 (1966)
37. Miyauchi, Y., Kwong, K. and Paton, B. C. 'Haemodilution perfusion in cyanotic dogs—physiological studies.' *Journal of Surgical Research*, **8,** 360 (1968)
38. Moffitt, E. A., White, R. D., Molnar, G. D. and McGoon, D. C. 'Comparative effects of whole blood haemodiluted and clear priming solutions on myocardial and body metabolism in man.' *Canadian Journal of Surgery*, **14,** 382 (1971)
39. Nahas, G. G., Malm, J. R., Manger, W. M., Verosky, M. and Sullivan, S. F. 'Controls of acidosis and the use of titrated ACD blood in open-heart surgery.' *Annals of Surgery*, **160,** 1049 (1964)
40. Neptune, W. B., Bougas, J. A. and Panico, F. G. 'Open-heart surgery without the need for donor blood priming in the pump oxygenator.' *New England Journal of Medicine*, **263,** 111 (1960)
41. Neville, W. E. 'Extracorporeal circulation.' In *Current Problems in Surgery*. Ed. W. E. Neville. Chicago: Yearbook Medical Publishers (1967)
42. Neville, W. E., Colby, C., Peacock, H. and Kronkowski, T. C. 'Superiority of buffered Ringer's lactate to heparinized blood as total prime of the large volume disc oxygenator.' *American Surgeon*, **165,** 206 (1965)
43. Neville, W. E., Faber, L. P. and Peacock, H. 'Total prime of the disc oxygenator with Ringer's lactate solution for cardiopulmonary bypass.' *Diseases of the Chest*, **45,** 320 (1964)
44. Neville, W. E., Kontaxis, A., Gavan, T. and Clowes, G. H. A. 'Post perfusion pulmonary vasculitis and its relationship to blood trauma.' *Archives of Surgery, Chicago*, **86,** 126 (1963)
45. Neville, W. E. and Talso, P. J. 'Postperfusion compartmental fluid alterations.' *Surgery*, **63,** 220 (1968)
46. Neville, W. E., Thomason, R. D. and Hirsch, D. M. 'Postperfusion hypervolaemia after haemodilution cardiopulmonary bypass.' *Archives of Surgery, Chicago*, **93,** 715 (1966)
47. Panico, F. G. and Neptune, W. B. 'A mechanism to eliminate the donor blood prime from the pump oxygenator.' *Surgical Forum*, **10,** 605 (1959)
48. Paton, B. C. and Rosenkrantz, J. 'Non-haemic priming fluids for extracorporeal circulation.' *Diseases of the Chest*, **18,** 311 (1965)
49. Perkins, H. A. 'Effects of extracorporeal circulation on blood.' *Transfusion*, **6,** 357 (1966)
50. Phillips, L. L. and Malm, J. R. 'Coagulation parameters following extracorporeal circulation using ACD blood buffered with THAM.' *Transfusion*, **7,** 185 (1967)
51. Phillips, L. L., Malm, J. R. and Deterling, R. A. 'Coagulation defects following extracorporeal circulation.' *Annals of Surgery*, **157,** 317 (1963)
52. Porter, G. A., Starr, A., Kimsey, J. and Lenertz, H. 'Mannitol haemodilution perfusion.' *Journal of Surgical Research*, **7,** 447 (1967)

53. Roe, B. B., Swenson, E. E., Hepps, S. A. and Bruns, D. L. 'Total body perfusion in cardiac operations with perfusate of balanced electrolytes and low molecular weight dextran.' *Archives of Surgery, Chicago*, **88,** 128 (1964)
54. Schechter, D. C. and Sarot, I. A. 'Hydrokinetics of haemodilution cardiopulmonary bypass.' *Diseases of the Chest*, **54,** 53 (1968)
55. Schechter, D. C. and Sarot, I. A. 'The potential hazards of immoderate haemodilution in cardiac surgery.' *Diseases of the Chest*, **55,** 94 (1969)
56. Sessler, A. D., Taswell, H. F., Moffitt, E. A. and Kirklin, J. W. 'Heparinized blood versus ACD blood for cardiopulmonary bypass.' *Transfusion*, **6,** 360 (1966)
57. Smith, W. W., Brown, I. W., Young, W. G. and Sealy, W. C. 'Studies of EDGLUGATE-Mg. A new donor blood anticoagulant-preservative mixture for extracorporeal circulation.' *Journal of Thoracic and Cardiovascular Surgery*, **38,** 573 (1959)
58. Stremmel, W., Schlosser, V. and Koehnlein, H. E. 'Effect of open-heart surgery with haemodilution perfusion upon insulin secretion.' *Journal of Thoracic and Cardiovascular Surgery*, **64,** 263 (1972)
59. Vasko, K. A., Riley, A. M. and Dewall, R. A. 'Poloxalkol® (Pluronic F-68): A priming solution for cardiopulmonary bypass.' *Transactions of the American Society for Artificial Internal Organs*, **28,** 526 (1972)
60. Zuhdi, N. 'Hypothermic and haemodilution techniques in cardiac surgery.' In *Cardiac Surgery* 2nd edn. Ed. J. C. Norman. Ch. 8, p. 159. New York: Appleton-Century-Crofts (1972)
61. Zuhdi, N., McCollough, B., Carey, J. and Greer, A. E. 'Double helical reservoir heart lung machine designed for hypothermic perfusion.' *Archives of Surgery, Chicago*, **82,** 320 (1961)
62. Zuhdi, N., McCollough, B., Carey, J., Krieger, C. and Greer, A. 'Hypothermic perfusion for open-heart surgical procedures: report on the use of a heart-lung machine primed with 5% dextrose in water inducing haemodilution.' *Journal of the International College of Surgeons*, **35,** 379 (1961)

9

Anaesthesia for Extracorporeal Circulation

V. Antony Grimshaw and
Michael D. Hargreaves

dimidum facti, qui coepit, habet

Introduction

Open-heart surgery, and the use of extracorporeal circulation for vital organ support, may be indicated for a broad range of conditions in patients of all ages from the very young to the very old. Within this broad span there are many influences on the anaesthetist in the way he approaches his task. The use of extracorporeal circulation itself adds its own constraints. The need to maintain anaesthesia without significantly reducing the concentration of oxygen in the fresh gas flowing to the artificial lung, which in all practical forms depends for its oxygenating capacity on a high gas-blood oxygen tension gradient, denying the anaesthetist the option to use nitrous oxide as part of an 'inhalational' technique, demonstrates the truth of this. When the perfusion technique includes the use of whole body mild or moderate hypothermia (with minimum body core temperatures of 28°C or 20°C respectively), the anaesthetist's task is, on balance, made easier, and the extracorporeal perfusion period is made safer for the patient. Other special techniques used with extracorporeal circulation, for example the use of profound hypothermia (with a minimum body temperature significantly below 20°C), or the use of local coronary perfusion with special solutions ('cardioplegia'), may increase the hazard for the patient and add to the problems of patient care for the anaesthetist and other members of the surgical team, but because they make it possible to extend the scope or quality of the surgical procedure, they are justified, even necessary, in clinical practice and must be accommodated in the anaesthetist's thinking. Such techniques may not have a direct influence on anaesthetic technique as such, but they often involve the anaesthetist, either directly, as in an additional role, for their provision, or through the anaesthetist's interest in and responsibility for the overall wellbeing of the patient.

Nonetheless, the dominant factors influencing anaesthetic practice during surgery with extracorporeal circulation come from the pathophysiological consequences of the condition of the patient, the disease itself, and the effects of surgery, especially during the perioperative and immediate postoperative periods. Against this background the anaesthetist must examine the different approaches open to him, the particular pharmacology of the drugs he chooses and the special circumstances in which he is working – the equipment, supporting staff and other facilities open to him, and the preferences of the surgeon. In any successful cardiac surgical team the anaesthetist must be able to work effectively with the surgeon. In the final analysis the methods used by anaesthetists in similar surgical procedures may differ not only because of differences in physical resources or in the emphasis placed on different aspects of the assessment of the patient, but also on personal preferences, depending on what an individual anaesthetist feels is best for him. Often in anaesthesia the safest technique is the one the anaesthetist knows from experience will best suit his circumstances and temperament.

As in other surgical disciplines, anaesthesia for extracorporeal circulation is influenced by the age and general health of the patient. In the old, the debilitated and particularly in the very young, although the underlying principles may be the same, even greater refinement of technique is often necessary.

These matters will be discussed in turn, beginning with the general approach of the anaesthetist to the cardiac patient, factors influencing the anaesthetist's assessment, and the broad choices of technique available to him. These general considerations will then be followed by an account of the authors' technique with observations on alternative methods available or in use in other centres. The chapter ends with a reference to the anaesthetist's role in postoperative care.

The anaesthetist's approach to the cardiac patient

General anaesthesia is essential. The anaesthetic objectives can be simply stated: to give peaceful oblivion to the patient; to provide optimal operating conditions for the surgeon; and to achieve these requirements within the paramount necessity of safety for the patient. It is also desirable that these objectives should be obtained with a high degree of certainty. This argues for a measure of standardization on a small number of proven techniques which require minimal modification from patient to patient.

The effects of serious heart disease on the circulation and hence on the function of other organ systems also, make early assessment and preparation of the patient essential. Only in the most extreme emergency can any departure from this rule be justified. The anaesthetist is perhaps fortunate that in cardiac surgery, more than in most other surgical disciplines, the surgeon (and the cardiologist) recognize the identity of interest which they have with the anaesthetist in ensuring an optimum preoperative condition for the patient.

In the immediate preoperative period, anxiety is likely to increase circulatory decompensation, and reduce the effectiveness of preoperative preparation. If the patient is positively motivated towards surgery, because the procedure has been fully explained to him, and perhaps because he recognizes the limited possibilities of other lines of treatment, he is likely to approach the actual operative day with less anxiety, even in some cases with enthusiasm. The anaesthetist has a major role in achieving this. He must establish a relationship with the patient at a preoperative visit and explain what the planned procedure involves, particularly in relation to the anaesthetic and postoperative intensive care unit. He must also be prepared to answer questions concerning the surgical treatment itself. The anaesthetist must therefore inform himself of the surgeon's intentions in sufficient detail to avoid any lack of patient confidence at this stage. The anaesthetist will confirm for himself the general condition of the patient and he should also arrange preoperative sedation and premedication for the day of operation and explain this to the patient also. During his examination of the patient the anaesthetist will assess the availability of peripheral vessels for induction drugs and monitoring lines and he will obtain early warning of any likelihood of airway or tracheal intubation problems.

Where the anaesthetist plays a direct role in the organization of perfusion techniques he will ensure that the relevant data are available for the calculation of blood flow during extracorporeal circulation.

Some physiological considerations

Venous return

Under normal circumstances venous return to the right atrium results from the combined effect of the onward flow of blood from the arterial side of the microcirculation into the peripheral veins, and the venous tone. This is aided, particularly in the erect posture, by the action of voluntary muscles compressing the valved veins intermittently, and by spontaneous inspiratory effort which tends to pull blood into the thorax by the same reduction of intrathoracic pressure which, transmitted to the alveoli, draws air into the lungs. This situation continues prior to the induction of anaesthesia and, although the muscle pump is likely to be less active in a premedicated patient, at least the recumbent posture reduces the effect of gravity on venous return from the dependent parts of the body.

At induction, the central and peripheral effects of general anaesthetics and some other drugs which may be used, such as analgesics, most intravenous inducing agents and the commonly used muscular relaxants (tubocurarine, for example) may reduce the peripheral vascular tone. Also, the use of neuromuscular blocking agents to facilitate intubation of the trachea and the control of respiration, by paralysing spontaneous muscular activity, removes the muscle pump effect and the intermittently reduced intrathoracic pressure of inspiratory effort. Respiration is maintained by the anaesthetist, usually by 'bag squeezing' on the anaesthetic breathing system, sometimes with a mechanical advantage to the hand which readily overcomes resistance to breathing by high positive pressures so that the mean intrathoracic pressure is raised, perhaps with a deleterious effect on venous return.

Careful choice of drugs and dosage, a reflex increase in peripheral venous tone, a small reduction of the mean volume of blood in the pulmonary circulation, as a result of the rise in mean alveolar pressure, and care in ventilation, are the principle means by which most patients show only a small reduction in blood pressure during induction. (The effects of drugs on the myocardium are considered below.)

During the maintenance period of anaesthesia, before and after extracorporeal circulation, the heart is operating under conditions of venous return close to those summarized by Linden[17]. The mediastinum is open, and controlled respiration by intermittent positive pressure continues. Under these circumstances, venous return depends upon the forward flow of venous blood, and perhaps upon the suction effect of blood leaving the ventricle. This statement requires reconsideration in the presence of diseased and abnormally functioning valves and may also be compromised by dysrhythmia and dyskinesia of the ventricle in coronary artery disease. Neglecting these reservations, the filling forces thus developed, the so-called *vis a fronte* and *vis a tergo*, arise from the pumping action of the heart itself, the whole movement of blood throughout the circulation depending on the momentum and cohesive property of the fluid. The only contribution which the peripheral muscles make, in the absence of any 'muscle pump' effect, is as part of their contribution to the general tissue tone surrounding the peripheral veins, which, acting in series with vascular wall tone, determines the total compliance 'seen' by the blood in the peripheral veins.

The effect of respiratory movement and intrathoracic pressure is minimal, in that, with the mediastinum and pericardium opened, atmospheric pressure is transmitted to the atrial surfaces. Intermittent positive pressure ventilation (IPPV), by raising the mean alveolar pressure significantly above atmospheric pressure, does influence pulmonary vascular resistance, tending to increase it. It also reduces pulmonary vascular volume and it moves the pulmonary perfusion/ventilation ratio further away from normal, although other factors, including reduced cardiac output and the effect of the open and surgically retracted thorax on local respiratory compliance, are also important in this. During IPPV under anaesthesia, passive diaphragmatic movement continues. The pressure changes in the abdomen are reflected in changes in pressure in the inferior vena cava and in the veins of the legs, but given the greater contribution of intramural smooth muscle to the tone of the latter, and applying Laplace's law to the different diameters of veins, including the inferior vena cava, the sum effect of increases in intra-abdominal pressure will be to return caval blood to the heart, rather than to the legs.

For a given cardiac output, venous return to the right heart depends on the vasomotor tone in the systemic veins, and thus on the sympathetic activity. Sympathetic drive may be high before induction of anaesthesia as a consequence of the low cardiac output, hypoxia or acidosis, which can result from the pre-existing disease. The propensity to a further augmentation of response is thereby reduced. Sympathetic activity can be unchanged, increased or decreased by anaesthesia, depending on the drugs and dosages used, and, in the case of inhalational general anaesthetic agents in particular, in a complex way, as a function of technique, 'depth' and duration of anaesthesia, and the surgical stimulus. In patients on drug therapy before anaesthesia, the drugs' own actions and their interactions with anaesthetic drugs should be considered. Where short-acting drugs are used in medical treatment it is often practicable to discontinue them a day or two before anaesthesia.

Although the baroreceptor and stretch receptor induced homeostatic reflexes usually continue to operate under general anaesthesia, they do so in a modified way and the response of the circulation to any anaesthesia or surgical challenge may be uncertain or unpredictable and inadequate. The influence of these factors on the choice of anaesthetic drugs and techniques is considered below.

The heart as a pump

Since, during anaesthesia, the mechanisms which maintain the venous return may be compromised, it is important for the anaesthetist to review the implications this has for the pump action of the heart. The two sides of the heart are separate pumps but their contraction is interrelated to the extent that, though the exact temporal relationship of the right and left ventricular systole may be modified, even if in dysrhythmia, the ventricular rates are the same. Over a period of time the output of the two sides must be equal.

The relationship between the force of contraction of a muscle fibre, and initial fibre length, has, since Starling stated his 'Law of the Heart'[29], been restated in various ways. For example, within limits, and if the gradient between ventricular end-diastolic pressure and the mean arterial pressure during the ejection phase is constant, stroke volume increases with ventricular end-diastolic volume. Thus an intrinsic mechanism exists, with others, by which the heart can adapt to changes in afterload and which determines, in part, the response to a reduced venous return, or ventricular filling pressure.

Ventricular filling is a function of the mean atrial pressures and of the compliance of the ventricle during diastole. In disease the resistance afforded by the atrioventricular (AV) valves is also significant. Ventricular compliance varies through diastole and, when the AV valve is closed during systole, the ventricular compliance as 'seen' by venous blood is essentially zero. The function of the atrium in matching the venous return to this changing compliance is likely to be significant, especially in the diseased heart, but the effect is probably more important at high outputs. Perhaps for this reason studies during anaesthesia have produced conflicting opinion on the subject. In clinical practice this 'reservoir' function of the atrium is not easily separated from the other effects of a normal atrial contraction—that is, the 'booster pump' effect on ventricular filling and the importance for effective closure of the AV valve of a correct relationship between atrial relaxation and the sharply rising ventricular pressure in early systole[20–22]. It has been suggested that slow supraventricular dysrhythmias arising during anaesthesia are benign[15]. We believe that it is a common experience in cardiac surgical units that, in the special case of the patient under anaesthesia for extracorporeal circulation, the general observation of Prys-Roberts is true: '. . . both atrial and AV junctional rhythms which arise *de novo* during anaesthesia can be extremely disruptive to the proper mechanical function of the heart'[26]. Where change from sinus to AV junctional rhythm occurs with little change in ventricular rate or filling time, the reduced cardiac performance evidenced by a fall in systemic arterial pressure demonstrates this.

During deep anaesthesia many anaesthetics have been implicated in the production of dysrhythmia. Although it is probable that most dysrhythmia associated with manipulation or surgery of the heart, or with the immediate postextracorporeal perfusion phase of the procedure are primarily caused 'on the table', for many agents even light anaesthesia must be assumed, on present evidence, to be a contributory cause, either directly or through the effects of hypoxia and ischaemia associated with any reduction in circulatory performance. Some hypotension is seen with light anaesthesia in some patients with heart disease either from peripheral circulatory effects, or direct myocardial depression.

Ventricular performance in patients requiring extracorporeal circulation is partly a function of filling and rhythm but mechanical (or anatomical) factors and the performance of heart muscle are also involved.

The gross mechanical effects of valvular dysfunction, congenital abnormality, myopathic or hypertrophied myocardium, aneurysmal dilatation and dyskinesia of a ventricular wall segment are normally subject to preoperative investigation and in most clinical circumstances the anaesthetist will have semiquantitative information available to him at the time of induction of anaesthesia. For this reason it is not proposed to discuss this aspect further.

For a given ventricle contracting from a given end-diastolic volume the energy imparted to the blood expelled during systole arises from the contraction of the myocardial fibres of the ventricle against the afterload provided by the arterial pressure.

Myocardial contractility is a term used in a number of different contexts to describe this fundamental property, and its definition has been confused by methodological problems in its measurement[27]. If contractility is defined in terms of the ability of the muscle fibre of a given initial length to do work—the greater the work the greater the contractility—then by the acceptance of the necessary simplifying assumptions, the definition can be extrapolated to refer to the whole ventricle, using only initial volume in place of initial fibre length and stroke work in place of fibre work. The intrinsic heterometric regulatory mechanism implicit in the Frank–Starling relationship[10, 29] can then be represented as a series of function curves plotting end-diastolic volume against stroke work. Within limits, increasing end-diastolic volume results in increasing work. Increased contractility, for example, produced by increased cardiac sympathetic nerve activity, or by inotropic drugs, displaces the function curve upwards and to the left, while a decrement in function as in failure, hypoxia, acidosis or exposure to drugs with negative inotropic actions, including many anaesthetic substances, displaces the curve downwards and to the right. In failure the slope of the function curve is also reduced, and in the range over which increased filling produced increased work there is but little increase in output for an increment of filling. In severe failure the gradient of the curve falls further, until, in the terminal phase, a negative gradient produces a falling output despite an increased end-diastolic volume[2, 3].

An increase in afterload also moves the function curve downwards but in the intact circulation there are complex interactions between the cardiac output, afterload and filling pressure[2, 16].

The Frank–Starling relationship holds true only over part of the ventricular function curve. There is an optimal length of the contractile elements (sarcomeres) for maximum force of contraction, related to the lateral relationship of the actin and myosin components of the contractile protein system. Leaving aside the possibility that extension of fibre length, by sliding of individual sarcomeres, or myofibrils may occur (with consequent reduction in the number of contractile elements operating across any section of muscle wall and proportionate loss of maximum contractile force), there comes a point during dilation of the ventricle where, on the generally accepted conceptual model of muscle contraction, sarcomere length exceeds the optimum (approximately 2.2 μm). Developed tension during contraction then decreases with further increase in end-diastolic volume. By Laplace's law, the intraventricular pressure developed for a given fibre tension also decreases with increasing end-diastolic volume. Even within the range where increased work results from increased filling, the gradient of the function curves fall as they are displaced downwards and to the right, so that increasing filling brings a smaller increase in work in failure as compared to the normal heart. Because the ventricular compliance curve, during filling, is non-linear, increasing increments of filling pressure are needed for each increment of end-diastolic volume. In respect of left side performance, the limit of acceptable filling pressure is influenced by the pulmonary consequences of high left atrial pressure. An acute rise in left atrial pressure, above 10–15 cm of water, will usually be associated with the development of pulmonary oedema. This may be delayed during the period of positive pressure respiration, due to the increase in alveolar pressure, unless a correspondingly higher left atrial pressure is reached. (*See also* 'pump lung' *below*.)

It is not intended to discuss in detail the biochemical factors which influence myocardial contractility during anaesthesia and surgery, but rather to mention some aspects of particular relevance to clinical practice. (The reader is referred to standard texts on clinical circulatory physiology for a full discussion and for information on the objective assessment of cardiac performance in the postoperative period.) Myocardial contraction depends on the removal of the inhibition of the troponin-tropomysin complex by the rapid increase in calcium ion concentration in the sarcoplasm which follows depolarization of the sarcolemma, and the availability of ATP and the ATP-ase activity of the myosin in the presence of magnesium ion. The high energy phosphate ATP is replaced from buffer stores of creatine phosphate, ADP through the action of myokinase or from the metabolism of a number of substrates aerobically or anaerobically. The enzyme systems by which the metabolism of free fatty acid, glucose glycogen lactate and other substrates are utilized by the healthy heart are subject to considerable modification in disease states and by hypoxia, ischaemia and by drugs. Repolarization and the redistribution of Ca^{++} to the sarcolemma and sarcoplasmic reticulum stores are energy consuming and ATP-ases variously activated by Ca^{++} and $Na^{+} - K^{+}$ are involved[27].

ATP concentration is high in well oxygenated heart muscle, and phosphate ion concentration is relatively low. Fatty acid is preferentially metabolized by the β-oxidation pathway to acetyl CoA and enters the tricarboxylic acid cycle. The levels of ATP and creatine phosphate are reduced in chronic failure and in ischaemia and hypoxia phosphate ion and ADP, AMP and adenosine are lost from the myocardium.

The chronotropic and inotropic effects of catecholamines, their role in glucose and glycogen metabolism and on insulin production, the stress effects of surgery on lipid metabolism at the expense of glucose utilization, and the associated rise in free fatty acid, which has deleterious effects on the myocardium, are all worthy of the anaesthetist's attention.

Catecholamines stimulate lipolysis and glycogenolysis, by modification of cyclic AMP mediated pathways. Hypoxia increases utilization of glucose and glycogen through this mechanism.

The inotropic effects of catecholamines are mediated at least in part by increasing the available intracellular Ca^{++}, probably independently of the action on the AMP mechanism. A similar explanation has been advanced for the inotropic action of cardiac glycosides, while the opposite mechanism has been invoked to explain the negative inotropic action of some anaesthetics[31].

Catecholamine levels in the myocardium are raised in early heart failure, but are later depleted. The depletion of myocardial stores of noradrenaline in low output failure and in hypertrophy is probably due to increased sympathetic nervous activity and a relative failure of synthesis. There is an associated reduction in myocardial contractility. It has been suggested that the mobilization of stored noradrenaline in hypoxic myocardium may be causally associated with the onset of dysrhythmia[24].

The coronary circulation

The oxygen supply to the myocardium depends upon the oxygen content and partial pressure in the arterial blood and on effective perfusion of myocardial capillaries.

While anaemia, haemodilution and anomalies of pulmonary function affect oxygen content a normal content may not ensure adequate myocardial oxygenation.

Although coronary perfusion occurs throughout the cardiac cycle, the distribution of blood to the myocardium is not uniform at all phases of ventricular contraction. The high intraventricular pressure of the left ventricle, and the consequent intramural pressure gradient in the left ventricular wall, together with the superficial distribution of the coronary arteries, cause the perfusion pressure to be highest in epicardial myocardium and least in the subendocardial myocardium, reducing, therefore, subendocardial perfusion virtually to zero during systole. Normally differential vasodilation in the subendocardial vessels allows the flow during diastole to 'catch up' with the more continuous perfusion of subepicardial myocardium. The vasodilation is produced by local metabolic products acting directly, and for the whole coronary circulation autoregulation is achieved, presumably by the same mechanism, in that the total flow remains relatively constant over a wide range of systemic pressure.

These mechanisms are impaired in failure and hypoxia, and oxygen demand is raised for a given output. The oxygen demand is also raised by an increased afterload. Relative ischaemia in hypertrophy or tachycardia or the absolute ischaemia in occlusive coronary artery disease, together with a raised oxygen demand, increase the likelihood of infarct. Under these circumstances, the subendocardial myocardium is particularly vulnerable.

Some specific conditions

Advanced mitral valve disease is associated with a history of atrial fibrillation, periods of cardiac failure, systemic embolization and, at least in *post mortem* cases, pulmonary embolism also. Cardiac output is low, with a cardiac index below 2 ℓ/min per m^2 at rest, and with very limited potential for increase due to valvular disease. There is a raised blood volume and haematocrit, raised peripheral resistance, chronic pulmonary congestion and chronic, irreversible changes in the pulmonary vasculature. Renal function is often found to be impaired.

The circulation is slow and a reduction in systemic vasomotor tone, by reducing venous return and peripheral resistance, can produce an abrupt reduction both in cardiac output and systemic arterial pressure which together may result in a critical reduction in coronary perfusion with further, and perhaps irreversible, deterioration in cardiac output.

The pulmonary dysfunction due to anatomical changes and the concomitant abnormality in ventilation/perfusion ratio, the low oxygen saturation of the mixed venous blood and the low cardiac output, by virtue of their effects on venous admixture, increase the effects of hypoventilation and a low inspired oxygen concentration on arterial blood-oxygen tension, thus making the patient very susceptible to further hypoxia or reduction of cardiac output.

Aortic valve lesions are commonly associated with a degree of coronary artery disease, occasionally calcification of the coronary ostia, ventricular hypertrophy and a high myocardial work rate for a low output at rest, and a low systemic diastolic pressure, resulting in myocardial ischaemia and hypoxia.

As with other patients with predominantly ischaemic disease, patients with aortic valve lesions are very susceptible to acute subendocardial ischaemia and myocardial infarction if, as often happens, systemic arterial pressure rises either before, or more commonly after, perfusion on extracorporeal circulation. The high risk of infarction during or immediately after anaesthesia in patients undergoing coronary artery surgery is increased in the months following a previous myocardial infarct[9]. The effects of medical treatment on biochemical and electrolyte changes have been discussed above.

The choice of anaesthetic agent for extracorporeal circulation

Nitrous oxide is an anaesthetic drug of low potency, such that even 80 per cent nitrous oxide cannot be relied upon to produce 'anaesthesia' but it is a useful analgesic in lower concentrations and it is widely used, typically as 60 per cent nitrous oxide in oxygen as a carrier gas for small concentrations of other more potent vaporizable anaesthetics or supplemented by intravenous agents[8]. It was thought that nitrous oxide had no significant myocardial effect but there is now considerable evidence that it does depress the myocardial function. Although the evidence is not unequivocal in clinical studies involving nitrous oxide and halothane in concentrations close to those which are used in cardiac surgical patients, it can be summarized thus: there is probably little effect on many patients with valvular disease but there may be a significant, even serious, reduction in cardiac performance in some, and in a greater proportion of patients with ischaemic heart disease. The cardiac effects of nitrous oxide are depressive, but it is also capable of α-adrenergic stimulation.

Halothane and the newer halogenated anaesthetics—methoxyflurane and enflurane—all produce myocardial depression. In addition, as with other halogenated anaesthetics, they increase the sensitivity of the myocardium to the dysrhythmic action of circulating catecholamines. The halogenated ethers, methoxyflurane and enflurane, are less likely to produce dysrhythmias, but methoxyflurane has nephrotoxicity which would disqualify its use in long operations, and in the presence of pre-existing renal dysfunction. The relative depressive action of halothane and enflurane has been the subject of debate and again there is some conflict in the evidence. Opinion is perhaps coming to accept the view of Prys-Roberts[25, 26], that for cardiac depressant activity there is little to choose between them—there is significant negative inotropic action in both agents.

Many anaesthetists in cardiac surgical centres have abandoned the use of inhalational agents other than nitrous oxide. Grey and Riding[13] used an oxygen–nitrous oxide induction followed by *d*-tubocurare in paralysing dosage, avoiding the circulatory depression recognized as a hazard of intravenous barbiturates. As has been observed, nitrous oxide is a myocardial depressant, although there is probably some increase in peripheral resistance and the arterial pressure is little changed. Curare is usually associated with a modest (10–15 per cent) fall in arterial pressure, due to autonomic ganglion blockade, and in a small number of patients significant falls in pressure and also bronchospasm, may occur, due to histamine release. Pancuronium does not produce ganglion blocade, and although it usually raises the arterial pressure for 10 to 20 minutes after intravenous injection, the increase is again usually acceptable clinically. We regard pancuronium as the muscle relaxant of choice for cardiac surgical patients.

Intravenous barbiturates have been given, safely, to all but the most decompensated patient with heart disease where maintenance of systemic venous tone is of critical importance and in such patients barbiturates are best avoided. In other patients it is perfectly satisfactory if the dose and rate of injection are controlled.

Diazepam in dosage sufficient to produce unconsciousness has very minimal effects on the myocardium or the blood pressure in the recumbent patient. It is a useful adjunct in the premedication of the anxious patient, but anaesthetic induction may be slow. It has been advocated for the decompensated patient[3].

Ketamine, alone, produces little change in overall circulatory performance. Usually an increase in cardiac output and heart rate are accompanied by a modest increase in blood pressure in the premedicated subject. The blood pressure may be higher in the unpremedicated patient and occasionally a severe rise in pressure occurs. Ketamine has been used for investigation before surgery, and in children, as an induction agent, since it can be given by intramuscular injection. It has useful analgesic properties and has been used during extracorporeal circulation in slow infusion. However, recovery of consciousness is rather abrupt if the dose is not exactly controlled and depression of sympathetic activity by other drugs unmasks the underlying myocardial depression of ketamine.

Etomidate appears to be a useful inducing agent, although it is relatively slow in action and usually causes some aching discomfort in the vein chosen for administration. It produces little or no change in arterial pressure, other than a small transient fall over an initial period of some 10 minutes. It has been reported that the cardiac output is not changed by its administration. Etomidate has no analgesic action[4].

Whereas an abrupt, severe or unpredictable fall in systemic vasomotor tone is undesirable since it will produce an acute fall in venous return and peripheral resistance, it is generally recognized that a moderate degree of vasodilation is desirable during cardiac surgery with extracorporeal circulation to improve tissue perfusion, reduce heart work and myocardial oxygen demand and to allow the retransfusion of patient blood and pump prime after bypass. While vasodilation usually accompanies the haemodilution which low blood primes produce during extracorporeal circulation, vasodilator drugs acting as autonomic ganglion blocks, α-adrenergic antagonists or direct depressants of vascular smooth muscle are widely used where necessary. In many centres the anaesthetic technique is designed to produce the required degree of vasodilation from early in the maintenance phase of anaesthesia. This objective cannot be reliably achieved by inhalational anaesthetics because at the concentrations required to produce vasodilation, myocardial depression is likely to be marked. It is doubtful if halothane, for example, produces as much reduction in peripheral vascular resistance at end-expired concentrations between 0.5 and 1 per cent as was once thought. The preferred methods use analgesic drugs in high dosage. The technique of neurolept-analgesia using fentanyl and droperidol is successfully used in patients undergoing cardiac surgery with extracorporeal circulation[6, 30]. Using fentanyl and droperidol, an initial dose of, typically, 10 mg of droperidol with 0.5–2 mg of fentanyl, in divided dosage, would produce a dissociated and deeply analgesic state amounting to unconsciousness in a few minutes. Further incremental dosage would be required for maintenance. The upper range of the initial dose of fentanyl quoted here is rather higher than has been advocated previously. Fentanyl is a powerful analgesic which is also used as an adjunct to other techniques and also in very high dosage as a development of the so-called 'Analgesic Anaesthesia' of de Castro[7]. Doses of fentanyl of up to 50 μg/kg have been used. Since fentanyl can produce muscle spasm it is necessary to use a muscle relaxant to control this. Fentanyl in normal dosage is short-acting but when used in high dosage over the period of major cardiac surgery the duration of action including respiratory depression is prolonged. The respiratory depression can be specifically antagonized with naloxone.

Droperidol and fentanyl each produce reduction in systemic vasomotor tone.

Morphine has also been used in high dosage (1–5 mg/kg). Unless given slowly—a maximum rate of 5 mg/min is suggested, with adequate fluid therapy to maintain atrial pressure—there is considerable risk of unacceptable hypotension[28]. Morphine alone does not depress the myocardium, but the addition of nitrous oxide does and therefore it should be omitted. This raises the possibility of awareness during surgery. Morphine also produces muscular rigidity.

Anaesthetic management

It is probably near the truth to say that most established techniques of general anaesthesia can be used in the patient about to undergo extracorporeal circulation, and many techniques have been described in this context in the literature[1, 3, 5, 6, 11, 23]. Success is only achieved by an understanding of the patient's circumstances and careful attention to all aspects of technique including dosage and rate of administration of drugs and oxygenation. It is proposed only to describe the authors' own technique. The description that follows has been adapted from a chapter by the present authors, M. D. Hargreaves and V. A. Grimshaw, in *General Anaesthesia* (Vol. 2, Ch. 10. Eds T. C. Grey, J. F. Nunn and J. E. Utting. London: Butterworths, 1980).

Most patients who are offered open-heart surgery have been fully investigated and prepared although this is obviously not the case in emergency situations which are particularly challenging to the clinical team. The patient will be readmitted a few days before the day of operation and final tests are made to confirm fitness for surgery. The patient's height and weight are measured so that the body surface area and blood flow during perfusion can be calculated.

At his preoperative visit, the anaesthetist checks that there has been no deterioration in the patient's condition. A useful guide to this can be obtained from the history of the exercise tolerance and general activity of the patient, but it is important to bear in mind that many patients so adapt their behaviour to their disability that superficial enquiry can be misleading. This point is of particular importance in the case of patients with limited preoperative investigation, as may be the case in patients with heart disease presenting with non-cardiac surgical problems.

Premedication

Effective doses of sedative drugs are safe in cardiac disease and in prepared patients full premedication is usual. Sedation helps to allay anxiety, which, especially in mitral valve disease, increases circulatory instability, pulmonary congestion and oxygen uptake. Induction is smoother in the well-premedicated patient, and total drug dosages during anaesthesia are reduced. In the severely ill and unprepared patient premedication may be omitted, but otherwise the writers' practice may be summarized as in *Table 9.1*. This produces a drowsy but co-operative patient, apparently indifferent to the prospect of surgery. By using hyoscine the incidence of

Table 9.1 Premedication for cardiac operation

2 hours before induction		*1 hour before induction*	
Body weight	*Pentobarbitone (orally)*	*Body weight*	*Papaveretum + hyoscine (intramuscularly)*
Over 50 kg	100 mg	20–30 kg	5 mg + 0.1 mg
25–50 kg	2 mg/kg	30–40 kg	10 mg + 0.2 mg
		50–50 kg	15 mg + 0.3 mg
		Over 50 kg	20 mg + 0.4 mg

arrhythmias, especially tachycardia, as with atropine, is reduced. Hyoscine controls secretions fully and contributes to the sedation. The use of an opiate provides full peripheral veins for venepuncture. Slight falls in blood pressure and in the arterial oxygen tension occur.

Nausea has not been a problem in the authors' practice[19]. Other premedication regimes use pethidine and promethazine, promethazine and atropine and trimeprazine with atropine or hyoscine. In anxious patients diazepam and latterly lorazepam have been advocated.

Induction of anaesthesia

All preparations are made before the patient is brought to the anaesthetic room, elevated on four pillows if there is any danger of pulmonary oedema supervening. Before induction the patient is preoxygenated for at least three minutes, at high flow. ECG electrodes are applied and the electrocardiogram is monitored continuously thereafter. A blood pressure cuff is applied and the pressure is checked. Two anaesthetists should be present, since in emergency one alone cannot continue anaesthetic management and carry our resuscitation. All necessary resuscitation equipment, including a defibrillator, must, of course, be immediately available.

Induction is accomplished by the slow intravenous injection of 2.5 mg/100 ml sodium thiopentone until the eyelash reflex is just abolished. A 23 gauge needle on a 20 ml syringe ensures slow injection. Total doses lie between 1.0 and 2.5 mg/kg. Some reduction in blood pressure is usual but only seldom is it sufficient to cause anxiety. Metaraminol 1 mg/ml and isoprenaline 2 μg/ml are always available, but are rarely used.

Relaxation is achieved with pancuronium bromide (0.1–0.15 mg/kg) and ventilation is begun with 60 per cent nitrous oxide in oxygen. Pancuronium produces satisfactory conditions for intubation in about two minutes in most patients. There is transient moderate increase in blood pressure and an increase in the heart rate. Tubocurarine does not increase heart rate but always reduces the blood pressure, occasionally severely, and adequate relaxation is delayed for at least four minutes. Suxamethonium can be used for intubation and it is certainly useful if difficulty is anticipated. An adult should receive at least 75 mg, as smaller doses produce unreliable relaxation in patients with very slow circulations. Coughing and straining are likely to produce circulatory disturbances and are probably more significant than the transitory changes in the electrocardiogram quite often seen at intubation. If the latter continue, or if suxamethonium produces a bradycardia, atropine (0.3 mg) is given with 100 per cent oxygen until a normal pattern is resumed.

Alternatively, especially where there is severe decompensation in the unprepared patient or in tamponade, diazepam up to 0.5 mg/kg or etomidate up to 0.3 mg/kg are used for induction. Etomidate is usually preceded by two minutes inhalation of 50 per cent nitrous oxide in oxygen and sometimes a 'normal' analgesic dose of fentanyl is given at a similar time before etomidate injection to obviate the discomfort often felt by the patient in the area around the vein chosen for administration. Intubation follows relaxation in the way already described. A double lumen nasogastric tube is now passed and an intra-oesophageal thermometer probe placed in the middle third of the oesophagus. Intravenous transfusion is established using a vein in the back of the hand and, after setting up closed bladder drainage by self-retaining catheter under sterile conditions, the patient is positioned on the operating table and taken into the operating theatre.

Maintenance of anaesthesia

In the operating theatre controlled ventilation is continued by a mechanical ventilator, with a humidifier, using 60 per cent nitrous oxide and 40 per cent oxygen. With hyperventilation moderate reductions in blood pressure often occur, due perhaps to a reduced cardiac output resulting from the lower $P\text{aco}_2$ or from the mechanical effects of intermittent positive pressure ventilation.

Hypoventilation is equally undesirable; the $P\text{aco}_2$ should be maintained at approximately 4.7 kPa (35 mmHg). A positive end-expiratory pressure (PEEP) may be helpful, especially when the pleurae are open, in preventing pulmonary collapse. The airway pressure should fall to between 0.5 and 1.0 kPa (5 and 10 cmH_2O).

Apart from additional doses of pancuronium given at the first sign of spontaneous diaphragmatic movement, supplements are often unnecessary in the preperfusion period. Sweating, lachrymation, or changes in heart rate or blood pressure associated with surgical stimulation, occasionally occur. Pethidine, in doses up to 0.2 mg/kg, or fentanyl, repeated as necessary, can be used. For most of our patients maintenance is achieved without the use of routine intravenous supplements although we have recently begun to use a high dose fentanyl regime with some success, (provided always that the short half-life of fentanyl in normal regimes is recognized as not applying in high dosage).

It has been suggested that some of the responses to surgical stress contribute to circulatory dysfunction during anaesthesia for major heart surgery, and that this can be prevented by high dose analgesic anaesthesia. Fentanyl has been quite widely used in this way in doses ranging from 10 μg to 50 μg per kilogram. Fentanyl reduces the coronary/arteriovenous difference for lactate and inorganic phosphate under acute ischaemic conditions. It reduces myocardial energy demand probably by a negative inotropic effect but in addition it is suggested that there is a beneficial reduction in heart rate and increased diastolic perfusion time[32].

The majority of patients receive small concentrations of halothane, usually 0.5 per cent added to a fresh gas flow of 4 ℓ/min with rebreathing between 2 and 4 ℓ/min in order to maintain a ventilation sufficient to keep $P\text{aco}_2$ at about 4.7 kPa (35 mmHg). Where hypotension is a problem or in decompensated patients, halothane is not used, or if started is discontinued. When hypertension occurs it can sometimes be controlled by a temporary increase in halothane concentration but we rarely add more than a nominal 1 per cent from a calibrated Fluotec Mk III* to the fresh gas.

Other inhalational agents have been used in cardiac surgery. Interest has been shown in enflurane, which is, like methoxyflurane, a halogenated ether. These substances have been associated with a lower level of anaesthetic-induced arrhythmia than halothane. However, contrary to initial reports it is probable that enflurane produces more impairment of cardiac function than any other volatile agent though this is not so clearly established at low MAC (minimum alveolar concentration) levels. Its effects on the circulation are most marked during artificial ventilation to normal or low $P\text{aco}_2$[25]. There is no doubt that halothane depresses the

*Cyprane Ltd., Keighley, UK

myocardium, but in low concentration—less than 1 per cent in the inspired gas—this effect is not often a problem. The inspired concentration can be varied as necessary and if there is evidence of untoward effect the vaporizer can be turned off.

Maintenance during heart-lung bypass

During bypass, the mechanical ventilation is discontinued and the lungs are inflated at an airway pressure of about 1 kPa (10 cm H_20). Formerly oxygen (20 per cent) in helium, had been used to avoid the development of absorption atelectasis in alveoli poorly ventilated after perfusion. Although theoretically sound this technique is not often used now, the lungs usually being held inflated with either the oxygen–nitrous oxide mixture during anaesthesia or with air. Since pulmonary blood flow is interrupted during bypass, anaesthesia can only be maintained by drugs added directly to the systemic circulation; in practice this usually means into the pump oxygenator system.

It is necessary to prevent any respiratory effort as the atria are being opened with the heart still beating but on partial bypass, as in mitral valve surgery, for example. This can be prevented by maintaining full muscle relaxation.

If there were no supplemental drugs in the priming fluid there would be an abrupt fall in the relevant tissue levels of these drugs when bypass begins. It is necessary to add a muscle relaxant for this reason, for example pancuronium bromide 2 mg to a 2 litre prime for an adult patient bypass. Nitrous oxide cannot be given via the oxygenator system – which will only function satisfactorily at high FIo_2. Where a potent volatile agent is to be used it can be added to the oxygenator gas, typically oxygen 97 per cent, CO_2 3 per cent (the CO_2 allows for the increased efficiency of a bubble oxygenator to extract CO_2 compared with its oxygenating function). In some centres 'intravenous' supplements are used; the authors occasionally use pethidine in this way before and during perfusion. Others have used morphine (in high dosage) or ketamine, as the main agent.

At the end of perfusion, pulmonary ventilation is recommenced as soon as pulmonary circulation is reinstated. The anaesthetic management may have to be modified by the need to maintain the circulation and initially 100 per cent oxygen is given. Nitrous oxide is introduced as soon as an arterial blood sample shows a satisfactory Pao_2 off perfusion. Relaxation is maintained as before, but caution is exercised as the end of the operation approaches. If pethidine is not repeated after perfusion rapid return to consciousness can be expected in the absence of cerebral complications.

General patient care

In addition to the management of anaesthesia, the anaesthetist plays an important role in the monitoring of respiratory and circulatory function, and the correction of such anomalies as are detected.

Monitoring preparations

Reference has been made to the use of an oesophageal thermometer probe. This is largely influenced by local cooling of the heart, when this is used, and the insertion of a rectal probe provides a useful indication of core temperature.

In the operating theatre a catheter is placed percutaneously in the femoral artery and catheters are inserted, through peripheral veins, into the inferior and superior vena cavae. Careful initial placement, using catheters of adequate size, is essential, since they become inaccessible later. Full sterility must be maintained. The catheters are connected by tubing of suitable length to electromanometers, the calibrated output of which is displayed on large oscilloscopes. Means of recording are also provided. Suitable taps are included in the system to allow for flushing with small volumes of heparinized saline, and for the withdrawal of blood samples. Continuous monitoring of the arterial pressure waveform, and of central venous pressure, is thus possible and serial blood samples are available for the estimation of the blood gases and the acid–base state of the patient. Facilities for making these latter measurements must be adjacent to the operating theatre. The blood pressure cuff is removed from the arm as soon as intra-arterial manometry is established.

During the early years of clinical perfusion most workers used simple EEG monitoring in an attempt to assess the adequacy of cerebral perfusion. This is much less used now, since not only are there difficulties in obtaining clean recordings in the theatre, but also the information which can be obtained without full electrode placements is very limited. A modified EEG amplifier ('Cerebral Function Monitor')*, is now available which makes interpretation easier[3].

The preperfusion period

This period in the management of open-heart surgery is often the most hazardous. The heart disease is uncorrected and the induction of anaesthesia may have further reduced cardiovascular performance.

When the mediastinum is opened and the heart and great vessels are manipulated, the effectiveness of myocardial action may be temporarily impaired. In the diseased heart particularly, arrhythmias are easily initiated by contact, especially when suction tubes are placed between the heart and the pericardium. Traction or swabs may obstruct the venous return or compress the pulmonary artery. During necessary temporary displacement of the heart the stroke volume may fall considerably with reduction in the arterial systolic pressure even to below 50 mmHg. Constant observation of the pressure waveforms and of the ECG is, therefore, essential. Except during such manipulations, however, a pressure similar to that seen before induction will usually be maintained during the preperfusion period. In some cases, especially in the presence of advanced heart disease, the blood pressure may be lower but provided it is stable and is accompanied by a good heart rate and rhythm it is rarely necessary to support the blood pressure. A mean arterial pressure of 60 mmHg is not uncommon in severe valvular

*Lectromed Ltd., St. Ouen, Jersey, Channel Islands

disease. Continuing urinary output should be sought as an index of adequate renal perfusion.

Cerebral circulation can be protected by allowing the $P\text{aCO}_2$ to rise to the upper end of the normal range, and by the careful management of the anaesthetic vapour concentration. If necessary, small doses of pressor agents may be used and are usually effective.

Arrhythmias of all types may be encountered, but are often only transient, resolving spontaneously when the cause is removed. Bradycardia, heart block and supraventricular and ventricular ectopic beats are the most common arrhythmias. Occasionally, ventricular tachycardia, flutter, or even fibrillation occur. Bradycardia may be due to hypoxia, which must be eliminated as a cause. Following median sternotomy there is much less risk of collapse unless one or both pleurae are inadvertently opened, when a further problem presents itself—that of seeing if the lung is re-expanded. Treatment of bradycardia with small doses of atropine is usually effective but in the absence of sinus rhythm, isoprenaline may be needed. Incomplete heart block is also treated with isoprenaline, 2–4 μg initially with further doses as necessary. Myocardial irritability may require the administration of potassium chloride, 0.5 g diluted and given very slowly. Lignocaine hydrochloride, 100 mg, is usually effective where potassium supplements do not produce the desired result. Very occasionally a metabolic acidosis may develop and since this contributes to the irritability of the heart, it should be treated with intravenous sodium bicarbonate.

Blood loss during this period is usually small but occasionally major haemorrhage occurs especially during reoperation and at the time of cannulation of the aorta and venae cava prior to perfusion, so that the anaesthetist must be prepared to transfuse blood rapidly. In the absence of such haemorrhage it is desirable to minimize the dilution of the patient's blood with transfused blood, and crystalloid solutions should be used cautiously also, especially when a non-haemic priming fluid is used. Thus the minimum of fluid, such as Hartmann's solution, needed to maintain the patency of the infusion catheters is often all that need be given. When, however, it is necessary, one of the venous pressure lines can be used temporarily to aid rapid transfusion. Perhaps 250 ml of blood loss can be accepted in the preperfusion stage without replacement, but this question must be considered individually for each patient.

Heparinization

Some four minutes before cannulae are introduced, the patient is heparinized (3 mg/kg body weight).

The perfusion period

Priming the pump oxygenator system

During perfusion the circulation is maintained by an artificial pump and oxygenator system, assembled from presterilized disposable components. Ethylene oxide sterilization is usually employed for the oxygenator system. After assembly the system is flushed with sterile 5 mg/100ml dextrose to remove toxic residues. It is then primed with the volume of fluid necessary to fill the 'arterial' side of the pump system, and to allow initial perfusion without the risk of air embolism. Usually about 1.7 to 2.6 litres of priming volume are required, depending on the system used. The composition of the priming fluid varies between centres but up to 30 ml/kg of non-haemic prime is accepted in most units, so that except in small children or anaemic patients blood is avoided and an isotonic electrolyte solution is used. During perfusion the haematocrit falls to between 20 and 25 per cent initially. Some redistribution of fluid from the circulation occurs, and urine output usually increases so that additional priming fluid must be added during perfusion. If the haematocrit falls below 20 per cent, consideration should be given to replacing lost perfusion volume with heparinized blood. Diuretics, for example mannitol (25 g, 20 mg/100ml solution), or frusemide (20–80 mg), are used if the urine output is unsatisfactory. Potassium is added to replace that lost in the urine. The replacement can best be regulated by serial measurement of serum potassium concentration, but an empirical regimen of potassium chloride, 4 g initially when perfusion is established, and 2 g/ℓ urine output thereafter, often gives acceptable serum levels. The potassium chloride solution must be added very slowly to the pump system, especially when the aorta is not cross-clamped, or if the coronary arteries are being perfused.

The perfusion period

The blood leaves the patient via vena caval cannulae or from a sump drainage system in the right atrium. In addition, blood from the coronary sinus will be aspirated by hand-held suckers, and blood reaching the left ventricle through the bronchial circulation or through an incompetent aortic valve will be removed by a left ventricular vent system. These ancillary systems and particularly the coronary suction, are traumatic to the blood and contribute to blood damage. The blood is returned to the patient through a cannula in the aorta or, in rare and special circumstances, in a femoral or external iliac artery.

The rate of flow is calculated on the basis of body surface area—2.4 litres of oxygenated blood per square metre provides adequate perfusion in euthermic patients. Initially the arterial blood pressure will be low, especially when haemodilution is high. During the first 15–20 minutes of perfusion the blood pressure tends to rise and urinary excretion recommences. In those patients in which urinary excretion does not occur spontaneously some improvements may be achieved, at the cost of increased blood destruction and perhaps a greater incidence of postoperative bleeding problems, by increasing the flow rate above 2.4 ℓ/m^2.

During heart surgery it is often necessary to cross-clamp the ascending aorta. This is obviously needed in aortic valve surgery but it is often advantageous in mitral valve surgery also by maintaining a bloodless field even in the presence of some degree of aortic incompetence. These operations can be carried out on the beating heart with a cross-clamped aorta. The empty beating heart does little work and has a low oxygen requirement. It can be maintained by intermittent coronary perfusion, removing the aortic clamp for a few minutes every 10 or 20 minutes. This technique was used for mitral valve surgery, but for aortic valve surgery artificial perfusion of the coronary arteries is necessary (*see below*). It is much more convenient to operate on an arrested heart but early methods of inducing elective arrest proved hazardous and were not all persisted with, but more satisfactory methods of inducing reversible arrest are now available. This has made possible bypass vein grafting to the coronary arteries, and has increased the precision of cardiac surgery generally.

Several methods are available for achieving these various objectives.

Hypothermia

General cooling (and subsequent rewarming) is most easily applied using a suitable heat exchanger system in the pump oxygenator, though surface cooling had been used, for example, to increase the time available to close an atrial septal defect without extracorporeal circulation. If mild hypothermia is used, with the body temperature not lower than 28°C, useful protection is obtained and the cardiac rhythm is usually slowed but not stopped. Moderate hypothermia with body temperature lowered to 20°C stops the heart and extends the safe cross-clamping time considerably. With mild total body hypothermia local cooling can be used to reduce the cardiac temperature to a lower figure (*see* Chapters 10 and 11).

Profound hypothermia with complete cessation of all circulation is used for intracardiac corrcction of complex congenital cardiac anomalies in small children and in infants (*see* Chapter 19).

Coronary perfusion

Arterial coronary perfusion can be achieved by inserting small self-retaining cannulae into the coronary ostia and perfusing them with blood from the oxygenator system, via accessory pumps. Often only the left coronary is perfused with some 200–350 ml blood per minute. Coronary perfusion is usually combined with some degree of mild hypothermia.

Induced cardiac arrest

The motionless heart has a smaller oxygen requirement than the beating heart and induced arrest has been used to achieve this. The use of potassium chloride leads to difficulties in inducing a normal heart beat after surgery while electrical fibrillation does not stop myocardial fibres from contracting individually. At the present time the technique of combined chemical and hypothermic cardioplegia is widely used. This combines the use of profound local cooling of the myocardium with a chemically induced arrest using a limited period of coronary perfusion with a suitable solution at 4°C. The technique used in the authors' experience is typical: some 10–15 ml/kg body weight of isotonic solution containing potassium (20 mmol/ℓ), magnesium (16 mmol/ℓ) and procaine (275 mg/ℓ) are used to perfuse the coronary circulation. Local surface cooling of the heart is applied simultaneously. The temperature of the cardiac muscle reaches about 18°C or less in the interventricular septum and the heart becomes completely flaccid. This gives at least 30 minutes of safe operating time, but the period of arrest can be extended by repeated infusions of cold cardioplegic solution.

Rewarming is accomplished by removing the aortic cross-clamp applied at the top of the ascending aorta before cardioplegia is induced, and allowing blood warmed in the pump oxygenator system to perfuse the patient, including the coronary circulation. The myocardium recovers in between 10 and 20 minutes.

Blood distribution control
Control of the distribution of blood between the patient and the heart-lung machine requires constant attention. If the blood volume in the patient is too low the great veins empty and collapse, reducing venous return to the pump. Excessive blood volume increases bleeding and the volume of blood returning through the left heart vent and the open-heart suction systems.

During heart-lung bypass the pressure in the arterial perfusion line and the coronary perfusion line should be monitored. An elevated pressure will detect inadequate flow due to obstruction of the perfusing cannulae, which may not be apparent to the operating team. The oxygen saturation in the blood leaving the oxygenator may be measured continuously or the Po_2 determined with a Clark electrode, but intermittent sampling is usually satisfactory.

The postperfusion period

Immediately before perfusion is discontinued ventilation of the lungs is recommenced. Where the cavae have been snared they are now released, allowing the blood to fill the heart and enter the lungs. The surgeon uses this blood to remove air from the left heart before allowing the systemic circulation to be maintained by left ventricular action. Sometimes cardiotonic drugs such as calcium gluconate (0.25 g) or isoprenaline (2–10 μg) may be needed to initiate adequate cardiac action. Cardiac filling is, of course, essential and the atrial pressures may need to be higher than in the preperfusion period with the left slightly higher than the right atrial pressure. The right atrial pressure may be increased slowly to say 2 kPa (15 mmHg) or until no further improvement in arterial pressure occurs. The pressure thus determined can be maintained with blood from the pump circuit or by intravenous infusion. Usually over a period of approximately 30 minutes the myocardium improves and a lower filling pressure is effective. However, further impairment may necessitate dopamine infusion.

Tachycardia, heart block and hypertension
Occasionally cardiac failure and tachycardia develop and may necessitate either electrical conversion or rapid digitalization with due regard to possible hypokalaemia when choosing the dosage.

In other patients bradycardia or various degrees of heart block may develop during the operation and should be treated by electrical pacing, using atrial or ventricular electrodes and an external stimulator. Often the block resolves spontaneously in the postoperative period.

Other patients develop systemic hypertension relative to the preperfusion pressure. This is most likely to occur after surgery for aortic valve disease or following direct myocardial revascularization for ischaemic heart disease. Apart from the increased bleeding and the risk of damage to suture lines in the aorta, the increase in heart work and the consequent rise in myocardial oxygen demand are particularly undesirable. If the circulating volume is high, hypertension is more likely to occur and the adjustment of the blood volume is the most direct method of dealing with this situation provided one of the venous cannulae is still *in situ*. Vasodilatation by intravenous antagonists, such as phentolamine (1 mg) or chlorpromazine (2.5–10 mg), or the use of sodium nitroprusside are usually effective in controlling the systemic hypertension, but it is important to avoid the severe hypotension produced by too large a dose of drugs given too quickly, or by a combination of unco-ordinated action by surgeon and anaesthetist.

Postperfusion bleeding

Control of bleeding is the major surgical task in the postperfusion period. While coagulation defects do occur, especially after traumatic or prolonged perfusions or where large volumes of homologous blood have been used, most bleeding problems in the postoperative period are due to surgical bleeding points. Coagulation defects can only be fully elucidated by prolonged laboratory examination but usually a clinical problem is resolved by empirical treatment or spontaneous improvement within 2–4 hours, before laboratory data are complete.

Perfusion does reduce clotting factors but usually not to critical levels. The loss of platelets is marked but recovers rapidly (in hours).

Platelet concentrates can be given. Fibrinolytic enzymes are released, in some patients in sufficient quantity to produce bleeding problems. Though this is rather uncommon, if it is suspected they may be inhibited by ϵ-aminocaproic acid 4 g intravenously repeated two- to four-hourly. Fresh blood, up to 6 units, fresh frozen plasma, vitamin K, 20 mg intravenously, and careful consideration of the adequacy of heparin neutralization are measures usually employed with success.

Closure of the thoracotomy and management of pulmonary ventilation

Before closure of the chest the surgeon may place pacing electrodes in the heart and if left atrial pressure is to be monitored postoperatively a suitable catheter will be introduced into the left atrium. Drainage tubes are placed in the mediastinum, and, after thoracotomy, in the pleural cavity. These tubes drain under continuous suction into graduated receivers, so that blood loss can be quantified.

Full inflation of the lungs is obtained with cautious manual control of the reservoir bag and expiratory valve. Cardiac output is very sensitive to prolonged high airway pressures at this stage.

Following completion of skin suturing the administration of nitrous oxide is discontinued. Spontaneous ventilation, if it is to be used postoperatively, is established. Alternatively, if controlled ventilation is to be maintained, consideration is given to the type of airway. Four choices exist. First, the standard endotracheal tube may be left in place at least overnight when a decision about the future respiratory management will be made. Secondly, a plastic nasal tube can be inserted with the possibility of maintaining artificial ventilation for a longer period with less discomfort. Since most patients require intubation and controlled ventilation for less than 24 hours, the writers adopt the former course. The third choice, to perform elective tracheostomy, is best avoided until longterm ventilator treatment is seen to be necessary. The fourth choice, the use of mask and airway, presents many problems of management and has not been successful in the writers' hands.

Respiration is maintained with oxygen during the relatively vulnerable period of transfer from the operating theatre to the intensive care unit. Monitoring during this period may be reduced to clinical observation, particularly palpation of the peripheral pulse or where necessary, of the cardiac impulse. However, portable monitoring equipment is available. A radiograph of the chest should be taken before leaving the operating theatre. This should demonstrate the full expansion of the lungs, the absence of pneumothorax and the position of drainage tubes and endotracheal cannula. It also serves as a reference against which later films can be assessed.

The patient is best transferred directly from the operating table to the bed to avoid excessive handling. A supine posture may be maintained until the left and right ventricular filling pressures have been assessed on the ward. Ultimately the patient will be raised to a semirecumbent posture when circulatory conditions allow.

Postoperative respiratory management

Postoperative care is ideally co-ordinated by one doctor who translates the consultations of many into nursing orders. The patient, the nurses and the house staff may well ask: 'Who decides when doctors disagree?'. The surgeon bears the ultimate responsibility for the outcome, and cannot delegate this. However, if the surgeon is not readily available, a trusted delegate may assume control of the postoperative management. With his responsibility the delegate must be given full authority to act.

During the early postoperative period, the patient usually needs intensive medical and nursing care. An intensive care unit staffed by specially trained nurses, and equipped with anaesthesia, ventilatory, monitoring and resuscitation equipment is ideal. X-ray facilities, clinical and chemical laboratory services and blood must be readily available. The most intensive care is required for the first 24 to 48 hours. After this immediate postoperative period, many patients no longer need concentrated attention. Others, however, may require intensive care for weeks.

The patient is brought directly to the intensive care unit from the operating theatre. Humidified oxygen is given. If mechanically ventilated, the apparatus is set up and adjusted for respiratory rate, tidal volume and oxygen concentration. Initially, the patient's ventilation is controlled entirely by the machine; later the machine may be adjusted to allow the patient to trigger each breath. The electrocardiographic leads are attached to the monitoring oscilloscope. Arterial blood pressure is taken by means of the percutaneous femoral artery catheter attached to a pressure transducer. The venous catheter, whose tip is in the superior cava, as well as the catheter placed in the left atrium, are attached to separate monitoring lines and transducers. Thermistors are placed in the rectum, on the dorsum of the foot and both central and peripheral temperatures are recorded. A double lumen nasogastric tube is already in the stomach and is attached to a continuous suction pump to prevent postoperative gastric distension. The mediastinal and/or pleural drainage tubes are attached to underwater suction. On arrival in the intensive care unit samples are sent to the laboratory for the estimation of blood gases, acid–base balance, haematological data, including coagulation parameters, blood glucose and blood and urine urea and electrolytes.

Postoperative respiratory problems are the summation of many factors which influence lung function. Extracorporeal perfusion reduces diffusing capacity and reduces gas volume in all compartments except the residual volume. Perfusion may reduce compliance or cause a severe lung injury. Anaesthesia, thoracotomy, incisional pain, preoperative lung function, blood volume, left heart performance, infection and the patient's ability to cough and co-operate, all influence pulmonary function postoperatively. These factors combine to produce varying degrees of hypoventilation, uneven alveolar ventilation or alveolar capillary diffusion block.

Sometimes the patient needs only humidified oxygen by mask, analgesics, turning, occasional pharyngeal aspiration and the services of a skilled chest physiotherapist. Most patients, however, require controlled positive pressure ventilation, and frequent arterial blood samples for gas analysis. Although in the immediate postoperative period, the patient may tolerate an endotracheal tube, a tracheostomy may be needed whenever the patient is unable to 'arterialize' his venous blood or when secretions cannot be satisfactorily removed beyond the initial 48 hours following the operation. Clinical observations of the amount and character of secretions, and of the quality and distribution of breath sounds and cyanosis of the buccal mucosa, must be made several times each hour. Portable chest radiographs and analysis of arterial blood gases and acid–base balance are done immediately after surgery, and then as often as the patient's respiratory function demands.

Arterial oxygen and carbon dioxide tension measurements evaluate overall lung performance. When the patient is allowed to breathe spontaneously, hypoventilation may ensue due to a multitude of factors acting in isolation or concurrently, such as residual anaesthesia and/or muscle relaxants, respiratory-depressing analgesics, incisional pain, respiratory muscle fatigue, decreased pulmonary compliance and compression of the lung by intrapleural blood, fluid or air. Hypoventilation in turn induces a decrease in both alveolar and arterial oxygen tension and an increase in alveolar and arterial carbon dioxide tension. Inhalation of 100 per cent oxygen masks the decrease in oxygen tension but does not prevent the rise in arterial $P\text{CO}_2$. An arterial $P\text{CO}_2$ above 50–60 mmHg is diagnostic of hypoventilation in the immediate postoperative period in patients allowed to breathe spontaneously. Assisted respiration via endotracheal intubation will sustain the patient until the cause of the hypoventilation is relieved.

Atelectasis, retained secretions, bronchial spasm, pulmonary congestion, pneumonia, and certain pre-existing diseases such as emphysema cause uneven alveolar ventilation. Groups of alveoli are sufficiently ventilated to fully arterialize the pulmonary blood perfusing them. Complete collapse of a lobe or lung produces a substantial right-to-left shunt. Arterial carbon dioxide tension may increase, remain normal or decrease, but it is often normal or low because the patient is usually hyperventilated. Clinical examination for collapse, atelectasis, retained secretions, or infection and/or serial chest radiographs, will detect the causes of uneven alveolar ventilation. Secretions are cleared by coughing, physiotherapy with postural drainage, bronchial dilator drugs, aspiration and, occasionally, bronchoscopy.

Thoracotomy, extracorporeal circulation, pulmonary oedema or alveolar infiltration secondary to haemolysis decrease oxygen diffusion across the alveolar-capillary membrane. Since inhalation of 100 per cent oxygen raises alveolar oxygen tension to over 600 mmHg, a sevenfold decrease in diffusion must occur before arterial haemoglobin saturation falls appreciably. This degree of alveolar-capillary diffusion block is occasionally encountered in massive pulmonary oedema or in the 'pump lung' syndrome. Positive pressure ventilation with PEEP using 40 per cent oxygen and aspiration of bronchial blood and fluid may control pulmonary oedema until the cause is relieved.

During cardiopulmonary bypass, the lungs may be damaged. This damage, once quite common, is now seen only rarely, since techniques of perfusion and patient care have improved. The term 'pump lung' has been used to describe a syndrome which originated perhaps in the damage to blood elements by traumatic early perfusion techniques. It is not caused by systemic hypotension, hypoxia or high left atrial pressure although these may contribute to the final picture in some cases. High left atrial pressure can produce alveolar damage and pulmonary oedema may develop but this is quite different to 'pump lung' characterized by congested lungs with periarteriolar haemorrhage. Platelets and white cells are seen adhered to pulmonary capillaries. The gross appearance of the lung at *post mortem* is congested and liver-red[18]. Blood and proteinaceous fluid may be aspirated from the airways. There is a rapid reduction in compliance and hypoxaemia develops in severe cases despite IPPV and high inspired oxygen. There is alveolar damage and the necessary use of high inspired oxygen may add to the problem by its effect after some 48 hours on the 'surfactant' production.

Embolization of microaggregates from the extracorporeal circulation or from the use of stored blood without micropore filtration may add to the problem but it does not cause it[12].

It is possible that vasoactive substances produced in the blood by trauma are primarily responsible but the aetiology of this syndrome is not really known. Treatment is largely supportive and though the use of corticosteroids has been advocated they appear to be ineffective in the established case. There may be some value in the prophylactic use of methyl prednisolone when given in high dosage.

Most patients undergoing open-heart surgery require an endotracheal tube postoperatively but often for less than 24 hours. Respiratory insufficiency, from hypoventilation, uneven ventilation, diffusion block or inability to control secretions, are adequate reasons for continued intubation in this period. In the majority of such patients IPPV will be continued in the immediate postoperative period. Machines which deliver a predetermined volume at known but varying airway pressures are superior to those delivering varying volumes of gas at a constant airway pressure. The best machines permit control of both peak respiratory and expiratory pressures as well as tidal volume and respiratory rate. The patient must be sedated initially to permit the machine to control his respirations. Opiates are often satisfactory, but occasionally the patient must be given pancuronium to overcome his respiratory effort. In time the patient may learn to co-operate with the machine, whether 'controlled' or 'triggered'. Prolonged mechanical ventilation may produce difficulties in weaning the patient from the machine. During mechanical ventilation reduced oxygen concentration should be used (less than 50 per cent) if the arterial oxygen tension is adequate.

Acid – base imbalance is common following extracorporeal perfusion with or without hypothermia. Hyperventilation, hypoventilation, low perfusion flow, arterial oxygen unsaturation, circulatory arrest, low cardiac output, acidotic blood transfusions, liver temperature, shivering, and overdosage of sodium bicarbonate are some of the many variables that influence acid–base balance. During surgery and the first few postoperative hours these factors, alone or in combination, may produce profound derangements in acid–base balance. The kidney has little time to compensate during this period. Therefore for practical purposes renal compensation need not be considered when treating acute acid–base changes during and immediately after open-heart surgery. Renal compensation and extracellular–intracellular ionic shifts must be appreciated if acid–base imbalance persists for beyond 24 hours.

Actual arterial blood pH and $Pa\text{CO}_2$ are routinely measured at intervals throughout the surgical and postoperative periods. In addition to the $Pa\text{CO}_2$, which reflects the respiratory contribution to the acid–base state, some measure of the contribution of the other, fixed, acids is necessary. Although various measures including 'buffer base', 'standard bicarbonate' and 'base excess/deficit' are used, we find that for acute changes in the acid–base state the determination of actual pH, actual $Pa\text{CO}_2$ and the inferred 'non-respiratory pH' afford a more rational approach to the problem[14]. The non-respiratory pH at any actual $Pa\text{CO}_2$ is defined as the pH which would be measured if the actual $Pa\text{CO}_2$ *in vivo* were 4.5 kPa (40 mmHg), which is assumed as the 'normal'. The calculation of non-respiratory pH is facilitated by assuming that a series of *in vivo* titration curves of $Pa\text{CO}_2$ against pH, obtained from the regression equations of experimentally determined data apply to the subject under investigation. Non-respiratory pH can then be obtained by plotting the actual pH and $Pa\text{CO}_2$ and following the interpolated titration curve to the 'normal' $Pa\text{CO}_2$ and reading the corresponding pH. In practice the curves fit well except in extreme haemodilution and then it is possible during anaesthesia to check a small part of the actual titration curve of the patient, measuring arterial pH at different steady state $Pa\text{CO}_2$ values obtained by appropriate choice of pulmonary ventilation or, where actual $Pa\text{CO}_2$ is close to the normal $Pa\text{CO}_2$, it is often possible, with experience, to approximate to non-respiratory pH intuitively.

Acidosis causes a direct decrease in myocardial contractility which results in low cardiac output and low blood pressure. The patient is ashen and may be cyanotic and the peripheral pulses are feeble. There is little or no urine output. The patient may be anxious and confused. Prolonged acidosis causes a vicious cycle of low cardiac output, causing poor tissue perfusion with associated anaerobic metabolism and non-respiratory acidosis which further decrease the cardiac output.

Non-respiratory acidosis is treated with sodium bicarbonate infusion intravenously. The non-respiratory pH may be titrated against repeated aliquots of 25 mmol bicarbonate given fairly slowly to avoid excessive urinary loss where, as often happens after haemodilution extracorporeal priming, a diuresis occurs. After administration of sodium bicarbonate, the cause of the acidosis should be sought and corrected. Common postoperative causes of non-respiratory acidosis include low cardiac output, shivering and arterial oxygen undersaturation.

Postoperative non-respiratory alkalosis is unusual, but occasionally occurs with overdosage of sodium bicarbonate, or when large volumes of citrated blood have been given. If the alkalosis is slight and if the patient's condition remains satisfactory, no treatment is necessary.

When a patient is breathing spontaneously respiratory acidosis implies hypoventilation. It occurs alone or in a combination with non-respiratory acidosis. Since the kidneys cannot compensate quickly, as already mentioned, the arterial pH decreases. Non-respiratory pH is normal (respiratory acidosis alone) or reduced (respiratory acidosis + non-respiratory—i.e. 'metabolic'—acidosis). The diagnostic finding is an elevated Pa_{CO_2}. Arterial Pa_{CO_2} above 6 kPa (45 mmHg) indicates hypoventilation, such that the patient requires respiratory assistance until the cause of hypoventilation is corrected. Intermittent use of a triggered 'respiratory assistor' may be sufficient. Analgesia and physiotherapy may also be indicated.

Primary hyperventilation usually occurs when respiration is controlled mechanically or during anaesthesia. It may occur if too much CO_2 is removed by the extracorporeal oxygenator during perfusion. Hyperventilation causes an increase in blood lactate and thus potentiates the development of non-respiratory acidosis during extracorporeal perfusion or hypothermia. Compensatory hyperventilation may occur in association with a primary non-respiratory acidosis. If either primary or compensatory hyperventilation is present, arterial P_{CO_2} will be low. Compensatory hyperventilation is treated by correction of the primary non-respiratory acidosis with sodium bicarbonate.

Primary hyperventilation or respiratory alkalosis may occasionally occur in the alert patient from pain or anxiety. This is properly treated by analgesics and sedatives.

Usually the patient with low arterial P_{CO_2} (below 3 kPa (25 mmHg)) may twitch and display increased reflexes. If the patient remains mechanically ventilated for several days, renal compensation occurs and bicarbonate is excreted. This will reduce the non-respiratory pH. Proper treatment requires reduction of the tidal volume and the rate of the breathing machine, or addition of small amounts of CO_2 to the ventilating gas, or an increase in the apparatus dead space by adding to the length of the endotracheal catheter mount tubing.

Serum electrolytes do not change significantly if the perfusion blood flows are adequate and if the urine volume is not excessive. Severe non-respiratory acidosis is accompanied by a shift of extracellular potassium and sodium into cells in exchange for hydrogen. Correction of the acute acidosis will raise both the serum potassium and sodium. Large urine volumes induced by mannitol, low molecular weight dextran, haemodilution perfusion or diuretics, may reduce serum potassium, sodium and chloride even though the urine is hypotonic. Low flow perfusions cause a decrease in serum calcium and magnesium in addition to a metabolic acidosis. If perfusion flows were adequate and the urine volume is not excessive, serum electrolyte determinations may be requested less often during the initial 24 postoperative hours.

On the first postoperative day a short trial of spontaneous breathing with the endotracheal tube in place will test the ability of the patient to sustain the effort of breathing spontaneously. Very often a straightforward clinical assessment will give the answer. Unfavourable signs in the spontaneously breathing patient are an increase in heart rate, the appearance of dysrhythmia, tachypnoea, sweating or restlessness. Measurement of the arterial blood-gas tension may also give an indication of the patient's condition. Should all these unfavourable factors be absent, the endotracheal tube can then be removed. If attempts of spontaneous respiration are not successful further assisted ventilation will be necessary until the patient's clinical state allows the resumption of spontaneous breathing.

Other aspects of postoperative care are dealt with elsewhere (Chapters 1, 12, 17 and 19).

References

1. Beard, A. J. W. 'Anaesthesia for open-heart surgery using extracorporeal circulation.' In *Thoracic Anaesthesia*. Ed. W. W. Mushin. Oxford: Blackwell (1963)
2. Bradley, R. D. *Studies in Acute Heart Failure*. London: Arnold (1977)
3. Branthwaite, M. A. *Anaesthesia for Cardiac Surgery and Allied Procedures*. Oxford: Blackwell (1977)
4. Volvin, M. P., Savege, T. M., Newland, P. E., Weaver, E. J. M., Waters, A. F., Brookes, J. M. and Inniss, R. 'Cardiorespiratory changes following induction of anaesthesia with etomidate in patients with cardiac disease.' *British Journal of Anaesthesia*, **5,** 551 (1979)
5. Conahan, I. J., Onimsky, A. J., Wollman, H. and Stroth, R. A. 'Prospective random comparison of halothane and morphine for open-heart anaesthesia.' *Anesthesiology*, **38,** 528 (1973)
6. Corssen, G., Chadoff, P., Domino, E. F. and Kahn, D. R. 'Neuroleptanalgesia and anaesthesia for open-heart surgery: pharmacologic rationale and clinical experience.' *Journal of Thoracic and Cardiovascular Surgery*, **49,** 901 (1965)
7. De Castro, J. and Parmentier, P. 'Pure analgesic anaesthesia and its limitations.' *VI World Congress of Anaesthesiology*, Mexico, **V (5),** 214 (1976)
8. Dundee, J. W., Brown, S. S., Hamilton, R. C. and McDowall, S. A. 'Analgesic supplementation of light general anaesthesia.' *Anaesthesia*, **24,** 52 (1969)
9. Föcx, P. 'Pre-operative assessment of patients with cardiac disease.' *British Journal of Anaesthesia*, **50,** 15 (1978)
10. Frank, O. 'Zur dynamik des Herzmuskels.' *Zeitschrift für Biologie*, **32,** 370 (1895)
11. Gilson, A. 'Anaesthesia for cardiac surgery.' *British Journal of Anaesthesia*, **43,** 221 (1971)
12. Giordano, J., Zimmer, M., Hobson, R. W. and Gervin, A. 'The effects of microaggregates in stored blood on canine pulmonary vascular resistance.' *Surgery*, **80,** 617 (1976)

13. Grey, T. C. and Riding, J. E. 'Anaesthesia for mitral valvotomy.' *Anaesthesia*, **12,** 129 (1957)
14. Kappagoda, C. T., Linden, R. J. and Snow, H. M. 'An approach to the problem of acid–base balance.' *Clinical Science*, **39,** 169 (1970)
15. Katz, R. L. and Biggar, J. T. 'Cardiac arrhythmias during anesthesia and operation.' *Anesthesiology*, **33,** 193 (1970)
16. Levy, M. N. 'The cardiovascular physiology of the critically ill patient.' *Surgical Clinics of North America*, **55,** 483 (1975)
17. Linden, R. J. 'Cardiac physiology'. In *General Anaesthesia. Vol. 1*. Eds C. T. Grey, J. F. Nunn and J. E. Utting. Ch. 31. London: Butterworths (1980)
18. Llamas, R. and Forthman, H. J. 'Respiratory distress syndrome in the adult after cardiopulmonary bypass.' *Journal of the American Medical Association*, **225,** 1183 (1973)
19. Lyons, S. M., Clarke, R. S. J. and Vulgarski, K. 'The premedication of the cardiac surgical patient.' *Anaesthesia*, **30,** 459 (1975)
20. Mitchell, J. H., Gilmore, J. P. and Sarnoff, S. J. 'The transport function of the atrium: factors influencing the relation between mean left atrial pressure and left ventricular end-diastolic pressure.' *American Journal of Cardiology*, **9,** 237 (1962)
21. Mitchell, J. H., Gupta, D. N. and Payne, R. M. 'Influence of atrial systole on effective ventricular stroke volume.' *Circulation Research*, **17,** 11 (1965)
22. Mitchell, J. H. and Shapiro, W. 'Atrial function and haemodynamic consequences of atrial fibrillation in man.' *American Journal of Cardiology*, **23,** 556 (1969)
23. Moffitt, E. A., Tarhan, S. and Lundborg, R. O. 'Anaesthesia for cardiac surgery.' *Anaesthesiology*, **29,** 1181 (1968)
24. Nayler, W. G. 'The ionic basis of contractility, relaxation and cardiac failure.' In *Modern Trends in Cardiology. Vol 3*. Ed. M. F. Oliver. London: Butterworths (1975)
25. Prys-Roberts, C. (Editorial). *British Journal of Anaesthesia*, **49,** 845 (1977)
26. Prys-Roberts, C. 'Ventricular performance.' In *The Circulation in Anaesthesia*. Ed. C. Prys-Roberts. Oxford: Blackwell (1980)
27. Smith, N. T. 'Myocardial function.' In *The Circulation in Anaesthesia*. Ed. C. Prys-Roberts. Ch. 3. Oxford: Blackwell
28. Stanley, T. H. and Grey, N. H. 'The effect of high dose morphine on blood and fluid requirements of open-heart operations.' *Anesthesiology*, **38,** 536 (1973)
29. Starling, E. H. '*The Linacre Lecture on the Law of the Heart*'. London: Longmans Green (1918)
30. Stoelting, R. K., Gibbs, P. S., Creasser, C. W. and Pearson, C. 'Hemodynamic and ventilatory responses to Fentanyl, Fentanyl-Droperidol and nitrous oxide in patients with acquired valvular heart disease.' *Anaesthesiology*, **42,** 319 (1975)
31. Symposium on myocardial metabolism. Ed. E. Braunwald. *Circulation Research*, **35,** (Suppl. III) (1974)
32. van de Vusse, G. J., van Belle, H., van Gerven, W., Kruger, R. and Reneman, R. S. 'Acute effects of Fentanyl on haemodynamics and myocardial carbohydrate utilisation and phosphate release during ischaemia.' *British Journal of Anaesthesia*, **50,** 927 (1979)

10

Intraoperative Myocardial Protection

Gerald D. Buckberg

ex vitio alterius, sapiens emendat suum

Introduction

Inadequate intraoperative myocardial protection results in cardiac muscle necrosis, which is most severe in the left ventricular subendocardial area. This complication is the most common cause of morbidity and death following otherwise technically successful cardiac surgery. At autopsy, as many as 90 per cent of hearts from patients dying in the perioperative period show varying degrees and combinations of gross, microscopic or histochemical subendocardial damage[19, 74, 95]. This form of myocardial infarction may develop in the absence of coronary artery obstruction. It may affect the entire inner left ventricular shell in patients with valvular and congenital heart disease, as well as regions of myocardium supplied by patent grafts in patients undergoing direct myocardial revascularization (*Figure 10.1*).

My fundamental hypothesis is that subendocardial necrosis is caused by an imbalance between subendocardial energy supply and energy demands. *Cardiac surgery is not a prerequisite for subendocardial necrosis, but perioperative events may catalyse its development.* Our understanding of the cause of this damage has been limited because we have only recently developed the methodology to study subendocardial oxygen (blood) supply[16], the primary fuel for energy production. By applying the knowledge gained from our experimental studies of the cause of subendocardial ischaemia, I hope to show the following: (1) that postoperative subendocardial necrosis reflects the *cumulative* damage caused by unfavourable alterations in the supply/demand balance before, during, and after extracorporeal circulation; (2) that it is seldom that a single factor (for example

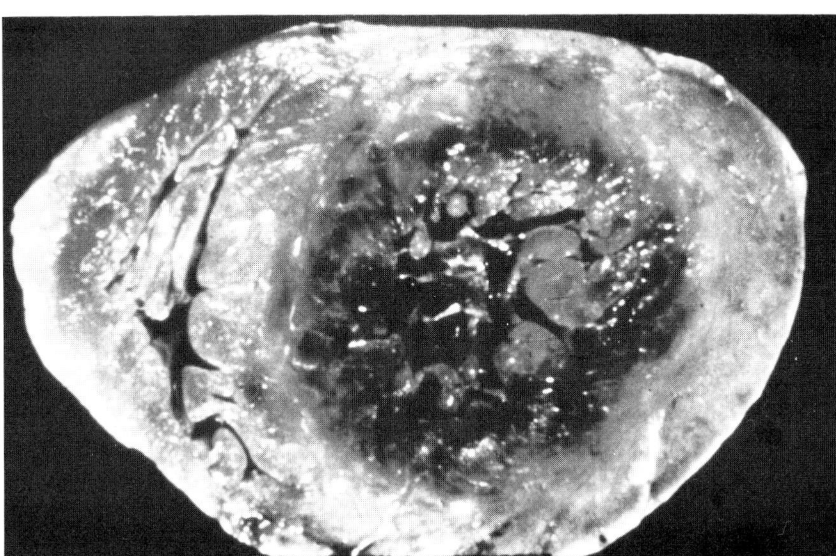

Figure 10.1 Cross-section through the heart of a patient who sustained severe intraoperative myocardial damage. This patient had aortic valve replacement while the fibrillating left ventricle was perfused continually with oxygenated blood. Note the extensive haemorrhagic necrosis of the entire inner shell of the left ventricle

cross-clamp time, ventricular fibrillation, temperature, etc.) is the only cause of subendocardial necrosis; (3) that rational decisions about ways to prevent or modify subendocardial necrosis can be made through a fuller understanding of how events before, during and after operation affect the subendocardial supply/demand balance; and (4) where future research into this problem ought to be directed.

Clinical manifestations

Severe subendocardial necrosis results in the inability to discontinue extracorporeal circulation because of arrhythmia, ineffective cardiac action, and, with extreme injury, development of the 'stone heart' (which is probably nothing more than ischaemic myocardial contracture). Moderate subendocardial damage results in the 'low-output syndrome', requiring

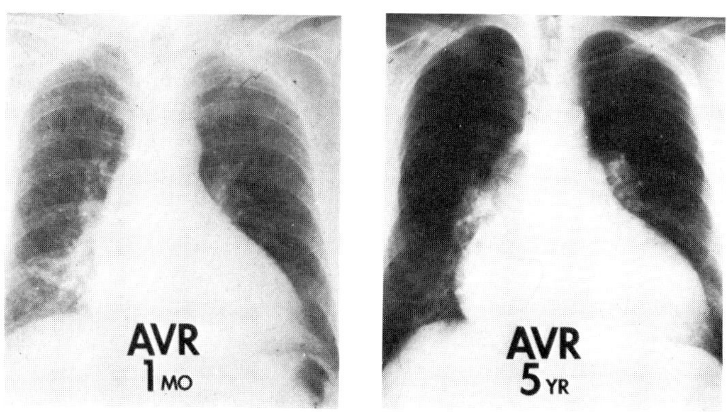

Figure 10.2 Chest radiograph one month (*left*) and 5 years (*right*) after aortic valve replacement in a patient who required inotropic cardiocirculatory drug support because of inadequate postoperative cardiac output. This patient underwent 64 minutes of ischaemic arrest with iced slush to produce topical cardiac hypothermia. The prosthetic valve continued to function normally five years postoperatively. Note the progressive cardiac dilatation despite perfect postoperative valve function. This probably reflects the healed result of intraoperative myocardial damage caused by inadequate myocardial protection

pharmacologic or mechanical circulatory assistance (balloon counterpulsation or left heart hypass) either in the operation room or early postoperatively. Milder damage may appear as congestive heart failure, developing before, or shortly after, hospital discharge. In some instances, the injury may escape clinical detection until the patient returns with cardiac failure secondary to myocardial fibrosis which has developed months to years after the operation (*Figure 10.2*).

The real incidence of subendocardial necrosis is unknown because most reports focus only on hospital mortality. The low-output syndrome and the use of inotropic drugs and intra-aortic balloon counterpulsation are considered routine postoperative problems. Furthermore, less severe myocardial damage is diagnosed only after careful study of postoperative electrocardiograms and myocardial specific enzymes[88] and, in addition, patients with more subtle heart muscle damage may develop delayed fibrosis despite an 'uneventful' postoperative course. In the past, follow-up left heart catheterization was not performed as a routine, so that only those patients who developed late, and often intractable, cardiac failure came to our attention. The current availability of non-invasive methods of evaluating myocardial function will allow better postoperative assessment of the present techniques of myocardial protection.

Vulnerability to ischaemic damage

In the working heart, the left ventricular subendocardial muscle is the most susceptible region of the left ventricle to ischaemia[49] because it can receive its blood (oxygen) supply only during diastole as the intramyocardial vessels are squeezed shut during systole. Conversely, the outer shell of the left ventricle and the normal right ventricle have lower compressive forces and can be perfused throughout the cardiac cycle. In normal hearts, coronary arteries can dilate and adjust the flow (autoregulate) to meet the oxygen needs. The reactive hyperaemic response following transient coronary artery occlusion provides evidence of this vasodilator reserve capacity. When subendocardial vessels dilate maximally, however, (in response to increased oxygen needs, reduced blood pressure or lowered oxygen content) blood supply to subendocardial muscle is determined by the diastolic coronary driving pressure (aortic diastolic minus left ventricular diastolic pressure) and the duration of diastole. We have shown previously[16] that the diastolic pressure time index or DPTI (the area between aortic diastolic and left atrial or pulmonary artery wedge pressure curves in diastole) provides a reasonable bedside and catheterization laboratory estimate of potential subendocardial flow, and that the product of DPTI × oxygen content predicts potential oxygen supply[8].

To assess the adequacy of blood flow, however, one must know not only how much oxygen is supplied (blood flow × oxygen content), but how much is needed. The area beneath the left ventricular systolic pressure curve (tension time index or TTI) is roughly proportionate to oxygen uptake[90]. This area underestimates oxygen demands by approximately 25–30 per cent when inotropic drugs are given[49]. The ratio DPTI/TTI allows a beat-to-beat guide to the adequacy of subendocardial oxygenation (how well demands are met) (*Figure 10.3*). Subendocardial ischaemia occurs if this ratio is less than 0.80 when the blood oxygen content is normal[16]. A higher ratio is obviously needed in patients with coronary artery disease because DPTI is lower beyond the stenotic lesion or during administration of inotropic drugs[74] (*Figure 10.4*). The usefulness of this index has been confirmed clinically[11, 38, 81] and its limitations established[49]. A low ratio (DPTI/TTI <0.8) before operation suggests an increased susceptibility to subendocardial necrosis. Balloon counterpulsation is, of course, ideally suited to improve the supply/demand relationship because it reduces myocardial

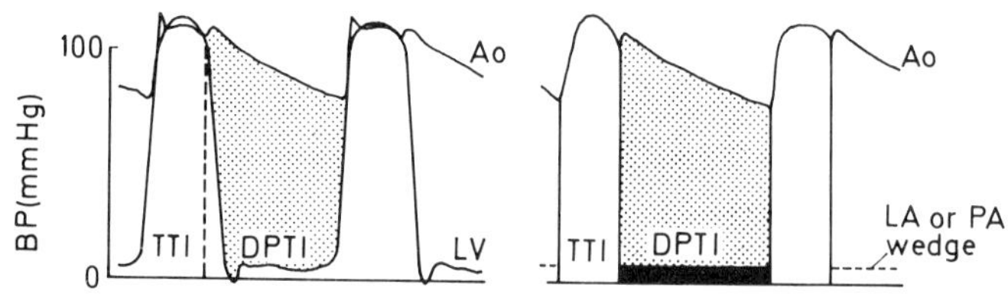

Figure 10.3 *Left panel*: superimposed phasic recordings of aortic (Ao) and left ventricular (LV) blood pressure and phasic left coronary blood flow (CBF). The stippled area in the pressure recording was used to calculate the diastolic pressure time index (DPTI), and the stippled area in the flow recording was used to calculate diastolic CBF. *Right panel*: shows how DPTI is calculated from the aortic and mean left atrial (LA) or pulmonary artery (PA) wedge pressures. (Right atrial pressure is used if it exceeds these.) The blackened area shows how these pressures affect DPTI. Similar markings are used in subsequent records. TTI = tension time index

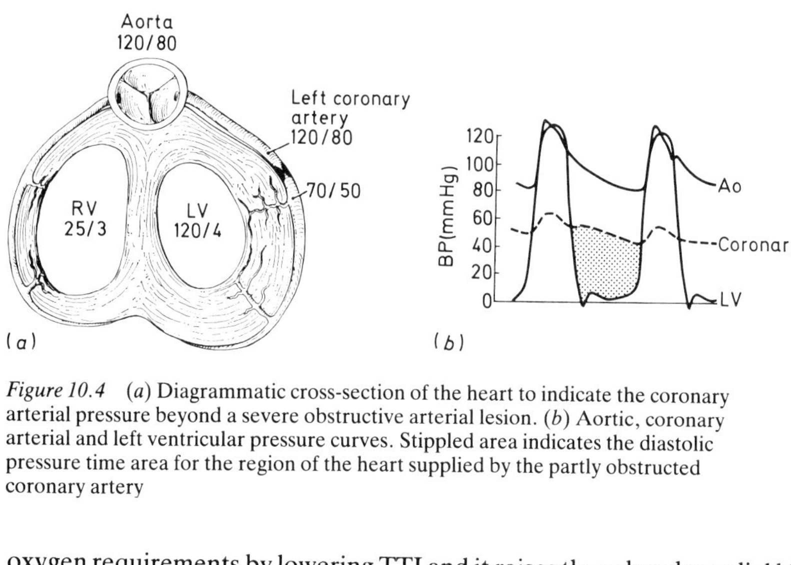

Figure 10.4 (*a*) Diagrammatic cross-section of the heart to indicate the coronary arterial pressure beyond a severe obstructive arterial lesion. (*b*) Aortic, coronary arterial and left ventricular pressure curves. Stippled area indicates the diastolic pressure time area for the region of the heart supplied by the partly obstructed coronary artery

oxygen requirements by lowering TTI and it raises the subendocardial blood supply by increasing DPTI.

The subendocardial muscle is in greatest jeopardy in patients with ventricular hypertrophy and/or coronary artery disease because both conditions cause resting vasodilatation and substantial reductions in the capacity of subendocardial vessels to dilate and regulate flow proportionate to changes in oxygen requirements. With ventricular hypertrophy, the coronary arteries must dilate to supply enough oxygenated blood to meet the raised oxygen demands of enlarged hearts[1] developing high intramyocardial tension (mitral insufficiency) or during increased pressure or volume work (aortic stenosis, systemic hypertension, aortic insufficiency) (*Figure 10.5*). In patients with coronary artery disease, the coronary driving pressure (DPTI) is low beyond the obstruction area so that relative exhaustion of vasodilator reserve may occur to ensure sufficient delivery of

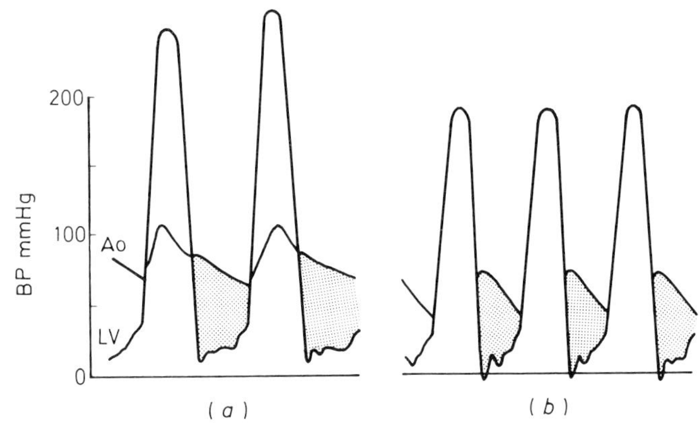

Figure 10.5 (*a*) Preoperative superimposed aortic (Ao) and left ventricular (LV) pressure recording from a patient with aortic stenosis. Note that DPTI (stippled area) is reduced by the raised LV diastolic pressure and the diastole is shortened because of prolonged ventricular ejection. TTI is increased due to high ventricular pressure and prolonged systole. (*b*) Preoperative recording from a patient with aortic insufficiency. Note that DPTI is reduced by the low aortic diastolic pressure and raised LV diastolic pressure and that the diastole is shortened by tachycardia. Both DPTI/TTI ratios are below 0.5. and each patient had electrocardiographic changes compatible with subendocardial myocardial ischaemia

oxygenated blood to the area supplied by the stenotic vessel under resting conditions. Myocardial ischaemia can develop, therefore, because of minor imbalances of oxygen supply and demand in these patients even before extracorporeal circulation is commenced.

Considerations before heart-lung bypass

Subendocardial ischaemia occurring before the institution of cardiopulmonary bypass is of particular concern because it may remain unrecognized except when severe; it is added to the inevitable ischaemia occurring during bypass and it may contribute substantially to the subendocardial damage which impairs postoperative myocardial performance. This ischaemia can be minimized by monitoring arterial blood pressure and pulmonary artery wedge pressure and optimizing the supply/demand balance (DPTI/TTI).

Hypotension should be avoided because subendocardial blood supply will decrease and ischaemia will occur in all hearts that have lost their autoregulatory capacity. Ischaemia may worsen, however, if appropriate decisions are not based on pulmonary artery wedge pressure recordings. Myocardial depression by anaesthetic drugs, for example, will reduce DPTI by lowering the arterial blood pressure and raising the left ventricular diastolic pressure. Treating this cause of hypotension with alpha-adrenergic drugs (Vasoxyl, Neosynephrine) may accentuate ischaemia by increasing the afterload which further raises the left ventricular diastolic pressure, while augmenting left ventricular oxygen needs (TTI) simultaneously. The rise in arterial blood pressure may be transient and followed by recurrent hypotension and the need to institute extracorporeal circulation prematurely.

Hypertension due to insufficient anaesthesia may, however, provide a false sense of security about the adequacy of subendocardial perfusion. High peripheral vascular resistance (increased afterload) raises the left ventricular oxygen requirements (TTI) markedly. The left ventricular

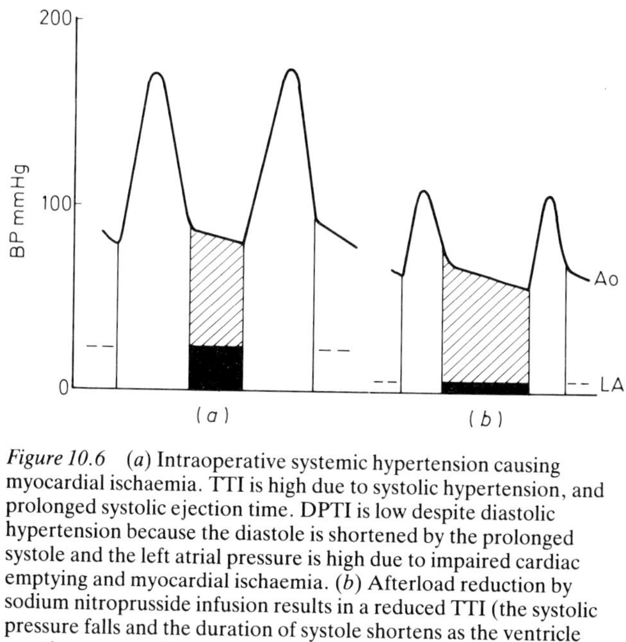

Figure 10.6 (*a*) Intraoperative systemic hypertension causing myocardial ischaemia. TTI is high due to systolic hypertension, and prolonged systolic ejection time. DPTI is low despite diastolic hypertension because the diastole is shortened by the prolonged systole and the left atrial pressure is high due to impaired cardiac emptying and myocardial ischaemia. (*b*) Afterload reduction by sodium nitroprusside infusion results in a reduced TTI (the systolic pressure falls and the duration of systole shortens as the ventricle empties more easily). DPTI increases as the left atrial pressure is lowered and the systole is shortened so that the diastolic filling period of the coronary arteries is prolonged. Note that DPTI/TTI increases despite reduction of the diastolic blood pressure

emptying becomes impaired, the left ventricular diastolic pressure increases, DPTI falls, and subendocardial flow becomes impeded. The administration of pharmacological vasodilators such as sodium nitroprusside or phentolamine may cause a marked improvement in the myocardial supply/demand balance despite lowering of the diastolic blood pressure[48] (*Figure 10.6*).

The effects of heart rate on the various disease states must be taken into account in order to optimize the heart rate before cardiopulmonary bypass. Tachycardia, for example, shortens the diastolic filling period of the coronary arteries and causes ischaemia in patients with coronary artery disease. Rapid heart rates should be avoided also in patients with aortic stenosis, since the diastolic interval is compromised even at slow heart rates because of the prolonged systolic ejection across the stenotic aortic valve. We have produced subendocardial ischaemia by tachycardia in experimental aortic stenosis[7]. Conversely, very slow heart rates are deleterious to subendocardial perfusion in patients with aortic insufficiency because during bradycardia more time is available for regurgitation. The DPTI is lowered markedly when the aortic diastolic pressure falls and the left ventricular diastolic pressure rises. Atrial pacing can substantially improve the adequacy of subendocardial perfusion in patients with aortic insufficiency[15].

The use of intra-aortic balloon counterpulsation has been advocated[38] to optimize the supply/demand balance prior to cardiopulmonary bypass. This is physiologically sound, but usually unnecessary if there is good monitoring and appropriate decision making. Pre-bypass ischaemia may cause severe hypotension, cardiac arrhythmia and even arrest, because patients with diseases such as aortic stenosis or left main coronary artery obstruction may not be able to repay the ischaemic debt satisfactorily until extracorporeal circulation reduces the oxygen demands and raises the perfusion pressure to ensure adequate blood supply.

Considerations during heart-lung bypass

Extracorporeal circulation, in itself, is thought to cause subendocardial necrosis because of reports showing the severity of subendocardial damage to be proportionate to the duration of cardiopulmonary bypass. Prolonged extracorporeal circulation can theoretically impair the subendocardial microcirculation, since all pump oxygenator systems do produce small particulate emboli which are directed preferentially to the subendocardium[99]. Such microembolization may account for the moderate reduction of ventricular compliance which accompanies continuous coronary perfusion for three or more hours of extracorporeal circulation. Despite this potential problem, up to three hours of extracorporeal circulation with adequate coronary perfusion does not cause detrimental changes in the coronary blood flow, its distribution, the myocardial metabolism, left ventricular performance[77] or obvious ultrastructural changes[94]. Rather, it is the inadequate protection against supply/demand imbalances during cardiopulmonary bypass that is the major cause of subendocardial necrosis. More myocardial injury occurs when the imbalance is prolonged during longer operation. Almost all the determinants of subendocardial oxygen supply and demand (such as the state of ventricular activity, temperature, blood oxygen content, coronary perfusion pressure and flow) are controlled during cardiopulmonary bypass. As the surgeons learn more about how various interventions during extracorporeal circulation affect the supply/demand balance, the ways in which this balloon has been unknowingly disrupted in the past become more apparent.

Surgical operations with the heart beating

Euthermia

Cardiopulmonary bypass reduces myocardial oxygen demands by approximately 50–70 per cent if the beating working left ventricle is converted to a beating empty state[54] by venting. The effectiveness of extracorporeal circulation on lowering oxygen needs is determined by: (1) the heart rate; (2) the adequacy of venting; and (3) the temperature (to be considered separately). Our studies have shown that during tachycardia, the vented euthermic heart requires almost as much oxygen as hearts doing external work at slower heart rates[14], since isometric tension (left ventricular pressure × radius) is a principal determinant of oxygen requirements.

When the aorta is not clamped, the bypassed heart is best protected against ischaemia when it is perfused continually at a satisfactory perfusion pressure (80–100 mmHg) with blood containing sufficient oxygen to meet the existing oxygen needs. In normal ventricles at 37°C, the coronary arteries dilate to ensure adequate oxygen delivery when the perfusion pressure is lowered to 50 mmHg[70]. In contrast, subendocardial underperfusion and ischaemia occur, despite the beating empty state in patients with hypertrophied hearts or in those with coronary artery stenosis, when the perfusion pressure is allowed to fall to 50 mmHg[4, 25, 70]. Such hearts may have expended their vasodilator reserve capacity even before bypass has begun (*see* previous section). Significant haemodilution worsens this ischaemia because oxygen delivery per ml of blood flow is reduced by lowering the blood oxygen content when compensatory vasodilation is not available. Haemodilution simultaneously decreases blood viscosity and makes it difficult to maintain the perfusion pressure at sufficiently high levels.

Hypothermia

Hypothermia protects the beating heart against ischaemic damage by slowing the heart rate, allowing more oxygen to be dissolved in the arterial blood, and by reducing the basal metabolic rate. The left ventricular oxygen uptake decreases by approximately 39 per cent at 28°C, and 50 per cent at 22°C[14]. Simultaneously, hypothermia may make the heart more vulnerable to ischaemia because of its inotropic effect (raising myocardial oxygen demands per beat), unfavourably shifting the oxyhaemoglobin dissociation curve to the left, therefore reducing the oxygen unloading at the tissue level, and reducing the coronary vascular reserve[2, 70] (the vasoactive ability to increase flow relative to needs). Coronary vascular resistance during maximum dilation is increased during hypothermia (flow is less at any given perfusion pressure) because (a) the blood viscosity is increased; (b) the diastole may be shortened despite bradycardia as the ventricular systole is prolonged; (c) muscular relaxation is less complete so that geometric distortion of subendocardial vessels may occur; (d) the diastolic wall tension is increased so that muscular impedance of subendocardial flow is greater; and (e) the autoregulatory mechanisms may become impaired.

The aforementioned potential limitations of adequate coronary perfusion during hypothermia are of major clinical importance since hypothermia is routinely used during most cardiac surgical operations, and it is therefore essential to establish whether the cold heart should be perfused continuously or stopped pharmacologically (*see* section on cardioplegia). Subendocardial ischaemia can be produced in continually perfused and cold (28°C) non-hypertrophied hearts with widely patent coronary arteries by (1) lowering the perfusion pressure to 50 mmHg[70] (a common perfusion pressure during clinical cardiopulmonary bypass) (*Figure 10.7*); (2) lowering the oxygen content by haemodilution[25] (haematocrit values between 15

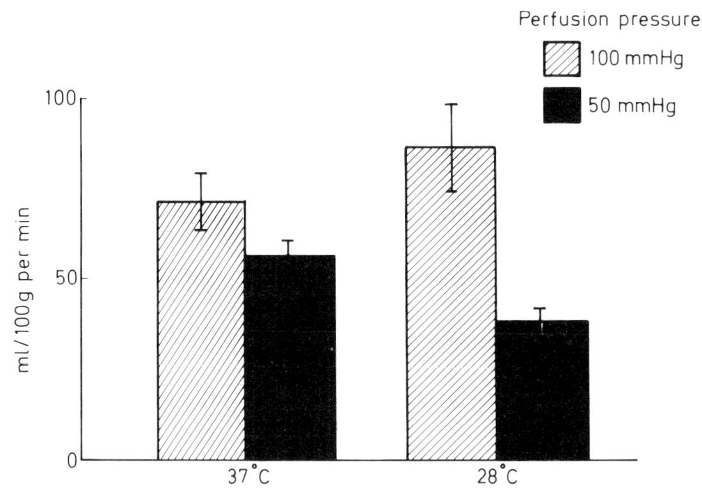

Figure 10.7 Graphic representation of left ventricular subendocardial blood flow (microspheres) with unobstructed coronary arteries in the beating empty heart when the perfusion pressure is reduced from 100 mmHg to 50 mmHg during euthermia and hypothermia. Note the maintenance of subendocardial perfusion at 37°C by coronary vasodilatation when the perfusion pressure is lowered and the pronounced subendocardial underperfusion when the perfusion pressure is lowered to 50 mmHg at 28°C

and 20 per cent are used during perfusion in many centres); and (3) preventing the expected bradycardia to occur[21] (tachycardia is caused by endogenous catecholamines and the administration of exogenous drugs, and may be even more severe with clinical surface body cooling). Tachycardia causes ischaemia in cold hearts by raising the oxygen demand per beat while hypothermia itself shortens the coronary diastolic filling period by slowing the process of cardiac relaxation[70]. It must be realized also that patients with coronary artery disease always have a reduced perfusion pressure beyond the stenotic coronary lesion, so that it may be impossible to perfuse their distal myocardium during hypothermia until all grafts are open and functioning (*Figure 10.8*).

The 'ideal' systemic pH during hypothermia may not be 7.40 as is customary during most cardiac operations. Clinical surface (whole body) cooling, usually carried out at pH 7.4, reduces the cardiac output and causes anaerobic metabolism and eventual ventricular fibrillation at temperatures around or below 28°C. Extracorporeal circulation is, of course, instituted

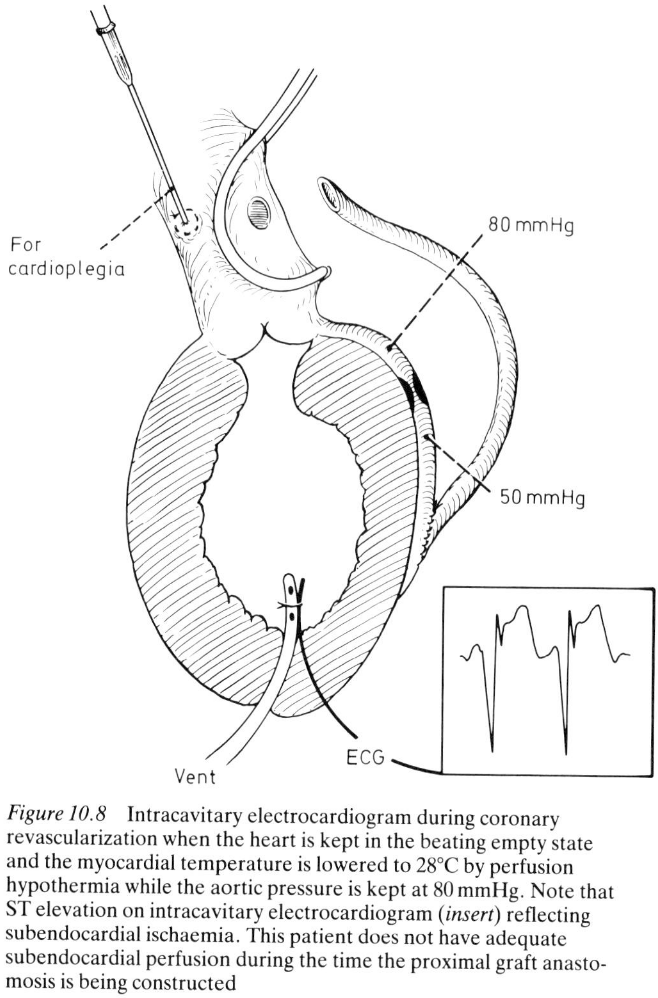

Figure 10.8 Intracavitary electrocardiogram during coronary revascularization when the heart is kept in the beating empty state and the myocardial temperature is lowered to 28°C by perfusion hypothermia while the aortic pressure is kept at 80 mmHg. Note that ST elevation on intracavitary electrocardiogram (*insert*) reflecting subendocardial ischaemia. This patient does not have adequate subendocardial perfusion during the time the proximal graft anastomosis is being constructed

immediately after this occurrence. Although the longterm effects of clinical body surface hypothermia on the myocardial structure are unknown, experimental immersion hypothermia may cause subendocardial necrosis even without cardiopulmonary bypass[89]. In contrast, poikilothermic animals, such as turtles, vary their pH with the temperature in concordance with changes in the pH of the water[55] and do not develop ventricular fibrillation while their body temperatures vary widely (*Figure 10.9*). Our preliminary studies at 28°C show subendocardial blood flow, myocardial metabolism, and ventricular performance, to be markedly better at pH 7.70 (the pH of poikilotherms at 28°C) than at pH 7.40[71]. These findings suggest that maintaining the blood pH at 7.40 during hypothermia (in either working or bypassed hearts) may impose an unphysiological constraint on the cardiovascular system on the one hand and may be neither normal nor ideal during surface cooling in infants or in adults undergoing routine extracorporeal circulation on the other. Further studies of the effects of pH changes during hypothermia on the regional flow and metabolism of other organs, especially the brain, are certainly warranted.

This section is intended to call attention to the mechanisms by which subendocardial ischaemia could occur in spite of maintaining continuous

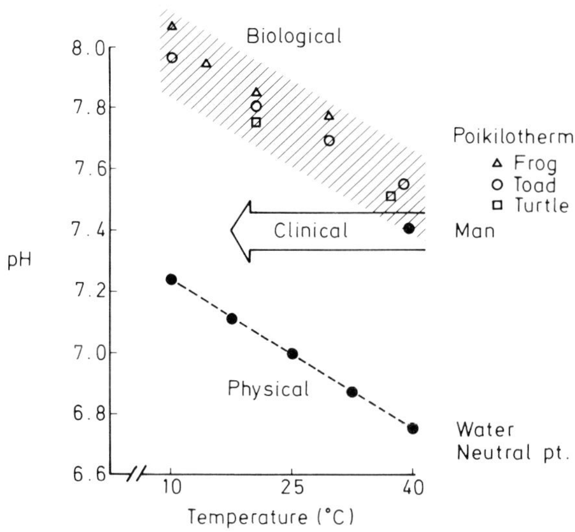

Figure 10.9 Changes in the pH of water in physical solution and of poikilothermic animals in nature when the temperature is lowered. Note how the clinical constraint of pH at 7.4 (arrow) is not in keeping with the naturally occurring phenomena in either physiochemical or biochemical systems

coronary perfusion with the heart beating and empty and the addition of hypothermia to reduce the metabolic needs. It is not intended to dissuade the clinical use of hypothermia, but rather to caution against the assumption that cardiac cooling ensures adequate protection against subendocardial necrosis even in the beating and decompressed heart.

Surgical operations with induced ventricular fibrillation

Euthermia

Ventricular fibrillation produces a quiet operative field, minimizes the risk of air embolism, and allows continuous coronary perfusion. Euthermic fibrillation achieves these goals at the expense of almost offsetting the effectiveness of cardiopulmonary bypass in reducing myocardial oxygen needs. At 37°C, the fibrillating left ventricle requires two- to threefold more oxygen than the beating empty heart and almost as much oxygen as the beating working heart[54] (*Figure 10.10*). These high oxygen demands occur because the asynchronously contracting myocardium develops tension at a rapid rate (both factors are primary determinants of oxygen demand). The subendocardial muscle develops the greatest intramural tension and needs

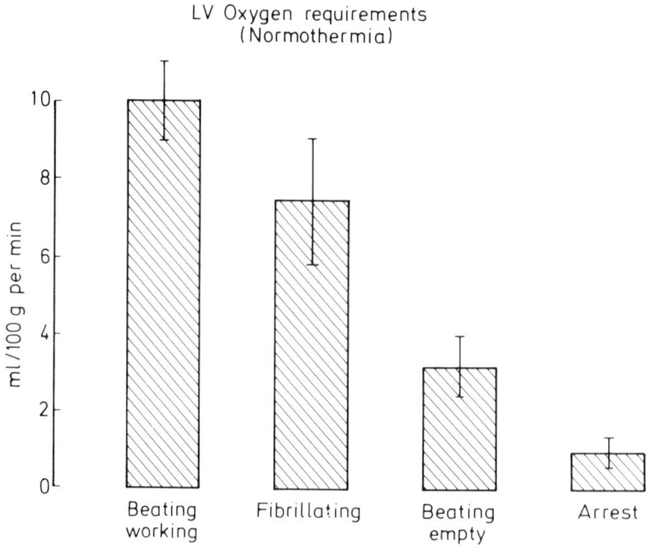

Figure 10.10 Myocardial oxygen uptake during euthermic perfusion of the beating working, beating empty, fibrillating and arrested heart. Note that at 37°C the fibrillating heart requires almost as much oxygen as the beating working heart. The beating empty heart (100 beats/min) requires only 30 per cent oxygen when compared with the beating working heart until the arrested heart requires only 10 per cent as much oxygen as the beating working heart

the largest amount of oxygen. A high subendocardial blood flow is necessary, therefore, to ensure adequate oxygenation during ventricular fibrillation[4,54].

Simultaneously, however, the fibrillating subendocardial muscle compresses its intramural coronary arteries and may throttle its own circulation by preventing sufficient flow from reaching it to meet metabolic needs. Ischaemia results when flow is not directed preferentially to the left ventricular inner shell[54]. This ischaemia is accentuated if the fibrillation is made more vigorous with a continuous electrical stimulus[51], or with administration of inotropic drugs[100], if the ventricle is not vented adequately[50], and if the perfusion pressure is reduced below 50 mmHg[9].

The deleterious effects of ventricular fibrillation are significantly greater in hypertrophied hearts (such as in patients with aortic or mitral valve disease, or with systemic hypertension) which are not protected against ischaemia even if the perfusion pressure is kept high and the ventricular venting is adequate[54] (*Figure 10.11*). Isom *et al.* reported that the enzymatic evidence of myocardial necrosis was more pronounced in hearts fibrillating during aortic valve replacement than in those kept beating[100]. McGoon reports a significantly higher postoperative mortality rate (7.3 per cent) in the 96 patients who fibrillated than in the 270 patients whose hearts were kept beating (1.5 per cent) in a consecutive series of 366 aortic valve replacements[72]. This was, however, a retrospective analysis in which the ventricles which fibrillated were allowed to continue to do so without any

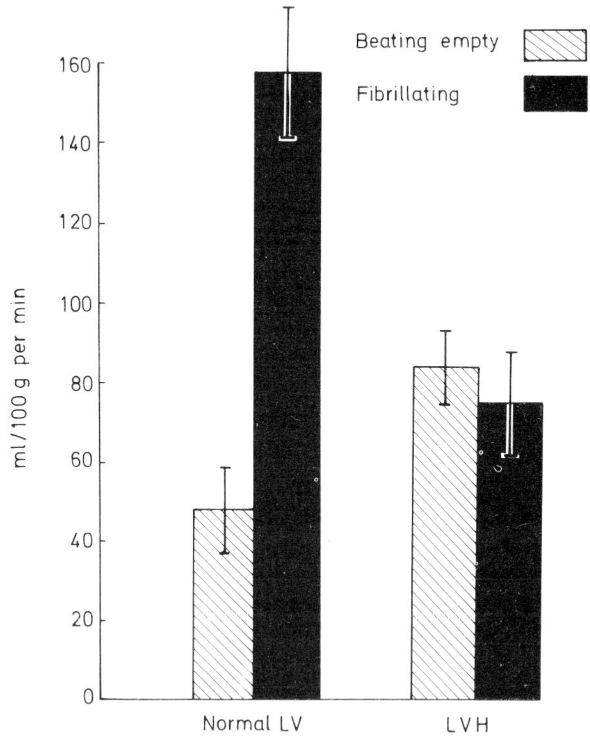

Figure 10.11 Graphic presentation of the subendocardial blood flow in the beating empty and the fibrillating normal and hypertrophied ventricle at 37°C. Note the marked increase in subendocardial perfusion in the normal left ventricle during fibrillation. This increased flow delivers the required oxygen to meet the raised metabolic demands of fibrillation. Note also the failure of expected increase in subendocardial perfusion in hypertrophied left ventricle. Metabolic evidence of ischaemia is present due to this failure to raise flow to meet the increased energy demands of ventricular fibrillation in thick walled ventricles

attempt at conversion. It is not, therefore, possible to know if the underlying problem causing their fibrillation, or the fibrillation itself, accounted for the higher mortality.

Mechanisms of myocardial ischaemia with ventricular fibrillation

There are several possible causes of ischaemic subendocardial damage during ventricular fibrillation[52]. First, the fibrillating muscle itself, especially if electrically or pharmacologically stimulated, seems to prevent the coronary flow from increasing sufficiently to meet the metabolic demands. The vigorously fibrillating myocardium may change its geometric configuration (ratio of left ventricular wall to lumen) and cause distortion of the subendocardial vessels[100]. A similar geometric distortion may occur with spontaneously fibrillating hypertrophied hearts and cause ischaemia. Second, distension of the fibrillating heart by inadequate venting adds a counterforce that opposes the coronary flow by reducing the driving pressure while increasing myocardial oxygen demands by an increased wall tension[50]. Third, fibrillation causes myocardial oedema which increases the extravascular resistance and further impedes blood flow. Both histologic studies[54] and the salutary effect of mannitol infusion[53] confirm the presence of oedema. Coronary perfusion pressure is the obvious counterforce to the impedance of myocardial flow offered by the fibrillating myocardium. Pulsatile perfusion (as created by the intra-aortic balloon) increases the safety margin of experimentally induced ventricular fibrillation[40], and minimizes, but does not avoid, lactate production in patients with coronary artery disease[78].

Hypothermia

Ventricular fibrillation becomes slower and less vigorous during hypothermia, presumably because the cold lowers the rate and force of tension developed by the myocardium. Left ventricular oxygen demands decrease by approximately 50 per cent at 28°C, and by 75 per cent at 22°C[14] (*Figure 10.12*). The myocardial wall tension (ventricular pressure × radius) which

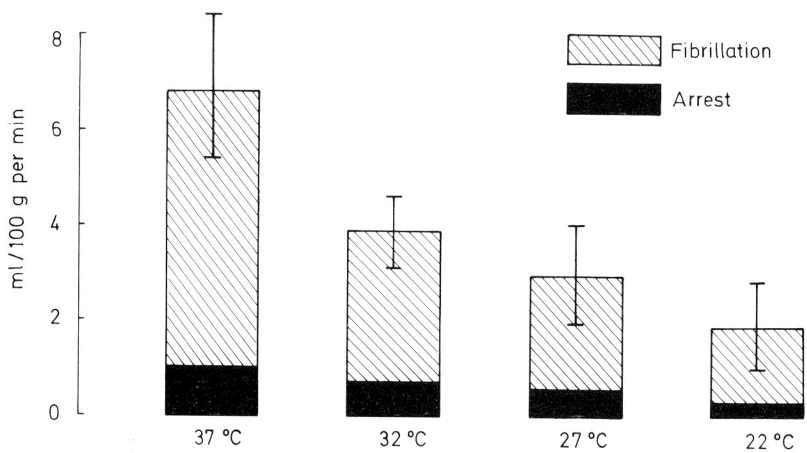

Figure 10.12 LV oxygen uptake in fibrillating and arrested heart. Note that oxygen uptake of the arrested heart is always significantly less than the fibrillating heart at any temperature. LVEDP = left ventricular end-diastolic pressure

determines the potential impedance to subendocardial blood flow, remains higher in fibrillating than in beating hearts at comparable temperatures. The clinical implications of these observations are that ventricular fibrillation may be less detrimental to subendocardial perfusion during hypothermia. Therefore, if the ventricle fibrillates (as may happen in patients with short left main coronary artery during aortic valve replacement) the myocardial temperature should be lowered substantially (22°C) in order to considerably reduce the oxygen demands of the heart, minimize the impedance to subendocardial blood supply and create near ideal operating conditions.

Hypothermia (28°C), despite lowering the oxygen demands, fails to protect the fibrillating heart with widely patent coronary arteries against subendocardial ischaemia when the perfusion pressure is reduced to 50 mmHg. Comparable ischaemia probably occurs with ventricular fibrillation in patients with coronary artery disease because a sufficiently high distal myocardial perfusion pressure cannot be maintained, even when the aortic pressure is kept at 80–100 mmHg (*Figure 10.12A*). Fibrillation induced ischaemia is worsened if the oxygen content of the blood is lowered by

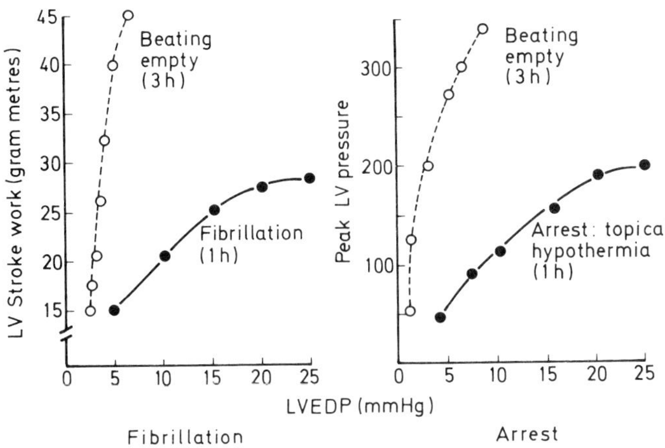

Figure 10.12A Comparable left ventricular functional depression occurring with either one hour or electrical fibrillation at 37°C, or one hour of ischaemic arrest with topical hypothermic protection. With ventricular fibrillation, there are increased demands and inadequate blood flow, while ischaemic arrest produces damage in the presence of reduced demands, because of absent coronary blood flow

haemodilution and also in the presence of ventricular hypertrophy. Furthermore, during the construction of the distal coronary anastomosis the oxygen requirements are higher in the myocardial territory supplied by the grafted vessel, while the local blood supply is interrupted. This may explain why, in patients with induced ventricular fibrillation during revascularization procedures, the myocardial lactate production is significantly raised[78] and perioperative myocardial infarction occurs despite patent grafts[23]. In this group of patients the need for postoperative inotropic support is reported to be high (65 per cent of 367 patients)[56] (*Figure 10.12A*).

In view of the multiple aforementioned hazards of ventricular fibrillation, it must be concluded that electric ventricular fibrillation should be avoided whenever possible during open-heart surgery.

Surgical operations with arrested heart

Cardiac operations are accomplished more rapidly and precisely when the heart is flaccid and bloodless. In clinical practice, these objectives are achieved by cross-clamping the aorta and inducing either ischaemic or pharmacological cardioplegia. The magnitude of subendocardial damage following aortic cross-clamping is determined by the duration and extent of the supply/demand imbalance, and this is more severe in hypertrophied hearts[58]. Based on the recognition that severe myocardial damage is caused by ischaemic arrest, most cardiac surgeons now use some form of chemical cardioplegia. A plethora of cardioplegic solutions are in current clinical use, many of them never having been tested experimentally. The search for the 'ideal' solution is ongoing, and has led to generalized confusion concerning what appear to be diametrically opposed views about the merits and deficiencies of the different clinical solutions which have been tested. This confusion stems, in large part, from the discrepancies between what appears to work quite well in clinical practice but has been shown to be deleterious in the experimental setting.

The purpose of this section is to (1) review my current understanding of chemical cardioplegia and why it is essential; (2) enumerate and discuss the principles which must underlie the development and use of clinical cardioplegic solutions; (3) explain why different clinical cardioplegic solutions may be equally safe and effective despite experimental evidence to the contrary; (4) demonstrate how the apparent conflict between clinical and laboratory results can be resolved by understanding the differences between clinical conditions and experimental models; and (5) point out where future studies in this area should be directed.

My fundamental hypothesis is that avoidance of ischaemic damage during aortic clamping is dependent upon sufficient myocardial energy being produced to meet energy demands. To understand the need for pharmacological cardioplegia, and the principles which must underlie the composition of any effective cardioplegic solution, I will review briefly the determinants

Table 10.1 Myocardial supply/demand balance during aortic cross-clamping

Supply	*Demands*
Non-coronary collaterals	Electromechanical activity
Intrinsic substrate stores	Wall tension
(glycogen)	
	Temperature (metabolic rate)

of energy supply and demand during aortic clamping and the pathophysiology of the ischaemic damage which occurs when sufficient energy supply is not available to meet cardiac energy demands (*Table 10.1*).

Supply

In the perfused heart, myocardial energy is produced by aerobic metabolism. The heart uses the oxygen supplied by the coronary flow to produce 36 moles of ATP for each mole of glucose metabolized. With aortic clamping, the heart is deprived of coronary blood flow and must derive its energy from the limited aerobic metabolism resulting from the small and inconstant supply of oxygen delivered through non-coronary collateral blood flow, and from the anaerobic metabolism of myocardial glycogen and glucose. Anaerobic metabolism produces only two to three moles of ATP but is the essential source of the energy needed to maintain cell viability when coronary blood flow is absent. The small energy output of anaerobiasis can maintain prolonged myocardial viability if such metabolism can continue unimpeded[12]. Factors to be dealt with which interfere with continued anaerobic energy production include (1) inadequate substrate (glucose or glycogen); (2) myocardial lactate accumulation; (3) inappropriate pH; and (4) metabolic inhibition of esseential enzymes (such as the inhibition of phosphofructokinase by massive amounts of citrate).

Demand

Energy demands are determined principally by myocardial electromechanical work and secondarily by wall tension and cardiac temperature. In the arrested state, very little energy production is needed to meet the basal requirements of maintaining the myocardial metabolic processes and membrane gradients intact. These low energy needs during cardiac arrest are reduced further by hypothermia (for example 1 cc O_2/100 g per min at 37°C versus 0.3 cc O_2/100 g per min at 22°C). In contrast, cold hearts which are allowed to perform electromechanical work require eight to ten times more energy (beating or fibrillating hearts at 22°C require approximately 2.0 cc O_2/100 g per min)[14] (*Figure 10.7*). When arrest is achieved by ischaemia, electromechanical work ceases only after the ischaemic fibrillating or beating heart expends the cardiac energy reserves sufficiently to render too little ATP available for continued electromechanical coupling and for energizing the sodium-potassium pump responsible for keeping intracellular potassium from crossing the cell membrane.

With pharmacological arrest, the cell membrane is depolarized chemically and the heart is placed in a state of sustained diastole. Consequently, vital energy stores are not expended in the performance of useless electromechanical activity. The small amount of energy needed during pharmacological arrest is used to maintain this diastolic state and is related to myocardial wall tension and temperature. Diastole occurs normally when the intracellular Ca^{++} which caused the previous contraction is pumped actively (sequestered) into the sarcoplasmic reticulum. The residual intracellular calcium concentration determines the diastolic wall tension. Calcium sequestration is an energy dependent process and is related directly to the concentration of intracellular calcium[66]. Hence, higher diastolic wall tensions raise the energy requirements of asystole (*see* discussion of cardioplegic drugs). Hypothermia lowers the basal metabolic requirements but also reduces the activity of the calcium pump. It is not surprising, therefore, that myocardial wall tension is slightly higher in cold than warm hearts during asystole.

Consequences of ischaemia

With ischaemia, the heart must revert to anaerobic metabolism with a consequent reduction in its net energy production from 36 moles of ATP (with aerobic glycolysis) to only 2–3 moles of ATP (with anaerobiosis) per mole of glucose metabolized. Continued glycolytic energy production relies upon substrate availability and a suitable environment for continued metabolism. The failure to produce more energy during ischaemia occurs because oxygen is necessary in order for the pyruvate produced by glycolysis to enter the citric acid cycle. In the absence of oxygen, pyruvate is converted to lactic acid. Unless lactate is washed away, it will accumulate and reduce the intracellular pH. Intracellular acidosis produces an unfavourable milieu for vital enzyme function and inhibits continued anaerobic production of ATP so that little or no energy is made available to keep the cell metabolic processes functioning.

The predominant effect of ischaemia and inadequate energy production is a disruption of the energy dependent cell membrane pumps which maintain transcellular gradients of sodium, potassium, calcium, and magnesium. The sodium pump is responsible for regulation of cell volume. Malfunction of this pump results in entry of extracellular sodium into the cell with consequent cell swelling. Simultaneously, the intracellular potassium leaves the cell and lowers the intracellular/extracellular concentration gradient, so that the cell membrane stays depolarized and the heart remains arrested. As extracellular potassium rises, the extracellular calcium increases wall tension and raises the metabolic demands because energy is needed to pump calcium back out of the cell (sequestration) and maintain the transcellular gradient. Failure to sequester intracellular calcium may lead to eventual myocardial contracture if intracellular calcium rises to extremely high levels[84]. Such contracture can occur *during* aortic clamping[65] and is worsened *following* reperfusion[92]. Magnesium, the second most predominant intracelular ion and essential co-factor for cellular respiratory enzyme function, leaves the cell during ischaemia. Intracellular hypomagnesaemia may restrict postischaemic energy availability.

Cardioplegia

The purpose of pharmacological cardioplegia is to offset the aforementioned consequences of ischaemia by producing an environment where myocardial energy demands are reduced while energy is produced to meet those demands. The principal prerequisites for the clinical use of a cardioplegic solution are (1) protection of the heart from ischaemic damage rather than producing damage by virtue of its composition; (2) distribution to all myocardial regions in amounts sufficient to produce the desired effects; (3) provisions for the solution's continued exertion of its protective effect for as long a period of aortic clamping as necessary; and (4) adequate laboratory testing of the solution under conditions which bear some resemblance to those encountered in clinical practice. Failure to adhere to the fourth principle has led to (1) most of the confusion existing today about current cardioplegic techniques; (2) persistent resistance to accept cardioplegia because of prior experiences with inadequately tested solutions; and (3) the fact that clinical results are neither as perfect nor as bad as those produced in the laboratory setting.

Background

Clinical cardioplegia was introduced by Melrose *et al.* in 1955 when he advocated the use of cold hypertonic (pH 7.8) potassium citrate blood to produce arrest and facilitate intracardiac operations[73]. Clinical results with the original Melrose solution were so erratic that clinical cardioplegia was abandoned for almost 20 years. The thoughtful studies of Brettschneider *et al.*[12], Kirsch, Rodewald and Kalmar[63] and Hearse, Stewart and Braimbridge[41] in Europe, and of Gay and Ebert[37] in the United States, have provided a solid framework for renewed use of cardioplegia. Recently, Tyers *et al.*[96] showed that the problem with the Melrose solution was inappropriate concentrations of its constituents rather than inappropriate composition. Our investigative studies lend full support to the original cardioplegic constituents of Melrose's solution and we currently use safe concentrations of alkaline, hypertonic, potassium citrate cold blood to stop the heart whenever we clamp the aorta in clinical open-heart surgery[33].

My interest in cardioplegia was stimulated by a dilemma occurring in our laboratory several years ago. Dr Colin Bayliss, a research colleague at UCLA, studied ways to allow prolonged storage of hearts destined for transplantation. Dr Bayliss reasoned, correctly, that the excised heart could be protected best if the myocardial temperature was reduced and the heart was stored in an environment where the ionic components of extracellular fluid were made to match those of the intracellular fluid so that no energy need be expended by cellular metabolic pumps to maintain or restore electrochemical gradients. He carefully designed a complex cardioplegic solution which protected excised hearts for up to 24 hours[5]. The dilemma arose when the same cardioplegic solution conferred no protection *in vivo* to hearts subjected to only two to three hours of aortic clamping.

Our laboratory dilemma reflects the classic problem of applying solid physiological principles to models which differ from those in which the principles were developed. In the excised heart, the cardioplegic solution fixes the extracellular environment and remains in place for as long as the aorta is clamped. In the *in vivo* heart, non-coronary collateral blood flow washes away all the carefully designed cardioplegic solutions and replaces them with systemic perfusate[10]. Consequently, the excised heart model is extremely useful for studying prolonged organ storage for transplantation, and for defining which cardioplegic additives may be detrimental. Conclusions based on such studies, however, may lead to serious problems if applied to the clinical setting where the contact of the cardioplegic solution with the myocardial cell is transient.

Non-coronary collateral flow

Non-coronary collateral flow is present to a variable degree in all hearts (*Figure 10.13*). This flow is highest during arrest, especially in hypertrophied hearts[10] and where there is coronary artery disease. While this source of nourishment cannot be relied upon to provide sufficient oxygen to meet even the low requirements of asystole, it will wash away whatever cardioplegic solution has been used to produce pharmacological arrest in every instance.

The presence of this blood supply (originating from mediastinal and bronchial vessels coursing through pericardial connections) has been quantified experimentally[10, 39] and is evident clinically. All cardiac surgeons have noted (1) blood coming from the coronary ostia during aortic valve replacement; (2) blood coming from the coronary arteriotomy during coronary revascularization when the aorta is clamped and flaccid; and (3)

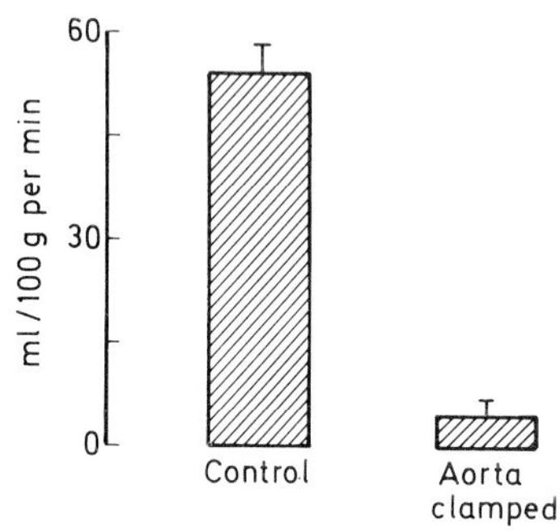

Figure 10.13 Left ventricular subendocardial blood flow (microspheres injected into the arterial line of the extracorporeal circuit) in the beating empty heart (*left panel*) and in the ischaemically arrested heart (*right panel*). Note that approximately 5 per cent of the control coronary blood flow reaches the arrested heart from non-coronary collateral sources while the aorta is clamped and the coronary blood flow is interrupted

the frequent recurrence of electromechanical activity (beating or fibrillating) in pharmacologically arrested hearts. Recurrence of fibrillation signifies that the cardioplegic solution is no longer in contact with the myocardial cells and that sufficient energy stores are available for electromechanical coupling. Conversely, ischaemically arrested hearts receive the same non-coronary collateral flow but can never resume electromechanical activity during aortic clamping because they have expended their high energy phosphate stores in the process of fibrillating or beating themselves to a halt.

The major beneficial aspect of the clinical presence of non-coronary collateral flow is that it washes away poorly conceived and untested cardioplegic solutions so that they cannot exert the continued deleterious effects which have been demonstrated experimentally. Secondarily, it reduces the clinical consequences of failing to include ingredients found 'vital' in the controlled environment of excised heart or tissue slice studies because the cardioplegic solution is replaced by the systemic perfusate (whose composition is probably comparable internationally). The realization of the transient nature of cardioplegic solutions in the clinical setting has allowed for the development of simple and safe solutions rather than those which are complex and costly and of strategies to counteract non-coronary collateral flow therefore allowing safer and more prolonged durations of aortic clamping.

Composition of cardioplegic solutions

The objectives of chemical cardioplegia are to stop the heart safely, to create an environment of continued energy production, and to counteract the deleterious effects of ischaemia. The principles (*Table 10.2*) which should underlie the chemical composition of any cardioplegic solution include (1) production of immediate arrest in order to lower energy demands and avoid energy depletion by ischaemic electromechanical work; (2) hypothermia in order to further reduce the energy demands and to prevent recurrence of electromechanical activity; (3) provision of substrate for continued anaerobic and/or aerobic energy production during aortic clamping; (4) buffering to counteract anaerobic acidosis and create a milieu for continued metabolism during hypothermia; (5) hyperosmolarity to reduce the oedema

Table 10.2

Principle	*Method*
Immediate arrest	K^+, Mg^{++}, Procaine
Hypothermia	15°–20°
Substrate	Glucose or oxygen
Appropriate pH (buffer)	THAM, bicarbonate, phosphate
Membrane stabilization	Ca^{++}, ? steroids, ? procaine
Avoid oedema	Osmolarity, onconicity

inevitably resulting from ischaemia and hypothermia; (6) membrane stabilization in the form of exogenous additives or avoidance of intentional hypocalcaemia; and (7) adequate testing under proper experimental conditions to ensure avoidance of iatrogenic, inappropriate concentration of ingredients[96].

Immediate arrest

By producing immediate arrest, the myocardial energy requirements are reduced so that the small energy output of anaerobic metabolism can be channelled towards maintenance of cell membrane integrity rather than being wasted on electromechanical work (beating or fibrillating). Recent studies by Wright *et al.*[102] show that substantial ATP stores can be expended during the brief period of electromechanical activity before pharmacological cardioplegia is produced by asanguinous solutions. To avoid this needless expenditure of energy stores, Brettschneider *et al.* have recommended the preceeding of the asanguinous cardioplegic infusions by a brief infusion of cold blood containing procaine in order to produce immediate arrest[12]. Other ways of minimizing this depletion of high energy stores before arrest include (1) mixing of the cardioplegic solution with blood so that the heart remains oxygenated while it is stopping[33]; (2) bubbling oxygen into asanguinous cardioplegic solutions[42]; (3) lowering the myocardial temperature with brief profound systemic hypothermia and giving rapid infusions of very cold (4–8° C) asanguinous solutions to hasten asystole. This last alternative is less physiological because ischaemic electromechanical activity is not avoided but only minimized.

I must preface the following discussion of the various methods of producing arrest by stating that I can find no current evidence of the superiority of any one technique of producing cardioplegia in the clinical setting.

Potassium

Potassium is the predominant intracellular ion and its concentration gradient is maintained by activity of the sodium-potassium pump. Extracellular hyperkalaemia causes asystole by depolarizing the cell membrane and producing a state of sustained diastole for as long as the extracellular potassium concentration remains high. The proper potassium concentration for producing cardioplegia is that amount required to cause asystole reliably. Hypothermia reduces the potassium concentration needed to produce cardioplegia. Hearse, Stewart and Braimbridge[42] report that only 13 mmol/ℓ are necessary at 24°C when an asanguinous vehicle is used. In our studies with blood cardioplegia, consistent production of asystole at 20°C required 28–30 mmol/ℓ of potassium[33]. Lower concentrations of potassium may be equally effective with more profound levels of hypothermia (4–8°C).

Clinical potassium concentrations should not probably exceed 40 mmol/ℓ, because higher levels of hyperkalaemia alter the cell membrane in a way that allows extracellular calcium to enter the cell and raise the energy demands[84]. Brettschneider *et al.*, for instance, found that the hearts perfused with high levels of potassium required nearly twice as much oxygen as the hearts stopped with lower amounts of potassium[12]. Studies by Rich and Brady[84] show that hyperkalaemic allowance of calcium entry into the cell results in an increased myocardial wall tension with consequent higher ATP breakdown during asystole and in myocardial contracture or 'stone heart' when the potassium concentration exceeds 100 mmol/ℓ.

Fortunately, non-coronary collateral flow is present in the clinical setting and may prevent many of the deleterious effects of the high levels of potassium used in some cardioplegic solutions. Because of the unpredictable and inconstant nature of the non-coronary collateral flow, however, this source of washout should not be relied upon to avert the potentially deleterious effects of inappropriate cardioplegic concentrations.

Magnesium

Magnesium is predominantly an intracellular ion which is a vital co-factor in respiratory enzyme function and also modulates muscular tension. Hypermagnesaemia produces cardioplegia by blocking the calcium entry into the cell. Magnesium (Mg^{++}) takes up calcium (Ca^{++}) receptor sites at the cell membrane. Hypermagnesaemia is not necessary to produce cardioplegia and there is considerable controversy about how much magnesium should be contained in the cardioplegic solutions.

Studies by Engelman *et al.*[24] suggest that there is no need for magnesium to be added to cardioplegic solutions since magnesium cardioplegia does not provide better myocardial protection than potassium cardioplegia during two hours of aortic clamping *in vivo* when the cardioplegic solution is replenished periodically. Conversely, Hearse, Stewart and Braimbridge[44], using an excised heart model, report the only comprehensive studies suggesting that hypermagnesaemia is a necessary adjunct to clinical cardioplegic solutions. These investigators established the potential dangers of perfusing hearts with either non-magnesium cardioplegic solutions or with extreme magnesium concentrations as occurs with the Kirsch solution[6].

They found the ideal cardioplegic magnesium concentration is 15 mmol/ℓ, a value equal to the intracellular concentration. In the isolated heart model, fixing the extracellular magnesium concentration equal to the intracellular magnesium concentration will abolish transcellular gradients, avoid Mg^{++} loss during ischaemia, and delay Ca^{++} entry into the cell. Such an ideal environment does not, however, occur in the clinical setting where non-coronary collateral flow always replaces the cardioplegic solution with blood containing normal magnesium concentration. This same cardioplegic washout diminishes the deleterious effects of extreme hypermagnesaemia. Such knowledge helps to explain why the good clinical results reported by Bleese *et al.*[6] could not be reproduced in the highly artificial setting used by Jynge, Hearse and Braimbridge in their laboratory[60].

Calcium

Extracellular hypocalcaemia produces cardioplegia by limiting the ionic calcium available to trigger myocardial contraction and thereby simultaneously lowers the energy requirements during asystole by reducing the amount of calcium which needs to be sequestered. Extreme hypocalcaemia, however, is deleterious since some calcium is necessary for cell membrane stabilization[36]. Recent studies show that myocardial perfusion for as little as five minutes with solutions containing less than 50 μmol of calcium caused severe sarcolemmic membrane damage[103]. This electron microscopic evidence of the danger of extreme hypocalcaemia has its functional counterpart in the studies of Jynge, Hearse and Braimbridge who found poor myocardial recovery of isolated hearts when calcium-free cardioplegic solutions were used[60].

These findings of the need to add some calcium to cardioplegic solution are in apparent contradiction with Engelman's conclusion that calcium addition is not necessary in the *in vivo* model[24]. This apparent conflict is resolved readily by realizing that the deleterious effects of calcium-deficient solutions are transient in the *in vivo* setting where normocalcaemic blood always replaces calcium-free cardioplegic solutions. The isolated heart studies do, however, emphasize the potential danger of excluding calcium from all cardioplegic solutions.

Normocalcaemic coronary perfusion is essential *only* when the heart must support the systemic circulation, but not during extracorporeal circulation. The ionic calcium of cardioplegic solutions should probably be lowered since hypocalcaemia hastens the occurrence of arrest and makes less calcium immediately available to enter the ischaemic cells. Ways to achieve safe hypocalcaemia include: (1) adding small amounts of ionic calcium to asanguinous solutions[31]; (2) chelating ionic calcium of blood with safe amounts of citrate[33]; and (3) blocking the calcium uptake pharmacologically with either verapamil[85] or nifedipine[20]. Citrate has the potential advantage of having a very transient effect, but its concentrations should be limited to amounts sufficient to produce approximately half-strength calcium concentrations. Extreme citrate concentrations interfere with aerobic and anerobic energy production[83] and produce dangerous levels of hypocalcaemia[36].

Studies by Robb-Nicholson, Currie and Wechsler[85], using verapamil and by Clark *et al.* using nifedipine[20] document that pharmacological hypocalcaemia enhances myocardial protection during hypothermic aortic clamping. These calcium-binding drugs provide the added dividend of preventing calcium from flooding into myocardial cells following aortic unclamping. Several studies also establish the value of keeping ionic calcium low during the initial phase of reoxygenation[20, 32]. One potential disadvantage of pharmacological hypocalcaemia with long-acting drugs is that post-bypass ventricular function may be depressed if the action of these drugs persists when the heart, rather than the extracorporeal circuit, is required to provide for the systemic circulation.

Procaine

Procaine is a local anaesthetic which produces cardioplegia when introduced into the heart in high concentrations. Procaine has been shown to stabilize the cell membrane but the mechanism by which procaine produces cardioplegia is uncertain. I suspect that its membrane stabilizing value may be through its cardioplegic effect. Our studies show that procaine cardioplegia produces as much myocardial protection as does the single-dose cardioplegia in the heart subjected to one hour of aortic clamping with topical hypothermia[27, 76].

The apparent conflict in the literature about the need for procaine can be explained by considering the experimental models. Kay *et al.* studied single-dose hypothermic cardioplegia and found that procaine added significantly to the protective effects of potassium cardioplegia during 90 minutes of aortic clamping[62]. Conversely, studies of multidose hypothermic cardioplegia for two hours showed that procaine does not add to the effects of potassium or magnesium cardioplegia if the solution is replenished every 15 to 20 minutes[24, 33, 34].

It is important to realize that the effects of procaine cardioplegia on the myocardial cell persist despite its washout by non-coronary collateral flow. Consequently, procaine may enhance the safety of single-dose cardioplegia by prolonging the duration of asystole through counteracting the return of the electromechanical activity which would otherwise recur when the cardioplegic solution is washed away by non-coronary collateral blood flow. Conversely, procaine is not needed with multidose cardioplegia because arrest is assured by the periodic replenishment of the cardioplegic solution.

We observed the prolonged cardioplegic effect of procaine in our earlier clinical experience when we added procaine to the plasma cardioplegic solution which we replenished each 20 minutes. We often had to wait 20–30 minutes for the heart to restart after the aortic clamp was removed. While no evidence of deleterious effects resulted, extracorporeal circulation was prolonged unnecessarily and the level of surgical anxiety was increased exponentially.

Hypothermia

Myocardial hypothermia reduces cardiac metabolism and it is therefore an important fact in extending the safety margin of aortic clamping of any duration. *Hypothermia is, however, only one of several essential elements of protection which must be addressed clinically and it cannot be relied upon as the major protective factor during ischaemia*. Complete reliance upon the absolute benefits of hypothermia has led to (1) a false sense of security about myocardial protection as long as the heart is kept cold; (2) an obstacle to the general acceptance, understanding, and interest in other aspects of the supply/demand balance which must be considered during aortic clamping; and (3) the use of clinical levels of hypothermia which have not been proven completely safe under experimental conditions.

The failure of hypothermia without cardioplegia to provide adequate myocardial protection is evident from various studies showing substantially more myocardial damage after topical hypothermic ischaemic arrest at left ventricular temperatures between 14° and 16°C than with single-dose cardioplegia where the mean left ventricular temperature averaged 26°C during one hour of ischaemia[39] (*Figure 10.14*). Furthermore, severe cardiac damage occurred after two hours of aortic clamping and intermittent

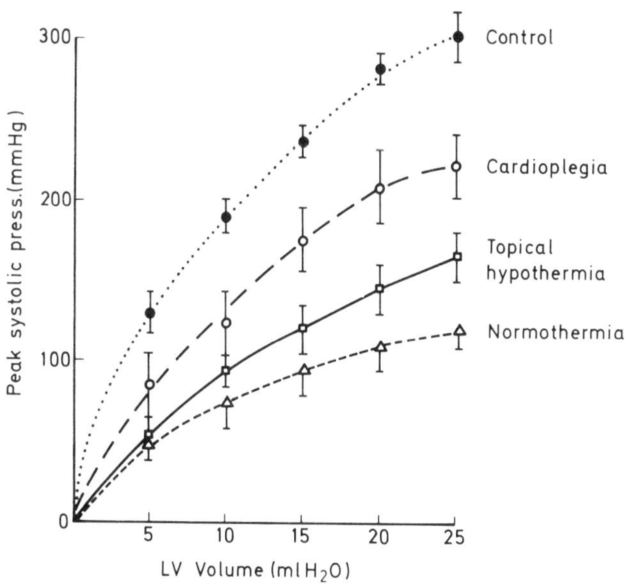

Figure 10.14 Left ventricular function after 60 minutes of euthermic, topical hypothermic, and cardioplegic arrest. Note the mild improvement offered by topical hypothermia, the increased protection offered by single-dose cardioplegia and the failure of cardioplegia to provide complete restoration of ventricular performance when it is only given as a single dose

infusion of blood at 20°C but without cardioplegic additives. On the other hand, multidose infusion of blood at 20°C with cardioplegic additives provided complete myocardial protection for two hours[34] (*Figure 10.15*).

At 22°C, the arrested heart requires only 0.31 cc of oxygen/100 g per min[14], an energy requirement which is extremely low and which is reduced to only 0.27 of O_2 cc/100 g per min by more profound cooling to 15°C[12]. The advantages of myocardial temperatures below 20°C include insurance of a

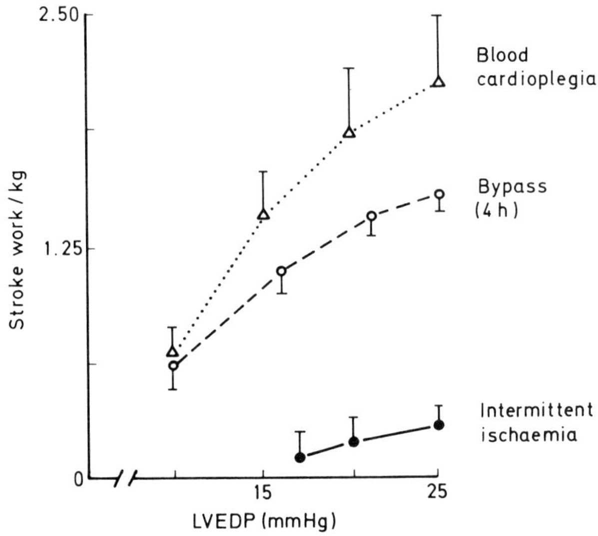

Figure 10.15 Left ventricular function curves after two hours of ischaemic arrest at 22°C (*bottom curve*), four hours of continuous euthermic coronary perfusion (bypass) and two hours of blood cardioplegic aortic clamping at 22°C (*top curve*). Note: (1) severe myocardial depression after cold ischaemic arrest with intermittent reinfusion of unmodified blood; (2) moderate depression after continuous coronary perfusion without ischaemia (reflecting a reduction in ventricular compliance); and (3) near normal myocardial function after two hours of aortic clamping with intermittent blood cardioplegia when compared with the control pre-ischaemic levels of performance. LVEDP = left ventricular end-diastolic pressure

longer period of cardioplegia with a single dose of any solution, and less potassium requirement to produce asystole.

The zeal and unfounded faith in profound hypothermia has led to recommendations for clinical use of cardioplegic solutions below 10°C despite experimental evidence that myocardial recovery from ischaemia is impaired when such profound hypothermic levels are tested in isolated hearts[97]. Studies by Tyers *et al.*[97] and more recently by Shragge, Digerness and Blackstone[93] show that myocardial glycogen does not fall in either ischaemic or perfused heart models cooled below 10°C. Such observations suggest that profound hypothermia may impair glycolysis and anaerobic energy production or utilization. Another potential deleterious effect of profound hypothermia is the possible sludging of red blood cells by rouleau formation which might impair subsequent reperusion of small myocardial segments.

While hypothermic levels below 10°C may be safe in the clinical setting, *in vivo* studies ought to be performed to prove this. It is unlikely, however, that persistent <10°C myocardial temperatures can be achieved and maintained persistently below 10°C under clinical conditions (despite the use of 4°C cardioplegic infusates) since all cardioplegic solutions are progressively replaced by non-coronary collateral flow which is at the same temperature as the extracorporeal circuit.

The level of clinical cardiac cooling is difficult to control because the presence of coronary artery disease makes perfusion hypothermia occur at unequal rates in different myocardial segments and because the septum may rewarm more rapidly than other myocardial areas since it is bathed with systemic venous return (unless the venae cavae are isolated and snared individually). Topical hypothermia, although cumbersome, enhances the action of the cardioplegic drugs in experimental studies of normal hearts left within the pericardial sac during the entire period of aortic clamping[76]. Topical hypothermia, however, produces differing and uneven rates of myocardial cooling especially at the level of the septum and the left ventricular subendocardial regions, specifically in patients with hypertrophied hearts. Furthermore, it is impossible to keep topical hypothermic contact with the heart during coronary operations where the heart must be removed from the pericardial sac during distal grafting of all but the left anterior descending branch and the very proximal segment of the right coronary arteries. Topical hypothermia is an excellent adjunct to cardioplegia during aortic valve replacement because the heart remains in the pericardial sac and the topical cold solution can be applied also to the inside of the ventricular cavity. A strong indication for adding topical hypothermia to cardioplegia is when the cardioplegic solution cannot be infused into the right coronary artery during aortic valve replacement, especially if there is coexistent mitral valve disease with right ventricular hypertrophy and/or hypertension.

The substrate

The current controversy about the need for and potential dangers of adding substrate to cardioplegic solutions arises principally from differences between experimental and clinical models rather than from scientific disagreement among investigators. I am sure that all investigators and clinicians agree that the ischaemic heart which is asystolic must continue to produce some energy in order to keep the cell metabolic processes intact and that the energy production requires the availability of substrate and the presence of an environment within which it can be metabolized.

In the laboratory setting, substrate depletion is rare in healthy hearts studied under controlled circumstances and in physiological environments. Conversely, during clinical open-heart surgery there are unavoidable episodes of hypo- and hypertension before the inception of extracorporeal circulation. Such episodes produce ischaemia, cause anaerobic glycolysis, and deplete the energy stores (especially in sick patients with cardiac disease). It seems apparent, therefore, that anaerobic energy production during aortic clamping might be either reduced or impaired unless some substrate is replenished.

The evidence supporting the avoidance of substrate enhancement is marshalled from studies of isolated hearts where postischaemic recovery is impaired when glucose is added to the perfusates, especially if insulin is used to enhance glucose uptake[45, 87]. Unquestionably, substrate enhancement stimulates glycolytic energy production with a consequent accelerated build-up of lactate and resultant intracellular acidosis. Anaerobic energy production is desirable, but the end products of this metabolism will impair subsequent glycolysis unless provisions are made to wash out lactate and counteract acidosis. Both Rovetto, Whitmer and Neely[87] and Hearse, Stewart and Braimbridge[45] found in their isolated heart studies that substrate enhancement is deleterious but neither of them made provisions to wash away the end products of anaerobiosis during the experiments. Conversely, Hewitt *et al.* provided for such washout in their study of *in vivo* hearts and found glucose and insulin to enhance markedly the effectiveness of cardioplegia[46]. In the clinical setting, non-coronary collateral blood flow and intermittent replenishment of a buffered cardioplegic solution washes away the acid metabolites.

In cardiac patients some substrate is provided continually by the glucose content of the non-coronary collateral blood flow. It is, however, probably advisable to add glucose and insulin to asanguinous (especially anoxic)

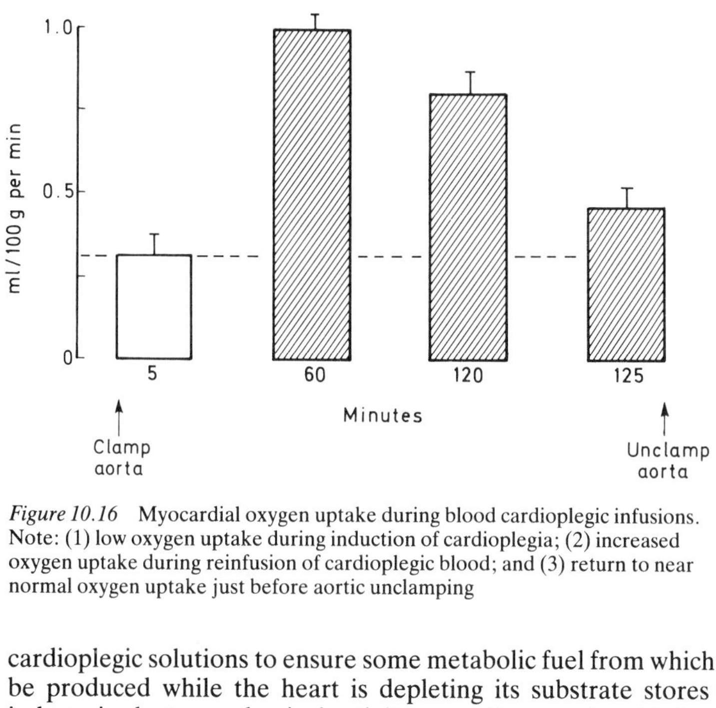

Figure 10.16 Myocardial oxygen uptake during blood cardioplegic infusions. Note: (1) low oxygen uptake during induction of cardioplegia; (2) increased oxygen uptake during reinfusion of cardioplegic blood; and (3) return to near normal oxygen uptake just before aortic unclamping

cardioplegic solutions to ensure some metabolic fuel from which energy can be produced while the heart is depleting its substrate stores during the ischaemic electromechanical activity preceding arrest and following cardioplegic washout. Substrate enhancement is apparently most helpful when the glycogen stores are raised by diet[46], glucose loading before aortic clamping[3], or glucose infusion during aortic clamping. Substrate enhancement is less important with oxygenated cardioplegic solutions since anaerobic energy stores are not depleted during the electromechanical activity preceding the arrest. The glucose content of the systemic perfusate (if used as the cardioplegic vehicle) may provide sufficient fuel for aerobic recharging of energy stores during multidose blood cardioplegia as cardiac oxygen uptake more than doubles with each blood cardioplegic replenishment[83] (*Figure 10.16*).

Buffering

Buffering the cardioplegic solution provides for an appropriate pH for continued metabolism at any myocardial temperature and counteracts the acidosis of ischaemia. As mentioned previously, the ischaemic heart relies upon continued anaerobic glycolysis to produce energy for basal metabolic needs. Such anaerobic energy production is inhibited by the intracellular acidosis and lactate production which results inevitably from glycolysis.

The ideal 'pH' for biological systems is described in the classic work of Peters and Van Slyke on acid–base balance published in 1932[80] and reviewed recently by Rahn, Reeves and Howell[82]. These authors stated that for a 'state compatible with life the reactions of the inner fluids must be slightly to the alkaline side of the neutral point'. The pH of water changes with temperature so that at 37°C, for example, the pH of water is 6.8 and the pH range of vertebrate blood is 7.35 to 7.45. It is not surprising, therefore, that when the pH of water rises to 7.2 at 20°C, poikilothermic vertebrates in their natural environment raise their pH to 7.8[4, 55]. It is only in the clinical setting, where the physician controls the pH, that some have persisted in constraining pH at 7.4 at all levels of temperature. The preceding biological and physical data suggest that this constraint is neither physiological nor ideal.

As mentioned previously, our experimental studies[71] show that the appropriate pH for myocardial metabolism at 28°C is 7.70, a value similar to that attained by poikilothermic animals at that temperature. It follows, logically, that cardioplegic solutions should be buffered to an even higher pH if their temperature is lowered below 28°C. Fortunately, blood pH during hypothermia is always more alkaline than when measured at 37°C. In all physical solutions, the pH rises 0.0134 units for each °C of hypothermia[86]. Consequently, pH 7.4 at 37°C becomes pH 7.67 at 17°C. This value is still considerably lower than the 8.0 to 8.1 level which is appropriate for optimal enzymatic function at 17°C.

Failure to provide an appropriate pH may impair continued anaerobic energy production despite availability of abundant substrates. The buffer of choice for cardioplegic solutions should be selected so that its optimal effects occur in the pH range most appropriate for the clinically-required myocardial temperature. For example, we chose THAM buffer because this intracellular and extracellular buffer exerts its optimum buffering effect between pH 7.8 and 8.1 at the 20°C myocardial temperature which we use. We have not tested other buffering systems, but suspect that other buffers would also be effective, depending upon the desired temperature. Lactate should not, however, be used because it is a poor buffer during hypothermia and it inhibits anaerobic glycolysis independent of pH[43].

Cardioplegic buffers and replenishment may assume added significance in the clinical setting where the body temperature is usually kept at 28°C and selective cardiac hypothermia is routinely practised. The systemic pH does not need to be adjusted much in excess of the naturally occurring physical rise to provide for an ideal systemic metabolism at 28°C, but such systemic perfusate blood replaces the buffered cardioplegic solutions with non-coronary collateral blood which is more acidotic than desirable. This problem would not, of course, occur during circulatory arrest in infants or be realized by those who make no effort to adjust the pH.

Membrane stabilization

It is becoming apparent that the cell membrane is the myocardial structure most vulnerable to ischaemic damage[36, 66, 103]. Consequently, a major effort should be made to avoid its injury during aortic clamping. It seems intuitively obvious that the cardioplegic solution itself should not cause cell membrane damage. The recent studies of Langer *et al.* show that such damage can be avoided by ensuring that any solution perfusing the heart contains some calcium[36] (*see* section on calcium).

Procaine and steroids are the two drugs used most often for membrane stabilization[6, 12] although the mechanism of action of either of them is uncertain. Our previous study of these drugs during one hour of topical hypothermic ischaemic arrest shows that they reduce the depression of postischaemic myocardial contractility, but fail to protect against postischaemic oedema and impaired compliance or allow for complete restitution of high energy phosphate stores[26]. Steroids also cause vasodilatation and result in higher postischaemic subendocardial flows[26]. Coronary hyperfusion cannot account for the protective action of steroids, since procaine-treated hearts recovered more completely, despite substantially less postischaemic flows[27].

Experimental studies show that complete myocardial protection is possible *without* membrane stabilization (i.e. procaine) when normal dog hearts are given multidose cardioplegia during two hours of aortic clamping[24, 32, 44]. Based on these studies we concluded that exogenous membrane stabilizing drugs were not necessary if the membrane was kept stable by a properly designed and correctly administered cardioplegic solution.

Our recent experience with cardioplegia in patients with coronary artery disease or in those with hypertrophied hearts, however, shows that the complete protection achieved in the experimental setting was attained in clinical practice[33]. While hearts treated with cardioplegia showed less enzymatic evidence of myocardial damage than those subjected to continuous coronary perfusion or short periods of ischaemic arrest, some enzymatic signs of injury were however observed. It is conceivable that membrane stabilization may have reduced this damage, but I believe that the problem lies more with the adequacy of cardioplegic delivery to all myocardial regions than with the chemical make-up of the cardioplegic solution (*see* section on limitations of pharmacological cardioplegia). In light of this discrepancy between laboratory and clinical findings, a controlled double-blind study on the adding of membrane-stabilizing drugs to established and effective cardioplegic protocols appears warranted.

Osmolarity

Myocardial oedema is a regular consequence of ischaemic damage and therefore it is essential that the cardioplegic solution should not compound this problem by causing myocardial swelling because of its inappropriate composition. To avoid producing iatrogenic cardiac oedema, the cardioplegic solution must contain sufficient osmotic and/or oncotic pressure to keep the fluid within the vascular space. In a recent study, we could produce myocardial oedema with clinical cardioplegic solutions which did not contain sufficient oncotic/osmotic ingredients to ensure reabsorption of water[28]. The amount of myocardial swelling and dehydration caused by different solutions was related to the fluid constituents, rather than their infusion pressures or volumes. Protein was *not* a necessary constituent (when ischaemia was limited to ten minutes) if the molarity of crystalloid solutions was raised sufficiently (to 370 mmol) with mannitol. This observation has clinical implications in that protein, a costly additive, does not appear necessary if sufficient mannitol is used. Our studies on cardioplegic oedema were, however, carried out with very short ischaemic intervals (10 minutes), and must be repeated with prolonged ischaemia before these results can be extrapolated to the clinical setting.

It is probably advantageous to make all cardioplegic solutions slightly hyperosmotic since myocardial oedema tends to accumulate while the aorta is clamped[31]. This ischaemic cardiac swelling may occur because both hypothermia and ischaemia impair transmyocardial fluid transport. The oedema develops in spite of only slight amounts of flows from non-coronary collateral sources. The ideal cardioplegic molarity has not been established, but should not exceed 400 mmol since several studies have shown that higher molarities produce myocardial damage in the absence of ischaemia[28] and, in addition, limit the effectiveness of cardioplegic solutions[96]. Conversely, 370 mmol cardioplegic solutions produce approximately 2 per cent myocardial dehydration and do not impair cardiac function[31].

Cardioplegic vehicle

The 'ideal' vehicle for the cardioplegic solution has not yet been established. I am, however, convinced that the vehicle should contain oxygen in order to prevent the useless expenditure of vital energy which might otherwise accompany the electromechanical work preceding the arrest, during the induction and replenishment of the cardioplegic solution. Oxygenation of the cardioplegic solution could be accomplished by either bubbling oxygen into asanguinous solutions, using blood from the extracorporeal circuit as the cardioplegic vehicle, or using stroma-free haemoglobin or some other oxygen carrier substance. I base this conclusion about the importance of

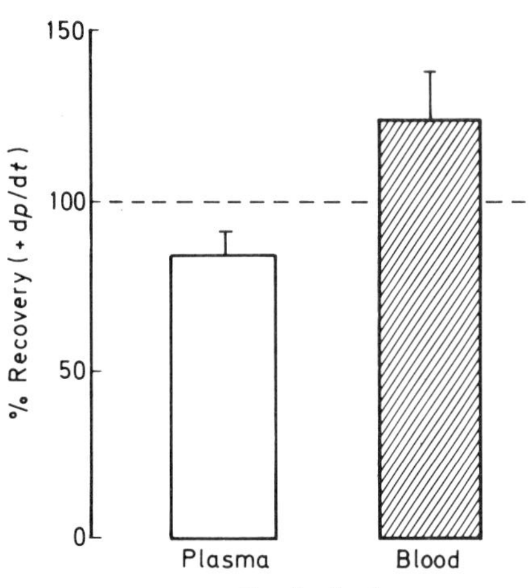

Figure 10.17 Volumetric left ventricular function (25 cc EDV), two hours following aortic clamping after infusion of the same cardioplegic solution given in either an asanguinous (plasma) or a sanguinous (blood) vehicle. Note: (1) slight myocardial depression when plasma vehicle is used; (2) complete recovery following blood cardioplegia. The slight augmentation above control values probably reflects the normal response to the catecholamines which were elaborated systemically during extracorporeal circulation

oxygenating the cardioplegic solution upon our studies which have demonstrated that the degree of myocardial protection during a period of two hours of aortic clamping, is better with blood cardioplegia than with plasma cardioplegia when the same cardioplegic additives were used in both solutions (*Figure 10.17*).

Limitations of pharmacological cardioplegia

Most clinical solutions which embrace the aforementioned principles of creating a favourable energy supply/demand balance will likely confer comparably good myocardial protection during ischaemia. In my view, the principal limitation of the effectiveness of pharmacological cardioplegia is with our ability to distribute and maintain the cardioplegic solutions to all myocardial segments in amounts sufficient to exert their protective effect. I base this conclusion on our studies showing that pharmacological arrest with one infusion of 500 ml of an asanguinous cardioplegic solution cooled at 4°C, embracing each factor which minimizes the supply/demand imbalance during aortic cross-clamping (for a period of 60 minutes), did not prevent mild but significant depression of myocardial compliance and function in normal hearts (*Figure 10.10*). Non-coronary collateral blood flow (3 ml/100 g per min) washed out the cardioplegic solution, rewarmed the heart (together with the ambient temperature) and restarted electromechanical activity[39]. We would expect more significant damage to occur in chronically

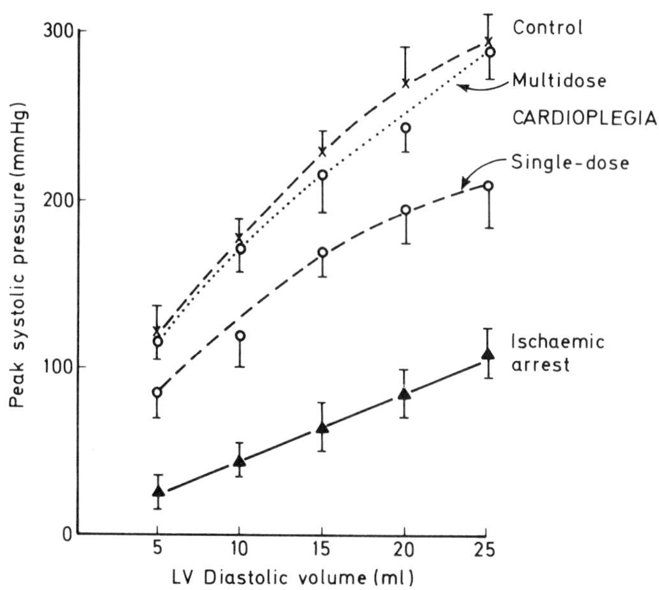

Figure 10.18 Left ventricular function after one hour of aortic clamping with ischaemic arrest at 22°C and perfusion hypothermia (*botton curve*), single-dose cardioplegia (*middle curve*) and multidose cardioplegia (*top curve*). Note: (1) profound depression of left ventricular function with cold ischaemic arrest; (2) 70 per cent recovery with single-dose cardioplegia; and (3) complete recovery following multidose cardioplegia

ischaemic or hypertrophied hearts subjected to a single dose of cardioplegia for a duration of 60 minutes or more.

This limitation of the single-dose cardioplegia was avoided, and the best protection against subendocardial damage achieved, when the cardioplegic solution was replenished periodically while the aorta was clamped for up to two hours (*Figure 10.18*). At this time, it is clearly established that the cardioplegic solution must be reinfused intermittently[24, 30, 31, 32, 75] (*Table 10.3*). The benefits of intermittent reinfusion of the cardioplegic solution include maintenance of arrest and of hypothermia, washout of acid metabolites, replenishment of substrate (oxygen or glucose for continued energy production), maintenance of an appropriate pH for hypothermic metabolic activity and treatment of evolving myocardial oedema. The ideal time for clinical reinfusion is uncertain because the chronically ischaemic and hypertrophied hearts of patients may have more non-coronary collateral flow than the normal dog hearts in which reinfusion at 20 minute intervals was found most appropriate. It is essential that care be taken to avoid air embolism during reinfusion, and to maintain the perfusion pressure at a low level in order to prevent the flaccid heart becoming oedematous.

Table 10.3 Advantages of multidose cardioplegia

Maintains arrest
Maintains hypothermia
Provides substrate
Maintains ideal pH
Washes out acid metabolites
Counteracts oedema

Non-homogeneous distribution of coronary blood flow is the principal limitation in patients with ischaemic heart disease. It is not surprising that this problem is also the principal limitation of the cardiac surgeon's ability to deliver any carefully designed cardioplegic solution to the hearts of patients with coronary artery disease. The frequent clinical observation that cold cardioplegic infusions in patients with coronary artery disease result in non-homogeneous ventricular cooling with occasional persistence of electromechanical activity in areas of obstructed coronary vessels has been reproduced by Hilton *et al.*[47] in the experimental setting. These investigators found that maldistribution of the cardioplegic solution causes localized postischaemic wall motion abnormalities which were not detectable when global myocardial function was tested. Such studies must be repeated in dogs with left ventricular hypertrophy (with and without coronary stenosis) to determine whether additional provisions should be made to ensure adequate delivery of cardioplegic solutions to hypertrophied hearts.

It is essential that we re-evaluate the way we deliver cardioplegic solutions in coronary patients. I am convinced that the current technique of infusing the cardioplegic solution through the proximal aorta in coronary patients is an unacceptable method because there is unreliable distribution to the distal areas of the myocardium. This problem can be cirvumvented by either making the proximal graft anastomoses before clamping the aorta and infusing the cardioplegic solution through the aortic root following the construction of each distal anastomosis, or by making the distal anastomoses first and delivering the solution through each sequential proximal and distal anastomosis to ensure delivery beyond the coronary stenoses. Obviously, the most critical myocardial regions should be revascularized first, rather than adhering strictly to any ritualistic procession from the left circumflex distribution to the right coronary distribution or vice versa.

The duration of ischaemia will be prolonged if all the anastomoses are made while the aorta is clamped. It should be remembered, however, that the degree of myocardial injury is determined by the quality of myocardial protection during the interruption of the coronary circulation, rather than by the duration of ischaemia. In our laboratory, for example, 15 minutes of euthermic anoxia causes more damage than 120 minutes of aortic clamping with multidose cardioplegia.

The systemic effects of admixture of cardioplegic solutions with the systemic perfusate must be considered when the solutions are allowed to recirculate. Potential problems with procaine include accentuation of heparin effects with possible consequent bleeding[69] and neurological complications if high systemic levels of this drug occur[98]. If, however, the more cumbersome technique of discarding the coronary venous effluent is employed, procaine addition may limit the number of times the cardioplegic solutions must be reinfused. One advantage of potassium cardioplegia is that the systemic effects of hyperkalaemia are well known and can be dealt with by using appropriate diuretic treatment (for example frusemide, mannitol) at the beginning of extracorporeal circulation. In children, however, we have encountered significant hyperkalaemia despite this precaution and now we discard the cardioplegic effluent in children and infants.

An untested but potential limitation of infusing various cardioplegic solutions is the possible vascular damage which might ensue when abnormally high concentrations of different ions come in contact with normal arteries and veins. Potassium, for example, is extremely irritating to peripheral veins when infused in concentrations which are customary during clinical cardioplegia. Hopefully, the short period of exposure of the coronary arteries and veins to high cardioplegic concentrations will minimize these potential effects, but longterm studies in the experimental setting are needed.

Clinical results may certainly be limited by using concentrations of ions proven deleterious in the experimental setting. Non-coronary collateral flow is always present, but it is too inconstant to be relied upon to minimize the known deleterious effects of inappropriate concentrations of cardioplegic constituents by washing them away before they cause damage. Nor should hypothermia be used as a substitute for the effectiveness of cardioplegic replenishment. While profound hypothermia may partially neutralize the effects of cardioplegic washout by delaying the recurrence of electromechanical activity during aortic clamping, cold alone will not counteract the progressive anaerobic lactate accumulation and build-up of metabolic products which may interfere with continued anaerobic energy production or the oedema developing in cold ischaemic hearts.

There may be serious implications of the false sense of security imposed by our current inability to detect subtle and potentially irreversible damage because of the relatively crude barometers of injury available in clinical practice. Schaper *et al.*, for example, showed severe ultrastructural damage in human hearts subjected to single-dose cardioplegia although none of these patients had apparent haemodynamic problems[91]. While such damage could possibly have been reduced by replenishing the cardioplegic solution in a multidose fashion, recent studies by Hearse and colleagues suggest that the solution used in those patients may have provided less than ideal protection[60]. The reversiblity of clinically undetectable intraoperative damage is not known, but irreversibility could account for the late fibrosis developing in the hearts of patients who had an 'unremarkable' early postoperative course[22].

Reperfusion injury

Haemorrhagic subendocardial necrosis can be produced experimentally without cardiopulmonary bypass by restoring blood flow to myocardial segments which have been made temporarily (40 minutes) ischaemic[59, 64]. *This experiment has its clinical counterpart in every operating room in the world where aortic cross-clamping is practised.*

Current evidence suggests that a major component of the damage induced by ischaemia occurs during the early phases of reoxygenation and that reperfusion damage can be avoided by appropriate modification of the blood delivered to the heart during immediate reperfusion[29, 30, 32, 35]. The reperfusion injury is characterized by intracellular calcium accumulation (leading to 'stone' or 'bone' heart when the condition is severe), explosive myocardial cell swelling which reduces postischaemic blood flow and depresses postischaemic compliance and ventricular function, and a marked inability of the postischaemic heart to utilize the delivered oxygen, even when coronary blood flow and oxygen content are quite ample[61, 68] (*Figure 10.19*). Preliminary studies show that this postischaemic reperfusion damage can be minimized (and often completely avoided) by maintaining

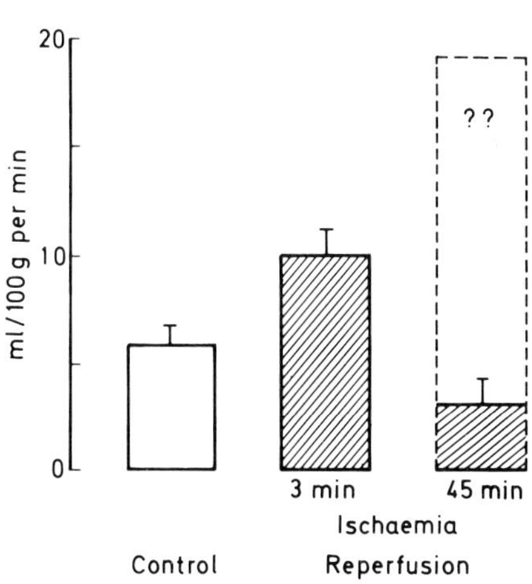

Figure 10.19 Oxygen uptake of the beating empty heart during the control period and after reversible (3 minute) and irreversible (45 minute) global ischaemia produced by aortic clamping. Note: (1) increased oxygen uptake above baseline levels during reperfusion after three minutes of ischaemia; (2) failure to show the expected increased oxygen uptake (*hatched line*) after prolonged ischaemia, with oxygen uptake actually falling below the resting requirements. In this instance, coronary blood flow was increased to 300 per cent above the control levels but the irreversible damaged heart failed to extract oxygen normally

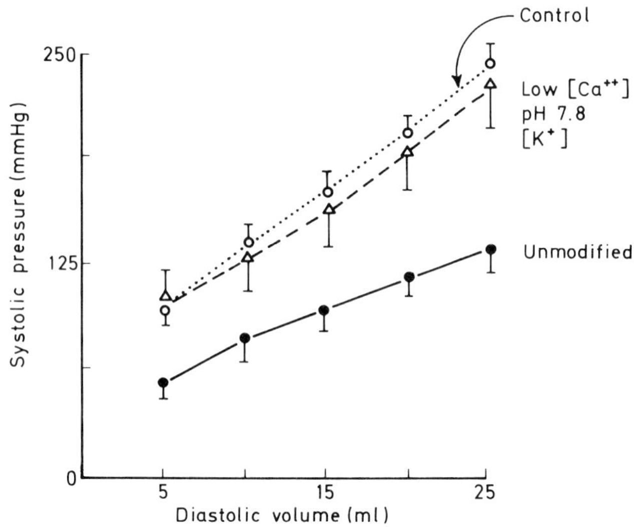

Figure 10.20 Postischaemic left ventricular function (following one hour of topical hypothermic ischaemia arrest) when the initial reperfusate blood (500 ml) was unmodified (*lower curve*) or where this initial reperfusate blood was made hypocalcaemic (with CPD), buffered to pH 7.8 (with THAM), and rendered moderately hyperkalaemic (KCI) to keep the heart arrested. Note the complete recovery when the postischaemic heart was kept arrested during reperfusion and reperfusate blood contained low calcium and high pH

cardioplegia during the immediate phase of reoxygenation while adjusting the pH, the calcium content and the molarity of reperfusate blood[32] (*Figure 10.20*). It is our concept that maintenance of cardioplegia during the initial phase of reperfusion allows as much of the delivered oxygen to be used for reparative work, rather than wasting it on useless electromechanical work (*Figure 10.21*). Such observations have immense clinical importance, since they suggest that many of the limitations of cardioplegia and its delivery may be counteracted, to a great extent, by appropriate reperfusion of the myocardium prior to aortic unclamping.

Considerations after heart-lung bypass

Impaired myocardial performance following discontinuation of extracorporeal circulation indicates that the heart, particularly the subendocardial muscle, has sustained ischaemic damage before and during bypass and that the injury has not yet been repaired[18]. If myocardial protection has been adequate, however, a technical problem must be suspected (malfunctioning heart valve prosthesis, occluded coronary artery, etc.). The diagnosis of supply/demand imbalance will become evident usually from a high left atrial pressure and low endocardial viability ratio (DPTI/TTI <0.8)[81]. Failure to optimize this ratio will accentuate ischaemia. The aims of the treatment are to reduce the oxygen demands and to increase the oxygen supply. The

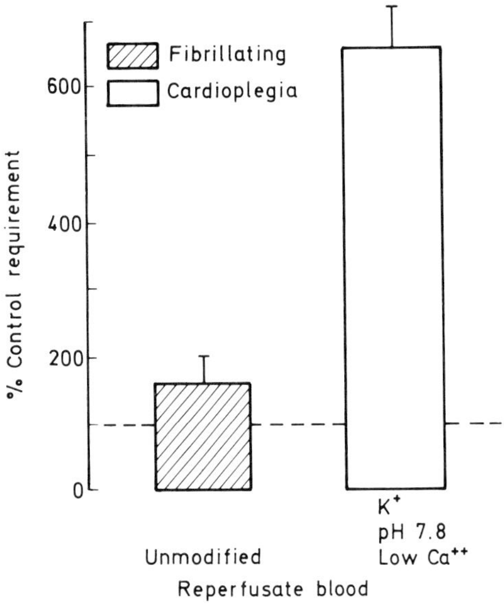

Figure 10.21 Left ventricular oxygen uptake during the initial reperfusion period (60 min 16°C ischaemic arrest) when the heart was allowed to fibrillate while being reperfused with unmodified blood (*left panel*) and when the heart was kept arrested and reperfused with hypocalcaemic, hyperkalaemic and alkalotic blood (*right panel*). Note: (1) hearts allowed to fibrillate during reperfusion consume approximately just as much oxygen as necessary to meet the basal requirements of fibrillation; and (2) hearts kept arrested consumed 500 per cent more oxygen than needed to meet the basal requirements of arrest

therapeutic options include: (1) resumption of *total* cardiopulmonary bypass or maintenance of partial heart-lung bypass (venoarterial, left atrial-aortic); (2) intra-aortic balloon counterpulsation; (3) briefly rearresting the post-ischaemic heart by inducing a *secondary cardioplegia*; and (4) manipulation of preload, afterload, heart rate and cardiac contractility.

Total versus partial heart-lung bypass

In the absence of extracorporeal circulation, interruption of myocardial oxygen supply causes an almost immediate depression of cardiac performance. Contractility does not recover completely until coronary reactive hyperaemia provides sufficient oxygen supply to restore the cellular metabolic processes to normal levels. It seems logical to assume that augmentation of myocardial oxygen demands during the reactive hyperaemia would accentuate the ischaemic damage. Conversely, it is not surprising that experimental studies show the ventricular performance to improve progressively when total cardiopulmonary bypass is prolonged following the ischaemic injury[68]. Thus, the energy stores become replenished, rather than further expended by premature external work.

Total heart-lung bypass markedly reduces the myocardial oxygen requirements by converting the heart to the beating empty state[68]. Simultaneously, subendocardial blood (oxygen) supply can be raised by increasing the aortic pressure and the red cell mass (especially if extreme haemodilution has been used). The use of inotropic drugs should be avoided during prolongation of total heart-lung bypass because they increase the oxygen demands unnecessarily at a time when no external cardiac work is required and the oxygen needs should be kept at a low level. Moreover, inotropic drugs can cause subendocardial necrosis even in normal hearts. Prolongation of total bypass may be needed after myocardial revascularization procedures despite only short ischaemic intervals, because maintenance of a satisfactory perfusion pressure to the distal myocardium is not possible until all aorta-to-coronary-artery grafts are functioning. The most severe subendocardial damage can be expected, therefore, in patients with coronary artery disease in whom complete myocardial revascularization has not been achieved.

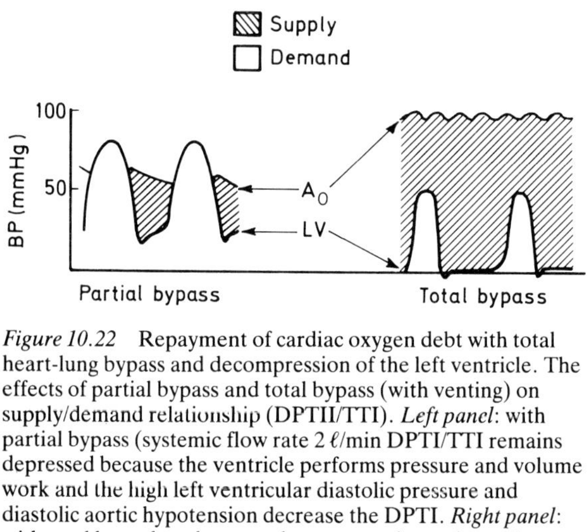

Figure 10.22 Repayment of cardiac oxygen debt with total heart-lung bypass and decompression of the left ventricle. The effects of partial bypass and total bypass (with venting) on supply/demand relationship (DPTII/TTI). *Left panel*: with partial bypass (systemic flow rate 2 ℓ/min DPTI/TTI remains depressed because the ventricle performs pressure and volume work and the high left ventricular diastolic pressure and diastolic aortic hypotension decrease the DPTI. *Right panel*: with total heart-lung bypass adequate venting reduces the oxygen demands and removes the impedence to subendocardial perfusion produced by high left ventricular diastolic pressure. The supply is optimized by elevation of the aortic blood pressure with increased extracorporeal flow rate and/or administration of a peripheral vasoconstrictive drug

The effectiveness of cardiopulmonary bypass in reducing ischaemia and relieving the work load of the heart is achieved only when the left ventricle is completely vented[79]. On the other hand, partial bypass (diverting 50–90 per cent of venous return) lowers left ventricular oxygen needs only slightly (10 per cent)[79] and may not improve oxygen supply. The partially bypassed heart must continue to perform both pressure and volume work and because of its impaired function it frequently has a high left ventricular end-diastolic pressure which reduces the coronary driving pressure and impedes subendocardial blood supply[17] (*Figure 10.22*).

Secondary cardioplegia

In the past, attention has been focused upon ways to improve oxygen delivery to the postischaemic myocardial cells. At present, it is obvious that the delivery of even abundant amounts of oxygen does not ensure that the cells can utilize this oxygen to repair ischaemic damage or reconstitute depressed energy stores. Our pilot studies show that some reversal of reperfusion damage is possible by rearresting the postischaemic heart with an oxygenated cardioplegic solution while the supportive extracorporeal circulation is prolonged[67]. Such secondary cardioplegia allows better myocardial recovery than is possible by prolongation of heart-lung bypass alone (*Figure 10.23*). Secondary cardioplegia is effective because it allows the limited oxygen uptake of a heart suffering from reperfusion injury to be

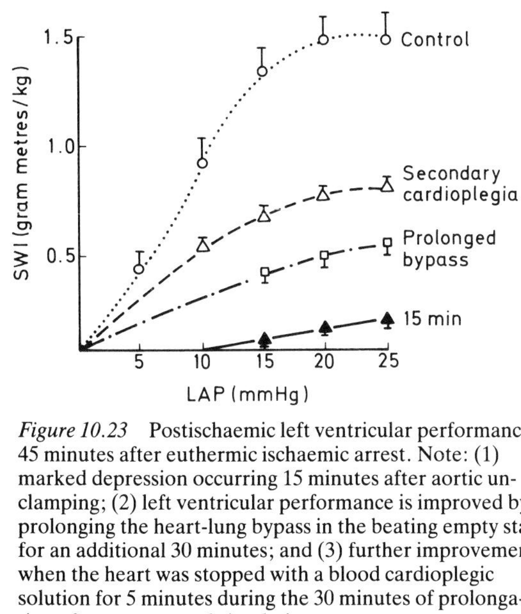

Figure 10.23 Postischaemic left ventricular performance 45 minutes after euthermic ischaemic arrest. Note: (1) marked depression occurring 15 minutes after aortic unclamping; (2) left ventricular performance is improved by prolonging the heart-lung bypass in the beating empty state for an additional 30 minutes; and (3) further improvement when the heart was stopped with a blood cardioplegic solution for 5 minutes during the 30 minutes of prolongation of extracorporeal circulation

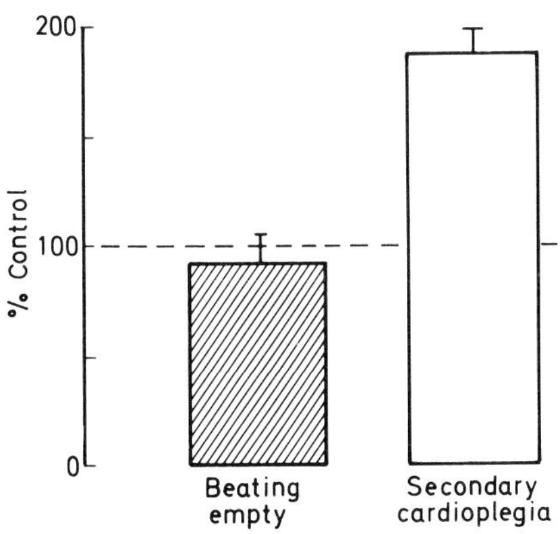

Figure 10.24 Myocardial oxygen uptake 15 minutes after aortic unclamping in the beating empty heart (*left panel*) and in the heart stopped by a continuous infusion of a blood cardioplegic solution for 5 minutes (*right panel*). Note the increased oxygen uptake in the heart stopped with blood cardioplegia. We presume this increased oxygen is used to promote cellular repair

channeled towards reparative processes rather than to be wasted in performing electromechanical work. The beating empty heart needs three to six times more oxygen than the arrested heart at 37°C[14] (*Figure 10.24*). As we learn more about the characteristics of reperfusion injury, it should be possible to develop cardioplegic solutions and reperfusates containing the appropriate ions, substrates, and possible co-factors which will completely avoid ischaemic and reperfusion damage.

Inotropic drugs

It is possible, in many patients who develop depressed myocardial performance shortly after aortic unclamping, to force the left ventricle to generate a normal cardiac output by the administration of inotropic drugs. In my view,

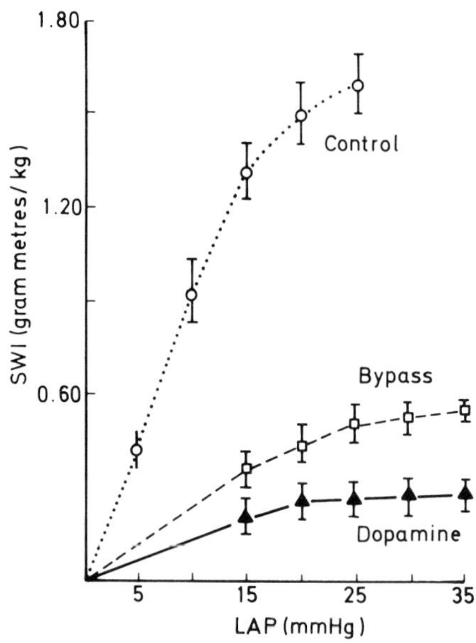

Figure 10.25 Postischaemic left ventricular performance in hearts subjected to 45 minutes of euthermic ischaemic arrest (45 min normothermic arrest). When ventricular performance was depressed 15 minutes after unclamping, the dopamine-treated hearts underwent a 15 minute infusion of this drug in order to discontinue the heart-lung bypass. The other group underwent prolongation of extracorporeal circulation for 30 additional minutes. The function curves were inscribed 15 minutes after the dopamine had been discontinued and the hearts had been replaced on extracorporeal circulation. Note that the function of hearts kept on extracorporeal circulation for a limited time interval is better than that of those treated with dopamine in order to discontinue the heart-lung bypass early after aortic unclamping

such premature administration of inotropic drug support provides the surgeon with a false sense of security about the adequacy of myocardial function and actually accentuates the ischaemic damage. Our studies have shown[68] that it is far better to rest the heart by prolonging the cardiopulmonary bypass while decompressing the heart chambers by venting for a limited duration of time than to discontinue the bypass and to stimulate the heart with inotropic drugs[68] (*Figure 10.25*).

Intra-aortic balloon counterpulsation

The use of the intra-aortic balloon is physiologically more sound than the use of inotropic drugs (which increase the oxygen needs). During the deflation phase of the balloon the oxygen demands are lowered while the inflation of the balloon augments the supply of oxygenated blood to the myocardium. Intra-aortic balloon counterpulsation does not, however,

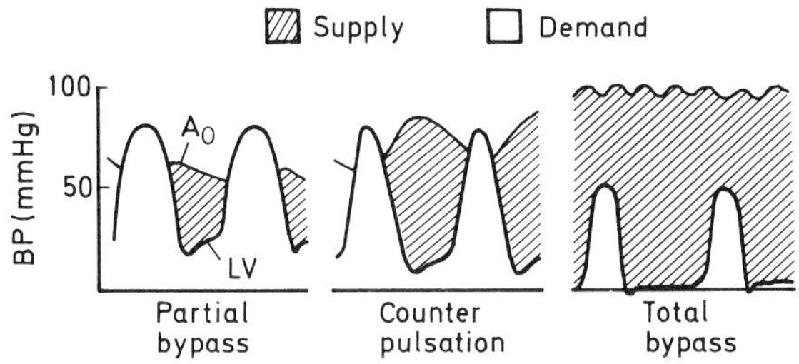

Figure 10.26 Effects of partial bypass, of diastolic aortic counterpulsation, and of total (vented) heart-lung bypass on supply/demand relationship. The cross-hatched area is the DPTI. The open area is the TTI. *Left panel*: with partial bypass, the supply/demand ratio remains depressed because the left ventricle performs pressures and volume work (increasing demands), and because there is high left ventricular diastolic pressure and aortic diastolic hypertension which decrease the supply. *Middle panel*: while counterpulsation increases markedly the 'supply' by raising the diastolic perfusion pressure and reduces TTI by lowering the systolic pressure with ventricular unloading, some volume and isometric ventricular pressure is still necessary. Note that the ventricular diastolic pressure remains elevated. *Right panel*: with total bypass, adequate venting reduces the oxygen demands and removes impedance to subendocardial perfusion by lowering the high left ventricular diastolic pressure. The supply is optimized by raising the aortic blood pressure with increased extracorporeal flow rate and/or administration of a peripheral vasoconstrictive drug

improve the supply/demand balance nearly as well as total cardiopulmonary bypass since the left ventricle must still perform pressure and volume work and retains a high diastolic pressure despite counterpulsation[4] (*Figure 10.26*). Intra-aortic counterpulsation may be helpful while total heart-lung bypass is prolonged because it increases subendocardial perfusion by augmenting the aortic diastolic pressure. Balloon counterpulsation is most effective when the supply/demand balance remains impaired (DPTI/TTI >0.8) after discontinuing total and/or partial bypass (*Figure 10.20*). Bregman[11], Phillips[81] and Goldman[38] and their associates report survival in patients who require balloon counterpulsation only when they can maintain a satisfactory supply/demand (DPTI/TTI >0.8) without mechanical support. The use of balloon counterpulsation has certainly extended our capacity to salvage patients who would have otherwise succumbed from severe subendocardial myocardial necrosis. It will be only through late follow-up studies of these ventricles that we will realize how much subendocardial damage has occurred.

Patients who sustain less severe left ventricular subendocardial injury exhibit a depressed cardiac performance in the early postoperative period and can usually be managed successfully by optimizing the supply/demand balance with adjustment of preload, afterload, heart rate and contractility to provide a satisfactory cardiac output[13] (*see* Considerations before bypass). The need for postoperative inotropic support implies, however, that a significant number of myocardial cells have been irreversibly damaged.

The degree of myocardial depression which requires mechanical or pharmacological circulatory support is encountered only in those patients who have sustained obvious and severe subendocardial necrosis. Sapsford *et al.* report an alarmingly high (more than 50 per cent) incidence of enzymatic evidence of myocardial necrosis in patients who did not need postoperative circulatory assistance[88]. The longterm effects of this more subtle form of subendocardial damage will not be known until we develop both the impetus and the simplified methodology for routine study of ventricular performance months-to-years after operation. I strongly suspect that through such studies we will find that delayed myocardial fibrosis reflects the healed result of perioperative subendocardial necrosis and I believe that the role of surgery in the natural history of congenital and acquired heart disease will not be established until perioperative subendocardial necrosis is prevented by adequate intraoperative myocardial protection.

References

1. Archie, J. P., Fixler, D. E., Ullyot, D. J., Buckberg, G. D. and Hoffman, J. I. E. 'Regional myocardial blood flow in lambs with concentric right ventricular hypertrophy.' *Circulation Research*, **34,** 143 (1974)
2. Archie, J. P. and Kirklin, J. W. 'Effect of hypothermic perfusion on myocardial oxygen consumption and coronary resistance.' *Surgical Forum*, **24,** 186 (1973)
3. Austen, W. G., Greenberg, J. J., Piccinini, J. C. 'Myocardial function and contractile force affected by glucose loading of the heart during anoxia.' *Surgery*, **67,** 839 (1965)
4. Baird, R. J., Dutka, F., Okumori, M., de la Rocha, A., Goldbach, M. D., Hill, T. J. and MacGregor, D. C. 'Surgical aspects of regional myocardial blood flow and myocardial pressure.' *Journal of Thoracic and Cardiovascular Surgery*, **69,** 17 (1975)
5. Bayliss, C. E. and Maloney, J. V., Jr. 'Shelf-storage of excised hearts by manipulation of transmembrane ionic gradients.' *Surgical Forum*, **21,** 194 (1970)
6. Bleese, N., Doring, V., Kalmar, P., Pokar, H., Polonius, M., Steiner, D. and Rodewald, G. 'Intraoperative myocardial protection by cardioplegia in hypothermia.' *Journal of Thoracic and Cardiovascular Surgery*, **75,** 405 (1978)
7. Brazier, J. R. and Buckberg, G. D. 'Effects of tachycardia on the adequacy of subendocardial oxygen delivery in aortic stenosis.' *American Heart Journal*, **90,** 222 (1975)
8. Brazier, J. R., Cooper, N. and Buckberg, G. D. 'The adequacy of subendocardial oxygen delivery: the interaction of determinants of flow, arterial oxygen content and myocardial oxygen need.' *Circulation*, **49,** 968 (1974)
9. Brazier, J. R., Cooper, N., McConnell, D. H. and Buckberg, G. D. 'Studies of the effects of hypothermia on regional myocardial blood flow and metabolism during cardiopulmonary bypass: III. Effects of temperature, time and perfusion pressure in fibrillating hearts.' *Journal of Thoracic and Cardiovascular Surgery*, **73,** 102 (1977)
10. Brazier, J. R., Hottenrot, C. and Buckberg, G. D. 'Non-coronary collateral myocardial blood flow.' *Annals of Thoracic Surgery*, **19,** 426 (1975)

11. Bregman, D., Parodi, E. N., Edie, R. N., Bowman, F. O., Jr., Reemtsma, K. and Malm, J. R. 'Intraoperative unidirectional intra-aortic balloon pumping in the management of left ventricular power failure.' *Journal of Thoracic and Cardiovascular Surgery*, **70,** 1010 (1975)
12. Bretschneider, J. H., Hubner, G., Knoll, D., Lohr, B., Nordbeck, H. and Spieckermann, P. G. 'Myocardial resistance and tolerance to ischaemia: physiological and biochemical basis.' *Journal of Cardiovascular Surgery*, **16,** 241 (1975)
13. Buckberg, G. D. 'Postoperative management of determinants of cardiac output and subendocardial oxygen supply and demand.' In *Second Henry Ford Hospital International Symposium on Cardiac Surgery*. Ed. J. C. Davila. Detroit: Appleton-Century-Crofts (1977)
14. Buckberg, G. D., Brazier, J. R., Nelson, R. L., Goldstein, S. M., McConnell, D. H. and Cooper, N. 'Studies of the effects of hypothermia on regional myocardial blood flow and metabolism during cardiopulmonary bypass. 1. The adequately perfused beating, fibrillating and arrested heart.' *Journal of Thoracic and Cardiovascular Surgery*, **73,** 84 (1977)
15. Buckberg, G. D., Fixler, D. E., Archie, J. P., Henney, R. P. and Hoffman, J. I. E. 'Variable effects of heart rate on phasic and regional left ventricular muscle blood flow in anaesthetized dogs.' *Cardiovascular Research*, **9,** 1 (1975)
16. Buckberg, G. D., Fixler, D. E., Archie, J. P. and Hoffman, J. I. E. 'Experimental subendocardial ischaemia in dogs with normal coronary arteries.' *Circulation Research*, **30,** 67 (1972)
17. Buckberg, G. D. and Kattus, A. A. 'Factors determining the distribution and adequacy of left ventricular myocardial blood flow.' In *Current Topics in Coronary Research*. Eds C. M. Bloor and R. A. Olsson, pp. 95–113. New York: Plenum Press (1973)
18. Buckberg, G. D., Olinger, G. N., Mulder, D. G. and Maloney, J. V., Jr. 'Depressed postoperative cardiac performance: prevention by adequate myocardial protection during cardiopulmonary bypass.' *Journal of Thoracic and Cardiovascular Surgery*, **70,** 974 (1975)
19. Buckberg, G. D., Towers, B., Paglia, D., Mulder, D. G. and Maloney, J. V., Jr. 'Subendocardial ischaemia after cardiopulmonary bypass.' *Journal of Thoracic and Cardiovascular Surgery*, **64,** 669 (1972)
20. Clark, R. E., Ferguson, B. A., West, P. N., Shuchleib, R. C. and Henry, P. D. 'Pharmacologic preservation of the ischaemic heart.' *Annals of Thoracic Surgery*, **24,** 307 (1977)
21. Cooper, N., Brazier, J. R., McConnell, D. H. and Buckberg, G. D. 'Studies of the effects of hypothermia on regional myocardial blood flow and metabolism during cardiopulmonary bypass: IV. Topical atrial hypothermia in normothermic beating hearts.' *Journal of Thoracic and Cardiovascular Surgery*, **73,** 195 (1977)
22. Daily, P. O. 'Discussion on myocardial protection with cardioplegia.' *Journal of Thoracic and Cardiovascular Surgery*, **73,** 370 (1977)
23. Ellis, R. J., Kilgfield, P., Gay, W. and Ebert, P. A. 'Distal coronary artery bypass: local occlusion *vs* ischaemic arrest.' *Surgery*, **78,** 424 (1975)
24. Engelman, R. M., Avvil, J., O'Donoghue, M. J. and Levitsky, S. 'Significance of multidose cardioplegia and hypothermia in myocardial preservation during ischaemic arrest.' *Journal of Thoracic and Cardiovascular Surgery*, **75,** 555 (1978)
25. Engelman, R. M., Spencer, F. C., Boyd, A. D. and Chandra, R. 'The significance of coronary arterial stenosis during cardiopulmonary bypass.' *Journal of Thoracic and Cardiovascular Surgery*, **70,** 869 (1975)

26. Fey, K., Follette, D. M., Livesay, J., Nelson, R. L. and Buckberg, G. D. 'Effects of steroid pre-treatment on left ventricular myocardial blood flow, compliance and performance after hypothermic ischaemic arrest.' *Surgical Forum*, **27,** 246 (1976)
27. Fey, K., Follette, D. M., Livesay, J., Nelson, R., Bugyi, H., DeLand, E. and Buckberg, G. D. 'Effects of membrane stabilization on the safety of hypothermic arrest after aortic cross-clamping.' *Circulation*, **56, (Suppl. II)**, 143 (1977)
28. Foglia, R. P., Steed, D. L., Follette, D. M., DeLand, E. C. and Buckberg, G. D. 'Creation and avoidance of myocardial edema by potassium cardioplegia.' *Surgical Forum*, **28,** 226 (1977)
29. Follette, D. M., Fey, K., Livesay, J., Maloney, J. V., Jr. and Buckberg, G. D. 'Studies on myocardial reperfusion injury. I. Favourable modification by adjusting reperfusate pH.' *Surgery*, **82,** 149 (1977)
30. Follette, D. M., Fey, K., Livesay, J., Nelson, R., Maloney, J. V., Jr. and Buckberg, G. D. 'The beneficial effects of citrate reperfusion of ischaemic heart on cardiopulmonary bypass.' *Surgical Forum*, **27,** 244 (1976)
31. Follette, D. M., Fey, K., Mulder, D. M., Maloney, J. V., Jr. and Buckberg, G. D. 'Prolonged safe aortic cross-clamping by combining membrane stabilization, multidose cardioplegia and physiological reperfusion.' *Journal of Thoracic and Cardiovascular Surgery*, **74,** 682 (1977)
32. Follette, D. M., Fey, K., Steed, D. L., Foglia, R. P. and Buckberg, G. D. 'Reducing reperfusion injury with hypocalcaemic hyperkalaemic, alkalotic blood during reoxygenation.' *Surgical Forum*, **29,** 284 (1978)
33. Follette, D. M., Mulder, D. G., Maloney, J. V., Jr. and Buckberg, G. D. 'Advantages of blood cardioplegia over continuous coronary perfusion or intermittent ischaemia.' *Journal of Thoracic and Cardiovascular Surgery*, **76,** 604 (1978)
34. Follette, D. M., Steed, D. L., Foglia, R. P., Fey, K. and Buckberg, G. D. 'Advantages of intermittent blood cardioplegia over intermittent ischaemia during prolonged hypothermic aortic clamping.' *Circulation*, **58 (Suppl. I)**, 200 (1978)
35. Follette, D., Steed, D., Foglia, R. P. *et al.* 'Reduction of postischaemic myocardial damage by maintaining arrest during initial reperfusion.' *Surgical Forum*, in press
36. Frank, J. S., Langer, G. A., Nudd, L. M. and Seraydarian, K. 'The myocardial cell surface, its histochemistry, and the effect of sialic acid and calcium removal on its structure and cellular ionic exchange.' *Circulation Research*, **41,** 702 (1977)
37. Gay, W. A., Jr. and Ebert, P. A. 'Functional, metabolic and morphologic effects of potassium-induced cardioplegia.' *Surgery*, **74,** 284 (1973)
38. Goldman, B. S., Gunstensen, J., Gilbert, B. W., Kelly, T. C., Scully, H., Williams, W. G. and Adelman, A. G. 'Increasing operability and survival with intra-aortic balloon pump assist.' *Canadian Journal of Surgery*, **19,** 69 (1976)
39. Goldstein, S. M., Nelson, R. L., McConnell, D. H. and Buckberg, G. D. 'Cardiac arrest after aortic cross-clamping: effects of conventional ischaemic *vs* pharmacologic techniques on myocardial supply/demand balance.' *Surgical Forum*, **26,** 271 (1975)
40. Habal, S. M., Weiss, M. B., Spotnitz, H. M., Parodi, E. N., Wolff, M., Cannon, P. J., Hoffman, B. F. and Malm, J. R. 'Effects of pulsatile and non-pulsatile coronary perfusion on canine left ventricular performance.' *Journal of Thoracic and Cardiovascular Surgery*, **72,** 5 (1976)
41. Hearse, D. J., Stewart, D. A. and Braimbridge, M. V. 'Cellular protection during myocardial ischaemia.' *Circulation*, **54,** 193 (1976)

42. Hearse, D. J., Stewart, D. A. and Braimbridge, M. V. 'Metabolic and myocardial protection during elective cardiac arrest.' *Circulation Research*, **36,** 481 (1975)
43. Hearse, D. J., Stewart, D. A. and Braimbridge, M. V. 'Myocardial protection during bypass and arrest: a possible hazard with lactate-containing infusates.' *Journal of Thoracic and Cardiovascular Surgery*, **72,** 880 (1976)
44. Hearse, D. J., Stewart, D. A. and Braimbridge, M. V. 'Myocardial protection during ischaemic cardiac arrest: importance of magnesium in cardioplegic infusates.' *Journal of Thoracic and Cardiovascular Surgery*, **75,** 877 (1978)
45. Hearse, D. J., Stewart, D. A. and Braimbridge, M. V. 'Myocardial protection during ischaemic cardiac arrest: possible deleterious effects of glucose and mannitol in coronary infusates.' *Journal of Thoracic and Cardiovascular Surgery*, **76,** 16 (1978)
46. Hewitt, R. L., Lolley, D. M., Adrouny, G. A. and Drapanas, T. 'Protective effect of glycogen and glucose on the anoxic arrested heart.' *Surgery*, **75,** 1 (1974)
47. Hilton, C. J., Teubl, W., Acker, M. and McEnany, M. T. 'Inadequate cardioplegic protection with obstructed coronary arteries.' *Annals of Thoracic Surgery*, in press
48. Hoar, P. F., Hickey, R. F. and Ullyot, D. J. 'Systemic hypertension following myocardial revascularization.' *Journal of Thoracic and Cardiovascular Surgery*, **71,** 859 (1976)
49. Hoffman, J. I. E. and Buckberg, G. D. 'Transmural variation in myocardial perfusion.' In *Progress in Cardiology*. Eds P. N. Yu and J. F. Goodwin, p. 38. Philadelphia: Lea and Febiger (1976)
50. Hottenrot, C. and Buckberg, G. D. 'Studies of the effects of ventricular fibrillation on the adequacy of regional myocardial flow: II. Effects of ventricular distension.' *Journal of Thoracic and Cardiovascular Surgery*, **68,** 626 (1974)
51. Hottenrot, C., Maloney, J. V., Jr. and Buckberg, G. D. 'Studies of the effects of ventricular fibrillation on the adequacy of regional myocardial flow: I. Electrical *vs* spontaneous fibrillation.' *Journal of Thoracic and Cardiovascular Surgery*, **68,** 615 (1974)
52. Hottenrot, C., Maloney, J. V., Jr. and Buckberg, G. D. 'Studies of the effects of ventricular fibrillation on the adequacy of regional myocardial flow: III. Mechanisms of ischaemia.' *Journal of Thoracic and Cardiovascular Surgery*, **68,** 634 (1974)
53. Hottenrot, C., Nelson, R. L., McConnell, D. H., Goldstein, S. M. and Buckberg, G. D. 'The effect of mannitol on the distribution and adequacy of coronary flow in ventricles made ischaemic by fibrillation or arrest during bypass.' *Surgical Forum*, **26,** 266 (1975)
54. Hottenrot, C. E., Towers, B., Kurkji, H. J., Maloney, J. F. and Buckberg, G. D. 'The hazard of ventricular fibrillation in hypertrophied ventricles during cardiopulmonary bypass.' *Journal of Thoracic and Cardiovascular Surgery*, **66,** 742 (1973)
55. Howell, B. J., Baumgardner, F. W., Bond, K. and Rahn, H. 'Acid–base balance in cold-blooded vertebrates as a function of body temperature.' *American Journal of Physiology*, **218,** 600 (1970)
56. Hutchinson, J. E., Green, G. E., Mekhijian, H. A. and Kemp, H. G. 'Coronary bypass grafting in 376 consecutive patients with three operative deaths.' *Journal of Thoracic and Cardiovascular Surgery*,**67,** 7 (1974)
57. Isom, O. W., Kutn, N. D., Falk, E. A. and Spencer, F. C. 'Patterns of myocardial metabolism during cardiopulmonary bypass and coronary perfusion.' *Journal of Thoracic and Cardiovascular Surgery*, **66,** 705 (1973)

58. Iyengar, S. R. K., Ramchand, S., Charrette, E. J. P., Iyengar, C. K. S. and Lynn, R. B. 'Anoxic cardiac arrest: an experimental and clinical study of its effects.' *Journal of Thoracic and Cardiovascular Surgery*, **66**, 722 (1973)
59. Jennings, R. B., Sommers, H. M., Smyth, G. A., Flack, H. A. and Linn, H. 'Myocardial necrosis induced by temporary occlusion of a coronary artery in the dog.' *Archives of Pathology*, **70**, 68 (1960)
60. Jynge, P., Hearse, D. J. and Braimbridge, M. 'Myocardial protection during ischaemic cardiac arrest.' *Journal of Thoracic and Cardiovascular Surgery*, **73**, 848 (1977)
61. Kane, J. J., Murphy, M. L., Bissett, J. K., de Soyza, N., Doherty, J. E. and Straub, K. D. 'Mitochondrial function, oxygen extraction, epicardial S–T segment changes and tritiated digoxin distribution after reperfusion of ischaemic myocardium.' *American Journal of Cardiology*, **36**, 218 (1975)
62. Kay, H. R., Levine, F. H., Fallon, J. T., Grotte, G. J., Butchart, E. G., Rao, S., McEnany, M. T., Austen, W. G. and Buckley, M. J. 'Effect of cross-clamp time, temperature and cardioplegic agents on myocardial function after induced arrest.' *Journal of Thoracic and Cardiovascular Surgery*, **76**, 590 (1978)
63. Kitsch, U., Rodewald, G. and Kalmar, P. 'Induced ischaemic arrest.' *Journal of Thoracic and Cardiovascular Surgery*, **63**, 121 (1972)
64. Kloner, R. A., Ganote, C. E., Whalen, D. A., Jr. and Jennings, R. B. 'Effect of a transient period of ischaemia on myocardial cells.' *American Journal of Pathology*, **74**, 399 (1974)
65. Kurkji, H., DeLand, E., Buckberg, G. D. and Maloney, J. V., Jr. 'Prevention of ischaemic myocardial contracture (stone heart).' *Surgical Forum*, **44**, 146 (1973)
66. Langer, G. A. 'The structure and function of the myocardial cell surface.' *American Journal of Physiology*, **235**, H461 (1978)
67. Lazar, H., Buckberg, G. D., Manganaro, A. J., Foglia, R. P., Becker, H., Mulder, D. G. and Maloney, J. V., Jr. 'Reversal of ischaemic damage with secondary blood cardioplegia.' *Journal of Thoracic and Cardiovascular Surgery*, **78**, 688 (1979)
68. Lazar, H. L., Foglia, R. P., Manganaro, A. J. and Buckberg, G. D. 'Detrimental effects of premature use of inotropic drugs to discontinue cardiopulmonary bypass.' *Surgical Forum*, **29**, 276 (1978)
69. Loomis, T. A., Jesseph, J. E. and Beyer, R. E. 'Prolongation of the anticoagulant action of heparin with procaine and butacaine conjugates.' *Journal of Pharmacology and Experimental Therapy*, **104**, 87 (1952)
70. McConnell, D. H., Brazier, J. R., Cooper, N. and Buckberg, G. D. 'Studies of the effects of hypothermia on regional myocardial blood flow and metabolism during cardiopulmonary bypass. II. Ischaemia during moderate hypothermia in continually perfused beating hearts.' *Journal of Thoracic and Cardiovascular Surgery*, **73**, 95 (1977)
71. McConnell, D. H., White, F., Nelson, R. L., Goldstein, S. M., Maloney, J. V., Jr., DeLand, E. C. and Buckberg, G. D. 'The importance of alkalosis in maintenance of 'ideal' blood pH during hypothermia.' *Surgical Forum*, **26**, 263 (1975)
72. McGoon, D. C. Personal communication (1975)
73. Melrose, D. G., Dreyer, B., Bantall, H. H. and Baker, J. B. E. 'Elective cardiac arrest.' *Lancet*, **2**, 21 (1955)
74. Najafi, H., Henson, D., Dye, W. S., Javid, H., Hunter, J. A., Callaghan, R., Eisenstein, R. and Julian, O. C. 'Left ventricular haemorrhagic necrosis.' *Annals of Thoracic Surgery*, **7**, 550 (1969)

75. Nelson, R. L., Fey, K. H., Follette, D. M., Livesay, J. J., DeLand, E. C., Maloney, J. V., Jr. and Buckberg, G. D. 'The critical importance of intermittent infusion of cardioplegic solution during aortic cross-clamping.' *Surgical Forum*, **27,** 241 (1976)
76. Nelson, R. L., Goldstein, S. M., McConnell, D. H., Maloney, J. V., Jr. and Buckberg, G. D. 'Improved myocardial performance after aortic cross-clamping by combining pharmacologic arrest with topical hypothermia.' *Circulation*, **53** and **54 (Suppl. III)**, 11 (1976)
77. Nelson, R. L., McConnell, D. H., Goldstein, S. M., Maloney, J. V., Jr. and Buckberg, G. D. 'The effects of profound topical cardiac hypothermia on myocardial blood flow, metabolism, compliance and function.' *Surgical Forum*, **26,** 261 (1975)
78. Pappas, G., Winter, S. D., Kopriva, C. J. and Steele, P. P. 'Improvement of myocardial and other vital organ functions and metabolism with a simple method of pulsatile flow (IABP) during clinical cardiopulmonary bypass.' *Surgery*, **77,** 34 (1975)
79. Pennock, J. L., Pierce, W. S. and Waldhausen, J. A. 'Quantitative evaluation of left ventricular bypass in reducing myocardial ischaemia.' *Surgery*, **79,** 523 (1976)
80. Peters, J. P. and Van Slyke, D. D. *Quantitative Clinical Chemistry*. p. 868. Baltimore: Williams and Wilkins (1932)
81. Philips, P. A., Marty, A. T. and Miyamoto, A. M. 'A clinical method for detecting subendocardial ischaemia after cardiopulmonary bypass.' *Journal of Thoracic and Cardiovascular Surgery*, **69,** 30 (1975)
82. Rahn, H., Reeves, R. B. and Howell, B. J. 'Hydrogen ion regulation, temperature and evolution.' *American Review of Respiratory Disease*, **112,** 165 (1975)
83. Randle, P. J., Denton, R. N. and England, P. J. 'Citrate as a metabolic regulator in muscle and adipose tissue.' In *Metabolic Roles of Citrate*. Ed. T. W. Goodman, pp. 87–103. London: Academic Press (1968)
84. Rich, T. L. and Brady, A. J. 'Potassium contracture and utilization of high-energy phosphates in rabbit heart.' *American Journal of Physiology*, **226,** 105 (1974)
85. Robb-Nicholson, C., Currie, W. D. and Wechsler, A. S. 'Effects of verapamil on myocardial tolerance to ischaemic arrest.' *Circulation*, **58 (Suppl. I)**, 119 (1978)
86. Rosenthal, T. B. 'The effects of temperature on the pH of blood and plasma *in vitro*'. *Journal of Biological Chemistry*, **173,** 25 (1948)
87. Rovetto, M. J., Whitmer, J. T. and Neely, J. R. 'Comparison of the effects of anoxia and whole heart ischaemia on carbohydrate utilization in isolated working rat hearts.' *Circulation Research*, **32,** 699 (1973)
88. Sapsford, R. N., Blackstone, E. H., Kirklin, J. W., Karp, R. B., Kouchoukos, N. T., Pacifico, A. D., Roe, C. R. and Bradley, E. L. 'Coronary perfusion versus cold ischaemic arrest during aortic valve surgery.' *Circulation*, **49,** 1190 (1974)
89. Sarajas, H. S. S. 'Myocardial damage induced by immersion hypothermia.' *American Journal of Cardiology*, **13,** 355 (1964)
90. Sarnoff, S. J., Braunwald, E. and Welch, G. H. 'Haemodynamic determinations of oxygen consumption of the heart with special reference to the tension time index.' *American Journal of Physiology*, **192,** 148 (1958)
91. Schaper, W., Schaper, J., Palmowski, J. *et al.* 'Ischaemia tolerance following cardioplegic arrest in human patients and in experimental animals.' *Journal of Cardiovascular Surgery*, **16,** 268 (1975)

92. Shen, A. C. and Jennings, R. B. 'Kinetics of calcium accumulation in acute myocardial ischaemic injury.' *American Journal of Pathology*, **67,** 441 (1972)
93. Shragge, B. W., Digerness, S. B. and Blackstone, E. H. 'Complete recovery of myocardial function following cold exposure.' *Circulation*, **58 (Suppl. II)**, 97 (1978)
94. Stemmer, E. A., McCart, P., Stanton, W. W., Jr., Thibault, W., Dearden, L. S. and Connolly, J. E. 'Functional and structural alterations in the myocardium during aortic cross clamping.' *Journal of Thoracic and Cardiovascular Surgery*, **66,** 754 (1973)
95. Taber, R. E., Morales, A. R. and Fine, G. 'Myocardial necrosis and the post-operative low cardiac output syndrome.' *Annals of Thoracic Surgery*, **4,** 12 (1967)
96. Tyers, G. F. O., Todd, G. J., Niebauer, I. M., Manley, N. J. and Waldhausen, J. A. 'The mechanism of myocardial damage following potassium citrate (Melrose) cardioplegia.' *Surgery*, **78,** 45 (1975)
97. Tyers, G. F. O., Williams, E. H., Hughes, H. C., Jr. and Waldhausen, J. A. 'Optimal myocardial hypothermia at 10 to 15°C.' *Surgical Forum*, **26,** 233 (1976)
98. Usubiaga, J. E., Wikinski, J., Ferrero, R., Usubiaga, L. E. and Wikinski, R. 'Anaesthesia and analgesia.' *Current Research*, **45,** 611 (1966)
99. Utley, J., Carlson, E. L., Hoffman, J. I. E., Martinez, H. M. and Buckberg, G. D. 'Total and regional myocardial blood flow measurements with 25μ, 9μ and filtered 1–10μ diameter microspheres and antipyrine.' *Circulation Research*, **34,** 391 (1974)
100. Utley, J. R., Michalsky, G. B., Treat, R. C., Mobin-Uddin, K. and Perlin, A. R. 'Effect of cardiotonic and vasoactive drugs on transmural flow distribution and ventricular volume in the fibrillating heart on cardiopulmonary bypass.' *Circulation*, **51, (Suppl. I)**, 1 (1975)
101. Wildenthal, K., Mierzwiak, D. S. and Mitchell, J. I. I. 'Acute effects of increased serum osmolality on left ventricular performance.' *American Journal of Physiology*, **216,** 898 (1969)
102. Wright, R. N., Levitsky, S., Holland, C. and Feinberg, H. 'Beneficial effects of potassium cardioplegia during intermittent aortic cross-clamping and reperfusion.' *Journal of Surgical Research*, **24,** 201 (1978)
103. Yates, J. C. and Dhalla, N. S. 'Structural and functional changes associated with failure and recovery of hearts after perfusion with Ca^{2+}-free medium.' *Journal of Molecular and Cellular Cardiology*, **7,** 91 (1975)

11

Myocardial Protection by Topical Hypothermia

Bruce A. Reitz, William A. Baumgartner and
Edward B. Stinson

abundans cautela non nocet

Introduction

In order to achieve the maximum chance for a successful outcome, the functional state of the myocardium must be maintained as well as possible during the conduct of a cardiac operation. Valvular replacement or repair, myocardial revascularization, or correction of congenital abnormality can be performed with minimum mortality and maximum longterm benefit to the patient if there is no myocardial cellular damage produced during the operation.

This clearly has been the goal of cardiac surgeons since the first intracardiac operations performed in the early 1950s. The fact that such a variety of methods for myocardial protection has been employed emphasizes that no perfect or universally accepted method has evolved. There is always some element of compromise between the minimum amount of myocardial cell damage and the optimum technical conditions for performance of the operative procedure. Under experimental conditions in animals, nearly complete preservation of myocardial structure and function during cardiopulmonary bypass can be achieved by continuous euthermic or mildly hypothermic perfusion of a beating, vented heart which is performing minimal external work[9]. However, most cardiac operations are facilitated by a quiet, flaccid myocardium and a bloodless field. Continuous coronary perfusion makes this impossible, and these conditions can only be provided by interrupting coronary blood flow and arresting the heart's mechanical activity. This chapter will review the technique of local profound cardiac hypothermia by the topical application of cold saline solution as it has been developed and applied at the Stanford University Medical Center. We have used this technique for over 18 years in nearly 10 000 cardiac surgical procedures. It provides a number of advantages for increased technical facility during the operative procedure and has resulted in consistently good clinical outcomes in a variety of cardiac operations. We will discuss the historical and laboratory background of the method, the technique as employed at present in a variety of procedures, and the clinical results expected. In addition, methods for applying this technique in conjunction with aortic root perfusion of hypothermic cardioplegic solutions will also be outlined.

Historical and laboratory development

Although hypothermia has been recommended as therapy for a variety of conditions since ancient times[38], it was not until the late 1940s that systematic evaluation was begun with the purpose of decreasing metabolic demand in order to perform direct-vision open-heart operations. The techniques for inducing total body hypothermia in order to achieve safe circulatory arrest were developed simultaneously with the techniques for total cardiopulmonary bypass using pump oxygenators. As a result of the studies by Bigelow and associates[5, 6], and Swan[39], hypothermia was shown to be effective in preserving organ structure and function following a limited period of ischaemia induced by circulatory arrest. The first open-heart procedure was performed by Lewis in 1952[23], consisting of repair of an atrial septal defect during five and a half minutes of circulatory arrest. This method was usable, and some remarkably good results were obtained, but when compared with the advantages of total cardiopulmonary bypass using pump oxygenators, it was cumbersome and time-limiting. After the first successful use of a pump oxygenator to repair an atrial septal defect by Gibbon in 1953[16], hypothermic circulatory arrest as the method of choice for performing open-heart operations was generally abandoned. The lesson of preservation obtained by hypothermia was not forgotten however, and in the late 1950s a number of surgeons turned to this modality in order to protect the heart during periods of aortic cross-clamping for the performance of intracardiac repairs.

Among the first investigators to suggest cardiac hypothermia as a method of myocardial preservation were Berne[4] and Cross[12]. They suggested the use of perfusion of the aortic root with cold blood after cross-clamping the aorta. Following initial laboratory studies in 1957, they reported several successful clinical cases. Lillehei applied the technique in 1958 during the first prosthetic replacement of an aortic valve[24]. Other surgeons who used perfusion hypothermia followed by a single external application of cold saline or ice slush were Kenyon[21], Urschel[41], and Hufnagel[19]. During this same period, Shumway and Lower reported in the *Surgical Forum* of 1959[35] experiments which showed the effectiveness in dogs of local profound cardiac hypothermia for myocardial protection. Their technique did not use either aortic root perfusion or saline slush, but rather consisted of continuous lavage of the pericardial well with ice-cold saline at 2–4°C. Myocardial temperatures were lowered to the range of 20–25°C, and provided up to 60 minutes of aortic cross-clamp time followed by consistently good myocardial function to allow routine survival. The one animal that failed to survive had an abnormally high bronchial return which was not removed by venting, and in this animal myocardial temperatures were in the range of 28–30°C. They also reported the first successful clinical application of this method in a 14-year-old patient with tetralogy of Fallot who underwent successful repair during 25 minutes of aortic cross-clamp time[36].

After this initial experience, other surgeons, notably Urschel[41], Hufnagel[19], Robicsek and Sanger[30–32], as well as Hurley[20], reported successful clinical results in a number of patients. Despite these reports, most centres around the world used the method of continuous coronary artery perfusion that was introduced simultaneously. The theoretical advantages of continuous coronary perfusion seemed to outweigh the technical disadvantages of this technique for most surgeons in the 1960s. There was, and continues to be, a vigorous debate concerning the relative merits and inadequacies of these various methods for myocardial protection.

After direct coronary artery bypass procedures were introduced in 1968, there was a rekindling of interest in this topic because it was clear that continuous coronary artery perfusion did not provide the kind of operating conditions that were most suitable for small-vessel anastomoses. Surgeons again turned to aortic cross-clamping and various methods of protecting the heart during this manoeuvre. Griepp and associates[17] reported a comparison of continuous coronary artery perfusion in the fibrillating, vented heart, and aortic cross-clamping combined with profound local hypothermia. In two comparable groups of patients undergoing coronary artery bypass, they showed a clear advantage for the group who had aortic cross-clamping and local profound hypothermia. Thus in the latter group the serum glutamic oxalacetic transaminase (SGOT) and lactic dehydrogenase (LDH) enzymes were lower in the postoperative period, the incidence of intraoperative myocardial infarction was drastically reduced, postoperative haemodynamics were not impaired, and the operative mortality rate was less than 1 per cent. Other surgeons reported similar experiences, and the majority of surgeons employed some type of aortic cross-clamping during the performance of distal coronary anastomoses.

Most recently, a variety of experimental and clinical studies have appeared in which various cardioplegic agents have been combined with hypothermia in order to provide myocardial protection during aortic cross-clamping. Although some advantage has been attributed to the cardioplegic agent[15], other studies support the concept that hypothermia is the major protective element[13]. The technique of local cardiac hypothermia induced and maintained by topical application of cold saline has proven itself to be the equal of any other method and can be used simultaneously with cardioplegic agents. It is simple and technically easy to implement, providing excellent operative conditions for a variety of procedures.

Effects of hypothermia

The basic premise underlying the application of topical cold saline is that *hypothermia reduces the metabolic rate and preserves the store of high-energy phosphate compounds, membrane integrity, and subcellular elements*. The metabolic requirements of cardiac tissue can be expressed by Van't Hoff's law: the logarithm of the rate of oxygen consumption is directly related to the logarithm of the absolute temperature. This has been shown to be true for isolated cardiac tissue *in vitro*[14, 40] and also for the whole heart when stored prior to transplantation[1].

The energy sources of the heart are glucose, lactate, pyruvate, free fatty acids, and amino acids. The proportional consumption of these nutrients in hearts cooled to 25°C appears to be unchanged when compared to the consumption of these nutrients at euthermic conditions[2]. When the heart has been arrested (by hyperkalaemia, cold, or ischaemia itself), the oxygen consumption is diminished, at 25°C, to 7 per cent of that at euthermic levels when the heart is beating[3]. Numerous investigators have shown that the pharmacologically arrested heart at euthermia consumes two to three times more oxygen than the heart arrested by cold alone, emphasizing that hypothermia is more efficient than pharmacological agents in reducing oxygen consumption[13, 22].

A number of experimental studies have been done to compare the protective effect of local cardiac hypothermia with euthermic anoxic arrest and also with cardioplegic arrest. These studies showed consistent survival of animals subjected to cardiopulmonary bypass and 60 minutes of aortic occlusion, but variable survival after 120 minutes, with the heart protected by the topical application of ice-cold saline alone[11, 29, 34–37]. Function and histology were well maintained after 60 minutes of ischaemia when the temperature was lowered to 15–18°C[37]. Other investigators have shown that a period of 60 minutes of myocardial ischaemia was accompanied by a significant increase of intracellular water, a decrease in myocardial compliance and contractile function, and more severe histological changes[26]. There is also good evidence that the period of time of resuscitation and the perfusion pressure during resuscitation are important factors in reducing the amount of cardiac dysfunction postoperatively[9].

Because of the logarithmic relationship between oxygen consumption, cellular reactions, and absolute temperature, the beneficial aspects of myocardial hypothermia are most pronounced during the initial 10–20°C of lowering of the temperature. It is incumbent upon the surgeon, therefore, to apply the method in a methodical and meticulous manner in order to achieve the most complete reduction of intramyocardial temperature that is possible. Those manoeuvres that we have found helpful in the clinical application of this technique are described in the next section.

Technique for myocardial protection by topical hypothermia

The various manoeuvres that we have found helpful for the implementation of this technique are summarized in *Table 11.1*. The technique requires that a pericardial well is fashioned by incising the pericardium in the shape of an inverted 'Y' and suturing its cut edges to the surgical drapes

Table 11.1 Important techniques for profound local hypothermia

(1) Continuous cold saline lavage during the entire period of aortic cross-clamping (100–150 ml/min at 2–4°C)

(2) Maintenance of an effective level of saline solution in the pericardial well (patient's head up to 30°, left tilt to 15°)

(3) Moderate systemic hypothermia (28–30°C during the period of aortic cross-clamping)

(4) Relatively low perfusion flows and pressures (30–50 ml/kg per min; 40–60 mmHg)

(5) Intracardiac lavage when possible (decreases temperature gradients and removes particulate debris)

(6) Removal of bronchial return with a pulmonary artery vent during aortic clamp interval (decreases cavitary warming and chamber distension)

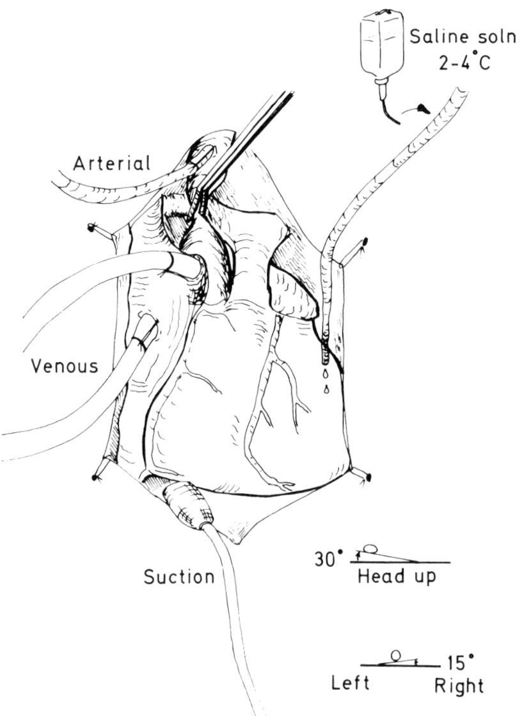

Figure 11.1 The operative field as seen during the use of topical hypothermia. A pericardial well is fashioned and a sterile nasogastric tube brought into the left side of the field. The cold saline is infused through this tube. A suction device is positioned to aspirate the fluid at a level just below the aortic or cardiac incision. The operating table is positioned as shown, with the head elevated to approximately 30° and the left side down 15°

following the standard median sternotomy. After routine cannulation of the ascending aorta and right atrium for cardiopulmonary bypass, a No. 18 French nasogastric tube is brought into the pericardium on the left side, as shown in *Figure 11.1*. This tube is attached to a 2 litre container of ice-cold saline solution placed outside the operating field. The saline is stored in the operating room in large refrigerators and kept at 4°C until immediately before use. Once cardiopulmonary bypass is established, the heart is either electively fibrillated before the application of the aortic clamp, or the aortic root is perfused with cold cardioplegic solution after emptying the heart and applying the aortic clamp. Cooling is initiated by the topical application of 2 to 3 litres of cold saline, directly into the pericardial well. Following this, the infusion of cold saline in the pericardial well is begun at the rate of 100–150 ml/min. This continuous high volume lavage of cold saline is necessary in order to maintain the lowest possible temperature of the perfusing medium. The containers of saline are changed by the circulating nurse as they are used.

A modified Salem sump tube is connected to wall suction and placed in the inferior aspect of the pericardial well to aspirate the solution at the desired level. The coolant is maintained at a level just below the incision in the heart, or just below the coronary artery which is being revascularized. When the heart is lifted out of the pericardial well and retracted to the right for the construction of anastomoses to the marginal branch of the circumflex artery, the saline line is held over the apex of the heart so that the coolant can continue to bathe the surface of the ventricles.

With the onset of cardiopulmonary bypass, mild to moderate systemic hypothermia is induced. The patient's temperature will be lowered to the range of 28–30°C, obtained by active cooling of the bypass prime. Once this temperature is reached the temperature of the prime is maintained at this level. The perfusion flows that are used at Stanford University are somewhat lower than those employed at other institutions. Our flows range from 30 to 50 ml/kg per min. These flows are quite adequate when used in conjunction with moderate systemic hypothermia. At such flow rates the perfusion pressures range between 40 and 60 mmHg. The advantage of low flow bypass is to reduce the amount of blood returning to the heart and therefore the amount of non-coronary collateral flow to the coronary arteries[7], thereby decreasing the tendency to both rewarm the heart and obscure the operative field. If the operation involves opening of the aorta or one of the cardiac chambers, intracardiac irrigation with cold saline solution is added when appropriate. This of course will lower the intramyocardial temperature as well as remove intracavitary particulate debris following valve excision.

In order to help maintain the major portion of the ventricles under the pool of cold saline, the patient's head is elevated by 30° and the operating table is tilted slightly to the left, as illustrated in *Figure 11.1*. Another adjunct for maintaining myocardial temperature at the lowest possible level is to insert a sump vent into the pulmonary artery and remove the bronchial blood return that would otherwise pass into the left side of the heart. Other surgeons have used a vent in the apex of the left ventricle for this purpose.

Approximately ten minutes before the anticipated removal of the aortic cross-clamp, the heat exchanger is activated in the cardiopulmonary bypass circuit and rewarming is begun. Following removal of the cross-clamp, electrical defibrillation is usually accomplished within five minutes, unless spontaneous return to rhythmic ventricular contraction has already occurred. The patient continues to be maintained on heart-lung bypass for approximately 15 to 30 minutes depending upon the length of the aortic cross-clamp duration. Particular attention is directed to removing all air from within the heart during this period. An adequate perfusion pressure of at least 50 mmHg is maintained in order to resuscitate the heart. This time period is mandatory to allow return of adequate ventricular function as well as to return the patient's temperature to euthermic levels.

Topical hypothermia combined with perfusion hypothermia with cardioplegic agent

A useful adjunct to more rapid attainment of profound myocardial hypothermia is the infusion in the aortic root of 500 ml of cold (4°C) electrolyte solution containing an increased amount of potassium. When this solution is infused at the beginning of the cross-clamp interval, the heart is arrested promptly and a significant reduction in the mean myocardial temperature can be obtained (perfusion hypothermia). This addition to the use of topical hypothermia has been employed in recent years by some surgeons at our institution. In order to test the efficacy of this approach, a randomized prospective study of two groups of patients was recently undertaken.

This study compared topical hypothermia alone with topical hypothermia combined with perfusion hypothermia with a cardioplegic solution (*Table 11.2*). The study was performed between November 1977 and April 1978, and included 113 patients undergoing elective myocardial revascularization operations. The patient characteristics of the two groups are outlined in *Table 11.3*. The groups were comparable with regard to preoperative functional classification, incidence of previous myocardial infarction and congestive heart failure, the category of diseased vessels and the number of dyssynergic segments as assessed by left ventricular angiography.

Table 11.2 Stanford cardioplegic solution

Component	*Concentration (per litre)*
Potassium	30 mmol
Sodium	25 mmol
Chloride	30 mmol
Bicarbonate	25 mmol
Dextrose	50 g
Mannitol	12.5 g
Molality	440 mmol
pH (at 4°C)	8.1–8.4

The operative procedures were standardized and differed only in the method for arresting the heart following the application of the aortic cross-clamp. In the first group the heart was arrested with a brief period of electrical stimulation to induce ventricular fibrillation. The heart was then bathed in cold saline and topical saline was used for myocardial protection during the cross-clamp interval. In the second group 500 ml of cold hyperkalaemic electrolyte solution were perfused through the aortic root after application of the cross-clamp. Subsequently, topical saline was used in the standard manner. The number of aortocoronary grafts that were placed was comparable in both groups, and so were the other operative

Table 11.3 Preoperative characteristics of patients undergoing coronary artery bypass with either topical hypothermia or topical and perfusion hypothermia

Characteristic	*Topical hypothermia*	*Topical and perfusion hypothermia*
Male	45	46
Female	7	15
Total	52	61
New York Heart Association classification		
1	3	0
2	16	16
3	31	37
4	2	8
Previous myocardial infarction		
by history	28	34
by electrocardiogram	20	26
Congestive heart failure	5	13
Category of diseased vessels		
Left main	8	6
Single vessel	5	7
Double vessel	19	17
Triple vessel	20	31
Left ventricular dysfunction assessed by angiography		
Segmental	18	17
Generalized	15	24

Table 11.4 Operative characteristics of patients undergoing coronary artery bypass with either topical hypothermia or topical and perfusion hypothermia

Characteristic	*Topical hypothermia*	*Topical and perfusion hypothermia*
Number of coronary grafts		
1	2	3
2	15	12
3	20	34
4	15	12
Coronary endarterectomy		
Right	9	8
Left	1	1
Need to defibrillate*	47	15
Perfusion time (min)†	103.5 ± 4.4	100.8 ± 3.7
Aortic cross-clamp time (min)†	55.5 ± 2.6	56.9 ± 2.4
Lowest patient temperature (°C)†	30.8 ± 0.2	30.7 ± 0.2

*$P<0.001$
†Values expressed as mean ± standard error

variables (*Table 11.4*). The only significant difference between the two groups in this respect was the need to defibrillate in only 15 of 61 patients (25 per cent) who received topical plus perfusion hypothermia, as compared to 47 of 52 (90 per cent) of those patients who received topical hypothermia alone. The other operative variable which was significantly different was the intraoperative temperature recorded in the two groups.

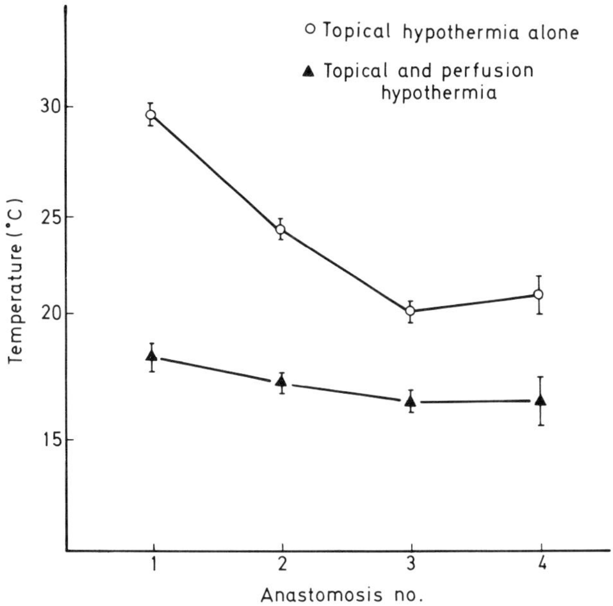

Figure 11.2 Group-averaged intramyocardial temperatures of the anterior interventricular septum measured immediately before the numbered anastomosis given (mean ± standard error)

Figure 11.2 illustrates group-averaged intramyocardial temperatures recorded in the anterior portion of the interventricular septum at intervals immediately before each of the distal anastomoses were made. The lowest mean myocardial temperature attained by topical hypothermia alone was 20.7°C while the lowest temperature attained by perfusion hypothermia combined with topical hypothermia was 16.6°C. Furthermore, the initial lowering of temperature was most effective by perfusion hypothermia in that the first reading was 18.8°C, as compared with 29.5°C for topical hypothermia alone.

The postoperative clinical courses of these two groups of patients were entirely comparable. There were no hospital deaths and the incidence of perioperative myocardial infarction was low in both groups (approximately 2 per cent). Serial enzyme determinations in the postoperative period were not significantly different for the two groups. The daily mean values for SGOT and LDH are shown in *Figure 11.3*.

In this randomized prospective study the application of topical hypothermia for myocardial protection was shown to be as good as topical hypothermia combined with perfusion hypothermia by a cardioplegic solution with regard to the hospital course and the rate of perioperative myocardial infarction. These results were obtained despite the fact that perfusion hypothermia resulted in substantially lower mean intramyocardial temperatures and a marked decrease in the percentage of patients who required cardiac electrical defibrillation. It is unlikely that the relative efficacy of either technique will be manifested by any striking difference in

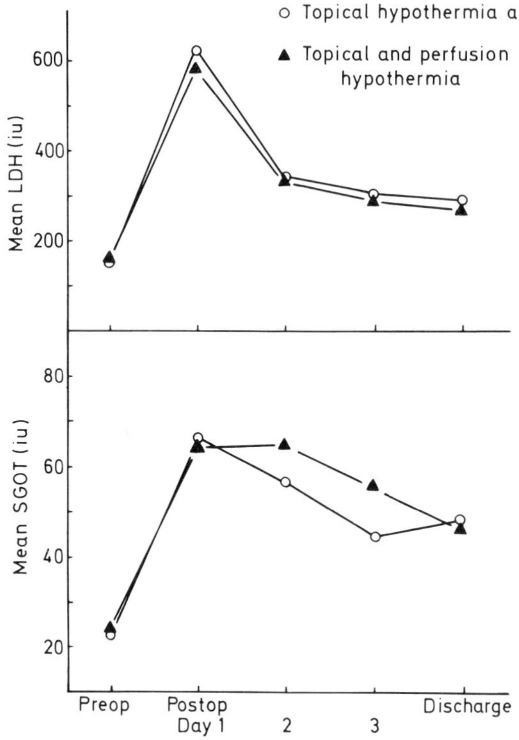

Figure 11.3 Mean serum enzymes of patients having coronary artery bypass operations with either topical hypothermia alone or topical and perfusion hypothermia. Lactic dehydrogenase (LDH) normal value, less than 300 International Units (iu). Serum glutamic oxalacetic transaminase (SGOT) normal value, less than 40 iu. No significant differences for any postoperative day were found.

operative mortality rate. The best method will probably be revealed by a subtle but definite difference in longterm postoperative ventricular function. We have not yet identified the marker that will prove the superiority of one method as compared to another. Since topical hypothermia is predicated upon the premise that protection of the myocardium is afforded by the hypothermia itself, the results of this study would indicate that initial perfusion with cold electrolyte solution is an important adjunct for the application of the technique. When a similar study was performed in animals, subendocardial fibrosis could be quantified and was found to be less when perfusion hypothermia was combined with topical hypothermia, than when compared with topical hypothermia alone[25]. If such careful histological studies could be performed in patients, it is likely that similar differences would be demonstrated in the late postoperative period.

Clinical results

After the initial clinical application of topical hypothermia in 1959, a series of 120 patients who had undergone a variety of surgical procedures for congenital lesions and acquired valvular disease was reported by Hurley in 1964[20]. The sole method of myocardial protection during the interval of ischaemic arrest was the application of continuous topical cold saline. There were four deaths (3.3 per cent), none of which could be attributed to the technique utilized.

Since this initial favourable experience, the technique has continued to be used routinely at Stanford University Medical Center in nearly 10 000 cardiac operations. The method provides a still, bloodless operative field with a flaccid myocardium. These operative conditions facilitate a quick and relatively atraumatic intracardiac operation.

Other surgeons who have been trained at Stanford and who have applied the technique as described here have reported excellent clinical results[8, 10, 18, 27, 28]. These are summarized in *Table 11.5* in which the mortality rates

Table 11.5 Clinical results obtained with myocardial protection by topical hypothermia

Procedure and source of reference	*Number of patients*	*Ischaemic time (min) Range (mean)*	*Mortality No (%)*
Coronary artery bypass[18]	89	16–96 (41)	1 (1.1)
Aortic valve replacement[10, 18, 27]	209	30–120 (58)	11 (5.3)
Mitral valve replacement[10, 18]	122	20–88 (47)	3 (2.5)
Multiple valve surgery[10, 18, 27]	72	31–138 (84)	4 (5.3)

for valve replacement and for myocardial revascularization procedures are seen to be quite low and comparable with any other series reported. Other surgeons, using modifications of this technique have reported excellent clinical results as well[30–32].

There is a clear clinical advantage to the topical hypothermia method when compared to continuous coronary artery perfusion, ventricular fibrillation, and left ventricular venting for coronary artery bypass graft procedures. This was demonstrated by Griepp[17] who compared two groups of approximately 150 patients each. Although mortality rates were similar in both groups, the incidence of perioperative infarction was 15 per cent in the unclamped group, and 8 per cent in the clamped group ($P<0.05$). Postoperative SGOT and LDH levels were significantly higher for the first four postoperative days in the unclamped group than in the clamped one.

Another comparison between coronary perfusion and topical hypothermia has been reported by Sapsford *et al*[33]. In a randomized study, 31 patients underwent aortic valve replacement with cannulation of the coronary arteries and continuous coronary perfusion, and were compared with 33 patients who had the same procedure during ischaemic arrest and topical hypothermia. There was no significant difference in the postoperative cardiac index, heart rate, left atrial pressure, and postoperative serum enzymes. There was a 27 per cent decrease in aortic occlusion time and a 21 per cent reduction in total cardiopulmonary bypass time for the topical hypothermia group. This emphasizes the improved operative conditions obtainable by the technique, and the authors concluded that for this reason it was preferable.

Summary

Satisfactory clinical results have consistently been obtained by the application of topical hypothermia for myocardial protection during periods of aortic cross-clamping. This method, introduced in 1959 by Shumway and Lower, verified in the laboratory, and used with consistently good results by a number of surgeons, offers certain technical advantages. The operative procedure is facilitated by a still and bloodless field provided by arrest of both mechanical activity of the heart and perfusion of the coronary arteries. It is known that ischaemic myocardial damage proceeds in a time-dependent manner, but is modified significantly by temperature. Intramyocardial temperatures of approximately 20°C can be maintained when the method of topical hypothermia is applied in a consistent and methodical fashion. Additional lowering of intramyocardial temperature can be produced by perfusion hypothermia using cold blood or electrolyte solution at the beginning of the aortic cross-clamp interval. Special manoeuvres which are helpful in providing the greatest degree of hypothermia have been detailed. The clinical results obtained at our institution as well as those reported by others have demonstrated that the method of topical hypothermia affords, when correctly used, satisfactory myocardial protection during periods of interruption of the coronary circulation.

References

1. Angell, W. W., Rikkers, L., Dong, E. and Shumway, N. E. 'Organ viability with hypothermia.' *Journal of Thoracic and Cardiovascular Surgery*, **58,** 619 (1969)
2. Bernard, W. F., Schwarz, H. F., Hug, G., Carroll, S. E. and Jokins, H. 'Alterations in myocardial metabolism subsequent to hypoxic and hypothermic cardiac arrest.' *Surgical Forum*, **12,** 171 (1961)
3. Bernard, W. F., Schwarz, H. F. and Mallick, N. P. 'Elective hypothermic cardiac arrest in normothermic animals.' *Annals of Surgery*, **153,** 43 (1961)
4. Berne, R. M., Jones, R. D. and Cross, F. S. 'Myocardial hypothermia in elective cardiac arrest.' *Journal of Applied Physiology*, **12,** 431 (1958)
5. Bigelow, W. G., Callaghan, J. C. and Hopps, J. A. 'General hypothermia for experimental intracardiac surgery.' *Annals of Surgery*, **132,** 531 (1950)
6. Bigelow, W. G., Lindsay, W. K. and Greenwood, W. F. 'Hypothermia: its possible role in cardiac surgery. An investigation of factors governing survival in dogs at low body temperatures.' *Annals of Surgery*, **132,** 849 (1950)
7. Brazier, J., Hottenrott, C. and Buckberg, G. 'Noncoronary collateral myocardial blood flow.' *Annals of Thoracic Surgery*, **19,** 426 (1975)

8. Brody, W. R. and Reitz, B. A. 'Topical hypothermic protection of the myocardium.' *Annals of Thoracic Surgery*, **20,** 66 (1975)
9. Buckberg, G. D. 'Left ventricular subendocardial necrosis.' *Annals of Thoracic Surgery*, **24,** 379 (1977)
10. Cohn, L. H. and Collins, J. J., Jr. 'Local cardiac hypothermia for myocardial protection.' *Annals of Thoracic Surgery*, **17,** 135 (1974)
11. Cohn, L. H., Fujiwara, Y., Kirk, E. and Collins, J. J., Jr. 'Effects of local cardiac hypothermia on the magnitude and distribution of coronary flow and on myocardial function and metabolism.' *Annals of Thoracic Surgery*, **19,** 10 (1975)
12. Cross, F. S., Jones, R. D. and Berne, R. M. 'Localized cardiac hypothermia as an adjunct to elective cardiac arrest.' *Surgical Forum*, **8,** 355 (1957)
13. Ellis, R. J., Pryor, W. and Ebert, P. A. 'Advantages of potassium cardioplegia and perfusion hypothermia in left ventricular hypertrophy.' *Annals of Thoracic Surgery*, **24,** 299 (1977)
14. Fuhrman, G. J., Fuhrman, F. A. and Field, J. 'Metabolism of rat heart slices with special reference to the effects of temperature and anoxia.' *American Journal of Physiology*, **163,** 642 (1950)
15. Gay, W. A., Jr. and Ebert, P. A. 'Functional, metabolic and morphological effects of potassium-induced cardioplegia.' *Surgery*, **74,** 284 (1973)
16. Gibbon, J. H. 'Application of a mechanical heart and lung apparatus to cardiac surgery.' *Minnesota Medicine*, **37,** 171 (1954)
17. Gricpp, R. B., Stinson, E. B., Oyer, P. E., Copeland, J. G. and Shumway, N. E. 'The superiority of aortic cross-clamping with profound local hypothermia for myocardial protection during aorto-coronary bypass grafting.' *Journal of Thoracic and Cardiovascular Surgery*, **70,** 995 (1975)
18. Griepp, R. B., Stinson, E. B. and Shumway, N. E. 'Profound local hypothermia for myocardial protection during open-heart surgery.' *Journal of Thoracic and Cardiovascular Surgery*, **66,** 731 (1973)
19. Hufnagel, C. A., Conrad, P., Schomo, J. and Pifarré, R. 'Profound cardiac hypothermia.' *Annals of Surgery*, **153,** 790 (1961)
20. Hurley, E. J., Lower, R. R., Dong, E., Pillsbury, R. L. and Shumway, N. E. 'Clinical experience with local hypothermia in elective cardiac arrest.' *Journal of Thoracic and Cardiovascular Surgery*, **47,** 50 (1964)
21. Kenyon, N. M., Litwak, R. S., Beck, H. J., Slonim, R. J., Spear, H. C. and Shibota, Y. 'Preliminary observations in isolated hypothermic cardiac asystole.' *Surgical Forum*, **10,** 567 (1959)
22. Levitsky, S. 'Intracoronary perfusates for myocardial protection.' *Annals of Thoracic Surgery*, **24,** 297 (1977)
23. Lewis, F. J. and Tauffic, M. 'Closure of atrial septal defects with the aid of hypothermia: experimental accomplishments and the report of one successful case.' *Surgery*, **33,** 52 (1953)
24. Long, D. M., Sterns, L. P., De Riemer, R. H., Warden, H. E. and Lillehei, C. W. 'Subtotal and total replacement of the aortic valve with plastic valve prosthesis: experimental investigation and successful clinical application utilizing selective cardiac hypothermia.' *Surgical Forum*, **10,** 660 (1959)
25. Myojin, K., Mee, R., Fishbein, M., Eldridge, R. and Cohn, L. H. 'Long-term effects of hyperkalaemic cardioplegia and local cardiac hypothermia on gross and microscopic structure of the left ventricle.' *Surgical Forum*, **29,** 267 (1978)
26. Nelson, R. L., Goldstein, S. M., McConnell, D. H., Maloney, J. V. and Buckberg, G. 'Studies of the effects of hypothermia on regional myocardial blood flow and metabolism during cardiopulmonary bypass. V. Profound topical hypothermia during ischaemia in arrested hearts.' *Journal of Thoracic and Cardiovascular Surgery*, **73,** 201 (1977)

27. Pupello, D. F., Blank, R. H., Bessone, L. N., Connar, R. G. and Carlton, L. M. Jr. 'Local deep hypothermia for combined valvular and coronary heart disease.' *Annals of Thoracic Surgery*, **21,** 508 (1976)
28. Pupello, D. F., Blank, R. H., Connar, R. G., Bessone, L. N., Shar, S. and Stevenson, A. 'Fifty-two consecutive aortic valve replacements employing local deep hypothermia.' *Annals of Thoracic Surgery*, **19,** 487 (1975)
29. Rao, K. S., Schatz, R., Feinberg, H. and Levitsky, S. 'Metabolic evidence that regional hypothermia induced by cold saline protects the heart during ischaemic arrest.' *Journal of Surgical Research*, **20,** 421 (1976)
30. Robicsek, F. 'Local cardiac hypothermia *in lieu* of coronary perfusion.' *Annals of Thoracic Surgery*, **19,** 605 (1975)
31. Robicsek, F., Sanger, P. W., Daugherty, H. K. and Lesage, M. A. 'Heart surgery in normothermic body perfusion, interruption of the coronary blood flow, and topical cardiac hypothermia.' *Annals of Thoracic Surgery*, **4,** 232 (1967)
32. Sanger, P. W., Robicsek, F., Daugherty, H. K., Gallucci, V. and Lesage, M. A. 'Topical cardiac hypothermia *in lieu* of coronary perfusion.' *Journal of Thoracic and Cardiovascular Surgery*, **52,** 533 (1966)
33. Sapsford, R. N., Blackstone, E. H., Kirklin, J. W., Karp, R. B., Kouchoukos, N. T., Pacifico, A. D., Rose, C. R. and Bradley, E. L. 'Coronary perfusion versus cold ischaemic arrest during aortic valve surgery. A randomized study.' *Circulation*, **49,** 1190 (1974)
34. Schraut, W., Lamberti, J. J., Kampman, K., Anagnostopoulos, C., Replogle, R. and Glagov, S. 'Does local cardiac hypothermia during cardiopulmonary bypass protect the myocardium from long-term morphological and functional injury?.' *Annals of Thoracic Surgery*, **24,** 315 (1977)
35. Shumway, N. E. and Lower, R. R. 'Topical hypothermia for extended periods of anoxic arrest.' *Surgical Forum*, **10,** 563 (1959)
36. Shumway, N. E., Lower, R. R. and Stofer, R. C. 'Selective hypothermia of the heart in anoxic cardiac arrest.' *Surgery, Gynecology and Obstetrics*, **109,** 750 (1959)
37. Stemmer, E. A., McCart, P., Stanton, W. W., Thibault, W., Dearden, L. S. and Connolly, J. E. 'Functional and structural alterations in the myocardium during aortic cross-clamping.' *Journal of Thoracic and Cardiovascular Surgery*, **66,** 754 (1973)
38. Swan, H. 'Clinical hypothermia: a lady with a past, and some promise for the future.' *Surgery*, **73,** 736 (1973)
39. Swan, H., Zeavin, I., Holmes, J. H. and Montgomery, V. 'Cessation of circulation in general hypothermia. I. Physiologic changes and their control.' *Annals of Surgery*, **138,** 360 (1953)
40. Tsifutis, A., Burton, R. M. and Goldring, D. 'The effect of hypothermia and anoxia upon oxygen consumption and contractility of human and rat heart muscle.' *American Heart Journal*, **79,** 88 (1970)
41. Urschel, H. C., Greenberg, J. J. and Hufnagel, C. A. 'Elective cardioplegia by local cardiac hypothermia.' *New England Journal of Medicine*, **261,** 1330 (1959)

12

Functional Disturbances following Extracorporeal Circulatory Support in Cardiac Surgery

Nicholas T. Kouchoukos and Robert B. Karp

Introduction

Extracorporeal support of the circulatory and respiratory systems required for the performance of surgical procedures on the heart, great vessels and coronary arteries results in physiological alterations of most of the organ systems. The majority of these alterations are transient, are not manifested clinically and require no specific therapy. Some, however, result in significant organ system dysfunction and can occasionally be lethal.

Some of the abnormalities resulting from the use of extracorporeal circulatory support are peculiar to the specific type of bypass system employed, and these have been enumerated in detail in the preceding chapters. The general abnormalities that occur following circulatory support with a non-pulsatile pumping system and any of the presently available oxygenators are primarily related to: (1) the degree of dysfunction of the various organ systems present preoperatively and the functional reserve of these systems; (2) the duration and adequacy of the period of extracorporeal support; and (3) the completeness of repair of the specific cardiac or vascular abnormalities. While precise and proper conduct of the operative procedure is essential for the achievement of an optimal surgical result, the detection and treatment of significant abnormalities in the function of various organ systems after operation are of equal importance.

Following a major cardiac surgical procedure, the patient may be considered as a complex system composed of a number of separate but interrelated 'sub-systems' (i.e. cardiovascular, pulmonary, renal, neurological, gastrointestinal and endocrine). The care of such a patient can be accomplished effectively utilizing a 'systems analysis' approach.

With this approach, as proposed by Kirklin (1970)[67], each organ sub-system is analysed separately by assessing all available information relative to 'the present performance of the system, the adequacy of this performance relative to the requirements of the patient as an integrated system, and the used and unused reserves of the sub-system'. Knowledge of the usual effects of extracorporeal circulatory support on a patient with a particular type of cardiac lesion, and of those abnormalities which are potentially life-threatening and will need therapy, is required to manage effectively the patient in the postoperative period. In this chapter, the major functional disturbances following the use of extracorporeal support will be emphasized, as well as the measures generally employed for their diagnosis and treatment.

Cardiovascular system

Impaired cardiac performance following open intracardiac operations, manifested chiefly by low cardiac output, is associated with a significant mortality and morbidity in the early postoperative period[5, 99]. When the patient is restless or agitated with cool, moist, cyanotic extremities, weak or absent peripheral pulses, and low urine flow early postoperatively, the diagnosis of low cardiac output can be made with relative certainty even in the presence of a normal blood pressure. Unfortunately, many patients with low cardiac output do not manifest these clinical signs. On the other

Table 12.1 Average cardiac index* after open intracardiac operations. (From Kirklin and Rastelli[68] by permission of Grune and Stratton Inc.)

Type of operation	*Cases*	*Cardiac index, mean (and range) after operation*			
		Chest open (½ hour after bypass)	*2 to 4 h*	*24 h*	*48 h*
Repair					
ASD with normal pulmonary vascular resistance	5	3.0 (2.1–3.9)	3.4 (2.4–4.4)	3.0 (2.3–4.0)	3.3 (2.9–3.7)
VSD with normal pulmonary vascular resistance	7	3.8 (3.2–5.3)	3.5 (2.9–4.2)	3.2 (2.7–4.4)	3.4 (2.7–4.4)
VSD with moderately elevated pulmonary vascular resistance	3	3.7 (3.4–4.0)	3.7 (2.9–4.4)	3.0 (1.9–3.6)	2.9 (2.3–3.5)
Tetralogy of Fallot	15	2.5 (2.0–3.5)	2.9 (2.0–5.5)	2.2 (1.6–3.7)	2.5 (1.7–5.2)
Replacement					
Aortic valve with S–E prosthesis	7	2.5 (1.6–3.1)	2.4 (1.4–3.8)	2.8 (2.0–4.5)	3.2 (2.3–4.1)
Mitral valve with S–E prosthesis	12	2.5 (1.1–4.1)	1.7 (1.0–2.6)	1.9 (0.9–3.0)	2.2 (1.2–3.5)

*Normal values = 3.5 (± 0.7) ℓ/min per m^2 of body surface area; ASD = Atrial septal defect; VSD = Ventricular septal defect; S–E = Starr–Edwards

Table 12.2 Low output syndrome after open intracardiac operations (25 patients). (Modified from Dietzman *et al.*[32] by courtesy of C. V. Mosby Co.)

Group no.	*No. of patients*	*Cardiac index* (l/min/m²)*	*Total peripheral resistance* (dynes/s/cm̄⁵)*	*Urine output* (ml/h)*	*Extremities (temperature colour)*	*Survivors No.*	*(%)*
I	9	2.90	930	55	warm, pink	9	(100)†
II	16	1.53	2254	7	cold, pale	9	(56)**

*$P<0.001$. Comparison of Groups I and II using Student's 't' test †There were two late deaths in Group I **There was one late death in Group II

hand, some patients with cool, cyanotic extremities and weak peripheral pulses may have an adequate cardiac output. Thus, actual measurement of cardiac output is required in most circumstances to assess accurately cardiac function. The range for cardiac output in normal resting adults is approximately 2.4 to 4.4 litres/minute per square metre (ℓ/min per m^2) of body surface area, with a mean of 3.5[12].

Mean values for cardiac output following a variety of open intracardiac operations are shown in *Table 12.1*[68]. These values vary with the type of operation.

The consequences of abnormally low cardiac output, particularly when there is evidence of increased sympathetic activity, are illustrated in *Table 12.2*[32]. In a series of 25 patients with early postoperatively measured cardiac indices of less than 3.0 ℓ/min per m^2, there was a significant difference in survival between patients with cardiac outputs between 2.0 and 3.0 ℓ/min per m^2, who had normal peripheral vascular resistances and adequate tissue perfusion, and patients with outputs of less than 2.0 ℓ/min per m^2, who had evidence of increased sympathetic activity (increased peripheral vascular resistance, reduced tissue perfusion, increased serum catecholamine levels). Even though cardiac output was abnormally low in the former group of patients, it was adequate to meet the metabolic requirements of the various organ systems. In other studies, deaths from acute cardiac failure have occurred most commonly in patients with a low value for mean cardiac output early postoperatively. In infants and small children following a variety of cardiac operations, an average, measured cardiac index of less than 2.0 ℓ/min per m^2 in the early postoperative period was associated with a greater than 10 per cent probability of death from acute cardiac failure (*Figure 12.1*)[99]. In adult patients following mitral valve replacement, a mean postoperative cardiac index of 1.5 ℓ/min per m^2 or less was associated with a 10 per cent or greater probability of death (*Figure 12.2*)[5]. The probability of death rose steeply in both groups at indices below these values.

In patients with low cardiac output and impaired left ventricular function, as evidenced by abnormally elevated mean left atrial and left ventricular end-diastolic pressures, the mortality and morbidity rates early after operation are also significantly increased. In *Figure 12.3* are shown the cardiac outputs and mean left atrial pressures of 30 adult patients in the first 4 hours following a variety of cardiac surgical procedures. These data were obtained during a period when low cardiac output was not systematically treated. Of 16 patients with cardiac indices of less than 2.2 ℓ/min per m^2 and left atrial pressures greater than 15 mmHg, 3 died within 24 hours after operation of irreversible ventricular arrhythmias, and 2 died within 2 weeks of operation of ventricular arrhythmias. Both of the latter patients continued to have low cardiac output during this period. Two additional patients had episodes of ventricular fibrillation but survived. Among the 14 patients with lower left atrial pressures and generally higher cardiac indices, there was only 1 postoperative death. Thus, evidence for the presence of impaired cardiac performance should be actively sought, particularly in the early period following operation, in order to institute appropriate therapeutic measures and minimize early mortality and morbidity rates.

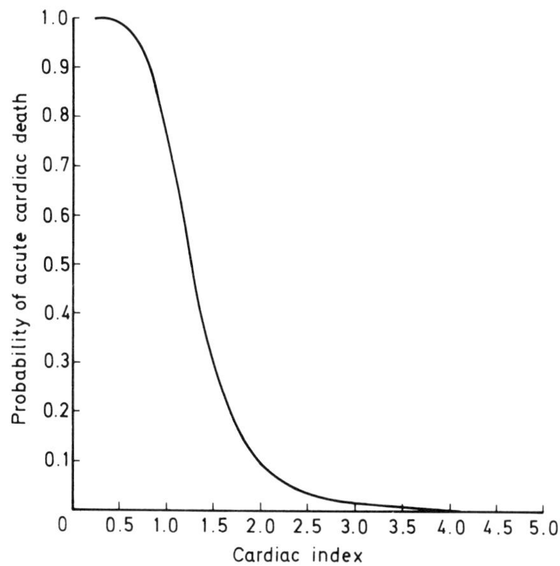

Figure 12.1 Probability of death from acute cardiac failure from the average cardiac index (ℓ/min per m^2) of 139 infants and children in the early postoperative period. (Modified from Parr, Blackstone and Kirklin[99] by courtesy of *Circulation*)

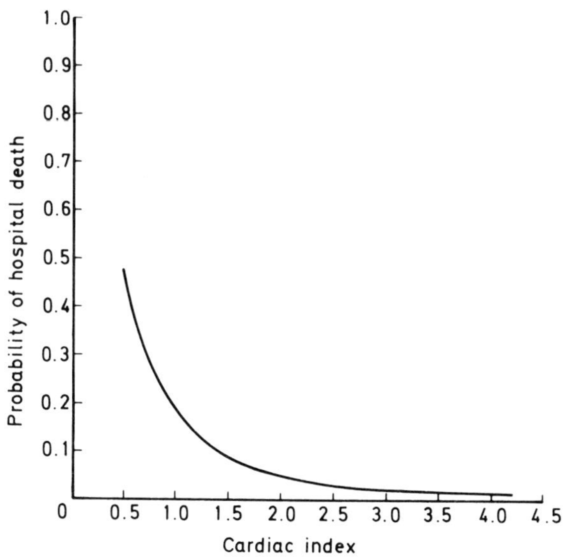

Figure 12.2 Probability of death from acute cardiac failure from the average cardiac index (ℓ/min per m^2) of 125 patients following mitral valve replacement. (Reproduced from Appelbaum *et al.*[5], by courtesy of *American Journal of Cardiology*)

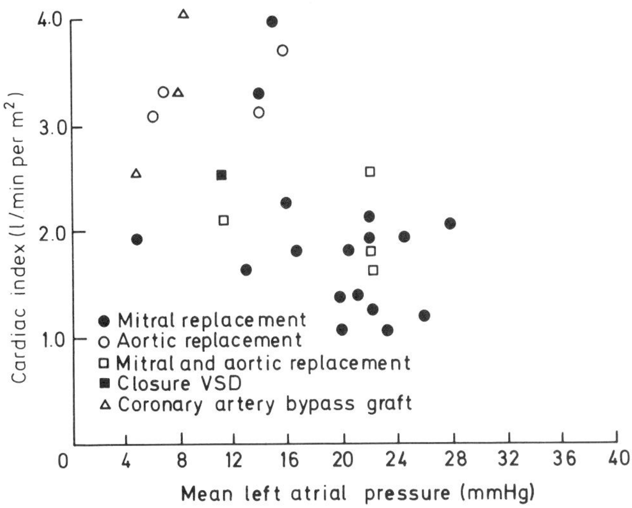

Figure 12.3 Comparison of cardiac index and mean left atrial pressure in 30 adult patients in the first 4 hours after open intracardiac operations

Routine maintenance measures

Certain parameters to assess the function of the cardiovascular system should be measured routinely in the early postoperative period. Arterial pressure is obtained with an indwelling catheter usually placed percutaneously in the radial (or alternatively, the femoral or brachial) artery. Heart rate and rhythm are determined from the electrocardiogram using electrodes attached to the chest wall. The left atrial and right atrial (central venous) pressures are determined from fine polyvinyl catheters placed at the time of operation. The arterial and atrial pressure catheters are connected to appropriate transducers and metering devices to record the pressures in millimetres of mercury. These measurements are obtained at 5–15 minute intervals in the first 24–48 hours following operation. The use of indwelling arterial and cardiac catheters for this period of time has been associated with an extremely low incidence of complications in our experience. They are utilized routinely in our hospital in all patients undergoing surgical procedures in which extracorporeal circulatory support is employed. The drainage from catheters placed in the mediastinum and the pleural and pericardial cavities, the volume of blood infused and the urine output from a urethral catheter are generally recorded at hourly intervals following operation. Arterial blood-gas analyses are obtained as often as necessary to ensure optimum gas exchange and acid-base balance (*see below*).

The cardiac output is generally determined by the indicator dilution technique–injecting indocyanine green dye into the left atrial catheter and sampling from the arterial catheter, or injecting dye into the right atrial catheter and sampling from a catheter placed in the pulmonary artery at the time of operation. The latter system is preferred when the left-sided cardiac chambers are large or the cardiac output is low, in order to minimize distortion of the dilution curves and errors in the calculated value for cardiac output. In infants and small children, dye is injected into the right atrium and blood is withdrawn from the radial or brachial artery to allow adequate time for stabilization of the absorption spectrum. Using appropriate densitometers and portable or large computers, cardiac output is calculated using the Stewart–Hamilton formula[113]. The thermal dilution technique employs cold saline as the indicator. This is injected into the right atrium with measurement of subsequent temperature change of the blood in the pulmonary artery using a thermistor-tipped catheter. This method allows repeated determinations of cardiac output without the need for withdrawal of blood[44]. The determination of stroke volume and cardiac output from the arterial pressure pulse has not, to date, proved reliable enough in the early postoperative period to supplant routinely the techniques outlined above[75]. All of the above-mentioned measurements can be obtained, analysed and displayed automatically with the use of a digital computer as shown in *Figure 12.4*[116]. The use of such an automated system has greatly facilitated the management of patients following cardiac surgical procedures[73]. It has provided data that can be retrieved more rapidly and that are more accurate than those obtained by conventional techiques[1].

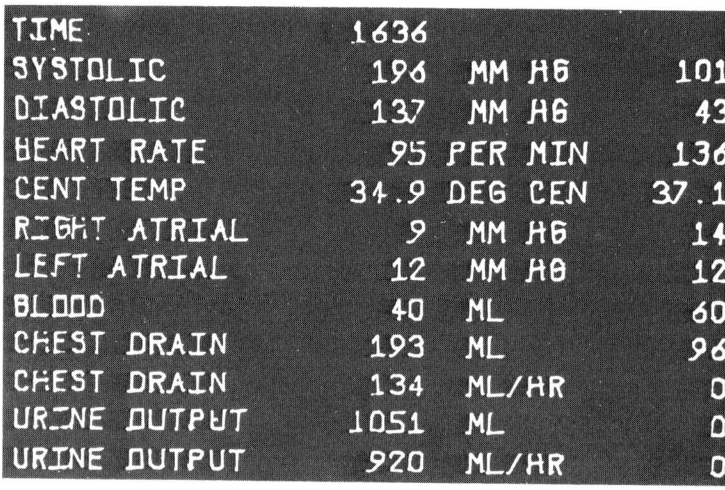

Figure 12.4 Oscilloscope display of medical data from a 3 second interval obtained from 2 patients connected to an automated monitoring system. Chest drainage and urine output are expressed as total millilitres and as millilitres for the previous clock hour. (Reproduced from Kouchoukos, Sheppard and Kirklin[73], by courtesy of the F. A. Davis Company)

The arterial pressure is generally considered to be a reliable indicator of cardiac function postoperatively. If arterial hypotension is present (systolic arterial pressure <70–80 mmHg), cardiac function is generally suboptimal. If the arterial pressure is normal or above normal, however, the cardiac output may be high, normal or low (*Figure 12.5*). The central venous (right atrial) pressure does not demonstrate a consistent relationship to cardiac output, blood volume deficit or the response to blood replacement

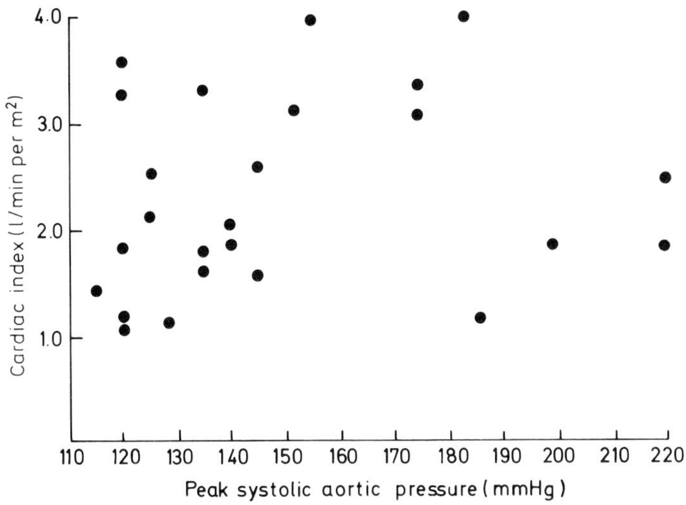

Figure 12.5 Comparison of cardiac index and peak systolic aortic pressure in 25 adult patients in the first 4 hours after open intracardiac operations

postoperatively[70]. In our experience, measurement (or estimate) of cardiac output combined with measurement of arterial pressure and mean left atrial pressure, which in the absence of either stenosis or incompetence of the mitral valve approximates left ventricular end-diastolic pressure, allows a more accurate assessment of cardiac function and the response to various therapeutic interventions than does the measurement of arterial and central venous pressures alone. If a left atrial catheter is not available, the pulmonary arterial wedge or diastolic pressure can be measured from a catheter placed in the pulmonary artery (Swan–Ganz), and this approximates the left ventricular filling pressure[43].

Aetiology of impaired cardiac performance

Hypovolaemia

Inadequate blood volume following procedures employing extracorporeal circulatory support is a frequent cause of impaired cardiac performance early postoperatively. The magnitude of the blood volume deficit present during this period depends on several factors, the most important being: (1) the adequacy of volume replacement at the termination of the operative procedure; (2) the degree of vasoconstriction present, particularly of the venous capacitance vessels; and (3) the volume of blood lost as mediastinal drainage relative to the volume of blood replaced. In general, blood is infused into the patient from the pump oxygenator at the termination of the perfusion to achieve a level of mean left atrial pressure of 14–18 mmHg in adults and 10–14 mmHg in children. This level of left atrial pressure results in optimal stretching of the sarcomeres (preload) and maximal stroke volume from the left ventricle by the Frank–Starling mechanism, but does not produce pulmonary congestion or oedema.

The left as well as right atrial pressures generally decrease to more normal levels in the early postoperative period[69]. The ultimate values for right and left atrial pressure postoperatively are determined primarily by the volume of blood in the respective central or pulmonary venous beds, the venous tone of the two systems and the pressure–volume characteristics of the right- and left-sided cardiac chambers. In adult patients with valvular heart disease, blood volume is decreased and whole body venous tone increased following operation[106]. These changes are maximal 24 to 48 hours following operation and approach the preoperative values by the fourth postoperative day.

As noted previously, the central venous (or right atrial) pressure does not demonstrate a consistent relationship to blood volume deficit or the response to blood replacement following operation. Measurement of left atrial pressure is the most reliable guide to the adequacy of volume replacement during this period. The effects of blood infusion on left atrial pressure and cardiac output early after surgical procedures for acquired heart disease are shown in *Figure 12.6*[72]. In 9 adult patients with normal

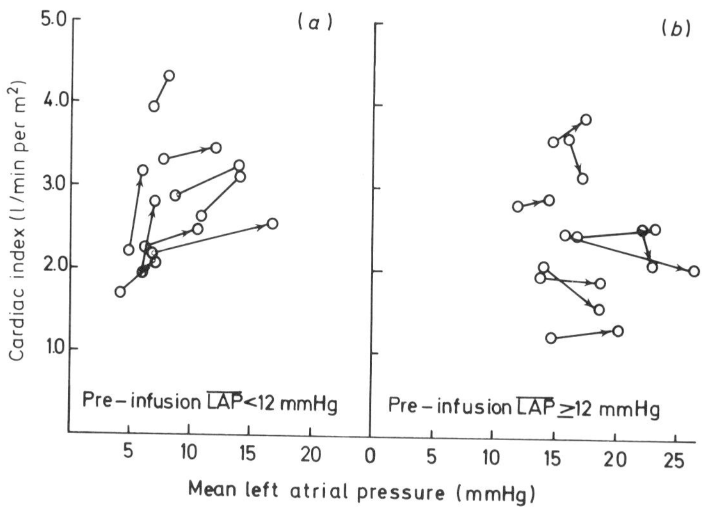

Figure 12.6 Effect of elevation of left atrial pressure by blood infusion on cardiac index in adult patients early after open intracardiac operations. (*a*) Nine patients with pre-infusion mean left atrial pressures (LAP) of less than 12 mmHg. (*b*) Nine patients with pre-infusion mean left atrial pressures of greater than 12 mmHg

mean left atrial pressures (less than 12 mmHg), infusion of blood to increase left atrial pressure an average of 3.4 mmHg produced a statistically significant increase in cardiac index (from 2.52 to 2.931 ℓ/min per m^2), while the heart rate remained constant. In 9 patients with mean left atrial pressures before blood infusion of greater than 12 mmHg (mean 15.6 mmHg), comparable increases in left atrial pressure by blood infusion were produced, but the cardiac index did not increase and the mean value actually decreased (from 2.58 to 2.41 ℓ/min per m^2). Thus, if cardiac output is low and left atrial pressure is low or normal (<12–14 mmHg) infusion of blood will generally increase the cardiac output early postoperatively, presumably by the Frank–Starling mechanism. If the left atrial pressure is already elevated above this level, further augmentation of blood volume and filling pressure will not usually increase the cardiac output.

Cardiac tamponade

Persistent bleeding into the pericardial cavity and mediastinum resulting in cardiac tamponade is a relatively uncommon but serious case of impaired cardiac performance following cardiac surgical procedures. Bleeding of sufficient quantity to require reoperation occurs in approximately 3 per cent of patients undergoing open-heart operations[53]. Cardiac tamponade generally becomes apparent in the early postoperative period but can be delayed in its presentation for up to 2 weeks following operation, particularly when anticoagulants are being administered[57]. The bleeding most commonly occurs from discrete sites such as suture lines of the heart or great vessels or from blood vessels such as the internal thoracic, which may be injured during the operative procedure. Less commonly, generalized bleeding sufficient to produce cardiac tamponade results from deficiencies in the clotting mechanism (*see* Chapter 15). A higher incidence of postoperative bleeding has been noted in patients with cyanotic heart disease and in those with right-sided cardiac failure, which presumably depresses the hepatic function and the synthesis of several clotting factors. Factors which may contribute to a generalized haemorrhagic diathesis following cardiac surgery include injury to platelets and red cells during perfusion, tissue trauma and the use of extravasated blood. All of these lead to the release of tissue thromboplastic and fibrinolytic activators[139]. Dilution of the patient's blood with priming blood or diluent deficient in various clotting factors (particularly platelets and factors V and VIII) and inadequate heparin neutralization may also contribute to impaired coagulation following operation[139].

The accumulation of fluid and clot within the pericardial cavity and mediastinal space results in an increase in intrapericardial pressure. This decreases the effective left ventricular end-diastolic pressure, end-diastolic volume and stroke volume. Although the cardiac output will initially remain at adequate levels because of an increase in heart rate, it gradually decreases and cardiac arrest ensues unless appropriate therapy is initiated.

The diagnosis of cardiac tamponade following operation may, at times, be difficult to establish with certainty. The presence of significant drainage from the mediastinal tubes, combined with a trend towards equalization and gradual increase of the right and left atrial pressures, strongly suggests the presence of tamponade. Subsequently, arterial hypotension and clinical evidence of low cardiac output may become apparent. A chest roentgenogram often demonstrates an increase in the mediastinal silhouette and adds support to the diagnosis. The above findings may not always be present, and bleeding must always be considered as a possible cause of impaired cardiac function.

The treatment of cardiac tamponade consists of urgent operation to evaculate the clot and identify and control the point or points of bleeding. If the bleeding is generalized, deficiencies of various clotting factors (platelets, factors V and VII, and fibrinogen) must be sought by the appropriate tests. The treatment consists of administration of fresh-frozen plasma, fresh whole blood, and platelet and plasma concentrates when deficiencies of these substances are demonstrated. The use of heparin for disseminated intravascular coagulation or epsilon aminocaproic acid for excessive fibrinolysis is generally not indicated since these abnormalities are generally self-limited.[139]

Myocardial dysfunction

Total cardiac performance can be significantly affected postoperatively by several mechanisms which result in impairment of cardiac muscular function.

Preoperative cardiac dysfunction Abnormalities of myocardial function may be present preoperatively in patients with acquired heart disease and may persist or actually become more severe postoperatively. These abnormalities can significantly affect cardiac performance following operation. In our experience with patients following mitral or multiple valve replacement, the severity of preoperative cardiac disability, as reflected by the functional class, clearly affects the hospital mortality rate (*Table 12.3*)[2, 123, 124]. Pre-existing myocardial dysfunction is probably an important contributing factor to the low cardiac output state observed following mitral valve replacement[5, 104].

Table 12.3 Hospital mortality following valve replacement according to preoperative functional class

Valve(s) replaced	*Preoperative functional class**	*No. of patients*	*Hospital deaths* No.	%
Mitral[2]	III	109	3	3
	IV	24	4	17
Aortic and mitral[122]	III	180	17	9
	IV	52	15	29
Aortic, mitral and tricuspid[124]	III	28	5	18
	IV	10	4	40

*New York Heart Association classification

Impairment of myocardial contractility has been demonstrated preoperatively in patients with aortic and mitral valvular disease[48, 56]. Significant left ventricular dysfunction has also been observed preoperatively in patients with coronary atherosclerotic heart disease, particularly those with predominant symptoms of congestive failure rather than angina pectoris. Higher operative and late mortality rates have been observed in such patients following myocardial revascularization in contrast to patients with more normal ventricular function[71, 121]. Follow-up studies of patients who have had valve replacement or coronary bypass surgery have demonstrated that the preoperative abnormalities in myocardial function often persist and may even become more severe in some patients, despite correction of the valvular or coronary arterial lesions[48, 56, 121].

Intraoperative myocardial injury Myocardial injury can occur during cardiopulmonary bypass and if severe, or if imposed upon a myocardium which is already abnormal (left ventricular hypertrophy, left ventricular fibrosis, coronary arterial occlusive disease) can significantly impair cardiac performance in the postoperative period. Ischaemia, haemorrhage and necrosis of the myocardium, particularly of the inner layers of the left ventricular wall, have been observed in patients who died after cardiopulmonary bypass, many of whom had low cardiac output postoperatively[19, 93, 128]. Studies of myocardial metabolism and measurement of specific enzymes to detect myocardial injury indicate that myocardial damage of varying degrees of severity occurs in many patients during or following operations in which cardiopulmonary bypass was employed, irrespective of the technique of myocardial preservation utilized during the procedure[51, 95, 111].

The presence of markedly hypertrophic left ventricular myocardium may predispose to severe ischaemic myocardial injury following cardiopulmonary bypass. A small, contracted left ventricle that does not eject effectively has been observed in patients of this type and has been termed the 'stone heart'[30]. Methods of myocardial preservation which have been observed as leading to this type of myocardial injury are euthermic cardioplegia[140] and, in our own experience, hypothermic coronary perfusion. The incidence of this complication had apparently been reduced following the use of hypothermic cardioplegia[140], suggesting that inadequate protection of the myocardium during cardiac surgical procedures plays an important role in the aetiology of this complication.

All of the currently utilized methods of myocardial preservation during cardiopulmonary bypass appear to produce injury to the myocardium. Recent studies suggest that myocardial perfusion under mild hypothermia and a beating heart is an adequate technique for myocardial preservation during cardiopulmonary bypass. Ventricular fibrillation at euthermic or mildly hypothermic levels is not advisable because of impairment of subendocardial perfusion. When arrest of the heart is necessary to ensure optimal operating conditions, hypothermic potassium-induced cardioplegia appears to be superior to euthermic cardioplegia[6] and to hypothermic ischaemic arrest[108].

Embolization of air into the coronary arteries can occur during operations in which the ascending aorta or left-sided heart chambers are opened, and it can impair the myocardial contractility[50]. Embolization of blood element aggregates into the coronary vessels may also affect myocardial function. Injury to the coronary arteries during the operative procedure (i.e. by direct cannulation, by inadvertent injury to the aberrant anterior descending coronary artery during repair of the tetralogy of Fallot or injury to the left circumflex coronary artery during replacement of the mitral valve) can produce myocardial infarction and severely impair the cardiac function.

Residual cardiovascular disease The presence of residual cardiovascular abnormalities may also contribute to impaired myocardial function following operations employing cardiopulmonary bypass. Examples of this include: the presence of significant tricuspid valvular incompetence following mitral or mitral and aortic valve replacement[70]; aortic valvular incompetence following mitral valve replacement[81]; coronary arterial occlusive disease following valve replacement[26, 88]; and the persistence of significant pulmonary arterial hypertension following correction of heart lesions with left-to-right shunt. Inadequate repair of various congenital and acquired cardiac lesions (i.e. incomplete relief of right ventricular outflow obstruction in tetralogy of Fallot, incomplete closure of ventricular septal defects, incomplete correction of valvular stenosis or incompetence, and perivalvular leaks) may also impair myocardial function postoperatively. Careful preoperative and intraoperative evaluation should allow detection and appropriate treatment of most cardiac and valvular lesions. When there is evidence for significant impairment of cardiac performance postoperatively, prompt reoperation should be considered in any patient in whom correctible residual lesions are present.

Impaired myocardial contractility If evidence for impaired myocardial contractility exists, the use of pharmacological agents to improve contractility is indicated. Isoproterenol is an effective agent since it exerts a chronotropic as well as inotropic action on the myocardium, and cardiac output may be augmented by both these mechanisms. In addition, it can produce peripheral vasodilation which may be beneficial if there is significant peripheral vasoconstriction. Tachycardia and ventricular arrhythmias can be produced with infusion of this drug and not infrequently they limit its use. Although isoproterenol can produce an increase in cardiac output postoperatively, the myocardial oxygen demand is also increased, and anaerobic myocardial metabolism may result[92].

Epinephrine is also a useful agent postoperatively, particularly when arterial hypotension is present. If infused in sufficient amounts, epinephrine increases myocardial contractility and peripheral vascular resistance and thus increases the cardiac output and arterial pressure. In smaller doses, it may actually result in a fall in peripheral vascular resistance due to the beta-adrenergic effect on blood vessels[42]. Epinephrine has been shown to augment cardiac output in patients following cardiac surgical procedures[25, 42]. Dopamine (Inotropin), a naturally occurring catecholamine with inotropic and chronotropic effects on the myocardium, has been shown to be effective in the management of some patients following cardiac operations[58, 59, 122]. It has a lesser chronotropic effect than isoproterenol in postoperative patients and may be the preferable agent because of this. The use of *l*-norepinephrine (Levophed) or metaraminol (Aramine) is only occasionally indicated when marked arterial hypotension is present. These drugs produce marked vasoconstriction and may significantly impair organ system function.

Digitalis preparations should be used postoperatively to improve myocardial contractility and to treat specific arrhythmias (*see below*). Rapidly acting digitalis preparations (digoxin, deslanoside, ouabain) should be administered postoperatively when there is evidence of impaired myocardial function and there are no contraindications to their use. Generally, these agents are used in conjunction with catecholamine infusions. As appropriate blood levels of digitalis are obtained, the catecholamine administration may be gradually reduced and discontinued. Digitalis preparations should be administered cautiously, taking into account the status of preoperative digitalization as well as the presence of hypokalaemia or alkalosis, which may increase the sensitivity of the patient to usual maintenance doses. We routinely discontinue digitalis preparations 48 hours before the operation in order to minimize the occurrence of intraoperative and postoperative arrhythmias.

Impedance to left ventricular ejection

Increased impedance to ventricular ejection which results in an increase in systolic wall tension (afterload) has been shown to reduce stroke volume and left ventricular stroke work in patients with diseased myocardium[109]. In postoperative patients with elevated mean arterial pressure, high peripheral vascular resistance and low cardiac output, an improvement in cardiac output has been achieved by reduction of arterial pressure[74]. In a group of patients with high mean arterial pressure (greater than 100 mmHg), and evidence of impaired cardiac performance (cardiac index less than 2.1 ℓ/min per m^2 and mean left atrial pressure greater than 15 mmHg), infusion of Arfonad (trimethaphan camsylate), a ganglion-blocking and vasodilating agent, produced a significant increase in stroke index and cardiac output (*Figure 12.7*). A comparable reduction of arterial pressure in patients with higher cardiac indices and lower left atrial pressures, suggesting more normal left ventricular function, resulted in a decrease in stroke volume, presumably as a result of decrease in left ventricular filling pressure (preload). Comparable effects on left ventricular function have been observed with sodium nitroprusside, a potent vasodilator in adult and paediatric cardiac surgical patients[4, 126]. Phentolamine (Rogitine) produces similar effects but may produce tachyarrhythmias. Phenoxybenzamine (Dibenzyline), an alpha-adrenergic blocking agent, has also been shown to improve cardiac performance in patients with low cardiac output postoperatively[32]. When administered intravenously, the maximal activity is not obtained for several hours and its effect may persist for several days. We prefer trimethaphan or nitroprusside because of their rapid onset and short duration of action. The infusion rates of these agents can be adjusted relatively easily to achieve the desired reduction in arterial pressure.

The use of vasodilating agents to reduce arterial pressure and impedance to left ventricular ejection should be considered in patients following open intracardiac operations when the cardiac index is low and the atrial and mean aortic pressures and the peripheral vascular resistance are elevated. The reduction of arterial pressure under these circumstance allows more effective emptying of the left ventricle and may, with reduction of left ventricular end-diastolic pressure, allow more efficient perfusion of the subendocardial myocardial layers. The reduction in left ventricular systolic pressure will also reduce myocardial oxygen consumption. If the cardiac output remains low following the administration of these vasodilating agents, the additional use of inotropic agents such as epinephrine or isoproterenol may be effective in increasing the cardiac output.

Assistance of the failing circulation with the intra-aortic balloon counter-pulsation device has been employed in patients in whom cardiopulmonary bypass cannot be discontinued without haemodynamic deterioration or in

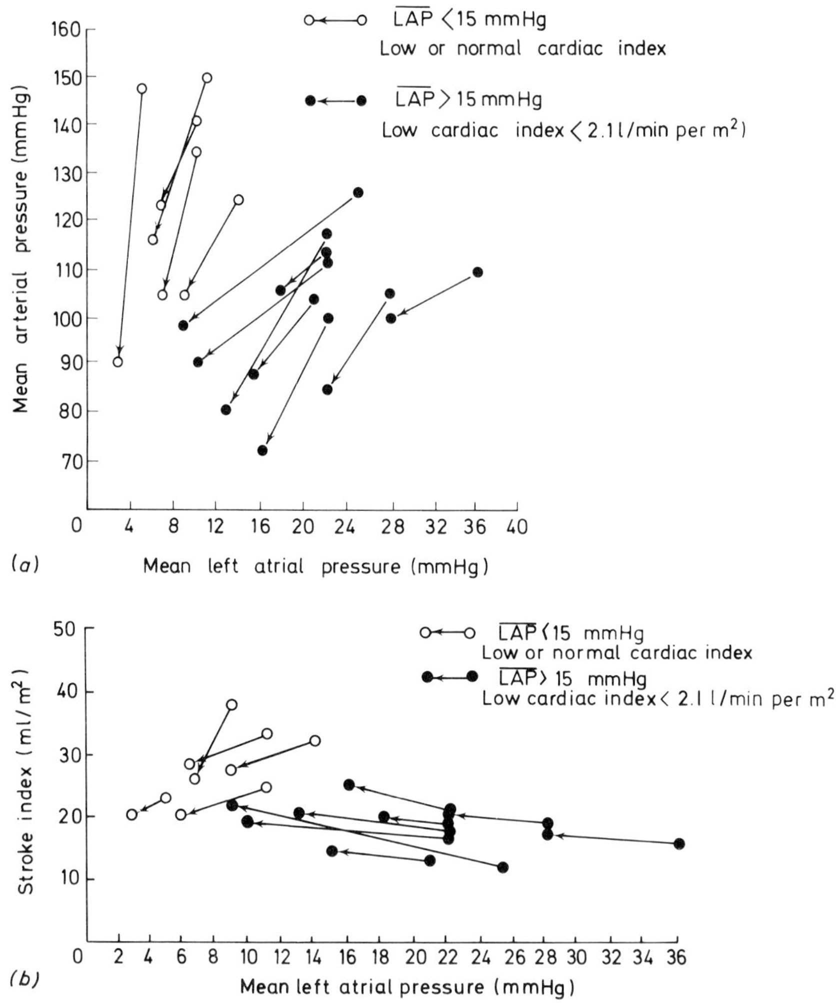

Figure 12.7 Response to infusion of trimethaphan (Arfonad) into patients within 6 hours after intracardiac operations. The 8 patients in the group with poor cardiac performance (cardiac index < 2.1 ℓ/min per m^2, mean left atrial pressure > 15 mmHg) had undergone mitral or mitral and aortic valve replacement. (*a*) Effect on mean arterial pressure and mean left atrial pressure. (*b*) Effect on mean left atrial pressure and stroke index. (From Kouchoukos, Sheppard and Kirklin[74], by courtesy of *Journal of Thoracic and Cardiovascular Surgery*)

patients who deteriorate later in the postoperative period. Intra-aortic balloon counterpulsation reduces left ventricular work and oxygen consumption and may improve myocardial perfusion. The majority of the patients in whom this device has been used have been those with severe coronary artery disease and evidence of severely impaired left ventricular function. It has also been applied in a small number of patients following other cardiac surgical procedures such as single or multiple valve replacement. The indications for use of this device are not completely defined, but in general it has been employed when there is evidence of deterioration of the haemodynamic state (mean aortic pressure less than 80 to 90 mmHg, mean left atrial or left ventricular end-diastolic pressure greater than 25 mmHg, and low cardiac output). The patients have usually received maximal pharmacological support. In patients of this type, the hospital mortality has ranged between 40 and 50 per cent, and 38 to 42 per cent of the patients were longterm survivors[20, 76, 98]. While these results are not optimal, it must be recognized that the majority of these patients would have died without the period of circulatory support. The favourable experience in these series may result in expanded use of the device postoperatively, possibly as a substitute for catecholamine support which may have detrimental effects, particularly in patients with ischaemic myocardium[92].

Acid–base and electrolyte abnormalities

Metabolic acidosis occurs infrequently following extracorporeal circulatory support with the currently utilized pump oxygenator systems and priming techniques (*see relevant chapters*). When metabolic acidosis is present postoperatively, it may reflect inadequate perfusion during bypass, particularly if the period of bypass was prolonged. More commonly, metabolic acidosis results from low cardiac output postoperatively with poor tissue perfusion. Since metabolic acidosis may adversely affect myocardial function[31], it should be treated vigorously in the postoperative period. Obviously, improvement in cardiac output is an important aspect of therapy. Vasopressor agents may be more effective in the treatment of low cardiac output if the acidosis is corrected[31]. Arterial hypoxaemia, if present, should also be corrected if possible, to ensure adequate oxygen delivery to the tissues.

The extracellular base deficit can be calculated from the arterial carbon dioxide tension ($P\text{CO}_2$), pH and haemoglobin levels using the Siggaard–Anderson nomograms and the patient's weight in kilograms[118]. If a base deficit of more than 3 mmol/ℓ exists, an initial dose of sodium bicarbonate of one-half the calculated extracellular base deficit (0.25 × weight in kg × deficit in mmol/ℓ) is administered. The arterial blood-gas analyses are repeated every two hours and additional sodium bicarbonate is administered as necessary using the same formula.

Alkalosis is more often present postoperatively than acidosis. Metabolic alkalosis may result from the citrate ion present in ACD blood and is often compounded by the respiratory alkalosis which occurs in many patients who are receiving assisted ventilation postoperatively. Patients who require ventilatory support should have careful control of the ventilator to avoid arterial carbon dioxide levels of less than 30 mmHg and arterial pH values above 7.6. Alkalosis above this level may impair myocardial contractility.[29]

Low serum potassium concentrations are frequently present following cardiopulmonary bypass and may result in arrhythmias which can significantly impair the cardiac performance (*see below*). Preoperative diuretic therapy may deplete total body potassium and potassium ion should be administered preoperatively in patients who have been on longterm diuretic therapy if the serum potassium concentration is low. The diuresis which occurs following cardiopulmonary bypass, particularly when haemodilution has been employed, promotes the urinary excretion of potassium. Respiratory alkalosis resulting from mechanical ventilation reduces the serum potassium concentration which may be further reduced by an increase in urinary potassium excretion.[41]

To minimize these potassium losses, we discontinue the diuretic therapy several days before operation. In addition, potassium chloride is administered postoperatively when the potassium levels are below 3.5 mmol/ℓ to minimize the occurrence of cardiac arrhythmias.

The calcium ion may exert a positive inotropic effect on the myocardium and if the serum calcium levels are low in the presence of low cardiac output, calcium ion should be administered. This is of particular importance when large amounts of citrated blood are being infused, since serum calcium may be inactivated by the citrate.

Abnormalities of heart rate and rhythm

Arrhythmias occur commonly following cardiac surgical procedures and although they are generally transient and well tolerated, they may, on occasions, significantly impair the cardiac performance. This is particularly true if there are other mechanisms operative which are also contributing to impaired cardiac function. Factors which predispose to the development of arrhythmias following cardiac procedures include electrolyte imbalance (particularly low serum potassium), metabolic acidosis, hypoxaemia, digitalis excess, surgical trauma and pre-existing cardiac disease.[55] Such abnormalities, when present early postoperatively, should be corrected promptly by appropriate therapeutic measures.

Arrhythmias affect cardiac performance chiefly by their effect on heart rate, one of the two determinants (with stroke volume) of cardiac output. Arrhythmias resulting in bradycardia will often produce a decrease in cardiac output even though there may be an initial compensatory increase in stroke volume. Ventricular extrasystoles may also occur at slow ventricular rates and further impair the cardiac function. Arrhythmias resulting in rapid heart rate (greater than 120–140 per minute) decrease the cardiac output by impairment of diastolic filling with resultant reduction in stroke volume. This may be an important factor following valve replacement, since the function of some prosthetic valves is significantly impaired at rapid heart rates. With very rapid heart rates, perfusion of the myocardium may be impaired, particularly the subendocardial layers, due to the reduction of coronary blood flow during diastole.

Placement of epicardial wires at the time of operation allows for accurate detection of arrhythmias postoperatively and for institution of therapy by electrical pacing[55, 133]. These wires should be placed both on the right atrium and the left or right ventricle and should preferably be placed in pairs one-half to one centimetre apart to allow accurate recordings to be made from them and to allow the use of low-current stimulation[135].

Supraventricular arrhythmias Sinus tachycardia not infrequently occurs following operation. It is generally transient and well tolerated if the myocardial function is normal. Occasionally, the heart rate may be excessively rapid (greater than 150–160 beats per minute) and under these circumstances, therapy may be required to improve the cardiac output.

Obvious causes for tachycardia (hypovolaemia, fever, pericardial tamponade) must be sought. Neostigmine (Prostigmin) in small doses (0.5–1 mg) may be successful in slowing the heart rate. Digitalis may also be effective, particularly if the tachycardia originates from an ectopic focus, since it should slow the rate of the ectopic pacemaker and prolong the atrioventricular (AV) conduction, thus slowing the ventricular rate[132]. Paroxysmal atrial tachycardia can often be interrupted by manoeuvres which increase the vagal tone (i.e. carotid massage, infusion of neostigmine, or elevation of the systolic blood pressure with vasopressor agents such as methoxamine (Vasoxyl) or phenylephrine hydrochloride (Neo-synephrine)). Atrial pacing at a rate faster than the spontaneous rate of paroxysmal atrial tachycardia can capture the atria and interrupt the arrhythmia. This should result in sinus rhythm when the artificial pacemaker is turned off, or the pacemaker rate can be decreased to a more normal rate once the atria are captured. Atrial flutter generally results in an atrial rate of 280 to 320 per minute, and the ventricular response is most often a fixed ratio of the atrial rate (i.e. 2 to 1 or 4 to 1). Pacing the atria at a faster rate is often successful in interrupting these arrhythmias[134]. It may be possible by electrical pacing to convert the flutter to atrial fibrillation which is an easier rhythm to control with digitalis. If the ventricular response with atrial fibrillation is slow, it can be best controlled by ventricular pacing particularly in the presence of ventricular extrasystoles. In addition to suppressing the ectopic beats, pacing under these conditions will improve the cardiac output[84].

Junctional arrhythmias If a junctional tachycardia is present, digitalis is contraindicated because it further enhances the automaticity of the AV junctional pacemaker. Intravenous lidocaine (Xylocaine) is the drug of choice under these circumstances since it suppresses the automaticity of the AV junctional pacemaker without significant effects on myocardial contractility or atrioventricular conduction. If the tachycardia is significantly impairing cardiac function with resulting hypotension, paired ventricular pacing to half the rate may occasionally be effective[132]. Junctional arrhythmias resulting in bradycardia can be effectively treated by atrial or ventricular pacing. This can often increase the cardiac output.[45]

Ventricular arrhythmias Ventricular extrasystoles may be treated by pacing either the atria or the ventricles at a slightly higher rate than the pre-existing ventricular rate in order to suppress the ectopic foci. When this is not successful, or if the ventricular rate is already rapid, the use of lidocaine or procainamide (Pronestyl) is generally effective. Ventricular tachycardia can occasionally be treated by pacing, but generally cardioversion combined with appropriate drug therapy (lidocaine or procainamide) is necessary. If hypokalaemia is present, it should be treated intravenously with potassium chloride.

Atrioventricular dissociation occurring postoperatively (either spontaneously or surgically induced) is usually transient, but should be treated by ventricular pacing if the ventricular rate is slow. If serious atrioventricular conduction abnormalities are present preoperatively or occur intraoperatively, permanent as well as temporary epicardial electrodes are placed on the right or left ventricular surface at the time of the cardiac procedure. The permanent electrodes are implanted in the subcutaneous layer of the anterior abdominal wall. If conduction disturbances persist in these patients early postoperatively, they are managed by the temporary wires. If use of a permanent pacer becomes necessary, a pulse generator can be connected to the implanted electrodes as a secondary procedure.

Detection and treatment of impaired cardiac performance

Based on the above information, we currently employ in our Intensive Care Unit a systematic approach to the detection and treatment of impaired cardiac performance following cardiac surgical procedures. Obviously, appropriate selection of patients for operation and precise and proper conduct of the operative procedure are the most important factors in preventing or minimizing the occurrence of impaired cardiac performance postoperatively.

As noted earlier, there may be clinical evidence of low cardiac output postoperatively. If the usual clinical signs of low cardiac output are not present, one may have good grounds for suspicion that the cardiac output is low if arterial hypotension, high left atrial pressure and metabolic acidosis are present. If low cardiac output is present preoperatively, the likelihood that it will be present postoperatively is high, and provision should be made to measure cardiac output postoperatively in such patients. Correctible factors contributing to low cardiac output, such as residual cardiac defects, excessive bleeding with cardiac tamponade and acid–base and electrolyte abnormalities should be systematically sought and appropriately treated (*Table 12.4*). If the heart rate is less than 80–90 beats per minute, the cardiac

Table 12.4 Mechanisms to improve cardiac performance following cardiac operations

(1) Correction of residual cardiac abnormalities
(2) Control of bleeding disorders and relief of cardiac tamponade
(3) Correction of acid–base and electrolyte disturbances
(4) Optimization of cardiac rate and rhythm
(5) Optimization of left ventricular preload and afterload
(6) Enhancement of myocardial contractility

output may be augmented by increasing the rate to 90–110 per minute with appropriate atrial or ventricular pacing. If the heart rate is rapid (greater than 130–140 beats per minute), the type of tachycardia should be accurately identified and treated appropriately.

Once these abnormalities have been identified and the appropriate measures taken to correct them, the cardiac output should be measured again, and if still low, interventions to improve directly the myocardial performance are indicated (*Table 12.5*). As noted previously, we have found that cardiac output, mean aortic pressure and left atrial pressure are the most reliable parameters to assess the cardiac function postoperatively.

Cardiac index less than 2.2 ℓ/min per m²

As noted earlier, a cardiac index of less than 2.2 ℓ/min per m^2 early postoperatively is associated with a high morbidity and mortality rate. If the cardiac index is below this level and the mean left atrial pressure is 14 mmHg or less, blood should be infused to augment the left atrial and left ventricular

Table 12.5 Logic for analysis and treatment of impaired cardiac performance early after operation

Mean left atrial pressure (mmHg)	*Mean arterial pressure (mmHg)*	*< 2.2*	*Cardiac index (ℓ/min per m²)* *2.2–3.0*	*> 3.0*
<7		Blood*	Blood*	Blood*
7–14		Blood*	Blood*	—
15–18	< 100	Epinephrine	—	—
	> 100	Epinephrine Dopamine† or Isoproterenol†	Trimethaphan** or Nitroprusside	—
> 18	< 100	Epinephrine Dopamine† or Isoproterenol†	—	—
	> 100	Epinephrine Dopamine† or Isoproterenol + Trimethaphan or Nitroprusside	Trimethaphan or Nitroprusside	

*Use albumin if haemoglobin concentration > 12 g/100ml
†If frequent premature contractions present or heart rate is above 120/min use Epinephrine.
**Optional in this category

end-diastolic pressures and to increase the cardiac output. If the haemoglobin level is greater than 12 g/100 ml, albumin rather than whole blood is used. Volume is administered under these circumstances regardless of the level of the mean aortic pressure. On occasions, if the arterial pressure is high with evidence of significant peripheral vasoconstriction, trimethaphan or sodium nitroprusside may be administered concomitantly to reduce the arterial pressure, particularly if bleeding is a potential problem, although as noted in *Figure 12.7*, this may further depress the cardiac output. If the mean left atrial pressure is between 15 and 18 mmHg, and the mean arterial pressure is less than 100 mmHg, epinephrine should be administered. If the mean left arterial pressure is greater than 100 mmHg, dopamine or isoproterenol may be used unless the heart rate is greater than 120 per minute or there is ventricular irritability in which case epinephrine should be used. If the mean left atrial pressure is greater than 18 mmHg, and the arterial pressure is less than 100 mmHg, epinephrine, dopamine or isoproterenol should be infused. If the mean arterial pressure is greater than 100 mmHg, trimethaphan or nitroprusside should be infused to reduce the arterial pressure and the left ventricular afterload, thereby reducing the resistance to ventricular ejection. Epinephrine, dopamine or isoproterenol is infused concomitantly to improve the myocardial contractility. The cardiac index should be measured at intervals during these interventions in order to assess the adequacy of therapy. An example of the use of this logic is shown in *Figure 12.8*. If the cardiac performance does not improve or

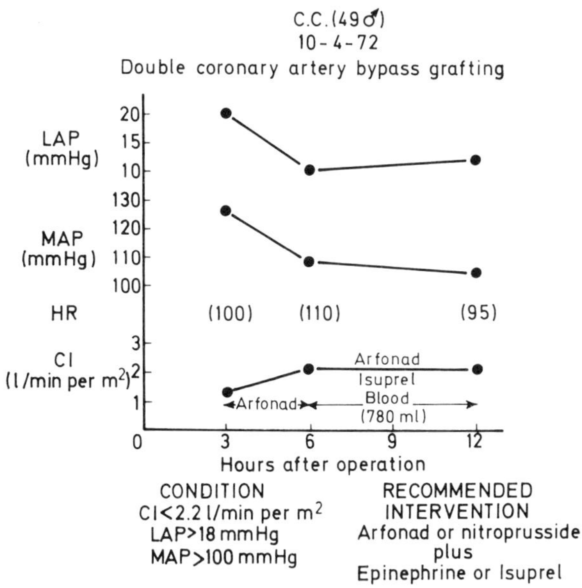

Figure 12.8 Haemodynamic data in a patient following coronary artery bypass grafting. Initial cardiac index (CI) was 1.3 ℓ/min per m^2; mean left atrial pressure (LAP), 22 mmHg; and mean arterial pressure (MAP), 128 mmHg. Recommended interventions are infusion of an impedance-reducing agent and an inotropic agent. After the infusion of Arfonad (trimethaphan), LAP decreased to 10 mmHg, MAP decreased to 108 mmHg, and CI increased to 2.3 ℓ/min per m^2. With the addition of Isuprel (isoproterenol) and infusion of blood (LAP fell below the limit of 14 mmHg), LAP rose slightly, MAP remained below 110 mmHg and CI remained above 2.2 ℓ/min per m^2

further deteriorates with this therapy, intra-aortic balloon pumping should be considered.

Cardiac index between 2.3 and 3.0 ℓ/min per m^2

If the mean left atrial pressure is less than 14 mmHg, blood or albumin should be infused to achieve a ventricular filling pressure which is optimal (12–14 mmHg). Other interventions are generally not necessary unless the mean arterial pressure is over 100 mmHg and the left atrial pressure is over 15 mmHg. Under these circumstances, trimethaphan or nitroprusside may be infused to reduce the arterial pressure.

Cardiac index over 3.0 ℓ/min per m^2

Under these conditions, no therapy is indicated except that blood may be infused if the left atrial pressure is less than 7 mmHg. This again ensures optimal left ventricular filling pressure.

Although not always successful, the above logic has resulted in a more precise analysis of impaired cardiac performance after intracardiac operations than previously utilized methods and has provided a systematic plan of treatment which alters left ventricular filling pressure (preload), resistance to ejection (afterload) and contractility. The logic is based upon data accumulated in adult patients, although similar information on infants and children has recently become available[4, 99].

Pulmonary system

This section will focus on the management of the pulmonary system following extracorporeal circulatory support, with comments on various factors important in the aetiology, identification and treatment of pulmonary complications requiring more than ordinary care in the postoperative period. Whether or not there is a distinct entity of pulmonary dysfunction routinely and uniquely associated with cardiopulmonary bypass has been questioned[3, 77]. Are there morphological and physiological differences in the lungs of patients exposed to cardiopulmonary bypass as compared to the lungs of patients operated on for general or non-cardiac thoracic surgical diseases? Does cardiopulmonary bypass produce changes in the lungs that are qualitatively different from those produced by other surgical procedures? There is ample information to suggest that the answer to these questions is a tentative 'yes'.

In most centres, some form of respiratory support is employed in the early postoperative care of patients after open intracardiac operations. This has usually involved some form of enrichment of inspired oxygen concentration, control of the airway, mechanical assistance or control of ventilation and monitoring of arterial blood gas tensions. Care of the pulmonary system demands criteria for identifying various parameters of pulmonary dysfunction, and the deviations from normal must be defined and quantitated. Prevention of pulmonary dysfunction requires information concerning the aetiological factors producing it. It is clear that the pulmonary function after cardiopulmonary bypass is related to the morphology of the preoperative cardiac lesion and the degree of haemodynamic disability. In addition, the preoperative presence of intrinsic pulmonary disease is correlated with the postoperative respiratory dysfunction. There are also many intraoperative events which have been implicated in the genesis of postoperative respiratory complications.

Pathophysiology of pulmonary dysfunction

That pulmonary complications after cardiopulmonary bypass exist in greater magnitude than after general surgical procedures was noted by various investigators soon after the development of open cardiac surgery[9, 34, 91]. These investigators characterized the pulmonary lesion physiologically as arterial desaturation, and pathologically as parenchymal congestion, perivascular haemorrhage and alveolar collapse. In lung biopsies of surviving patients taken 1 to 4 hours after cardiopulmonary bypass, several groups have demonstrated a rather consistent pathological change in pulmonary ultrastructure[7, 27, 105]. Interstitial oedema of some degree was always present and the capillaries appeared congested. There were accumulations of leucocytes and their degranulation products, and there was focal endothelial damage. Endothelial cell changes consisted of swelling of the cytoplasm, of the matrix compartment of the mitochondria and of the endoplasmic reticulum. The pericapillary space showed dispersion in almost

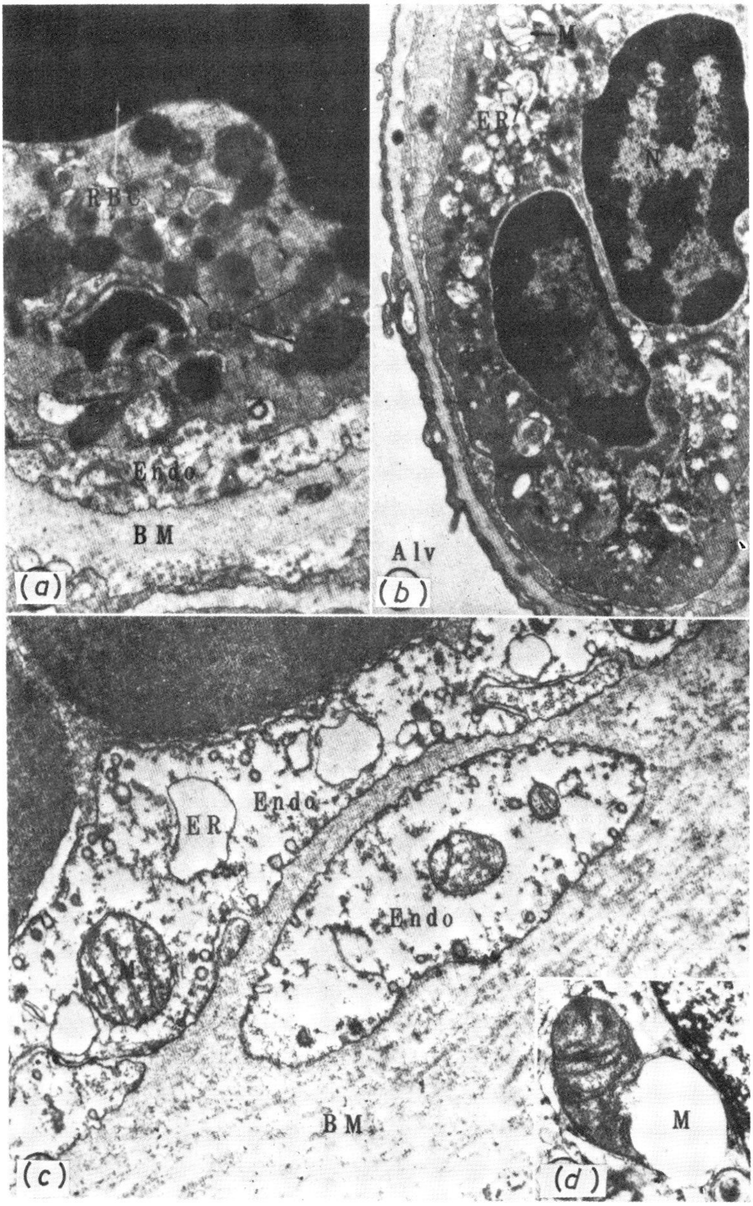

Figure 12.9 Postperfusion human lung biopsy specimens. (*a*) Granules (GR) from polymorphonucleocyte floating freely in the lumen of a septal capillary. (*b*) Abnormal polymorphonucleocyte filling the lumen of a septal capillary. There is swelling of endoplasmic reticulum (ER) and mitochondria (M). (*c*) Marked endothelial alteration with swelling of cytoplasm, endoplasmic reticulum and mitochondria. (*d*) Marked mitochondrial matrical swelling. (From Ratliff *et al.*[105], by courtesy of *Journal of Thoracic and Cardiovascular Surgery*)

all biopsies (*Figure 12.9*). The Type I and Type II pneumocytes at times showed necrosis and sloughing, and there was vacuolization and decrease in the number of laminated inclusion bodies of the granular Type II alveolar cells. These ultrastructural abnormalities have been correlated with the duration of perfusion and the presence of preoperative pulmonary hypertension[7, 105].

Andersen and Ghia[3] have shown quite conclusively that the pulmonary performance after cardiopulmonary bypass differs quantitatively and qualitatively from the pulmonary performance after other operations. They were able to relate the expected respiratory course to the preoperative functional cardiac classification. Patients in the more severe functional

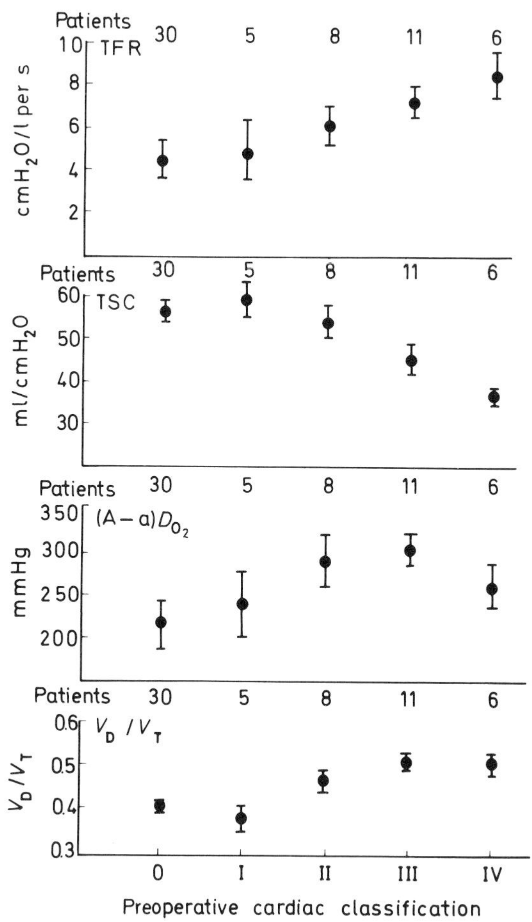

Figure 12.10 The relation between cardiac status (New York Heart Association functional class) and pulmonary function tests in patients scheduled for open intracardiac operations. O = general surgical procedure; TFR = total flow resistance; TSC = total static compliance; (A–a)D_{O_2} = alveolar-arterial oxygen difference; V_D/V_T = wasted ventilation. (From Andersen and Ghia[3], by courtesy of *Journal of Thoracic and Cardiovascular Surgery*)

categories of heart disease had more pronounced preoperative abnormalities in pulmonary function (*Figure 12.10*). Others have also shown a linear relationship between the degree of cardiac abnormality and the pulmonary dysfunction preoperatively[13, 86].

After cardiopulmonary bypass, most patients manifest some degree of pulmonary dysfunction. This is usually characterized by increased work of breathing[23, 47], arterial hypoxaemia (breathing air) with increased alveolar-arterial differences for oxygen[3, 38, 85, 97] and increased fluid in the tracheobronchial tree[66]. McClenahan, Young and Sykes[85] measured significant differences in alveolar-arterial oxygen tensions ($(A\text{–}a)D_{O_2}$) between patients submitted to cardiopulmonary bypass and those who had intrathoracic surgery without cardiopulmonary bypass. Other investigators have found similar differences[38]. Laver, Hallowell and Goldblatt[77], however, have questioned whether there is any significant difference in the degree of pulmonary dysfunction in such patients. They measured pulmonary arteriovenous shunting Q_S/Q_T in patients after cardiac operations with and without extracorporeal circulatory support and the values were similar in the two groups (12 and 14 per cent, respectively). The fact remains that after open intracardiac operations there is a significant shunt due to both venous admixture (physiological shunt) and alveolar collapse (anatomical shunt). Andersen and Ghia[3] measured the mechanical properties of the lungs in patients before and after cardiopulmonary bypass and in patients submitted to non-cardiopulmonary bypass procedures. Total air-flow resistance increased in the bypass patients and showed no change in non-bypass patients. Total static compliance was unchanged in both groups. However, several other groups have found changes in compliance after cardiopulmonary bypass[16, 37]. These changes in the mechanical properties of the lungs have been ascribed in part to an increase in extravascular lung water.

The accumulation of increased extravascular lung water offers an attractive unifying hypothesis to explain the various disturbances of lung function after cardiopulmonary bypass. There is increased mismatching of ventilation and perfusion ($V_A Q$). This may be attributed to either collapsed alveoli, compressed alveoli or fluid-filled alveoli (all conceivably the result of interstitial oedema). In its more pronounced manifestations, the accumulation of lung water leads to excess tracheobronchial secretions, increased airway resistance and decreased lung compliance. McCredie[86] has demonstrated that the extravascular lung water is elevated in patients with cardiac disease, and the elevation is linearly related to the severity of the disease, as assessed by the New York Heart Association functional classification. The presence of elevated extravascular lung water postoperatively as part of a cardiopulmonary bypass lesion has not been conclusively demonstrated. O'Connor *et al.*[94], using the double-indicator dilution technique of Chinard[22], found increases in extravascular water in some patients. In other studies, increases in lung water were not demonstrated[97]. The latter studies did, however, demonstrate an increase in pulmonary vascular resistance and an increase in wasted ventilation (V_D/V_T), suggesting areas of compressed or occluded capillaries. Thus, the Chinard method, which is dependent upon open, perfused capillaries, would be unreliable in a situation where capillary flow might be compromised[127].

Fishman[40] has suggested that the Starling equation for fluid flux across a membrane applies to the lungs. Almost certainly there are influences after cardiopulmonary bypass which would turn the equation towards fluid accumulation outside the pulmonary capillary. These would include elevation of left atrial pressure (the result of increased left ventricular end-diastolic pressure) and the decrease in plasma oncotic pressure which has been demonstrated to occur after cardiopulmonary bypass[39, 136].

The compliance or distensibility of the pulmonary vascular bed is also modified with severe degrees of heart disease. Yu *et al.*[141] found restricted pulmonary vascular distensibility in patients with mitral valve disease, decompensated aortic valve disease or cardiomyopathy. In dogs, Kerr and Kirklin[65] noted that the pulmonary venous compartment is much less distensible than the systemic venous compartment. These observations coincide with those initially made by Berglund[15] and suggest that a small augmentation of central blood volume either before or after cardiopulmonary bypass in patients with severe heart disease may increase the capillary distending pressure markedly. By the Starling law of fluid flux across a membrane, this could lead to interstitial oedema and lung dysfunction.

Downs *et al.*[35] have evaluated the acute respiratory failure in infants following cardiovascular surgery and have isolated a group of patients who are likely to develop respiratory complications. These are children with marked pulmonary arterial hypertension due either to pulmonary venous hypertension or large left-to-right shunts. There are two other considerations which make the infant or child more susceptible to pulmonary dysfunction than the adult. The first is that the infant's lung seems immature as regards a greater tendency to leak fluid across the alveolar capillary membrane. Levine, Rodriguez-Martinez and Mellins[82] found an increase of the filtration coefficient of 1 to 2 orders of magnitude greater in puppies than in more mature experimental animals. Gomes *et al.*[52] have implied that the same phenomenon occurs clinically in infants and suggest that the left atrial pressure should be kept only moderately elevated or low at all times following operations to correct total anomalous pulmonary venous return. The second factor is that the lungs of infants are much smaller than those of adults. The pressures in the pulmonary artery may be viewed as hydrostatic columns of water such that left atrial or pulmonary artery pressures of equal magnitude in adults and children will have a much greater hydrostatic effect in the smaller lungs of children[61].

Barratt-Boyes, Simpson and Neutze[11] state that the use of profound hypothermia and circulatory arrest has diminished the pulmonary complications in their series of infants having intracardiac surgical procedures. The assumption here is that the shorter period of cardiopulmonary bypass gives a smaller dose of whatever causes postoperative pulmonary dysfunction. However, this has not been noted in other series[125].

It is well recognized that the most important intraoperative factor influencing the postoperative pulmonary function is the oxygenator system. Lee *et al.*[79] have shown that plasma proteins become denatured by oxygenators in which there is a blood-gas interface. The membrane oxygenator eliminates the blood-gas interface and reduces protein denaturation and the tendency to form microaggregates. However, most membrane oxygenators are less efficient than other oxygenators now in routine clinical use.

Microaggregates have been demonstrated in the pulmonary capillaries after cardiopulmonary bypass[7, 28, 105]. It may be assumed that these microaggregates occlude capillaries and may also damage the capillary endothelium. This could lead to fluid and protein extravasation and, finally, perivascular haemorrhage. The use of Dacron wool filters with conventional oxygenators has been shown to decrease the number of microaggregates found in the lung after cardiopulmonary bypass[8, 27]. It is still unclear as to whether a decrease in the incidence and severity of pulmonary dysfunction parallels the diminution of microaggregates found in the lung. The age of the blood used for the pump prime is also important. Larger quantities of microaggregates have been found in old blood as compared to fresh blood[28,90].

Finally, there is the possibility that cardiopulmonary bypass may lead to a degree of pulmonary parenchymal cell death. This might result from ischaemia during bypass, chemical or molecular changes in the perfusate, or perhaps hypothermic injury to the pulmonary parenchyma. Elevation of several serum lysosomal fractions has been demonstrated after cardiopulmonary bypass[107]. Parker *et al.*[96] found a significant decrease in serum complement after bypass and suggested a possible relationship between this and the pulmonary cellular dysfunction. Depletion of lung surfactant may be one manifestation of this reaction.

Surfactant depletion has been implicated as a causative factor for the pulmonary dysfunction seen after cardiopulmonary bypass. Occlusion of a pulmonary artery in dogs results in an alteration in alveolar surface forces and elevation of the surface tension of the lung with depletion of surfactant[36, 60]. Interruption of pulmonary blood flow during extracorporeal circulatory support may, as with pulmonary arterial occlusion, result in increased surfactant removal from the lung and/or decreased metabolism of the surfactant in the lung[89]. In the experiments on pulmonary ligation mentioned above, surfactant depletion was noted, but only in localized areas of haemorrhagic atelectasis and only after several days. These experiments suggest that ischaemia may have some influence on the production of haemorrhagic atelectasis. Other investigators, however, have found that when one lung was kept ischaemic by clamping of the pulmonary artery during bypass it did not develop microscopic changes, whereas the lung whose pulmonary artery was left open did develop such changes[80]. These authors observed, however, that when the ischaemic lung was subsequently perfused, it developed similar changes to those in the contralateral lung. Gardner, Finley and Tooley[46] noted somewhat similar findings in the lungs of dogs infused with blood that had been circulated for several hours in an isolated extracorporeal system. These studies suggest that a circulating factor or factors may be responsible for the microscopic and physiological lesions observed in the lungs after cardiopulmonary bypass.

In addition to primary pulmonary injury (this includes direct injury and toxic products brought to the lung by the circulation), other factors may contribute to postoperative pulmonary dysfunction. A low cardiac output influences the pulmonary performance in several ways. It magnifies the

(A–a)D_{O_2} and modifies the distribution of blood flow in the gravitational field of the lung (*see below*). Other extrapulmonary factors affecting pulmonary function are upper airway obstruction and chest wall deformities.

The position of the oxyhaemoglobin dissociation curve during the operation and shortly thereafter may have profound effects on the oxygen uptake and transport. Hypothermia shifts the oxyhaemoglobin dissociation curve to the left. The dissociation curve is also influenced by the state of red blood cell 2, 3-diphosphoglycerate (DPG), the presence of acidosis and the arterial carbon dioxide tension. Although congestive heart failure results in an increase of 2,3-DPG, it has been shown that after cardiopulmonary bypass there is a decrease in 2, 3-DPG[17, 114]. The latter situation will decrease the oxygen transfer at cellular level. Bordiuk *et al.*[17] found an increased red cell affinity for oxygen after bypass, but this was less than would be expected relative to the demonstrated 2, 3-DPG decrease. The significant effects of the alteration of 2, 3-DPG during and after cardiopulmonary bypass are as yet unclear. However, the integrity of red blood cell function during and after bypass may be important, as very high tensions of oxygen in plasma may be deleterious to the lung.

Although there have been many studies concerning ventilation during extracorporeal circulatory support, the results have not been consistent. There are data to suggest, however, that the method of ventilation during operation affects the pulmonary mechanics[14]. Some authors have advocated static lung inflation during cardiopulmonary bypass in order to minimize pulmonary injury[137].

In summary, the important intraoperative factors contributing to postoperative pulmonary dysfunction are the type of oxygenator used and the effect of the blood-gas interface on proteins and formed elements of the blood. There is probably formation of microaggregates which results in some degree of pulmonary capillary occlusion and endothelial disruption. The lack of pulmonary blood flow may cause changes in the metabolic properties of the lung, leading to decreased surfactant production and changes in the metabolic activity of the Type I and II pneumocytes.

Postoperative management

The management of the pulmonary system postoperatively depends on the following considerations: (1) adequate alveolar ventilation and the use of mechanical ventilators and other forms of assisted ventilation; (2) satisfactory matching of ventilation and perfusion based on knowledge of cardiac output, diffusion problems, pulmonary vascular resistance and the pressure of atelectasis; (3) satisfactory oxygen delivery based on adequate red cell function, haemoglobin concentration and cardiac output and knowledge of the metabolic requirements; and (4) analysis of the final satisfactory function of the lungs by means of arterial blood gas measurements.

After open intracardiac operations, most patients are kept intubated and are mechanically ventilated for a period of time. Access to the tracheobronchial tree is via an orotracheal tube in adults and a nasotracheal tube in infants. Generally, the patient is mechanically ventilated until the following criteria are fulfilled: (1) there is satisfactory alveolar ventilation as indicated by acceptable arterial carbon dioxide tension ($P_{CO_2}<55$ mmHg) and absence of hypoxaemia ($P_{O_2}>110$ mmHg) on 40 per cent inspired oxygen concentration; (2) cardiac performance is judged satisfactory and adequate to sustain the increased work of breathing which would be expected after extubation; (3) cardiac arrhythmias are absent or under control; and (4) reoperation for bleeding will not be required.

In our unit the type of respiratory support used for adults differs from that used in babies and young children. In adults the ventilation is controlled early postoperatively using a volume ventilator (Emerson). The mechanically controlled ventilation is maintained for a period of about 4 to 12 hours in patients who have no severe cardiac or pulmonary dysfunction. Gradually controlled volume cycled ventilation is changed to intermittent mandatory ventilation (IMV). Arterial blood-gas analyses are performed intermittently during this period. This analysis includes measurement of arterial oxygen and carbon dioxide tensions, oxygen saturation and pH, and calculation of base deficit and standard bicarbonate. The frequency of IMV is decreased over a 6 to 12 hour period. After the rate is decreased to 6 per minute, the patient is extubated. Generally, three arterial blood-gas analyses are obtained, one shortly after the patient is brought from the operating room, the second approximately 6 hours later, and the third shortly before anticipated extubation. A subsequent blood-gas analysis is performed 30 minutes after extubation.

There are certain specific considerations which apply to patients maintained on controlled ventilation. A frequency of between 9 and 14 breaths per minute is generally satisfactory. For the average adult patient, tidal volumes range between 650 and 900 ml. It appears that there are chest wall reflexes which produce a feeling of dyspnoea in patients who have adequate arterial oxygen saturation but low tidal volumes. Increasing the tidal volume often obviates the feeling of breathlessness and produces a sense of relative wellbeing. This coincides with an arterial P_{CO_2} of between 28 and 34 mmHg, and produces a moderate alkalaemia. Certain objections to this range of carbon dioxide tensions are noted below (*see below*). Muscle relaxants and paralysing agents are not generally used, and morphine is only infrequently used to allow control of ventilation. The fraction of inspired oxygen (F_{IO_2}) is generally adjusted to 40 per cent. If there is a large (A–a)D_{O_2} with resulting arterial oxygen tensions of less than 110 mmHg, the F_{IO_2} is increased. In addition, in most cases of persistent postoperative hypoxaemia, the intermittent positive pressure is changed to continuous positive pressure using from 5 to 10 mmHg end-expiratory pressure.

We prefer a volume-controlled ventilator for most patients because the F_{IO_2} may be adjusted to any level. In many cases, however, a pressure-cycled ventilator should be equally satisfactory. With the Bird ventilator, however, the F_{IO_2} cannot be easily regulated, and with higher flows and pressures, the F_{IO_2} may increase to 80 per cent. It has an advantage in that it can be used in an assist mode, and the P_{CO_2} will tend to be more normal rather than in the hypocapneic range. In patients with pulmonary dysfunction, volume control is the more satisfactory mode. In such patients the lung mechanics are disturbed, the compliance is diminished and the airway resistance is elevated; the functional residual capacity is usually decreased, and the alveolar distending pressures, both during inspiration and expiration, are inadequate; the alveolar volume is decreased, and collapsed, compressed or fluid-filled alveoli must be opened. The pressure-cycled ventilators are unsuited to this application, but volume-cycled ventilators are highly satisfactory and may generate pressures at the endotracheal tube of 60 to 100 centimetres of water.

The levels of arterial blood-gas tensions in 16 adult patients following aortic valve replacement are illustrated in *Table 12.6*. These patients were in no respiratory distress prior to operation and had little or no pulmonary

Table 12.6 Gas exchange studies. [Modified from Parker *et al.*[97], by courtesy of the American Heart Association]

	Preoperative	*Postoperative*			
		4 hours	*20 hours*	*44 hours*	*8 days*
$(A\text{–}a)D_{O_2}$ (air) (mmHg)	14.5 ±11.1	18.9 ±9.7	32.5 ±10.2 (<0.002)	29.0 ±9.5 (<0.001)	25.1 ±9.3 (<0.005)
$(A\text{–}a)D_{O_2}$ (100% O_2)	58.6 ±41.0	82.6 ±41.0 (<0.05)	135.6 ±71.6 (<0.001)	194.2 ±58.9 (<0.001)	114.8 ±44.4 (<0.005)
Q_S/Q_T(%)	2.9 ±2.1	3.4 ±1.4	5.4 ±2.6 (<0.005)	9.8 ±2.4 (<0.001)	4.7 ±1.7
V_D/V_T	0.20 ±0.12	0.29 ±0.10 (<0.05)	0.39 ±0.07 (<0.05)	0.44 ±0.10 (<0.001)	—

$(A\text{-}a)D_O$ = alveolar arterial oxygen difference; Q_S/Q_T = per cent intrapulmonary shunt; V_D/V_T = fraction wasted ventilation.
± Value is ± standard deviation. Numbers in parenthesis represent significance of change (*P value*) from preoperative study.

dysfunction two days after operation. Postoperatively, there was a significant $(A\text{–}a)D_{O_2}$, suggesting the presence of perfused but non-ventilated alveoli. Wasted ventilation was increased, suggesting ventilated but non-perfused alveoli. Thus, it is reasonable to state that one of the earliest and mildest forms of pulmonary dysfunction after cardiopulmonary bypass is a mismatching of ventilation and perfusion.

In our experience, neither pressure- nor volume-regulated respirators nor early extubation without respiratory support have been routinely satisfactory in the management of infants after open intracardiac operations[125]. It is often difficult to maintain an infant properly on a mechanical respirator. Early extubation does not allow control of the airway in the infant who may need assistance in clearing tracheobronchial secretions or who may require intermittent ventilatory support. Continuous positive airway pressure (CPAP), as described by Gregory *et al.*[54], has been used in our unit for infants and children undergoing cardiac surgical procedures since 1971. The apparatus employed is shown in *Figure 12.11*. The system contains no valves, and continuous positive airway pressure is maintained by a high gas inflow and a screw clamp on the exit port of the reservoir bag. The infant is allowed to breathe spontaneously with intermittent manual ventilation. Rebreathing is prevented by using a flow rate of gas into the system which exceeds twice the respiratory minute volume of the infant. The patient may

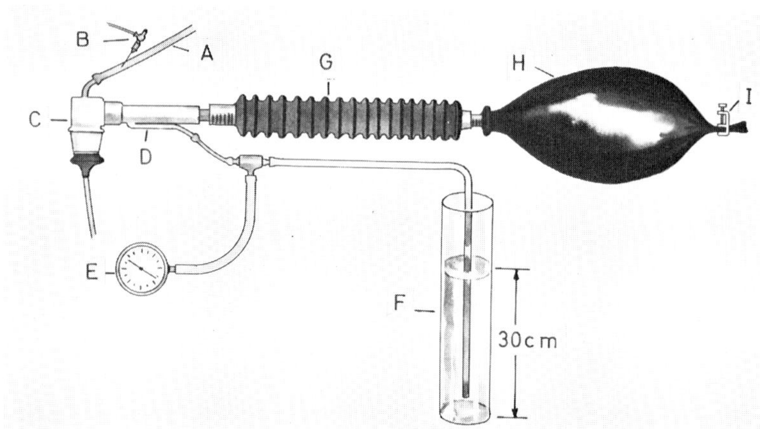

Figure 12.11 Continuous positive airway pressure system. A = Source of gas inflow; B = sampling site for inspired oxygen concentration; C = Norman elbow; D = Sommer's T piece; E = Aneroid manometer; F = Safety valve; G = tubing; H = reservoir bag; I = Hoffman screw clamp. (Redrawn from Gregory *et al.*[54], by courtesy of *New England Journal of Medicine*)

remain on this system for 12 to 72 hours. The inspired oxygen concentration is gradually decreased to 40 per cent. Following this, the positive airway pressure is gradually decreased in increments of 1 millimetre of mercury from 6 to 1, as long as the arterial P_{O_2} is maintained above 70 mmHg. The patient is then extubated and placed in an atmosphere of high oxygen and high humidity. If the arterial blood gases remain satisfactory there is no need for reintubation or ventilatory assistance.

The continuous positive pressure airway system probably increases the work of breathing. However, this apparent disadvantage is outweighed by an increase in functional residual capacity, a probable lengthening and widening of the small narrow airways and attainment of a greater opening pressure in a larger number of alveolar units. These effects presumably oppose airway collapse and atelectasis, maintain adequate surfactant activity and decrease airway resistance. It is likely that the lungs of the infants are highly sensitive to small changes in the parameters of the Starling equation for fluid flux across a membrane, and following cardiopulmonary bypass, the baby may be thought of as having interstitial pulmonary oedema. An explanation for the beneficial effect of continuous positive airway pressure in this situation might be obtained from the analysis of the work of Sharp *et al.*[115] (*Figure 12.12*). In the presence of pulmonary oedema, positive pressure breathing increases pulmonary compliance, whereas in normal lungs it does not.

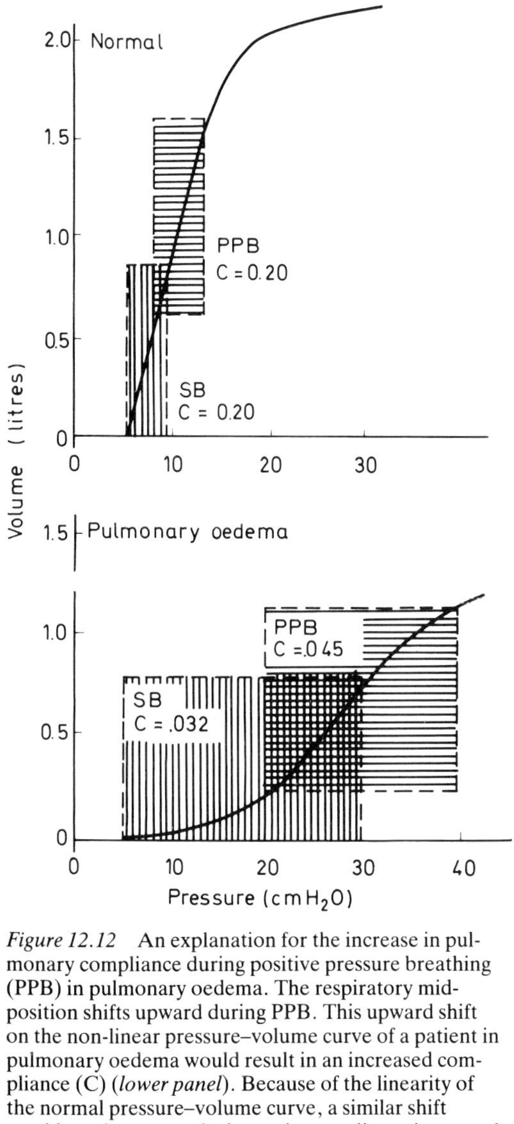

Figure 12.12 An explanation for the increase in pulmonary compliance during positive pressure breathing (PPB) in pulmonary oedema. The respiratory mid-position shifts upward during PPB. This upward shift on the non-linear pressure–volume curve of a patient in pulmonary oedema would result in an increased compliance (C) (*lower panel*). Because of the linearity of the normal pressure–volume curve, a similar shift would produce no such change in compliance in normal subjects (*upper panel*). (From Sharp *et al.*[115], by courtesy of *Journal of Clinical Investigation*)

In patients with established pulmonary dysfunction we have found continuous positive pressure ventilation helpful in maintaining adequate arterial oxygen saturation. This technique has been useful in the management of pulmonary dysfunction accompanying other respiratory distress syndromes[101, 102, 131]. Cheney and Martin[21] suggest that the optimal arterial oxygen tensions during pulmonary oedema are related to the mean airway pressure rather than to the tidal volume. Uzawa and Ashbaugh[131], Pontoppidan, Geffin and Lowenstein[101] and Cheney and Martin[21] have shown a significant difference in arterial oxygen tension using continuous positive pressure ventilation as compared to intermittent positive pressure ventilation. Positive end-expiratory pressure may act in a number of ways to improve the pulmonary performance. In the majority of patients with respiratory distress syndromes, the most significant finding is a decrease in functional residual capacity (FRC). Continuous positive pressure breathing increases FRC and thus increases the number of alveolar units remaining open and ventilated. The immediate effect of this may be an increase in $P\text{O}_2$ (alveolar and arterial) which secondarily leads to a decrease in pulmonary artery pressure. A third effect might be a reversal of the shift of fluid into the alveolar spaces, and stabilization of the surfactant system. As noted above for continuous positive airway pressure, continuous positive pressure breathing by a ventilator may also increase lung compliance in conditions of interstitial pulmonary oedema.

In our unit, continuous positive pressure ventilation is instituted when a large $(\text{A–a})D\text{O}_2$ exists and when there is arterial desaturation while using a volume ventilator. A positive end-expiratory pressure between 8 and 13 mmHg is used. Some investigators have noted a decreased cardiac output during positive pressure breathing. This has not been the case in our experience, most likely because the filling pressures of the left and right sides of the heart were monitored by atrial catheters and could be manipulated by fluid or blood influsion. Shugerman, Rogers and Miller[117] have suggested that those very patients who have decreased lung compliance benefit most from continuous positive pressure ventilation in that the depressant effect on cardiac output of continuous positive pressure is not as great as in normals. They suggest that the high airway pressures are not transmitted to the pleural space, being dissipated by the elevated forces tending to close the alveoli, and thus have little effect on atrial filling.

For the purposes of this discussion, it may be stated that the ultimate assessment of pulmonary performance postoperatively rests in the analysis of the arterial blood-gas profile. Most intensive care units are not equipped to measure the work of breathing and this is admittedly a drawback. However, in actual practice, arterial blood-gas determinations combined with the clinical assessment of work of breathing allow the development of a useful patient management programme. The arterial blood is usually sampled from an indwelling radial artery catheter. The results of the analysis can be available within 5 minutes, and adjustments in the management programme may be made.

There are complex interactions between ventilation, perfusion, the effects of gravity, pulmonary vascular resistance, carbon dioxide tension and cardiac output on the one hand and arterial oxygen tension on the other. Philbin *et al.*[100] noted a clear relationship between cardiac index and arterial oxygen saturation in patients with pulmonary arteriovenous shunting. A decrease in cardiac index produced a decrease in arterial oxygenation when the shunt fraction remained constant (*Figures 12.13a, 12.13b*). A similar relationship had been noted in anaesthetized patients[64]. However, Sanders *et al.*[110] noted an increase in arteriovenous shunting in preoperative cardiac patients treated with isoproterenol or epinephrine to increase the cardiac output. These authors believed that the rise in cardiac output increased the ventilation–perfusion abnormalities in their patients resulting from greater

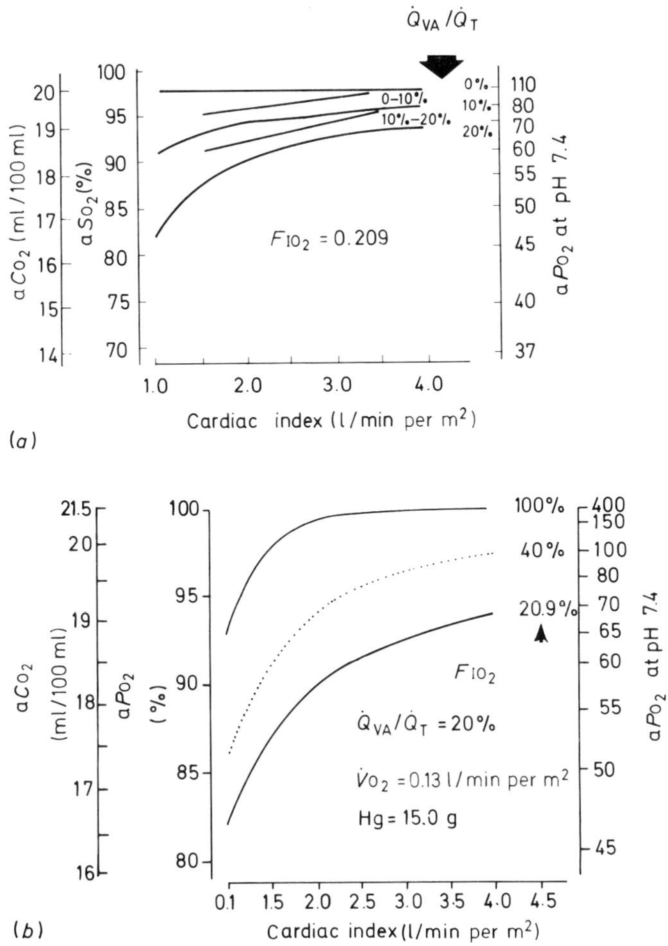

Figure 12.13 (*a*) Relationship of measured values of cardiac index to arterial oxygen content (aC_{O_2}), arterial saturation (aS_{O_2}) and arterial tension (aP_{O_2}) compared with calculated curves. The straight lines represent linear regressions for measured values of venous admixture. (*b*) Relationship (calculated) of cardiac index to aC_{O_2}, aS_{O_2} and aP_{O_2} for 20 per cent venous admixture ($Q_{VA}Q_T$) when inspired O_2 concentration is 20.9, 40 and 100 per cent. (From Philbin *et al.*[100], by courtesy of *Anesthesiology*)

perfusion of non-ventilated alveoli. The conclusions of Philbin *et al.*[100] seem more applicable to the postoperative cardiac patient, and the increase in arterial oxygenation subsequent to a rise in cardiac output may be attributed to an increase in mixed venous oxygen tension.

We have noted that an occasional patient ventilated with either 50 per cent or 100 per cent oxygen will have a higher shunt fraction when 100 per cent oxygen is used. This may be explained by the tendency for oxygen to close poorly ventilated alveoli and produce an anatomical area of venous admixture. The vasodilating effect of 100 per cent oxygen may improve the flow to marginally ventilated or poorly ventilated alveoli and in this way also increase the calculated shunt fraction.

Some investigators have noted an effect of carbon dioxide tension on arterial oxygen tension[88, 129]. Trimble *et al.*[129] stated that hypocarbia may aggravate the post-traumatic pulmonary insufficiency by inducing bronchial constriction, which may cause increased maldistribution of ventilation, heightened airway resistance and an increased work of breathing. In anaesthetized man, Prys Roberts *et al.*[103] noted a reciprocal relationship between alveolar-arterial oxygen difference and cardiac output which was related to changes in P_{CO_2} (*Figure 12.14*). Breivik *et al.*[18] showed that in

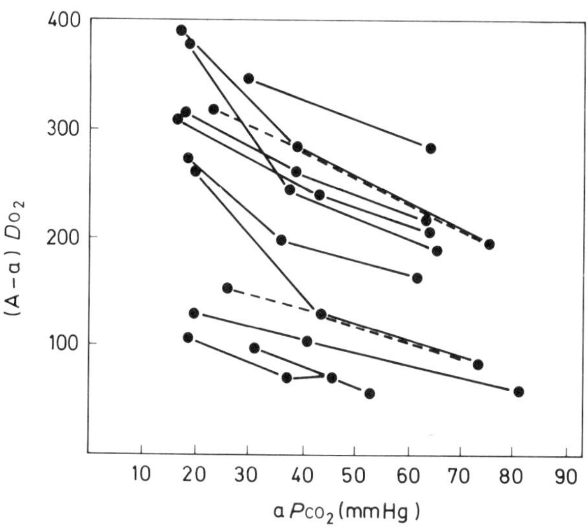

Figure 12.14 Relation between alveolar-arterial difference for oxygen and arterial carbon dioxide tension (aP_{CO_2}) during artificial ventilation. (From Prys Roberts *et al.*[103], by courtesy of *Journal of Applied Physiology*)

patients with progressive pulmonary consolidation during controlled mechanical ventilation, the normalization of a low arterial P_{CO_2} increased the arterial P_{O_2}, the cardiac output and the oxygen transport. They further stated that the beneficial circulatory effects of increasing low P_{CO_2} levels offset, in part, the circulatory depressant effects of positive end-expiratory pressure. The increase in arterial P_{O_2} resulting from the normalization of the P_{CO_2} allowed a lowering of inspired oxygen concentrations from toxic to non-toxic levels.

The effect of hypocapnia on lung mechanics was analysed by Monkcom and Patterson[88] (*Figure 12.15*). They demonstrated that airway hypocapnia increased airway resistance, decreased pulmonary compliance and increased (A–a)D_{O_2}. These changes were reversed when only the inspired carbon dioxide tension was increased. Presumably the (A–a)D_{O_2} changes in these experimental animals were the result of changed lung mechanics altering the distribution of ventilation.

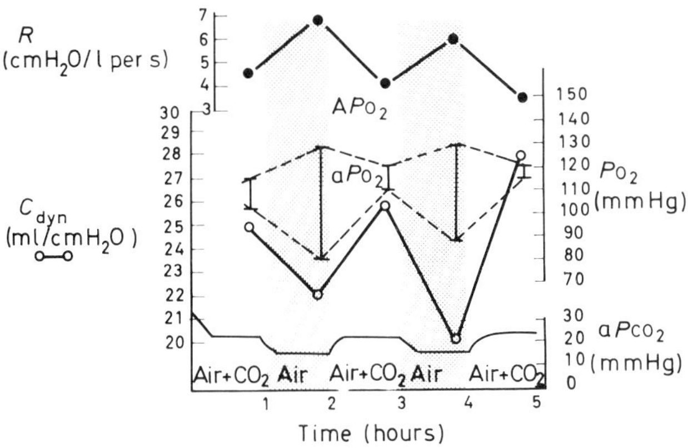

Figure 12.15 Changes in respiratory mechanics and alveolar-arterial oxygen differences as the ventilating mixture is alternated at hourly intervals between room air and room air with 3 per cent carbon dioxide added. R = airway resistance. C_{dyn} = dynamic compliance. (From Monkcom and Patterson[88], by courtesy of *Journal of Thoracic and Cardiovascular Surgery*)

Oxygen toxicity

In a review of acute respiratory failure in the adult, Pontoppidan, Geffin and Lowenstein[101, 102] have stated that the 'role of pulmonary oxygen toxicity in patients with severe respiratory failure requiring high concentrations of inspired oxygen is still uncertain.' Nevertheless, they have marshalled sufficient evidence to imply that a high inspired oxygen tension may be one of a number of deleterious factors producing atelectasis, consolidation, perivascular haemorrhage, exudation and finally fibrotic proliferation in the lungs of patients with acute respiratory insufficiency. In normal man, the breathing of oxygen causes a rapidly progressive fall in vital capacity after 60 hours of exposure. Oxygen leads to resorption atelectasis which probably precedes the toxic effect of oxygen on cell function by hours or days. Depletion of surfactant activity in dogs breathing oxygen for 24 hours has also been observed[78]. Absorption atelectasis and surfactant depletion may be prevented by mechanical ventilation. Indeed, Singer, Wright and Stanley[119] found no difference in the pulmonary function of patients mechanically ventilated for 24 hours exposed to either 100 per cent or 50 per cent oxygen. However, Barber, Lee and Hamilton[10] found a marked increase in $(A–a)DO_2$ in patients ventilated with oxygen as compared to those ventilated with air. Morphological changes attributable to oxygen toxicity have been noted by Kapanci *et al.*[63] in 6 patients given 60 per cent to 100 per cent oxygen for from 14 hours to 13 days. The changes included a decrease in endothelial volume suggesting direct endothelial cell injury by oxygen. Thus, although the dose–time course of oxygen toxicity in man has not been completely defined, oxygen toxicity must be considered as one factor leading to respiratory failure in postoperative patients. The ability to control and monitor FIO_2 in ventilated patients thus assumes great importance. In our unit this is done with an inexpensive paramagnetic analyser (Beckman).

Special measures

Laryngeal and tracheal injury secondary to airway intubation have received increased attention in recent years[49]. Injury to vocal cords, the subglottic larynx and the trachea is primarily attributable to pressure phenomena (i.e. inflation of the balloon cuff, angulation of the tracheostomy or endotracheal tube, impingement of the tip of the tube on the posterior or anterior wall of the trachea and movement of the tip of the tube). Laryngotracheal injury occurs in three clinical circumstances: (1) in patients who require prolonged respiratory support; (2) in patients with low cardiac output or shock; and (3) in infants and children. Presently, we prefer the Portex rather than the rubber endotracheal tubes. Adults are intubated by the oral–tracheal route and children by the nasotracheal route. In children, an effort is made to keep the tube loose fitting in the trachea. Tubes are securely fixed at the lips or the nares and motion against the firm arm of the ventilator is avoided, thus preventing a rocking action at the tip of the endotracheal tube. Inspired gas is at all times humidified and suctioning on the endotracheal tube is performed as necessary by the nursing staff. Tracheostomies are assiduously avoided in infants and children and infrequently performed on adults. With these techniques, the incidence of laryngeal and tracheal stenosis has been extremely low in our experience.

Maintenance of a patent airway is assisted by frequent suctioning of the endotracheal tube, humidification of the inspired gas, saline lavage and occasional use of acetylcysteine (Mucomyst). As noted above, the use of continuous positive pressure ventilation in adults and continuous positive airway pressure in infants probably contribute to the patency of large- and medium-size airways.

In patients with moderate pulmonary dysfunction and excessive tracheobronchial secretions who have no other indications for intubation, chest physiotherapy is quite important. Peroral or nasotracheal aspiration is utilized infrequently since there is a certain risk of producing arterial oxygen desaturation and vasovagal reflexes with this manoeuvre. Bronchoscopy is also used infrequently.

The ventilation perfusion relationships are markedly affected by gravity as observed by West[138]. Clauss *et al.*[24] have extended West's observations to measurements of oxygen tension in 13 patients after cardiac valve replacement. Changing position from supine to lateral increased the oxygen tension in every case. They suggest that this effect is due to an increase in the efficiency of ventilation with the attainment of better VA/Q ratios. Patients should thus be turned frequently while being ventilated.

In patients requiring ventilatory support for longer than 2 days, an increasing $(A\text{–}a)D\text{O}_2$ may be observed. This has been called respiratory lung and, alternatively, oxygen toxicity. Sladen, Laver and Pontoppidan[120] have observed this in association with fluid retention. They noted a marked decrease in the $(A\text{–}a)D\text{O}_2$ and clearing of the chest roentgenogram following the use of potent diuretic agents. Thus, even in the absence of frank congestive heart failure, a major element of pulmonary dysfunction may be reversed after cardiopulmonary bypass by the use of diuretics such as frusemide, often by a single dose.

Prolonged ventilatory support is generally required when there is low cardiac output postoperatively. The measures noted above–airway care, avoidance of high $F\text{IO}_2$ and use of diuretics–are especially important in these seriously ill patients in addition to measures used to improve the cardiac function. Respiratory support can be discontinued only when cardiac output has progressed to levels adequate to sustain the work of breathing in addition to the metabolic demands of other systems. Thus, weaning from mechanical ventilators under these circumstances should be based both on blood-gas analysis and direct or indirect analysis of cardiac performance.

Renal system

With the currently utilized techniques of extracorporeal circulatory support in which moderate or severe haemodilution is employed, acute tubular necrosis and renal failure are infrequent complications following cardiac operations. The majority of patients in whom these complications occur have significant impairment of cardiac and renal function preoperatively and often have evidence of low cardiac output postoperatively.

In patients undergoing open cardiac operations with extracorporeal circulatory support, urine flow decreases progressively during induction of anaesthesia and thoracotomy. Anuria is generally present during the early period of cardiopulmonary bypass even when haemodilution of the perfusate is employed. During the first few hours after operation the urine output is significantly higher in patients in whom haemodilution was used[87]. This is probably related to the osmotic diuretic effects of the glucose or mannitol used in the perfusate. The urine output then declines to more normal levels (30–50 ml per hour). High urine flow rates produced by osmotic diuresis have been shown experimentally to prevent pathological renal tubular changes that occur following extracorporeal circulatory support associated with low urine flow[112].

If low urine output occurs following operation, low cardiac output may be present, and appropriate measures should be taken to detect and treat it as outlined in the previous section. If urine output continues to be low (less than 15 ml per hour) for 2 consecutive hours, additional therapy is indicated. If the mean left atrial pressure is less than 15 mmHg, 25 grams of mannitol may be infused over a 1 hour period. This dosage can be repeated after 3 to 4 hours if the urine output remains low. If the mean left atrial pressure is greater than 15 mmHg, 20 to 40 mg of frusemide (Lasix) should be given intravenously. This agent produces a marked diuresis but may increase urinary potassium losses. Serum potassium concentrations should thus be monitored closely when this drug is used. In addition to its diuretic effect, frusemide can reduce the left ventricular filling pressure in patients with chronic heart failure by vasodilation of the pulmonary vasculature, by increase in peripheral venous pooling, or by both these mechanisms. These effects occur before the onset of significant diuresis[33]. With use of haemodilution and diuretic therapy as outlined, postoperative renal failure in the absence of severe cardiac failure and low cardiac output has been encountered rarely in our experience.

Central nervous system

Central nervous system dysfunction following extracorporeal circulatory support is usually manifested as diffuse or localized neurological deficits or as behavioural abnormalities. Air embolization is an important cause of neurological dysfunction following operation and is usually preventable. The predisposing factors and the prevention of intraoperative air embolism have been discussed in other chapters. However, it should be re-emphasized that prevention or minimization of air embolization is based on rigorous adherence to a routine protocol for venting the heart during operation and for evacuation of air from the cardiac chambers when cardiopulmonary bypass is discontinued. Embolization of particulate matter such as calcium, fat, microaggregates and fibrin may also cause neurological injury. The use of filters and of oxygenators which contain filters in the extracorporeal circuit has to a great extent lessened the incidence of embolization of particulate matter. In our own experience, the incidence of fibrin embolization has been appreciably reduced by a change from the disc oxygenator to a bubble oxygenator containing a filter (Bentley-Temptrol).

Neurological deficits may also result from inadequate cerebral perfusion in the absence of particulate embolization. Javid *et al.*[62] studied 100 consecutive patients who had open intracardiac operations and analysed the incidence of neurological deficits and behavioural changes. These patients were all adults in whom a disc oxygenator was employed. There were three specific groups of patients with a high incidence of neurological dysfunction. These were patients who had periods of hypotension during perfusion (mean arterial blood pressure below 50 mmHg), patients in whom long periods of cardiopulmonary bypass were employed and patients who were over 50 years of age (*Table 12.7*). The incidence of neurological deficits or behavioural changes was quite high in the total group of patients. This may be attributable to the use of the disc oxygenator and to the fact that these patients were evaluated very carefully in the postoperative period.

Table 12.7 Factors affecting neurological function following cardiac operations using extracorporeal circulatory support. (Modified from Javid *et al.*[62] by courtesy of the C. V. Mosby Co and from Tufo, Ostfeld and Shekelle[130] by courtesy of the American Medical Association)

	Incidence of neurological deficit or behavioural abnormality postoperatively (%)
Age of patient	
< 50 years	39
> 50 years	69
Duration of cardiopulmonary bypass	
< 120 minutes	37
> 120 minutes	63
Mean perfusion pressure	
> 50 mmHg	34
< 50 mmHg	60

The central nervous system can be evaluated in a superficial way early after operation. The patient is asked to respond to verbal commands. Motor function can be assessed by asking the patient to move each extremity and visual acuity can be assessed by any convenient, simple method. Agitation in the early postoperative period can result from hypoxaemia, low cardiac output or central nervous system injury. Not infrequently, marked improvement in restlessness and agitation is observed following the treatment of hypoxaemia and low cardiac output. If agitation is present in the absence of these factors, or if it persists despite appropriate therapy, neurological injury may be present.

Whatever the cause of the neurological dysfunction and whether it results in specific neurological deficits or behavioural changes, the signs and symptoms improve or disappear in many patients in the postoperative period. Thus, even though there may be a severe neurological deficit initially, careful attention to the haemodynamic state of the patient and the usual supportive measures may lead to satisfactory and often complete neurological recovery late after operation.

Behavioural changes may manifest themselves early after operation or in the later postoperative period. These include changes in effect, periods of confusion or disorientation, or frank delirium. Many patients complain of insomnia. A number of patients develop signs of depression and children may frequently have nightmares. Most of these changes are benign and self-limited. The treatment consists of reassurance of the patient and his family, active involvement of the family in the needs of the patient and optimal nursing care. Neurological deficits should be treated aggressively by the physician and physiotherapist. The knowledge that many of these neurological deficits improve should cause all concerned to maintain an optimistic outlook and to manage these deficits positively.

References

1. *A Review of the Patient-monitoring System at the University of Alabama Medical Center, Appendix C, March, 1973.* Cambridge Mass. Arthur D. Little, Inc (1973)
2. Allen, W. B., Karp, R. B. and Kouchoukos, N. T. 'Mitral valve replacement: Starr–Edwards cloth-covered composite-seat prosthesis.' *Archives of Surgery*, **109,** 642 (1974)
3. Andersen, N. B. and Ghia, J. 'Pulmonary function, cardiac status and post-operative course in relation to cardiopulmonary bypass.' *Journal of Thoracic and Cardiovascular Surgery*, **59,** 474 (1970)
4. Appelbaum, A., Blackstone, E., Kouchoukos, N. T. and Kirklin, J. W. 'Afterload reduction and cardiac output in infants early after intracardiac surgery.' *American Journal of Cardiology*, **39,** 445 (1977)
5. Appelbaum, A., Kouchoukos, N. T., Blackstone, E. H. and Kirklin, J. W. 'The early risks of open mitral valve surgery.' *American Journal of Cardiology*, **37,** 201 (1976)
6. Archie, J. P., Jr. and Kirklin, J. W. 'Myocardial blood flow and cardiac surgery.' In *Advances in Cardiovascular Surgery*. Ed. J. W. Kirklin, Ch. 15. New York: Grune and Stratton (1973)
7. Asada, S. and Yamaguchi, M. 'Fine structural changes in the lung following cardiopulmonary bypass.' *Chest*, **59,** 478 (1971)

8. Ashmore, P. G., Swank, R. L., Gallery, R., Ambrose, P. and Pritchard, K. H. 'Effect of Dacron-wool filtration on the microembolic phenomenon in extracorporeal circulation.' *Journal of Thoracic and Cardiovascular Surgery*, **63,** 240 (1972)
9. Baer, D. M. and Osborn, J. J. 'The post-perfusion pulmonary congestion syndrome.' *American Journal of Clinical Pathology*, **34,** 442 (1960)
10. Barber, R. E., Lee, J. and Hamilton, W. K. 'Oxygen toxicity in man: a prospective study in patients with irreversible brain damage.' *New England Journal of Medicine*, **283,** 1478 (1970)
11. Barratt-Boyes, B. G., Simpson, M. and Neutze, J. M. 'Intracardiac surgery in neonates and infants using deep hypothermia with surface cooling and limited cardiopulmonary bypass.' *Circulation*, **43** and **44 (Suppl. II)**, 25 (1971)
12. Barratt-Boyes, B. G. and Wood, E. H. 'Cardiac output and related measurements and pressure values in the right heart and associated vessels, together with an analysis of the haemodynamic response to the inhalation of high oxygen mixtures in healthy subjects.' *Journal of Laboratory and Clinical Medicine*, **51,** 72 (1958)
13. Bates, D. V. and Christie, R. V. *Respiratory Function in Disease*. Philadelphia: W. B. Saunders (1964)
14. Bendixen, H. H., Hedley-Whyte, J. and Laver, M. B. 'Impaired oxygenation in surgical patients during general anaesthesia with controlled ventilation. A concept of atelectasis.' *New England Journal of Medicine*, **269,** 991 (1963)
15. Berglund, E. 'Ventricular function. VI. Balance of left and right ventricular output. Relation between left and right atrial pressures.' *American Journal of Physiology*, **178,** 381 (1954)
16. Blair, E., Hedstrand, V., Westerholme, C. J. and Björk, V. O. 'Effect of total cardiopulmonary bypass on human lung elastic properties.' *Circulation*, **35** and **36 (Suppl. I)**, 206 (1967)
17. Bordiuk, J. M., McKenna, P. J., Giannelli, S., Jr. and Ayres, S. M. 'Alterations in 2,3-DPG and O_2 hemoglobin affinity in patients undergoing open heart surgery.' *Circulation*, **43** and **44 (Suppl. I)**, 141 (1971)
18. Breivik, H., Grenvik, A., Millen, E. and Safar, P. 'Normalizing low arterial CO_2 tension during mechanical ventilation.' *Chest*, **63,** 525 (1973)
19. Buckberg, G. D., Towers, B., Paglia, D. E., Mulder, D. G. and Maloney, J. 'Subendocardial ischaemia after cardiopulmonary bypass.' *Journal of Thoracic and Cardiovascular Surgery*, **64**, 669 (1972)
20. Buckley, M. J., Graver, J. M., Gold, H. KJ., Mundth, E. D., Daggett, W. M. and Austen, W. G. 'Intra-aortic balloon pump assist for cardiogenic shock after cardiopulmonary bypass.' *Circulation*, **47** and **48 (Suppl. II)**, 90 (1973)
21. Cheney, G. W., Jr. and Martin, W. E. 'Effects of continuous positive pressure ventilation on gas exchange in acute pulmonary oedema.' *Journal of Applied Physiology*, **30,** 378 (1971)
22. Chinard, F. P. 'Capillary permeability.' *Bulletin of Johns Hopkins Hospital*, **88,** 489 (1951)
23. Christlieb, I., Dammann, J. R., Jr., Thungs, N. S. and Muller, W. H. 'Post-operative care in cardiac surgery. A frequent determinant of success or failure.' *Diseases of the Chest*, **44,** 47 (1963)
24. Clauss, R. H., Scalabrini, B. Y., Ray, J. F. and Reed, G. E. 'Effects of changing body position upon improved ventilation–perfusion relationships.' *Circulation*, **37** and **38 (Suppl. II)**, 214 (1968)
25. Coffin, L. H., Ankeney, J. L. and Bekeler, E. M. 'Experimental and clinical use of epinephrine for treatment of low cardiac output syndrome.' *Circulation*, **33 (Suppl. I)**, 78 (1966)

26. Coleman, E. H. and Soroff, L. A. 'Incidence of significant coronary artery disease in rheumatic valvular heart disease.' *American Journal of Cardiology*, **25,** 401 (1970)
27. Connell, R. S., Page, U. S., Barley, T. D., Bigelow, J. C. and Webb, M. C. 'The effect on pulmonary ultrastructure of Dacron-wool filtration during cardiopulmonary bypass.' *Annals of Thoracic Surgery*, **15,** 217 (1973)
28. Connell, R. S. and Swank, R. L. 'Pulmonary microembolism after blood transfusion: an electron microscopic study.' *Annals of Surgery*, **177,** 40 (1973)
29. Cook, W. A., Webb, W. R. and Unal, M. O. 'Myocardial function capacity in response to compensated and uncompensated respiratory alkalosis.' *Surgical Forum*, **16,** 186 (1965)
30. Cooley, D. A., Reul, G. J. and Wukasch, D. C. 'Ischaemic contraction of the heart: "Stone Heart."' *American Journal of Cardiology*, **29,** 575 (1972)
31. Darby, T. D., Aldinger, E. E., Gadsden, R. H. and Thrower, W. B. 'Effects of metabolic acidosis on ventricular isometric systolic tension and the response to epinephrine and levarterenol.' *Circulation Research*, **8,** 1242 (1960)
32. Dietzman, R. H., Ersek, R. A., Lillehei, C. W., Castenada, A. R. and Lillehei, R. A. 'Low output syndrome: recognition and treatment.' *Journal of Thoracic and Cardiovascular Surgery*, **57,** 138 (1969)
33. Dikshit, K., Vyden, J. K., Forrester, J. S., Chatterjee, K., Prakash, R. and Swan, H. J. C. 'Renal and extra-renal haemodynamic effects of furosemide in congestive failure after acute myocardial infarction.' *New England Journal of Medicine*, **288,** 1087 (1973)
34. Dodrill, F. D. 'The effects of total body perfusion upon the lungs.' In *Extracorporeal Circulation*. Ed. J. G. Allen, pp. 327–335. Springfield: Thomas (1958)
35. Downs, J. J., Nicodemus, H. F., Pierce, W. S. and Waldhausen, J. A. 'Acute respiratory failure in infants following cardiovascular surgery.' *Journal of Thoracic and Cardiovascular Surgery*, **59,** 21 (1970)
36. Edmunds, L. H., Jr. and Huber, G. L. 'Pulmonary artery occlusion I. Volume–pressure relationships and alveolar bubble stability.' *Journal of Applied Physiology*, **22,** 990 (1967)
37. Ellison, L. T., Duke, J. F., III and Ellison, R. G. 'Pulmonary compliance following open-heart surgery and its relationship to ventilation and gas exchange.' *Circulation*, **35** and **36 (Suppl. I)**, 217 (1967)
38. Eltringham, W. K., Schroder, R., Jenny, M., Matloff, J. R. and Zollinger, R. M., Jr. 'Pulmonary arteriovenous admixture in cardiac surgical patients.' *Circulation*, **37** and **38 (Suppl. 2)**, 207 (1968)
39. English, T. A. H., Kirklin, J. W. and Digerness, S. 'Changes in colloid osmotic pressure during and shortly after open intracardiac operation.' *Journal of Thoracic and Cardiovascular Surgery*, **61,** 338 (1971)
40. Fisherman, A. P. 'Pulmonary oedema: the water exchanging function of the lung.' *Circulation*, **46,** 39 (1972)
41. Flemma, R. J. and Young, W. G. 'The metabolic effects of mechanical ventilation and respiratory alkalosis in post-operative patients.' *Surgery*, **56,** 36 (1964)
42. Fordham, R. M. M. and Resnekov, L. 'Comparison of haemodynamic effect of intravenous isoprenaline and adrenaline after aortic valvular homograft replacement.' *British Heart Journal*, **32,** 393 (1970)
43. Forrester, J. S., Diamond, G., Ganz, W., Danzig, R. and Swan, H. J. C. 'Right and left heart pressures in the acutely ill patient.' *Clinical Research*, **18,** 306 (1970)

44. Forrester, J. S., Ganz, W., Diamond, G., McHugh, T., Chonette, D. W. and Swan, H. J. C. 'Thermodilution cardiac output determination with a single flow-directed catheter.' *American Heart Journal*, **83,** 306 (1972)
45. Friesen, W. G., Woodson, R. D., Ames, A. W., Herr, R. H., Starr, A. and Kassebaum, D. G. 'A haemodynamic comparison of atrial and ventricular pacing in post-operative cardiac surgical patients.' *Journal of Thoracic and Cardiovascular Surgery*, **55,** 271 (1968)
46. Gardner, R. E., Finley, T. N. and Tooley, W. H. 'The effect of cardiopulmonary bypass on surface activity of lung extracts.' *Bulletin of the Society of Internal Surgery*, **5,** 542 (1962)
47. Garzon, A. A., Seltzer, B., Lichtenstein, S. and Karlson, K. E. 'Influence of open-heart surgery on respiratory work.' *Diseases of the Chest*, **52,** 392 (1967)
48. Gault, J. H., Covell, J. W., Braunwald, E. and Ross, J., Jr. 'Left ventricular performance following correction of free aortic regurgitation.' *Circulation*, **42,** 773 (1970)
49. Geffin, B., Grillo, H. C., Cooper, J. D. and Pontoppidan, H. 'Stenosis following tracheostomy for respiratory care.' *Journal of the American Medical Association*, **216,** 1984 (1971)
50. Goldfarb, D. and Bahnson, H. T. 'Early and late effects on the heart of small amounts of air in the coronary circulation.' *Journal of Thoracic and Cardiovascular Surgery*, **46,** 368 (1963)
51. Goldschlager, N., Gerbode, F., Osborn, J. J. and Cohn, K. E. 'Patterns of myocardial oxygen and lactate extraction in patients undergoing cardiopulmonary bypass.' *American Heart Journal*, **83,** 167 (1972)
52. Gomes, M. M. R., Feldt, R. H., McGoon, D. C. and Danielson, G. K. 'Total anomalous pulmonary venous connection. Surgical considerations and results of operation.' *Journal of Thoracic and Cardiovascular Surgery*, **60,** 116 (1970)
53. Gomes, M. M. R. and McGoon, D. C. 'Bleeding patterns after open-heart surgery.' *Journal of Thoracic and Cardiovascular Surgery*, **60,** 87 (1970)
54. Gregory, G. A., Kitterman, J. A., Phibbs, R. H., Tooley, W. H. and Hamilton, W. 'Treatment of the idiopathic respiratory distress syndrome with continuous positive airway pressure.' *New England Journal of Medicine*, **284,** 1333 (1971)
55. Harris, P. D., Malm, J. R., Bowman, F. O., Jr., Hoffman, B. F., Kaiser, G. A. and Singer, D. A. 'Epicardial pacing to control arrhythmias following cardiac surgery.' *Circulation*, **37** and **38** (**Suppl. II**), 178 (1968)
56. Hildner, F. J., Javier, R. P., Cohen, L. A., Samet, P., Nathgan, M. J., Yahr, W. Z. and Greenberg, J. J. 'Myocardial dysfunction associated with valvular heart disease.' *American Journal of Cardiology*, **30,** 319 (1972)
57. Hill, J. D., Johnson, D. C., Miller, G. E., Jr., Kerth, W. J. and Gerbode, F. 'Latent mediastinal tamponade after open-heart surgery.' *Archives of Surgery, Chicago*, **99,** 808 (1969)
58. Holloway, E. L., Stinson, E. B., Derby, G. C. and Harrison, D. C. 'Action of drugs in patients early and after cardiac surgery I. Comparison of isoproterenol and dopamine.' *American Journal of Cardiology*, **35,** 656 (1975)
59. Holzer, J., Karliner, J. S., O'Rourke, R. A., Pill, W. and Ross, J. R., Jr. 'Effectiveness of dopamine in patients with cardiogenic shock.' *American Journal of Cardiology*, **32,** 79 (1973)
60. Huber, G. L. and Edmunds, L. H., Jr. 'Pulmonary artery occlusion II: morphologic studies.' *Journal of Applied Physiology*, **22,** 1002 (1967)
61. Iliff, L. D., Greene, R. E. and West, J. M. B. 'Effect of interstitial oedema on distribution of ventilation and perfusion in isolated lung.' *Journal of Applied Physiology*, **33,** 462 (1972)

62. Javid, H., Tufo, H. M., Najafi, H., Dye, W. S., Hunter, J. A. and Julian, O. C. 'Neurological abnormalities following open-heart surgery.' *Journal of Thoracic and Cardiovascular Surgery*, **58,** 502 (1969)
63. Kapanci, Y., Tosco, R., Eggermann, J. and Gould, V. E. 'Oxygen pneumonitis in man. Light- and electron-microscopic morphometric studies.' *Chest*, **63,** 162 (1972)
64. Kelman, G. R., Nunn, J. F., Prys Robert, C. and Greenbaum, R. 'The influence of cardiac output on arterial oxygenation. A theoretical study.' *British Journal of Anaesthesiology*, **39,** 450 (1967)
65. Kerr, A. R. and Kirklin, J. W. 'Effect of rapid increase of blood volume on atrial pressures and pulmonary blood volume: an experimental study.' *Annals of Surgery*, **172,** 278 (1970)
66. Kirklin, J. W. 'Pulmonary dysfunction after open-heart surgery.' *Medical Clinics of North America*, **48,** 1063 (1964)
67. Kirklin, J. W. 'Systems analysis in surgical patients.' From the *Macewen Memorial Lectures*, **15,** Glasgow: University of Glasgow (1970)
68. Kirklin, J. W. and Rastelli, G. C. 'Low cardiac output after open-heart intracardiac operations.' *Progress in Cardiovascular Disease*, **10,** 117 (1967)
69. Kirklin, J. W. and Theye, R. A. 'Cardiac performance after open intracardiac surgery.' *Circulation*, **28,** 1061 (1963)
70. Kloster, F. E., Bristow, J. D., Starr, A., McCord, C. and Griswold, H. E. 'Serial cardiac output and blood volume studies following cardiac valve replacement.' *Circulation*, **33,** 528 (1966)
71. Kouchoukos, N. T., Doty, D. B., Buettner, L. E. and Kirklin, J. W. 'Treatment of postinfarction cardiac failure by myocardial excision and revascularization.' *Circulation*, **45,** (**Suppl. I**), 72 (1972)
72. Kouchoukos, N. T., Kirklin, J. W., Sheppard, L. C. and Roe, P. 'Effect of left atrial pressure by blood infusion on stroke volume early after cardiac operations.' *Surgical Forum*, **22,** 126 (1971)
73. Kouchoukos, N. T., Sheppard, L. C. and Kirklin, J. W. 'Automated patient care following cardiac surgery.' In *Cardiovascular Clinics*, Vol. 3, No. 3. Ed. A. N. Brest, p. 109. Philadelphia: F. A. Davis Company (1971)
74. Kouchoukos, N. T., Sheppard, L. C. and Kirklin, J. W. 'Effect of alternations in arterial pressure on cardiac performance early after open intracardiac operations.' *Journal of Thoracic and Cardiovascular Surgery*, **64,** 563 (1972)
75. Kouchoukos, N. T., Sheppard, L. C., McDonald, D. A. and Kirklin, J. W. 'Estimation of stroke volume from the central arterial pressure contour in postoperative patients.' *Surgical Forum*, **20,** 180 (1969)
76. Lamberti, J. J., Cohn, L. H., Lesch, M. and Collins, J. J., Jr. 'Intra-aortic balloon counterpulsation. Indications and longterm results in post-operative left ventricular power failure.' *Archives of Surgery*, **109,** 766 (1974)
77. Laver, M. B., Hallowell, P. and Goldblatt, A. 'Pulmonary dysfunction secondary to heart disease.' *Anesthesiology*, **33,** 161 (1970)
78. Lee, C. J., Lyons, J. H., Konisberg, S., Morgan, F. and Moore, F. 'Effects of spontaneous and positive pressure breathing of ambient air and pure oxygen at one atmosphere pressure on pulmonary surface characteristics.' *Journal of Thoracic and Cardiovascular Surgery*, **53,**759 (1967)
79. Lee, W. H., Jr., Krumhaar, D., Fonkalsrud, E., Schjeide, O. A. and Maloney, J. V., Jr. 'Denaturation of plasma proteins as a cause of morbidity and death after intracardiac operations.' *Surgery*, **50,** 29 (1961)
80. Lesage, A. M., Tsuchioka, H., Young, W. G. and Sealy, W. C. 'Pathogenesis of pulmonary damage during extracorporeal perfusion.' *Archives of Surgery, Chicago*, **93,** 1002 (1966)

81. Levine, F. H. and Copeland, J. G. 'Prosthetic replacement of the mitral valve. Continuing assessment of the 100 patients operated upon during 1961–1965.' *Circulation*, **47,** 518 (1973)
82. Levine, O. R., Rodriguez-Martinez, F. and Mellins, R. B. 'Fluid filtration in the lung of the intact puppy.' *Journal of Applied Physiology*, **34,** 683 (1973)
83. Linhart, J. W. and Wheat, M. W. Jr. 'Myocardial dysfunction following aortic valve replacement. The significance of coronary artery disease.' *Journal of Thoracic and Cardiovascular Surgery*, **54,** 259 (1967)
84. Litwak, R. S., Kuhn, L. A., Gadboys, H. L., Lukban, S. J. and Sakurai, H. 'Support of myocardial performance after open cardiac operations by rate augmentation.' *Journal of Thoracic and Cardiovascular Surgery*, **56,** 484 (1968)
85. McClenahan, J. B., Young, W. E. and Sykes, M. K. 'Respiratory changes after open-heart surgery.' *Thorax*, **20,** 545 (1965)
86. McCredie, M. 'Measurement of pulmonary oedema in valvular heart disease.' *Circulation*, **36,** 381 (1967)
87. Meilke, J. E., Hunt, J. C., Maher, F. T. and Kirklin, J. W. 'Renal performance during clinical cardiopulmonary bypass with and without haemodilution.' *Journal of Thoracic and Cardiovascular Surgery*, **51,** 229 (1966)
88. Monkcom, W. and Patterson, R. W. 'Ventilation–perfusion inequalities resulting from hypocapnic changes in lung mechanics.' *Journal of Thoracic and Cardiovascular Surgery*, **63,** 577 (1972)
89. Morgan, T. E. 'Pulmonary surfactant.' *New England Journal of Medicine*, **284,** 1185 (1971)
90. Moseley, R. V. and Doty, D. B. 'Changes in the filtration characteristics of stored blood.' *Annals of Surgery*, **171,** 329 (1970)
91. Mueller, W. H., Jr., Littlefield, J. B. and Dammann, J. F., Jr. 'Pulmonary parenchymal changes associated with cardiopulmonary bypass.' In *Extracorporeal Circulation*. Ed. J. G. Allen. pp. 336–341. Springfield: Thomas (1958)
92. Muller, H., Giannelli, S., Jr., Ayres, S. M., Conklin, E. F. and Gregory, J. J. 'Effect of isoproterenol on ventricular work and myocardial metabolism in the post-operative heart.' *Circulation*, **37.** (**Suppl. II**), 146 (1968)
93. Najafi, H., Henson, D., Dye, W. S., Javid, H., Hunter, J. A., Callaghan, R., Eisenstein, R. and Julian, O. C. 'Left ventricular haemorrhagic necrosis.' *Annals of Thoracic Surgery*, **7,** 550 (1969)
94. O'Connor, N. E., Sheh, J., Bartlett, R. H. and Gazzaniga, A. B. 'Changes in pulmonary extravascular water volume following mitral valve replacement.' *Journal of Thoracic and Cardiovascular Surgery*, **61,** 342 (1971)
95. Oldham, H. N., Jr., Roe, C. R., Young, W. G., Dixon, S. H., Jr. and Sabiston, D. C. Jr. 'Intraoperative detection of myocardial damage during coronary artery surgery by plasma creatinine phosphokinase isoenzyme analysis.' *Surgery*, **74,** 917 (1973)
96. Parker, D. J., Cantrell, J. W., Karp, R. B., Stround, R. M. and Digerness, S. B. 'Changes in serum complement and immunoglobins following cardiopulmonary bypass.' *Surgery,* **71,** 824(1972)
97. Parker, D. J., Karp, R. B., Kirklin, J. W. and Bedard, P. 'Lung water and alveolar and capillary volumes after intracardiac surgery.' *Circulation*, **45** (**Suppl. I**), 139 (1972)
98. Parker, F. B., Neville, J. F., Hanson, E. L. and Webb, W. R. 'Intra-aortic balloon counterpulsation and cardiac surgery.' *Annals of Thoracic Surgery*, **17,** 144 (1974)
99. Parr, G. V. S., Blackstone, E. H. and Kirklin, J. W. 'Cardiac performance and mortality early after intracardiac surgery in infants and young children.' *Circulation*, **51,** 867 (1975)

100. Philbin, D. M., Sullivan, S. F., Bowman, F. O., Malm, J. R. and Papper, E. M. 'Postoperative hypoxaemia; contribution of the cardiac output.' *Anesthesiology*, **32,** 136 (1970)
101. Pontoppidan, H., Geffin, B. and Lowenstein, W. 'Acute respiratory failure in the adult.' *New England Journal of Medicine*, **287,** 743 (1972)
102. Pontoppidan, H., Geffin, B. and Lowenstein, W. 'Acute respiratory failure in the adult.' *New England Journal of Medicine*, **287,** 799 (1972)
103. Prys Roberts, R. C., Kelman, G. R., Greenbaum, R., Kain, M. L. and Bay, J. 'Haemodynamics and alveolar-arterial $P\text{O}_2$ differences at varying $P\text{aCO}_2$ in anaesthetized man.' *Journal of Applied Physiology*, **25,** 80 (1968)
104. Rastelli, G. C. and Kirklin, J. W. 'Haemodynamic state early after replacement of mitral valve.' *Circulation*, **34,** 448 (1966)
105. Ratliff, N. B., Young, W. G., Hackel, D. B., Mikat, E. and Wilson, J. W. 'Pulmonary injury secondary to extracorporeal circulation.' *Journal of Thoracic and Cardiovascular Surgery*, **65,** 425 (1973)
106. Reid, D. J., Digerness, S. B. and Kirklin, J. W. 'Changes in whole body venous tone and distribution of blood after open intracardiac surgery.' *American Journal of Cardiology*, **22,** 621 (1968)
107. Replogle, R. L., Gazzaniga, A. B. and Gross, R. E. 'Use of corticosteroids during cardiopulmonary bypass. Possible lysozome stabilization.' *Circulation*, **33** and **34** (**Suppl. I**), 86 (1966)
108. Richardson, J. V., Kouchoukos, N. T., Wright, J. O. and Karp, R. B. 'Combined aortic valve replacement and myocardial revascularization: results in 220 patients. *Circulation*, **59,** 75 (1979)
109. Ross, J., Jr. and Braunwald, E. 'The study of left ventricular function in man by increasing resistance to ventricular ejection with angiotensin.' *Circulation*, **29,** 739 (1964)
110. Sanders, C. A., Harthorne, J. W., Heitman, H. and Laver, M. B. 'Effect of vaso-pressor administration on blood-gas exchange in mitral disease.' *Clinical Research*, **13,** 351 (1965)
111. Sapsford, R. N., Blackstone, E. H., Kirklin, J. W. Karp, R. B., Kouchoukos, N. T., Pacifico, A. D., Roe, C. R. and Bradley, E. L. 'Coronary perfusion versus cold ischaemic arrest during aortic valve surgery.' *Circulation*, **44,** 1190 (1974)
112. Schuster, S. R., Kakvan, M., Vawter, G. F. and Narter, N. 'An experimental study of the effect of mannitol during cardiopulmonary bypass.' *Circulation*, **29** (**Suppl. I**), 72 (1964)
113. Sekelj, P., Tait, G. R. and Nathanson, M. M. 'Studies on dye dilution curves using a digital computer.' *IEEE Transactions on Bio-medical Engineering*, **13,** 32 (1966)
114. Shappell, S. D. 'Haemoglobin affinity for oxygen 2,3-DPG and cardiovascular disease.' *Cardiology Digest*, **9,** (Dec.) (1972)
115. Sharp, J. T., Bunnell, I. L., Griffith, G. T. and Greene, D. G. 'The effects of therapy on pulmonary mechanics in human pulmonary oedema.' *Journal of Clinical Investigation*, **40,** 665 (1961)
116. Sheppard, L. C., Kouchoukos, N. T., Kurtts, M. A. and Kirklin, J. W. 'Automated treatment of critically ill patients following operation.' *Annals of Surgery*, **168,** 596 (1968)
117. Shugerman, H. J., Rogers, R. M. and Miller, L. D. 'Positive end-expiratory pressure (PEEP): indications and physiologic considerations.' *Chest*, **62,** (**Suppl. 2**), 865 (1972)
118. Siggaard-Anderson, O. 'Titratable acid on base of body fluids.' *Annals of the New York Academy of Science*, **133,** 41 (1966)

119. Singer, M. M., Wright, F. and Stanley, K. 'Oxygen toxicity in man: a prospective study in patients after open-heart surgery.' *New England Journal of Medicine*, **283,** 1473 (1970)
120. Sladen, A., Laver, M. B. and Pontoppidan, H. 'Pulmonary complications and water retention in prolonged mechanical ventilation.' *New England Journal of Medicine*, **279,** 448 (1968)
121. Spencer, F. C., Green, G. E., Tice, D. A., Wallsh, E., Mills, N. L. and Glassman, E. 'Coronary artery bypass grafts for congestive heart failure. A report of experience with 40 patients.' *Journal of Thoracic and Cardiovascular Surgery*, **62,** 529 (1971)
122. Stephenson, L. W., Blackstone, E. H. and Kouchoukos, N. T. 'Dopamine vs. epinephrine in patients following cardiac surgery: randomized study.' *Surgical Forum*, **27,** 272 (1976)
123. Stephenson, L. W., Kouchoukos, N. T. and Kirklin, J. W. 'Triple-valve replacement: an analysis of eight years' experience.' *Annals of Thoracic Surgery*, **23,** 327 (1977)
124. Stephenson, L. W., Kouchoukos, N. T., Kirklin, J. W., Karp, R. B. and Pacifico, A. D. 'Combined aortic and mitral valve replacement. Results in 251 patients.' *Circulation*, **51** and **52 (Suppl. II)**, 31 (1975)
125. Stewart, S., III, Edmunds, L. H., Jr., Kirklin, J. W. and Allarde, R. R. 'Spontaneous breathing with continuous positive airway pressure after open intracardiac operations in infants.' *Journal of Thoracic and Cardiovascular Surgery*, **65,** 37 (1973)
126. Stinson, E. B., Holloway, E. L., Derby, G., Oyer, P. E., Hollingsworth, J., Criepp, R. B. and Harrison, D. C. 'Comparative haemodynamic responses to chlorpromazine, nitroprusside, nitroglycerin and trimethaphan immediately after open-heart operations.' *Circulation*, **51** and **52 (Suppl. I)**, 126 (1975)
127. Sugg, J. H., Karp, R. B. and Kirklin, J. W. 'Effect of pulmonary capillary occlusion on extravascular lung water in pulmonary oedema.' *Surgical Forum*, **23,** 216 (1972)
128. Taber, R. E., Morales, A. R. and Fine, G. 'Myocardial necrosis and the postoperative low cardiac output syndrome.' *Annals of Thoracic Surgery*, **4,** 12 (1967)
129. Trimble, C., Smith, D. E., Rosenthal, M. H. and Fosburg, R. G. 'Pathophysiologic role of hypocarbia in post-traumatic pulmonary insufficiency.' *American Journal of Surgery*, **122,** 633 (1971)
130. Tufo, H. M., Ostfeld, A. M. and Shekelle, R. 'Central nervous system dysfunction following open-heart surgery.' *Journal of the American Medical Association*, **212,** 1333 (1970)
131. Uzawa, T. and Ashbaugh, D. G. 'Continuous positive pressure breathing in acute haemorrhagic pulmonary oedema.' *Journal of Applied Physiology*, **26,** 427 (1969)
132. Waldo, A. L. and Kaiser, G. A. 'Electrophysiological considerations for the cardiac surgical patient.' In *Preoperative, Operative and Postoperative Care of the Cardiac Surgical Patient*. Eds R. S. Litwak and R. Juanado. New York: Intercontinental Medical Book Corporation (1973)
133. Waldo, A. L., MacLean, W. A. H., Cooper, T., Kouchoukos, N. T. and Karp, R. B. 'Use of temporarily placed epicardial atrial wire electrodes for the diagnosis and treatment of cardiac arrhythmias following open-heart surgery.' *Journal of Thoracic and Cardiovascular Surgery*, **76,** 500 (1978)
134. Waldo, A. L., MacLean, W. A. H., Karp, R. B., Kouchoukos, N. T. and James, T. N. 'Sustained rapid atrial pacing to control supraventricular tachycardias following open-heart surgery.' *Circulation*, **51** and **52 (Suppl. II)**, 13 (1975)

135. Waldo, A. L., Ross, S. M. and Kaiser, G. A. 'The epicardial electrogram in the diagnosis of cardiac arrhythmias following cardiac surgery.' *Geriatrics*, **26,** 108 (1971)
136. Webber, C. E. and Garnett, E. S. 'The relationship between colloid osmotic pressure and plasma proteins during and after cardiopulmonary bypass.' *Journal of Thoracic and Cardiovascular Surgery*, **65,** 234 (1973)
137. Weedn, R. J., Coalson, J. L. and Greenfield, L. J. 'Effects of oxygen and ventilation on pulmonary mechanics and ultrastructure during cardiopulmonary bypass.' *American Journal of Surgery*, **120,** 584 (1970)
138. West, J. B. 'Regional differences in gas exchange in the lung of erect man.' *Journal of Applied Physiology*, **17,** 893 (1962)
139. Wisch, N., Litwak, R. S., Luckban, S. B. and Glass, J. L. 'Haematologic complications of open-heart surgery.' *American Journal of Cardiology*, **31,** 282 (1973)
140. Wukasch, D. C., Reul, G. L., Milam, J. D., Hallman, G. L. and Cooley, D. A. 'The "stone heart" syndrome.' *Surgery*, **72,** 1071 (1972)
141. Yu, P. N., Murphy, G. W., Schreiner, B. F., Jr. and James, D. H. 'Distensibility characteristics of the human pulmonary vascular bed.' *Circulation*, **35,** 710 (1967)

13

Blood Loss Following Extracorporeal Circulation for Heart Valve Surgery

Marian I. Ionescu, Anand P. Tandon, Michele F. Roesler and David A. S. Mary

facile est inventis addere

Introduction

During the past 20 years, through experimental and clinical research, extracorporeal circulation became established as a routine technique for the temporary support of the circulation and respiration.

The objective of extracorporeal circulation in cardiac surgery is to provide optimal conditions for intracardiac surgical operations, while maintaining essentially physiological tissue and organ perfusion and oxygenation for limited periods of time, with complete return to functional integrity of all parameters of homeostasis after the procedure.

Despite considerable progress and refinement in materials, techniques and knowledge, the artificial perfusion of the body is far from being a perfect substitute for the normal circulation and respiration.

Extracorporeal circulation, even when used for short periods of time, for intracardiac operations results in functional alterations of most of the organ systems. In the majority of cases these alterations are transient or clinically undiscernible and require little or no specific treatment.

These abnormalities induced during cardiac operations performed with the aid of extracorporeal circulation are due to several factors.

The severity of the functional abnormality depends on the magnitude of its cause or interrelated causes.

The degree of preoperative pathological changes in different organ systems and the functional reserve of these organs are the prime causes of postoperative abnormalities.

The completeness of the surgical repair of the specific cardiac lesions is a *sine qua non* condition for minimizing the postoperative disturbances.

The duration and adequacy of anaesthesia and extracorporeal circulation are important factors in the development of postperfusion abnormalities.

The presence and degree of functional disturbances following the use of extracorporeal circulation are to a certain extent a guide to the adequacy of perfusion.

In general the adequacy of extracorporeal circulation can be assessed in simple terms of survival of the patient and return to normal of cardiovascular, pulmonary, neurological and renal functions.

There are also other ways of assessing the adequacy of perfusion by a multitude of more subtle and complex clinical and laboratory investigations.

Considering that the indication for surgical correction of a particular cardiac lesion in a given patient was correct and that the operative procedure was complete, the only remaining major determinant of the postoperative evolution lies in the duration and quality of the extracorporeal circulatory and respiratory support.

Among other potential disturbances following open-heart surgery under total body perfusion is the continued and excessive postoperative haemorrhage.

The most important single factor contributing to increased postoperative bleeding is trauma inflicted on the blood during and immediately after the heart-lung bypass.

The artificial heart-lung machine consists of reservoirs, pumps and circuits very different in their physical and chemical properties from the natural cardiovascular system. These materials traumatize the formed elements and the proteins of the blood by direct contact. The non-pulsatile flow, the unphysiological gas exchange and the unnatural velocity and pressure gradients inside the extracorporeal circuit produce additional injury to the circulating volume. Indirectly the trauma inflicted upon the blood affects all tissues and organ systems, enhancing the propensity for increased haemorrhage.

Because all conventional extracorporeal circuits are traumatic, it seems logical to reduce the time of exposure of the blood to the artificial heart-lung machine and to reduce temporarily the quantity of blood exposed to trauma by haemodilution or complete non-haemic prime. A smooth perfusion with large-bore cannulae, gentle and controlled open-heart suction, smooth cooling and rewarming of the perfusate, and gentle handling of the tissues are some of the conditions for a less traumatic perfusion.

A smooth perfusion prevents pathological blood flow distribution and metabolic and acid–base changes, and reduces blood trauma and individual organ alterations.

In addition to the deleterious effects of the pump oxygenator, the transfusion of large quantities of stored blood accounts for some of the postperfusion complications. The rapid infusion of large amounts of citrated blood reduces the level of circulating ionized calcium and this may impair myocardial activity[40]. The pH of stored blood is low and the anaerobic glycolysis which continues to take place may further reduce it[42]. Metabolic acidosis may develop, especially in patients already underperfused. Several hours later, the metabolism of the citrate may produce metabolic alkalosis[25]. The potassium concentration of the stored blood increases gradually due to a failure of the active transport mechanism in the red cells[27].

The capacity of the red cells to release oxygen deteriorates with storage by losing 2,3-diphosphoglycerate[4].

The survival rate of platelets is considerably reduced in blood stored over 48 hours in ACD (acid-citrate-dextrose) solution[24]. Stored blood is also deficient in clotting factors V and VIII.

One of the factors which has improved the overall results of cardiac surgery with extracorporeal circulation is the dilution of the circulating blood with either partial or total non-haemic prime of the heart-lung machine. The haemodilution technique reduces the amount of blood used, reduces the viscosity of the blood, improves the microcirculation, preserves the clotting factors[34], reduces the haemolysis[34], and decreases the amount of postoperative bleeding[32].

The use of fresh blood at the conclusion of extracorporeal circulation obviates the disadvantages related to infusion of stored blood and adds the clotting factors required at that particular moment in time.

The present study was undertaken in order to evaluate the relative roles of some of the factors considered responsible for the prolonged or excessive postoperative blood loss. Correlation was sought between postoperative haemorrhage on the one hand and the type of oxygenator and priming solutions and the duration of heart-lung bypass on the other. Several other factors were also analysed in an attempt to establish their role in postoperative bleeding.

Clinical materials and methods

This study includes 428 patients operated upon for heart valve disease between July 1965 and December 1973 and a separate group of patients operated upon for heart valve replacement between 1977 and 1978 in which moderate total body hypothermia, cardioplegia and a different oxygenator-heat exchanger* were used[38]. All patients included in this report had their operation through a median sternotomy incision and with the aid of extracorporeal circulation.

Nineteen patients required reoperation for excessive bleeding and were not included in this study. *Table 13.1* gives details of the age, sex and type of heart valve surgery performed in these patients and shows the 8 main groups of patients divided according to the type of oxygenator and priming solutions used.

Mitral valve repair was undertaken in 27 patients while the remaining 401 had valve replacement with either prostheses or tissue valves. The extracorporeal circulation was standardized in all cases of a particular group as shown in *Tables 13.2* and *13.3*.

The technique of heart-lung bypass was essentially similar in all groups except for the use of different oxygenators and priming solutions. The temperature of the perfusate was continuously maintained around 35–36° in all patients except for the Melrose and the more recent Shiley oxygenator groups. In the Melrose oxygenator group mild hypothermia (31–33°C) was used. Since January 1977 moderate total body hypothermia (26–29°C) with cold cardioplegia and topical hypothermia were used for all patients in conjunction with the Shiley oxygenator which is described and discussed in Chapter 6. Two separate venous cannulae were used for gravity drainage of the caval blood into the oxygenator. The arterialized blood from the heart-lung machine was returned to the patient through a large-bore plastic cannula inserted in the ascending aorta. Two cardiotomy suction lines, connected to roller pumps were used for the aspiration of intracardiac and intrapericardial blood. The left heart cavities were decompressed by a vent tube inserted into the left ventricle through the left atrium and across the mitral valve.

Until January 1977 for isolated mitral valve replacement the aorta was cross-clamped once or twice for a duration of 15 to 20 minutes each and the heart was intermittently bathed with ice-cold saline; while for isolated aortic or for multiple-valve replacement the main left coronary artery was continuously perfused using a separate roller pump. The left coronary perfusion flow averaged 200 ml/min (range 70 to 300 ml/min) and the line pressure was maintained below 120 mmHg.

From January 1977, all single or multiple-valve replacements have been carried out using moderate total body hypothermia (26–29°C) with cold cardioplegia and topical hypothermia.

Until May 1970 acid-citrate-dextrose (ACD) blood, 3 to 14 days old, was used for priming the heart-lung machine and for postoperative transfusion. Since then only fresh ACD blood has been used for transfusion in the post-bypass period.

*Shiley Inc, Irvine, California, USA

Table 13.1 Details of patients and the types of open-heart valve surgery performed using different oxygenators and priming solutions

Group	Oxygenators and priming solutions	Mean age (years) (range)	Sex		Valve surgery						
			m	*f*	*M*	*T*	*A*	*M + T*	*M + A*	*M + A + T*	*Total*
1	*Melrose*: Haemodilution prime with dextrose 5%	42.6 (12–52)	10	10	13	—	5	1	1	—	20
2	*Kay–Cross*: Haemodilution prime with dextrose 5% and Dextran 40	48.8 (35–53)	6	6	4	—	7	—	1	—	12
3	*Kay–Cross*: Haemodilution prime with dextrose 5%	45.2 (30–57)	10	8	2	—	16	—	—	—	18
4	*Kay–Cross*: Haemodilution prime with Travenol and Hartman's solutions	44.8 (22–62)	15	13	28	—	—	—	—	—	28
5	*Travenol*: Haemodilution prime with Travenol and Hartman's solutions	48.0 (35–68)	21	26	42	1	3	1	—	—	47
6	*Travenol*: Non-haemic prime with Travenol and Hartman's solutions	47.6 (10–69)	60	68	62	2	36	19	8	1	128
	(a) Before December 1971	49.1 (24–62)	19	17	19	—	8	6	3	—	36
	(b) Between January and September 1972	47–3 (10–63)	23	34	31	2	11	11	1	1	57
	(c) Between September 1972 and August 1973	43.5 (17–69)	18	17	12	—	17	2	4	—	35
7	*Temptrol*: Non-haemic prime with Travenol solution	45.5 (9–61)	20	17	19	1	7	4	5	1	37
8	Shiley oxygenator with Leeds pump priming solution	47.5 (14.70)	66	72	51	—	45	6	31	5	138
	Total	46.8 (9–69)	208	220	221	4	119	31	46	7	428

m = males; *f* = females; *M* = mitral; *T* = tricuspid; *A* = aortic

Table 13.2 Details of extracorporeal circulation and blood infusion

Group	Type of oxygenator	Priming solutions	Priming volume (litres)	Perfusion flow (ℓ/min per m²)	Blood transfusion in the operating room after heart-lung bypass (litres)
		Haemodilution			
1	Melrose rotating disc/drum	50% stored ACD blood plus 50% dextrose in water*	3.0–3.5	3.0–3.5	0.5–3.0 stored ACD blood
2	Kay–Cross rotating disc	60% stored ACD blood 26.7% Dextran 40, plus 13.3% dextrose in water*	3.0–4.5	3.0–3.5	0.5–3.0 stored ACD blood
3	Kay–Cross rotating disc	60% stored ACD blood plus 40% dextrose in water*	3.0–4.5	3.0–3.5	0.5–3.0 stored ACD blood
4	Kay–Cross rotating disc	60% stored ACD blood plus 40% Travenol and Hartman's solutions†	3.0–4.5	3.0–3.5	0.5–3.0 stored ACD blood
5	Travenol miniprime disposable	25–50% stored ACD blood plus 50–75% Travenol and Hartman's solution†	2.0	2.3–2.6	0.5–1.5 stored ACD blood
		Non-haemic prime			
6	Travenol miniprime disposable	Travenol and Hartman's solutions†	2.0	2.3–2.6	0–1.5 fresh ACD blood
7	Temptrol disposable	Travenol solution	2.0	2.3–2.6	0–1.5 fresh ACD blood
8	Shiley disposable with incorporated heat exchanger	Leeds pump priming solution	1.8	2.3–2.6**	0–1.5 fresh ACD blood

* Five per cent dextrose in distilled water
† Equal volumes of Travenol and Hartman's solutions have been used
** At various times during heart-lung bypass, as, for example, at the end of the open-heart procedure, the perfusion flow was temporarily increased up to 3.2 ℓ/min per m²

Table 13.3 Composition of priming solutions

Components	*Hartman's solution (mmol/ℓ)*	*Travenol solution (mmol/ℓ)**	*'Leeds' priming solution (mmol/ℓ)**
Sodium	131	102	101.2
Potassium	5	5	5
Calcium	4	5	2.5
Magnesium	–	2	0.8
Chloride	111	107	105.8
Phosphate	–	2	1.2
Bicarbonate (as lactate)	29	–	–
Gluconate	–	5	2.5
Dextrose	–	25 (g/l)	25 (g/l)

* Various amounts of sodium bicarbonate were added to the extracorporeal circuit depending on the acid–base balance

At the beginning of the heart-lung bypass, heparin was administered in a dose of 2.5 mg per kilogram body weight. This was neutralized at the end of the perfusion with protamine sulphate using twice the amount of heparin.

None of the patients studied was found to have coagulation abnormalities. In patients treated preoperatively with long-acting anticoagulants, these were discontinued 3 to 5 days prior to the operation. In patients with previously inserted prosthetic valves and in those with a clear history of systemic embolism, the long-acting anticoagulants were replaced with intravenous heparin 2 to 3 days preoperatively. The heparin administration was discontinued 6 hours prior to the operation. Anticoagulation, when indicated, was resumed 24 to 72 hours postoperatively. The postoperative blood loss through drainage tubes was measured in millilitres per square metre of body surface area (ml/m^2) at 6 hours and at 24 hours. In the majority of cases the drainage tubes were removed at or about 24 hours following the operation.

The patients were divided into different groups according to the type of oxygenator and priming solutions used, the duration of heart-lung bypass, postoperative platelet count, type of heart valve surgery, number and location of extracorporeal circuit filters, prophylactic use of epsilon aminocaproic acid (EACA) and preoperative anticoagulant treatment (*Tables 13.4* to *13.11*). The amount of postoperative blood loss in each group was established and its clinical significance was analysed using standard statistical methods.

Results

Postoperative blood loss related to the oxygenators and priming solutions

The postoperative blood loss was analysed in 8 groups of patients divided according to the types of oxygenators and priming solutions used. In order to assess the bleeding pattern in the different groups independent of the influence of perfusion time, the durations of cardiopulmonary bypass of the various groups were also compared (*Table 13.4*). There was no statistically significant difference in the length of perfusion or in the mean postoperative blood loss between the Melrose (group 1) and the Kay–Cross (groups 2 and 3) disc oxygenators. Although the use of 5 per cent dextrose and Dextran 40

Table 13.4 Postoperative blood loss related to the oxygenators and priming solutions

Group	*Type of oxygenators and priming solutions*	*No. of patients*	*(Blood loss (ml/m²)** *6 hours*	*24 hours)*	*Perfusion duration* (minutes)*
1	*Melrose*: Haemodilution prime with dexrose 5%	20	435 ± 58	896 ± 112	95 ± 8
2	*Kay–Cross*: Haemodilution prime with dextrose 5% and Dextran 40	12	514 ± 97	1039 ± 183	93 ± 10
3	*Kay–Cross*: Haemodilution prime with dextrose 5%	18	420 ± 52	748 ± 90	75 ± 6
4	*Kay–Cross*: Haemodilution prime with Travenol and Hartman's solutions	28	384 ± 47	738 ± 83	50 ± 5
5	*Travenol*: Haemodilution prime with Travenol and Hartman's solutions	47	298 ± 25	583 ± 38	58 ± 4
6	*Travenol*: Non-haemic prime with Travenol and Hartman's solutions	128	192 ± 10	348 ± 15	69 ± 3
	(a) Before December 1971	36	217 ± 16	417 ± 29	61 ± 4
	(b) Between January and September 1972	57	198 ± 16	349 ± 22	71 ± 4
	(c) Between September 1972 and August 1973	35	150 ± 14	276 ± 22	83 ± 6
7	*Temptrol*: Non-haemic prime with Travenol solution	37	175 ± 17	338 ± 23	74 ± 5
8	*Shiley*: Non-haemic prime with 'Leeds' priming solution	138	128 ± 15	279 ± 21	71 ± 7

	Group	*P*	*P*	*P*
	1 and 2	NS	NS	NS
	1 and 3	NS	NS	NS
	2 and 3	NS	NS	NS
	4 and 5	NS	NS	NS
Statistical comparison of data amongst the various groups	5 and 6	< 0.001	< 0.001	< 0.05
	6(a) and (b)	NS	< 0.05	NS
	(b) and (c)	< 0.05	< 0.05	NS
	(a) and (c)	<0.01	<0.001	< 0.02
	6 and 7	NS	NS	NS
	6(c) and 7	NS	NS	NS
	6 and 8	< 0.05	< 0.05	NS
	6(c) and 8	NS	NS	NS
	7 and 8	< 0.05	< 0.05	NS

* Results are expressed as mean ± standard error of the mean
P = statistical probability; NS = not significant

as priming solutions (group 2) appeared to be associated with increased postoperative blood loss, this was not statistically significant, when compared with the mean values of groups 1 and 3. The relative influence of the disc oxygenator and bubble oxygenator on postoperative blood loss was assessed by comparing the mean values of groups 4 (Kay–Cross disc oxygenator) and 5 (Travenol disposable bubble oxygenator). Identical priming solutions were used in both groups and the perfusion durations were very similar. There was no statistically significant difference in postoperative bleeding between these two groups, although the mean blood loss in the Travenol group was lower than that in the Kay–Cross group.

Patients in groups 6 (Travenol bubble oxygenator with non-haemic prime), 7 (Temptrol bubble oxygenator with non-haemic prime) and 8 (Shiley bubble oxygenator with non-haemic prime) had a significantly lower postoperative blood loss than the rest of the patients in this series. These three groups differed from the others in two important aspects: no blood was added to the prime and fresh blood instead of old stored blood was used at the end of the heart-lung bypass and during the first 24 hours postoperatively. There was no significant difference in the postoperative bleeding between groups 6 and 7 using different bubble oxygenators but both employing non-haemic priming solutions and having comparable perfusion durations. The effects of non-haemic prime on postoperative blood loss were analysed by comparing the bleeding patterns of groups 5 and 6. The oxygenators employed in both these groups were identical (Travenol disposable bubble oxygenator) but the priming solutions were different, haemodilution prime being used in group 5 and non-haemic prime in group 6. A significantly lower postoperative blood loss was noted in group 6 in spite of longer perfusion durations. A marginally significant difference was also noted in the blood loss between groups 6 and 8 as well as 7 and 8 though there is no difference in the postoperative blood loss between groups 6 and 8, most likely due to the increased care being taken in the operating theatre in controlling the bleeding and in the use of fresh blood. Generally speaking, there is no significant difference in the postoperative blood loss in patients operated upon with various types of bubble oxygenators.

Analysis of additional factors with possible influence on postoperative blood loss

To permit appraisal of various factors with possible influence on the postoperative blood loss within a relatively homogeneous group, the analysis that follows was based on the largest single group of 128 patients undergoing open-heart surgery with the Travenol disposable oxygenator and non-haemic prime. Between 1977 and 1978, when the Shiley oxygenator had been regularly used with non-haemic prime, 138 patients underwent primarily single or multiple-valve replacement. They have also been analysed and the results are presented herein.

Duration of cardiopulmonary bypass

The duration of heart-lung bypass ranged from 22 to 180 minutes with a mean of 69 minutes in the Travenol group and 71 minutes in the Shiley group. Bleeding patterns were analysed in the two groups of patients according to the duration of perfusion and are detailed in *Table 13.5*. No

Table 13.5 Postoperative blood loss related to the duration of perfusion

Group	Perfusion duration (min)	Travenol group No. of patients	Travenol group Blood loss (ml/m²)* 6 hours	Travenol group Blood loss (ml/m²)* 24 hours	Shiley group No. of patients	Shiley group Blood loss (ml/m²)* 6 hours	Shiley group Blood loss (ml/m²)* 24 hours
A	< 60	53	196 ± 14	343 ± 22	51	123 ± 11	267 ± 24
B	60–90	45	181 ± 16	335 ± 23	47	127 ± 13	284 ± 26
C	90–120	23	202 ± 24	384 ± 45	31	137 ± 19	295 ± 31
D	> 120	7	195 ± 63	349 ± 76	9	131 ± 27	282 ± 39
		Group	*P*	*P*	*Group*	*P*	*P*
	Statistical comparison between the highest and lowest mean values	B and C	NS	NS	A and C	NS	NS

* See Table 13.4

Table 13.6 Postoperative blood loss related to platelet counts

Group	Platelet counts (per mm³)	Travenol group No. of patients	Travenol group Blood loss (ml/m²)* 6 hours	Travenol group Blood loss (ml/m²)* 24 hours	Shiley group No. of patients	Shiley group Blood loss (ml/m²)* 6 hours	Shiley group Blood loss (ml/m²)* 24 hours
A	< 100 000	42	214 ± 20	372 ± 29	46	142 ± 14	301 ± 23
B	100–150 000	64	194 ± 14	354 ± 22	69	129 ± 11	282 ± 15
C	> 150 000	22	132 ± 11	262 ± 21	23	116 ± 9	265 ± 17
		Group	*P*	*P*	*Group*	*P*	*P*
	Statistical comparison	A and B	NS	NS	A and B	NS	NS
		B and C	< 0.05	NS	B and C	NS	NS
		A and C	< 0.01	< 0.05	A and C	< 0.01	< 0.01

* See Table 13.4

significant difference in the postoperative blood loss was observed amongst the various subgroups of patients with perfusion duration up to 90 minutes. The number of patients having perfusion duration over 120 minutes was, however, small for adequate comparison. These results are at variance with our previous study[11], when a significantly higher blood loss was observed in patients with a perfusion duration longer than 90 minutes. The policy of using clear prime during cardiopulmonary bypass and fresh blood in the post-bypass period, instead of haemodilution and stored blood, which were used in the majority of patients previously reported[11], provides the probable explanation for the observed difference.

Postoperative platelet count

In this series the preoperative platelet count ranged from 120 000 to 250 000/mm^3 with a mean of 185 000/mm^3. Postoperatively the platelet count ranged from 15 000 to 200 000/mm^3 with a mean of 115 000/mm^3 (a reduction of 37 per cent when compared with the mean preoperative value). The platelet counts were performed approximately 2 hours after the conclusion of cardiopulmonary bypass, and by this time the patients would have received up to 2 units of fresh blood. The postoperative blood loss was analysed in the various subgroups of patients who were divided according to the postoperative platelet count (*Table 13.6*). The mean blood loss was lowest in group C and increased in inverse relation to the platelet counts, reaching statistical significance in group A, which had the highest mean postoperative blood loss.

Type of heart valve surgery

The postoperative blood loss following 41 mitral valve replacements, 30 aortic valve replacements and 18 multiple-valve replacements in the Travenol group and 51, 45 and 42 patients with mitral, aortic and multiple-valve replacements, respectively, in the Shiley group was analysed (*Table 13.7*). There was no statistically significant difference in the mean postoperative blood loss amongst the three groups although the mean blood loss following multiple-valve replacement was higher than in the other two groups. Similarly no significant difference was noted in the mean postoperative blood loss between patients who had previous valve surgery and those who underwent open-heart valve surgery for the first time (*Table 13.8*) although the mean values in the former group were higher, probably reflecting an insignificant increase in bleeding from intrathoracic adhesions.

The use of filters in the heart-lung machine

Swank filters were used in all cardiopulmonary bypass operations until 1974. In the Travenol group of patients, two parallel arterial filters were used in 102 patients, one filter each in the arterial and in the cardiotomy suction line were used in 16, and one arterial filter in only 10 patients (*Table 13.9*). The latest group of 138 patients who were operated upon with the Shiley oxygenator had only one filter inserted in the cardiotomy suction line and their mean postoperative blood loss is also presented in *Table 13.9*.

Table 13.7 Analysis of postoperative blood loss according to the type of valve surgery

		Travenol group			Shiley group		
			Blood loss (ml/m²)*			Blood loss (ml/m²)*	
Group	Operation	No. of patients	6 hours	24 hours	No. of patients	6 hours	24 hours
A	Mitral valve replacement	41	185 ± 19	324 ± 25	51	122 ± 13	259 ± 21
B	Aortic valve replacement	30	182 ± 20	353 ± 33	45	126 ± 19	278 ± 19
C	Multiple-valve replacement	18	210 ± 31	382 ± 53	42	146 ± 17	306 ± 21
	Statistical comparison	Group	*P*	*P*	Group	*P*	*P*
		A and B	NS	NS	A and B	NS	NS
		B and C	NS	NS	B and C	NS	NS
		A and C	NS	NS	A and C	< 0.05	< 0.05

* *See Table 13.4*

Table 13.8 Postoperative blood loss related to previous valve surgery

	Travenol group					Shiley group				
	No. of patients	Postoperative blood loss (ml/m²) 6 hours	24 hours	Perfusion duration* (min)	Platelet counts* (× 10³/mm³)	No. of patients	Postoperative blood loss (ml/m²) 6 hours	24 hours	Perfusion duration* (min)	Platelet counts* (× 10³/mm³)
Previous valve surgery	37	200 ± 15	359 ± 25	67 ± 5	116 ± 8	45	139 ± 19	293 ± 23	74 ± 7	121 ± 9
No previous valve surgery	91	190 ± 12	336 ± 18	72 ± 3	121 ± 4	93	123 ± 11	272 ± 17	69 ± 4	133 ± 4
Statistical comparison of the data		*P* NS	*P* NS	*P* NS	*P* NS		*P* NS	*P* NS	*P* NS	*P* NS

* *See Table 13.4*

Table 13.9 Influence of filters used during cardiopulmonary bypass on postoperative blood loss

Group	*Filters*	*No. of patients*	*Postoperative blood loss (ml/m²)** *6 hours*	*24 hours*
A	Two arterial filters in parallel	192	198 ± 12	360 ± 18
B	One arterial filter and one cardiotomy suction filter	16	175 ± 25	315 ± 34
C	One arterial filter	10	173 ± 15	306 ± 26
D	Shiley oxygenator with one cardiotomy filter	138	128 ± 15	279 ± 21
		Group	*P*	*P*
	Statistical comparison	A and B	NS	NS
		B and C	NS	NS
		A and C	NS	NS
		A and D	<0.001	<0.001

* *See Table 13.4*

There was no statistically significant difference in the mean postoperative blood loss between the first three groups of patients. All these patients (Groups A, B and C in *Table 13.9*) were perfused with circuits comprising at least one arterial filter. Although the comparison is not entirely satisfactory because of the large disparity in the number of patients in the different groups, the use of more than one arterial line filter does not appear to have any advantage in relation to the postoperative blood loss.

On the other hand, there was a statistically significant difference in postoperative blood loss between patients perfused with the Travenol oxygenator and two arterial filters in parallel and the patients operated upon with the Shiley oxygenator and one cardiotomy filter only (Groups A and D of *Table 13.9*).

Most recent data, as discussed in Chapter 7, shows that the use of filters in the arterial line is not beneficial and filtration of the cardiotomy suction blood is sufficient in extracorporeal circuits containing a bubble oxygenator.

Table 13.10 Effect of prophylactic treatment with EACA on postoperative blood loss

	No. of patients	*Postoperative blood loss (ml/m²)** *6 hours*	*24 hours*
With EACA treatment	33	240 ± 23	398 ± 31
Without EACA treatment	95	174 ± 10	333 ± 17
		P	*P*
Statistical comparison		< 0.01	NS

* *See Table 13.4*

Postoperative blood loss related to the use of EACA

Thirty-three of the 128 patients operated upon with the Travenol disposable bubble oxygenator (Group 6, *Tables 13.1* and *13.4*) received prophylactically 75 to 100 mg of EACA per kilogram of body weight (*Table 13.10*). The difference in postoperative blood loss was statistically significant at 6 hours after the operation but not significant at 24 hours. Unexpectedly, patients who received EACA bled more in the first 6 postoperative hours than those who did not receive this treatment.

Postoperative blood loss related to preoperative anticoagulant treatment

Ten patients from the Travenol group and 23 patients from the Shiley group were treated preoperatively with anticoagulants (warfarin sodium). The treatment was discontinued 3 to 5 days before the operation. The duration of the heart-lung bypass and the platelet counts in these and the control patients were similar (*Table 13.11*). The difference in postoperative blood loss between these two groups of patients was not significant.

Reduction in the postoperative blood loss as a function of time

Between 1965 and 1978 the postoperative blood loss decreased from the highest recorded mean values of 514 ml/m^2 at 6 hours and 1039 ml/m^2 at 24 hours to 128 ml/m^2 at 6 hours and 279 $\pm$ 21 ml/m^2 at 24 hours as noted in groups 2 and 8 respectively (*Table 13.4*). Two basic recognizable factors in the technique of the extracorporeal circulation and postoperative management might have contributed to this significant change: the use of non-haemic prime and transfusions of fresh blood at the end of perfusion and during the first 24 hours of the postoperative period. It is speculative whether a more meticulous haemostasis in recent years has played a role in reducing the postoperative blood loss. It is, however, not possible to exclude the contribution of improvements in surgical skill and tissue handling coincident with the length of experience.

Discussion

The haematological changes contributing to the deranged haemostasis following open-heart surgery include inadequate neutralization of heparin, inappropriate use of protamine sulphate, intravascular coagulation, fibrinolysis, hypofibrinogenaemia, deficiency of factors V, VIII and IX and thrombocytopenia[8–10, 13–15, 22, 23, 36, 43]. Although the relative importance of the induced deficiencies of the individual coagulation factors is controversial, trauma to the blood elements due to surface contact during the passage of blood through the components of the extracorporeal circuit, and in particular due to shearing forces at the blood-gas interface during oxygenation, remains the central point in precipitating a cascade of events. The destruction of platelets and red cells releases thromboplastic material, enhancing intravascular coagulability which is further aggravated by the development of acidosis due to vasoconstriction and decreased capillary

Table 13.11 Postoperative blood loss related to preoperative anticoagulant therapy

	Travenol group					*Shiley group*				
	No. of patients	*Postoperative blood loss (ml/m²)** *6 hours*	*24 hours*	*Perfusion duration* (min)*	*Platelet counts* (× 10³/mm³)*	*No. of patients*	*Postoperative blood loss (ml/m²)** *6 hours*	*24 hours*	*Perfusion duration* (min)*	*Platelet counts* (× 10³/mm³)*
Patients with preoperative anticoagulant therapy	10	174 ± 25	314 ± 35	69 ± 12	114 ± 10	23	123 ± 27	269 ± 22	65 ± 11	123 ± 12
Control group	118	192 ± 10	348 ± 15	69 ± 3	120 ± 4	115	129 ± 11	281 ± 16	72 ± 7	130 ± 5

* *See Table 13.4*

blood flow commonly associated with extracorporeal circulation. The intravascular coagulation thus induced results in consumption of factors V, VIII and fibrinogen with consequent reduction in their blood levels. Intravascular coagulation in turn promotes the action of plasminogen activators, which convert plasminogen to the fibrinolytic enzyme plasmin. A full defibrination syndrome may occasionally be established with continued thromboplastic production, disseminated intravascular coagulation and activation of fibrinolytic systems[9,10,13,22,33]. In addition, depletion of certain coagulation factors, such as factor IX, may occur due to protein denaturation as a result of trauma to the liquid constituents of the blood at the blood-gas interface during oxygenation[22,26,36]. The effects of the blood coagulation are further influenced by certain measures commonly undertaken as an integral part of cardiopulmonary bypass. Heparin, if administered in insufficient amounts, facilitates the development of intravascular coagulation and consumptive coagulopathy and when inadequately neutralized with protamine sulphate would cause excessive bleeding by its direct action. Protamine sulphate on the other hand, if given in excess, has an anticoagulant effect[36]. Based upon the consideration of the need for accurate neutralization of heparin, protamine titration has been advocated[36]. Old, stored blood, being more vulnerable to trauma[39], is liable to initiate intravascular coagulation when used during cardiopulmonary bypass. As it is deficient in factors V, VIII and platelets[16,41], when infused in large amounts it may dilute the blood levels of these clotting factors and aggravate the haemorrhage.

Besides the haematological derangements produced during cardiopulmonary bypass, some patients may have pre-existing bleeding diathesis. It is recognized that patients with cyanotic congenital heart disease and secondary polycythaemia have a propensity to increased postoperative haemorrhage because of associated thrombocytopenia, impaired clot retraction and hypofibrinogenaemia[17,21]. Patients with acquired heart disease may also have coagulation abnormalities due to depressed liver function as a result of chronic hepatic congestion[22]. In addition to the coagulation abnormalities, capillary damage from hypoxaemia due to disturbances in the microcirculation following hypotension, inadequate perfusion flow and corpuscular aggregation during cardiopulmonary bypass may be an important factor which would elude detection by known laboratory procedures[23]. Difficulties in ascertaining the influence of various aspects of surgical procedures on postoperative blood loss stem from the fact that the variables are multitudinous and often interrelated[17].

In order to maintain homogeneity and to ensure valid comparisons of the effects of different aspects of cardiopulmonary bypass on postoperative blood loss amongst the various groups, associated relevant factors were taken into consideration in this study as far as possible. Data obtained for the analysis were from those patients who underwent heart valve surgery for acquired valve disease. The cases with congenital heart disease and ischaemic heart disease (with revascularization procedures) in the absence of valvular disease were excluded. None of the patients in the study had preoperative coagulation abnormalities, as indicated by normal bleeding, clotting and prothrombin times and normal platelet counts. The operations were performed in all patients using a standard midsternal incision and the methods of administration of heparin and its neutralization with protamine sulphate were uniform throughout the series. Data on postoperative blood loss following different heart valve operations were compared and shown to be similar. The groups for subsequent analysis were therefore considered homogeneous in these respects.

In the evaluation of the influences of different types of oxygenators on postoperative haemorrhage the nature of the priming solutions used and the duration of cardiopulmonary bypass were taken into account. Although observed blood loss in the groups that underwent operations with the Melrose and Kay–Cross disc oxygenators was higher than in those employing Travenol, Temptrol and Shiley bubble oxygenators, when the results were further analysed with comparable perfusion durations and type of priming solutions used, no significant difference in blood loss could be demonstrated between the groups using the disc and the bubble oxygenator. There was, however, a slight difference in favour of the Shiley oxygenator. Assuming that blood trauma is the major determinant of postoperative haemorrhage, this was not an altogether unexpected finding. Lee *et al.*[26] in their experimental studies observed no significant differences in denaturation of plasma proteins using disc, bubble and screen oxygenators. Anderson and Kuchiba[1] by using the rates of haemolysis and platelet loss as indices of blood trauma found the Temptrol, Travenol U310 and Rygg bubble oxygenators to be less traumatic to the blood than the disc oxygenators, while the Travenol 6LF oxygenator gave varying results, producing the highest as well as the lowest blood trauma. The results with the Travenol 6LF oxygenator were influenced by the variation of oxygen flow and the degree of turbulence occurring in the individual oxygenator. The Travenol 6LF type of bubble oxygenator used in our series and the postoperative blood loss following its use was similar to that occurring with the use of the Temptrol oxygenator. Although the Shiley oxygenator has been used more recently and therefore the results are not strictly comparable, the postoperative blood loss resulting from its use was slightly lower than that observed with the other bubble oxygenators.

The nature of the priming solutions on the other hand appears to play a more important role in determining postoperative blood loss. In the present study the use of non-haemic prime in the Travenol oxygenator group produced a lower postoperative blood loss when compared with the haemodilution group using the same type of oxygenator and comparable perfusion durations. Similar conclusions were reached in the studies of Moffitt *et al.*[31] who compared the effects of whole blood and haemodilution priming of the vertical screen oxygenator with the clear prime (with 5 per cent dextrose) of the bubble oxygenator. Cooley, Beall and Grondin[5] in their clinical and experimental studies used 5 per cent dextrose in water as the priming solution in bubble oxygenators. They concluded that this method was superior to the use of blood prime so far as postoperative bleeding and cerebral, renal and pulmonary complications were concerned, besides being technically simpler to operate. Studies on the effects of using 5 per cent dextrose in water for definitive priming of the heart-lung machine have shown normal blood clotting at the end of the operation with no significant alteration of coagulation[11]. The reasons for improved results with non-haemic prime may be related to the omission of stored blood which is commonly used in haemodilution prime and also to the fact that clear prime reduces the haematocrit and blood vsicosity, improves capillary blood flow and reduces the propensity to intravascular coagulation and sludging of corpuscles[18].

Besides the use of non-haemic prime, concurrent additional measures which appeared to have contributed to the reduction of the amount of postoperative blood loss in these groups of patients in our study was the use of flesh blood instead of stored blood at the end of cardiopulmonary bypass. The beneficial effect of fresh blood is probably due to its normal content of factors V, VIII and viable platelets which become depleted during the cardiopulmonary bypass and which stored blood fails to restore.

Following the use of low molecular weight dextran in the priming for extracorporeal circulation there has been a reported increase in postoperative haemorrhage[19,20], which might be attributable to its heparin-potentiating effect[2] and its property of decreasing intravascular aggregation of blood cells and increasing the fluidity of blood[12]. The experience has, however, not been uniform[28,37]. In the present study when low molecular weight dextran was used for haemodilution prime, postoperative blood loss, although comparatively higher, was not statistically significant.

In our previous study[11], where haemodilution prime was used in the majority of the patients, postoperative haemorrhage was significantly higher with perfusion durations longer than 90 minutes. As shown in the present analysis the correlation did not seem to hold true up to 120 minutes of perfusion duration when non-haemic prime was utilized. The apparent discrepancy may be explained on the basis of increased vulnerability to trauma of the stored blood invariably utilized for haemodilution prime.

After open-heart surgery 20 to 65 per cent depletion of platelets occurs which may persist up to a week after the operation. This has been attributed to the loss of platelets by destruction, by adhesion to the components of the extracorporeal circuit, by heparinization, by platelet sequestration and by transfusion of large volumes of blood with damaged or non-viable platelets[7,9,10,22,29,35]. The postoperative platelet count correlates well with postoperative haemorrhage. In the present series a significantly higher blood loss was observed when the platelet count was below 100 000 per cubic millimetre. However, platelet deficiency represents only one aspect of clotting abnormalities induced by cardiopulmonary bypass and it is uncertain whether infusion of platelet concentrates reduces the bleeding diathesis. Woods *et al.*[43] compared postoperative blood loss between a control group and a group receiving platelet concentrates. The blood loss was not significantly different in the two groups except for the cyanotic patients who had less bleeding following infusion of platelet concentrates. The favourable results obtained in our patients who received transfusions of fresh blood indicate that the restoration of the associated deficiencies of the other factors involved in the coagulation process[14,36] are of equal importance.

In the control of postoperative haemorrhage the role of EACA, which inhibits plasminogen activators, remains controversial. Gans and Krivit[9] in a matched series of patients, found decreased fibrinolytic activity in the group pretreated with EACA and observed marked reduction in bleeding in a few instances following administration of this drug. Beall *et al.*[3] on the other hand did not find evidence of fibrinolysis in the majority of the patients who had undergone cardiopulmonary bypass, although the presence of plasminogen activators was observed. Midell *et al.*[30] reported a significant reduction in postoperative blood loss by prophylactic administration of EACA. Deysine and Clifton[6] found it useful in the majority of patients with severe postoperative haemorrhage, although laboratory evidence of fibrinolysis was lacking in most of the cases. In the present series the beneficial effects of EACA were however not apparent as has also been reported by others[17].

Previous anticoagulant therapy was not associated with an increase in the postoperative bleeding in this study. This was probably related to the policy of withdrawal of long-acting anticoagulants 3 to 5 days before the operation so that the pharmacological action of these drugs was not evident at the time of surgery.

In the assessment of postoperative haemorrhage the 'manner of surgery'[14, 17] has to be taken into account and is the most difficult factor to standardize. Besides the consideration of the types of patients, methods of extracorporeal circulation employed, the length and trauma of the procedures, the use of blood and blood substitutes and the use of anticoagulants and haemostatic agents, the surgeon's approach to meticulous haemostasis still remains the most essential single measure in reducing postoperative blood loss. This aspect became apparent in our study of three groups of patients analysed in chronological sequence between December 1971 and August 1973. During this period, although other variables were more or less constant, a progressive reduction in postoperative blood loss was observed due to particular attention being paid to haemostasis in a conscious attempt to minimize postoperative haemorrhage. The important points raised by this observation are the limitations of this and other similar clinical studies. The analysis and conclusions of the clinical correlates of postoperative blood loss are therefore to be viewed in this perspective. It seems, nevertheless, that the change from haemodilution prime and the use of old banked blood to non-haemic prime and transfusion of only flesh blood has resulted in significantly reduced postoperative blood loss in recent years. The use of different oxygenators on the other hand has not had a significant influence. The duration of cardiopulmonary bypass beyond 90 minutes has been an important factor contributing to increased postoperative bleeding when haemodilution prime was employed. With the recent use of non-haemic prime a perfusion duration of up to 120 minutes has not been associated with a significantly greater blood loss. Postoperative platelet count below 100 0000 per cubic millimetre correlated with increased propensity to bleeding. No correlation was however observed between postoperative haemorrhage and either the type of valve surgery performed or the use of preoperative anticoagulants. The prophylactic use of EACA produced paradoxical results, although the blood loss was not significantly higher than in the control group.

Conclusion

The evolution of techniques for the artificial maintenance of circulation and respiration over the past 20 years has followed the general line of development seen in many other fields of scientific advancement. Improved knowledge and understanding of biological phenomena have created the instruments and apparatus for the practical application of the newly acquired information. As soon as the need for large scale, routine use of a particular technique arose, the necessity for simplification became apparent.

In the field of extracorporeal circulation the evolution has been from complex to simple, from the electronically controlled, automatic Gibbon–Mayo heart-lung machine towards the simple, disposable bubble oxygenator. Similarly, from whole blood supplemented with human albumin, the ingredients for priming the heart-lung machine have evolved towards haemodilution and finally to complete non-haemic, clear solutions for adult perfusions. The simplification and standardization of techniques and procedures for extracorporeal circulation have been followed by improved results and by a wider application of these techniques to other medical fields than open-heart surgery.

The improvement during the past few years in postoperative blood loss following intracardiac surgery with the aid of a heart-lung machine is such an example.

The use of simple, low-volume oxygenators has allowed the utilization of complete non-haemic prime which has contributed to the reduction in postoperative blood loss. This in itself has reduced the amount of blood required for postoperative transfusion and consequently fresh blood could be obtained for routine open-heart surgery. As evidenced in this study, the two factors which have influenced significantly the amount of postoperative blood loss have been the use of non-haemic prime during the extracorporeal circulation and the transfusion of fresh blood after the operation.

References

1. Anderson, M. N. and Kuchiba, K. 'Blood trauma produced by pump oxygenators.' *Journal of Thoracic and Cardiovascular Surgery*, **57,** 238 (1969)
2. Atik, M. 'Dextrans, their use in surgery and medicine.' *Anaesthesiology*, **27,** 425 (1966)
3. Beall, A. C., Jr., Strawn, J. R. Tillerty, W. V. and Cooley, D. A. 'Effects of extracorporeal circulation on fibrinolytic activity in man.' *Clinical Research*, **14,** 238 (1966)
4. Burn, H. F. and Jandl, J. D. 'Control of haemoglobin function within the red cell.' *New England Journal of Medicine*, **282,** 1414 (1970)
5. Cooley, D. A., Beall, A. C., Jr. and Grondin, P. 'Open-heart operations with disposable oxygenators, 5 per cent dextrose prime, and normothermia.' *Surgery*, **52,** 713 (1962)
6. Deysine, M. and Clifton, E. E. 'Mechanism of action of epsilon aminocaproic acid in the control of haemorrhage.' *Annals of the New York Academy of Science*, **115,** 291 (1964)

7. Gadboys, H. L., Slonim, R. and Litwak, R. S. 'Homologous blood syndrome. I. Preliminary observations on its relationship to clinical cardiopulmonary bypass.' *Annals of Surgery*, **156,** 793 (1962)
8. Galletti, P. M. and Brecher, G. A. *Heart Lung Bypass*. Ch. XVII, p. 264, New York: Grune and Stratton, Inc. (1962)
9. Gans, H. and Krivit, W. 'Problems in haemostasis during and after open-heart surgery. VI. Overall changes in blood coagulation mechanism.' *Journal of the American Medical Association*, **179,** 145 (1962)
10. Gans, H. and Krivit, W. 'Problems in haemostasis during open-heart surgery. IV. On the changes in blood clotting mechanism during cardiopulmonary bypass procedures.' *Annals of Surgery*, **155,** 353 (1962)
11. Garcia, J. B., Pakrashi, B. C., Mary, D. A., Tandon, A. P. and Ionescu, M. I. 'Postoperative blood loss after extracorporeal circulation for heart valve surgery.' *Journal of Thoracic and Cardiovascular Surgery*, **65,** 487 (1973)
12. Garzon, A. A., Fink, L. H., Sheffano, G. W. and Karlson, K. E. 'Blood loss associated with low molecular weight dextran.' *Journal of Thoracic and Caradiovascular Surgery*, **48,** 873 (1964)
13. Gibbon, J., Jr. and Camishion, R. C. 'Problems in haemostasis with extracorporeal apparatus.' *Annals of the New York Academy of Science*, **115**, 195 (1964)
14. Gollub, S. 'Unexplained bleeding in cardiothoracic operations.' *Annals of the New York Academy of Science*, **115,** 199 (1964)
15. Gollub, S. 'Variables affecting haemostasis in cardiopulmonary bypass.' *Annals of the New York Academy of Science*, **115,** 278 (1964)
16. Goldstein, R., Bunker, J. P. and McGovern, J. J. 'The effect of storage of whole blood and anticoagulants upon coagulation factors.' *Annals of the New York Academy of Science*, **115,** 195 (1964)
17. Gomes, M. R. and McGoon, D. C. 'Bleeding patterns after open-heart surgery.' *Journal of Thoracic and Cardiovascular Surgery*, **60,** 87 (1970)
18. Haraway, R. M., III. *Syndrome of Disseminated Intravascular Coagulation*, Ch. 16, p. 333. Springfield: Thomas (1966)
19. Hellstrom, G. and Björk, V. O. 'Haemodilution with rheomacrodex total body perfusion.' *Journal of Thoracic and Cardiovascular Surgery*, **45,** 395 (1963)
20. Hara, M., Maris, M., Crumpler, J., Corn, B. and Perkins, W. H. 'Effect of various priming solutions upon red cell mass, plasma volume, and extracellular fluid volume of dogs following haemodilution technique of extracorporeal circulation.' *Journal of Thoracic and Cardiovascular Surgery*, **53,** 354 (1967)
21. Jackson, D. P. 'Haemorrhagic diathesis in patients with cyanotic congenital heart disease: preoperative management.' *Annals of the New York Academy of Science*, **115,** 235 (1964)
22. Kendall, A. G. and Lowenstein, L. 'Alterations in blood coagulation and haemostasis during extracorporeal circulation. Part I.' *Canadian Medical Association Journal*, **87,** 786 (1962)
23. Kendall, A. G. and Lowenstein, L. 'Alterations in blood coagulation and haemostasis during extracorporeal circulation. Part II.' *Canadian Medical Association Journal*, **87,** 859 (1962)
24. Kissmeyer-Nielson, F. and Madsen, C. H. 'Platelets in blood stored in untreated and siliconized glass bottles and plastic bags.' *Journal of Clinical Pathology*, **14,** 626 (1961)
25. Laufman, H. and Erichson, R. B. *Haematological Problems in Surgery*. Philadelphia: W. B. Saunders (1970)
26. Lee, W. H., Jr., Krumharr, D., Fonkalsrud, E. W., Schjeide, O. A. and Maloney, J. F., Jr. 'Denaturation of plasma proteins as a cause of morbidity and death after intracardiac operation.' *Surgery*, **50,** 29 (1961)

27. Leveen, H. M., Schatman, B. and Falk, G. 'Cardiac arrest produced by massive transfusions.' *Surgery, Gynecology and Obstetrics*, **109,** 502, (1959)
28. Long, D. M., Sanchez, L., Varco, R. L. and Lillehei, C. W. 'The use of low-molecular-weight dextran and serum albumin as plasma expanders in extracorporeal circulation.' *Surgery*, **50,** 12 (1961)
29. McKenzie, F. N., Dhall, D. P., Arfords, K. E., Norlund, S. and Matheson, N. A. 'Blood platelet behaviour during and after open-heart surgery.' *British Medical Journal*, **2,** 795 (1969)
30. Midell, A. I., Grady, L. H., Bloodwell, R. D., Beall, A. C., Yasher, J. J. and Cooley, D. A. 'Epsilon aminocaproic acid for bleeding after cardiopulmonary bypass.' *Annals of Thoracic Surgery*, **11,** 577 (1971)
31. Moffitt, E. A., White, R. D., Molnar, G. D. and McGoon, D. C. 'Comparative effects of whole blood, haemodiluted and clear priming solutions on myocardial and body metabolism in man.' *Canadian Journal of Surgery*, **14,** 382 (1971)
32. Neville, W. E., Maben, H., Colby, C. and Peacock, H. 'Total prime of the large volume disc oxygenator.' *Annals of Thoracic Surgery*, **1,** 575 (1965)
33. Nilsson, I. M., and Swederg, J. 'Coagulation studies in cardiac surgery with extracorporeal circulation using a bubble oxygenator.' *Acta chirurgica Scandinavica*, **117,** 47 (1959)
34. Peirce, E. C., II. *Extracorporeal Circulation for Open-Heart Surgery*, Ch. 4, p. 47. Springfield: Thomas (1969)
35. Perkins, H. A., Osborn, J. J. and Gerbode, F. 'The effect of heparin on the platelet count *in vitro*.' *American Journal of Clinical Pathology*, **30,** 397 (1958)
36. Perkins, H. A., Osborn, J. J. and Gerbode, F. 'The management of abnormal bleeding following extracorporeal circulation.' *Annals of Internal Medicine*, **51,** 658 (1959)
37. Raison, J. C. A. 'Report of the use of low-molecular-weight dextran in a rotating oxygenator.' *Thorax*, **17,** 338 (1962)
38. Roesler, M. F., Bull, C. and Ionescu, M. I. 'Clinical and laboratory evaluation of the Shiley S-100A oxygenator heat exchanger.' *Journal of Cardiovascular Surgery*, **21,** 271 (1980)
39. Rothnie, N. G., Norman, A. G., Steele, M. and Kinmonth, J. B. 'Changes in blood coagulation due to perfusion for cardiac surgery', *British Journal of Surgery*, **48,** 272 (1960)
40. Salzman, E. and Britten, A. F. H. *Haemorrhage and Thrombosis*. Boston: Little, Brown and Co. (1965)
41. Strumia, M. M. and Strumia, P. V. 'Alterations in banked blood, with special reference to haemostasis.' *Annals of the New York Academy of Science*, **115,** 443 (1964)
42. Wintrob, M. M. *Clinical Hematology* (6th edn). Philadelphia: Lea and Febiger (1967)
43. Woods, J. E., Taswell, H. F., Kirklin, J. W. and Owen, C. A. 'The transfusion of platelet concentrates in patients undergoing open-heart surgery.' *Mayo Clinic Proceedings*, **42,** 318 (1967)
44. Zuhdi, N., Carey, J. M. and Greer, A. E. 'Haemodilution and coagulation factors in extracorporeal circulation.' *Journal of Thoracic and Cardiovascular Surgery*, **43,** 816 (1962)

14

Haematological Aspects of Extracorporeal Circulation

Marc R. de Leval, J. Donald Hill and
C. Harold Mielke

acu rem tetigisti

Introduction

Denaturation of blood remains one of the major factors limiting the development of improved techniques of extracorporeal circulation. Besides the deleterious effects of the pump oxygenators, other factors, such as the nature of the solutions used to prime the extracorporeal circuit, massive blood transfusion, administration of heparin and its neutralization after bypass, account for the haematological problems encountered during and after extracorporeal circulation. The most immediate consequence of these disturbances is postoperative haemorrhage. The mechanisms responsible for postoperative haemorrhage will be considered in the present chapter. The particular problems related to longterm extracorporeal circulation, as well as the role of microemboli and their removal by blood filtration, will also be discussed.

Haematological effects of extracorporeal circulation for open-heart surgery

Although many patients have a normal clotting mechanism before surgery[68], postoperative bleeding is a threat in all open-heart operations. As Salzman and Britten[59] pointed out, the magnitude of the defect in particular components of the haemostatic mechanism correlates poorly with the severity of the haemorrhagic syndrome observed. A patient may have severe postoperative haemorrhage while laboratory measurements of haemostasis demonstrate only mild abnormalities. This situation is quite different from other haemorrhagic diseases in which a specific deficiency state can be identified, the correction of which is associated with a return of normal haemostasis.

Pump prime and massive blood transfusion

The nature of the perfusate varies greatly from institution to institution. Currently, either partial or total haemodilution is being used by most surgeons. Balanced electrolyte solutions with an antacid (bicarbonate, lactate or Tris buffer*) constitute the usual basis of the priming volume. The addition of low molecular weight dextran or other solutions such as mannitol is less often used. It has been demonstrated in dog experiments that haemodilution does not produce serious haematological derangements[30]. On the contrary, haemodilution appears to be beneficial since it saves blood, reduces the viscosity of the blood and improves the microcirculation, reduces the haemolysis[55], seems to preserve the blood-clotting mechanisms[55], and decreases the postoperative bleeding[50].

Total haemodilution without any blood replacement is sometimes used in patients of a religious group[27]. However, a rapid loss of the diluent from the vascular compartment with a progressive reduction in blood volume can decrease the venous return[49], overload the body and cause transient

* THAM, Tris, Trihydroxymethylaminomethane

neurological disturbances[57]. On the other hand, even if total haemodilution is used for the bypass and if all the pump perfusate is reinfused after the termination of perfusion[15], some blood loss is inevitable until after protamine has been administered. Therefore, most patients who undergo open-heart surgery require several units of blood, and the necessity of infusing large volumes of blood to cope with unexpected blood losses and bleeding problems is an inherent danger of this type of surgery.

For adult patients it is not necessary to prime the extracorporeal circuit with fresh blood[9]. Stored blood in acid-citrate-dextrose (ACD) which is heparinized and recalcified is widely used. In infants whose liver capacity to handle a load of citrate is limited[62] and where the blood volume is but a small fraction of the pump–patient circulation, one prefers to prime with fresh heparinized blood whenever it is possible.

Massive transfusion of ACD blood used as priming volume or to restore the blood volume after bypass is a common situation the heart surgeon has to deal with during the postoperative period. Several metabolic and haematological problems can be related to the composition of that stored blood: each unit of blood contains 120 ml of acid-citrate-dextrose anticoagulant solution. In spite of the body's capacity for prompt metabolism of citrate, the rapid administration of large volumes of citrated blood can reduce the circulating level of ionized calcium. In some cases the calculated value may fall below 0.5 mmol/ℓ, a level incompatible with myocardial activity[59]. A good prophylactic measure is the administration of 10 ml of 10 mg/ml calcium gluconate or of calcium chloride for each 2.5 litres of blood transfused. The pH of the blood collected in ACD falls immediately to 6.9–7.1. Anaerobic glycolysis continues to take place in the blood cells which may reduce the pH to as low as 6.5 after 21 days' storage[69]. Infusion of such blood can can lead to metabolic acidosis especially if the patient is already poorly perfused. Howland Schweizer and Boyan[36] suggested the administration of sodium bicarbonate when large amounts of blood are transfused. After several hours, the acidosis may be replaced by a metabolic alkalosis due to metabolism of the citrate with a resultant excess of sodium ions (16 mmol in 500 ml of ACD blood[47]). The alkalosis reaches its peak on the third post-transfusion day[44]. The potassium concentration increases gradually in stored blood and may reach 25 mmol/ℓ in 15 days. This appears to follow a failure of active transport mechanisms in the erythrocyte membrane and is not the result of haemolysis[46]. Since blood is being stored at 4°C, rapid transfusion of large amounts of cold blood may lower the body temperature.

Haematological alterations of ACD blood should also be considered. The erythrocytes survive storage fairly well with the average life being approximately 75 per cent of normal[44]. However, the capacity of red cells to release oxygen deteriorates with storage by losing 2,3-DPG (diphosphoglycerate)[10]. Within 48 hours, 5 per cent of the segmented leukocytes disappear and platelet survival is drastically reduced in blood stored more than 48 hours at 4°C in ACD solution[41]. Thrombocytopaenia can be expected in all patients who receive more than 8 units of ACD blood in a short period of time[71] and the frequency of bleeding rises as the transfused volume increases[42]. In practice, 1 unit of blood less than 24 hours old should be given with each 2 to 4 units of older bank blood if the total transfused volume is likely to exceed 8 units in order to supply the patient with viable platelets[59]. Stored blood is also deficient in the more labile clotting factors: factor V and factor VIII. A deficiency in these factors may be expected in patients whose blood volume has been replaced with bank blood.

In order to save blood and to avoid the side-effects of massive transfusions, several surgeons reinfuse the pump perfusate into the patient at the end of the bypass or even during the postoperative period[67].

Alterations of the blood in the extracorporeal circuit

As it circulates in the extracorporeal circuit, the blood is subjected to an abnormal physical and chemical environment. The blood trauma includes both cell and plasma denaturation.

Damage to the red cells

The haemolytic index, which is the amount of haemoglobin released by a pump into the plasma, and the trauma index, which is the amount of haemoglobin released by a pump performing a fixed number of strokes, have been defined to assess the deleterious effects of the pumps. Significant haemolysis can also occur in the oxygenators especially where large surface tension forces develop between the gas bubbles and the red cells. Membrane oxygenators have greatly reduced the amount of haemolysis. Levels of free haemoglobin as low as 20 mg/100 ml were observed after 9 days of perfusion at a flow rate of 3 to 4 litres/minute using the Bramson membrane oxygenator. The amount of free haemoglobin reached during the actual perfusion is moderated by the ability of the patient to remove it. Normally the retriculoendothelial system is able to remove approximately 0.1 mg haemoglobin/kg per minute (more or less 5 mg/100 ml per hour of haemoglobin for an adult patient[5]). Haemoglobinuria due to filtration of haemoglobin by the kidneys occurs when the plasma level rises above 100 mg/100 ml but the actual renal damage is probably produced only when very high levels, in the order of 3000 mg/100 ml or more, are reached[11].

Several bio-engineering studies have been carried out in relation to the factors influencing erythrocyte destruction in artificial organs. Bernstein *et al.*[5,6] demonstrated the haemolytic effect of the shear forces resulting from sudden dimensional changes in tubing and cannulae and from the jet forces at velocities of 2000 cm/second. According to Blackshear, Dorman and Steinback[7], shear stresses must reach the level of 10^4 dynes/cm^2 to induce significant lysis. More recently, it was pointed out that haemolytic mechanisms are mostly surface related[64]. Negative pressures also produce haemolysis when they fall below one-third atmosphere[5,6].

Besides immediate lysis of red cells, perfusion leads to increased mechanical cell fragility[21]. Postperfusion anaemia[43] and shortened red blood cell life[38] are both related to delayed haemolysis. According to Bernstein *et al.*[6], the sublethal trauma is more important than the immediate haemolysis; for each red cell lysed, 500 cells would be altered. The magnitude of delayed haemolysis in the first 24 hours after perfusion may be 5 times that of the immediate haemolysis. This haemolysis in paralleled by a rise of plasma lactic dehydrogenase (LDH) released from the red cells[5].

Damage to the leukocytes

There is little data available on the effect of extracorporeal circulation on white cells. In general, the leukocytes decrease with the onset of perfusion and rise as the perfusion is prolonged more than 1 or 2 hours. Subsequently, leukocytosis occurs and persists in the absence of infection for over a week[44].

Damage to the platelets

The decrease in platelet count during cardiopulmonary bypass is well documented. However, the mechanisms responsible for this are not clearly defined. We have studied various aetiological factors considered to be responsible for the reduction as well as for the return towards normal of the number of platelets in a simple reproducible model of venoarterial bypass in dogs[14]. Transfusions of ^{51}Cr-labelled platelets prior to instituting bypass made it possible to follow the same blood elements during and after the perfusion.

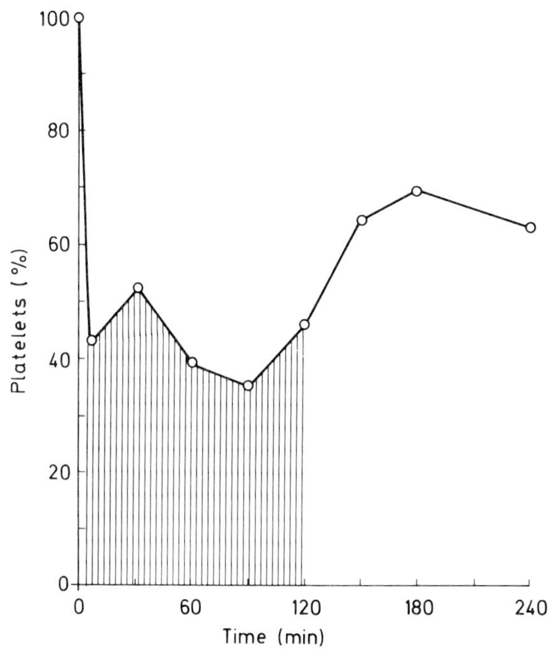

Figure 14.1 Platelet count during and after a 2-hour partial bypass using the Temptrol bubble oxygenator. (From de Leval *et al.*[14] by courtesy of *Transactions of the American Society for Artificial Internal Organs*)

These experiments have shown that 60 to 70 per cent of the circulating platelets disappear as soon as the bypass starts (*Figure 14.1*). The level then stabilizes or slightly decreases. After perfusion, the platelet count rises in 2 hours to reach a plateau, the level of which depends on the conditions of the experiment. The fact that the curves of the radioactivity of the blood parallel the curves of the platelet counts (*Figure 14.2*) indicates a reversible sequestration of the platelets during extracorporeal circulation. Measuring

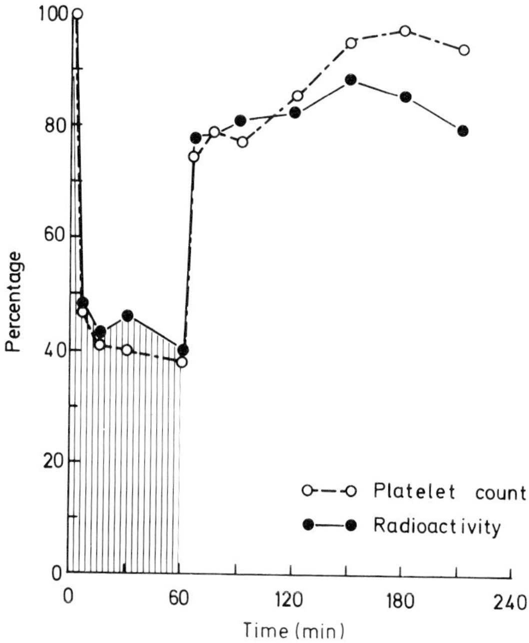

Figure 14.2 Parallelism of the radioactivity curve (platelet radioactivity) and the platelet count during and after a 1-hour partial bypass using the Bramson membrane oxygenator. These data indicate that the same platelets disappear and come back in the circulation. (From de Leval *et al.*[14] by courtesy of *Transactions of the American Society for Artificial Internal Organs*)

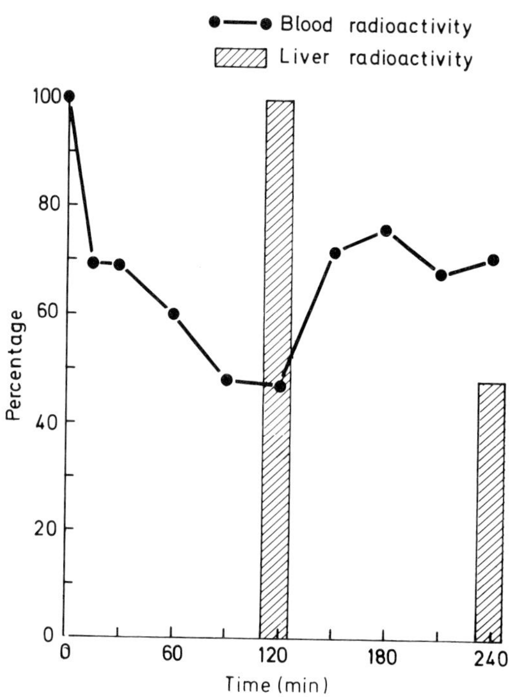

Figure 14.3 Blood radioactivity and liver radioactivity during and after a 2-hour partial bypass. A high liver radioactivity corresponds to a low blood radioactivity at the end of the bypass. Two hours later, more than 50 per cent of the liver radioactivity disappeared while the blood radioactivity had increased

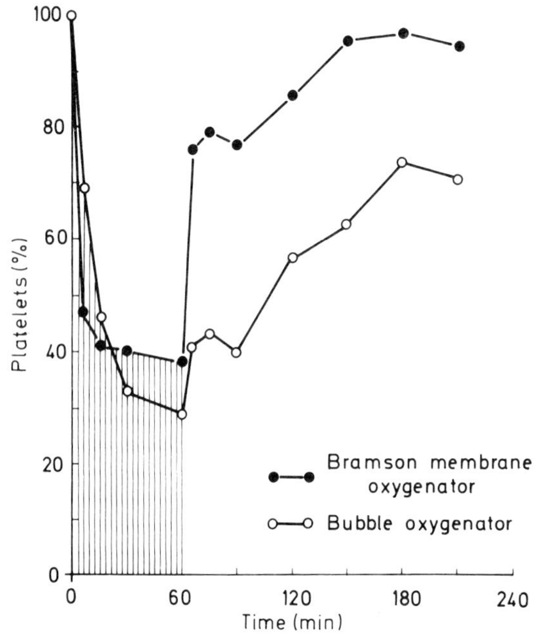

Figure 14.4 Comparison of the effect of the Bramson membrane oxygenator and Temptrol bubble oxygenator on the platelets during and after a 2-hour partial bypass (From de Leval *et al.*[14], by courtesy of *Transactions of the American Society for Artificial Internal Organs*)

organ radioactivity we demonstrated that a reversible sequestration of platelets occurs in the liver (*Figure 14.3*). In addition to this reversible sequestration there is also a permanent platelet loss indicated by the difference between platelet counts pre-bypass and 2 hours post-bypass. As illustrated in *Figure 14.4*, the platelet loss after a 2 hour bypass is minimal (± 5 per cent) with the Bramson membrane oxygenator and reaches 30 per cent with a bubble oxygenator. The use of the cardiotomy suction further decreases the platelet count as indicated in *Figure 14.5*, where the effects of the pump, the bubble oxygenator and the cardiotomy suction are compared. Blood-gas interface seems, therefore, to be responsible for the damage.

We have also found a decrease in platelet adhesiveness and aggregation during extracorporeal circulation. These changes return to normal within 2 hours after the bypass. The life span of these platelets measured by radioactive technique is normal. These findings indicate that the platelets are submitted to an all-or-none process during extracorporeal circulation. These observations differentiate the reactivity of the platelets and the red cells, the latter being subjected to lethal and sublethal damage.

Because platelets influenced by the extracorporeal circulation disappear into the body where they seem to recover before they return to the circulation, the importance of *in vivo* studies is enhanced. The spontaneous reversibility of some of the changes encountered has to be kept in mind when new drugs such as antiaggregating agents are evaluated.

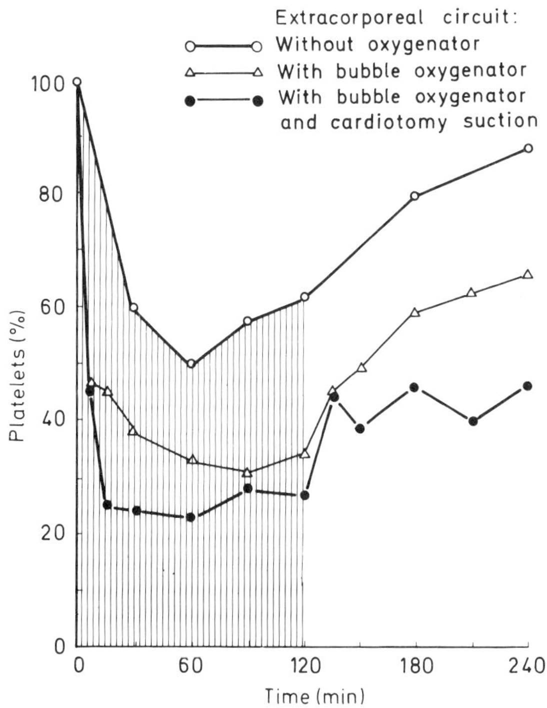

Figure 14.5 Comparison of the effects of the pump, the bubble oxygenator and the cardiotomy suction on the platelets during a 2-hour bypass. (From de Leval *et al.*[14], by courtesy of *Transactions of the American Society for Artificial Internal Organs*)

Alterations in coagulation and fibrinolytic systems

Interpretation of coagulation tests during and after extracorporeal circulation is complicated by the use of heparin and protamine and by the great variations in the nature of the priming volume and the amount or age of blood transfused. A patient receiving bank blood equal to 1 blood volume has only 34 – 40 per cent of his own blood left for clotting and after 2 replacement transfusions, he is left with about 13 per cent of his own blood[61]. The impact that this has upon the clotting mechanism becomes increasingly apparent since normal haemostasis requires a minimum blood content of approximately 20 per cent of any clotting factor[44].

Preoperative coagulation disorders should also be considered. Children with cyanotic congenital disease not infrequently display haemostatic defects[18]. Defective clot retraction, prolonged bleeding time, prolonged prothrombin time, prolonged partial thromboplastin time or thromboplastin generating time, hypofibrinogenaemia and accelerated fibrinolysis have all been noted.

Congestive hepatic dysfunction can also account for mild coagulation defects producing a prolonged prothrombin time in some cardiac patients. Although their liver disease may impair their ability to restore depleted clotting factors after bypass, these patients do not seem to bleed excessively[59]. They appear analogous to patients who are receiving oral anticoagulants, in whom it is not necessary to correct the drug-induced haemostatic abnormality before surgery if the prothrombin activity is over 25 per cent. Besides, they receive an exchange transfusion during the extracorporal perfusion, which tends to correct the abnormality[59].

A reduction in factor I (fibrinogen), factor II (prothrombin), factor V (proaccelerin) and factor VIII (antihaemophilic globulin) are usual findings after open-heart surgery[70].

Factor V and VIII deficiency and decrease in fibrinogen associated with thrombocytopaenia are consistent with a consumption coagulopathy. However, the thrombocytopaenia is mainly due to a platelet sequestration and destruction[14] and the administration of heparin during the bypass inhibits or limits the development of the disseminated intravascular coagulation (DIC) syndrome[29].

Activation of the fibrinolytic system during extracorporeal circulation is well documented[51,25]. The generation of plasmin is accompanied by a non-competitive binding of plasmin by antiplasmin[17]. Because the reserve of antiplasmin is not completely exhausted during bypass[19], this would explain why major haemorrhagic complications due to fibrinolysis are rather rare after open-heart surgery. According to the same authors, the preoperative antiplasmin level would be the critical factor which determines whether the activation of the fibrinolytic mechanism will result in haemostatic failure.

Neutralization of heparin by protamine is widely used to achieve adequate haemostasis at the conclusion of cardiopulmonary bypass[37]. The initial dose of heparin usually employed varies between 200 and 400 units/kg and 100 units or more/kg per hour are subsequently added. The correct dose of protamine has been difficult to estimate clinically and has been reported from 0.75 to 4 times the total dose of heparin[37,41]. Recurrence of bleeding after the administration of protamine has been frequently reported. Various reasons have been given for the cause of this 'heparin rebound'. A secondary rise of free heparin after its initial neutralization has been suggested[11]; however, an insufficient dose of protamine would most likely be the cause[56]. Protamine itself acts as an anticoagulant. When it is administered alone (3 mg/kg) it will prolong the clotting time threefold[1]. Protamine acts as an antithromboplastin producing a deficiency in factor VIII, a decrease in fibrinogen and in platelets[23]. Fortunately, the anticoagulant effects depend on the concentration of protamine in excess of heparin[60]. However, some findings suggest that the cause of post-bypass bleeding could be related to intravascular coagulation which follows the neutralization of heparin[24]. According to these authors, during cardiopulmonary bypass, in the absence of clotting, the extent of fibrinolysis appears to be negligible. In the presence of clotting, fibrin is broken down to a variable degree with a release of fibrin split products which can exert marked anticoagulant activity. Such bleeding could be prevented by the administration of an antiproteinase but at the expense of the development of a hypercoagulable state. The latter might be responsible for an increased tendency towards thrombus formation[24] and be harmful for the patient.

Besides its haematological effects, protamine has cardiovascular effects including a systemic arterial hypotension, a reduction of myocardial contractility, d*p*/d*t*, left ventricular pressure and cardiac output[26]. Adequate transfusion[28] and slow infusion of the protamine obviates these side-effects.

Haematological effects of prolonged extracorporeal circulation

The development of membrane oxygenators for prolonged periods of assisted circulation has re-emphasized the importance of blood trauma in the pump oxygenators. Although acute thrombosis in the membrane oxygenators appears to be a major problem[20] we have never seen thrombogenesis in the Bramson membrane oxygenator which we used in 15 patients with respiratory insufficiency[33]. The potential for internal and external bleeding has been the principal risk of clinical prolonged extracorporeal oxygenation. Anticoagulation of the patient, alteration of platelets

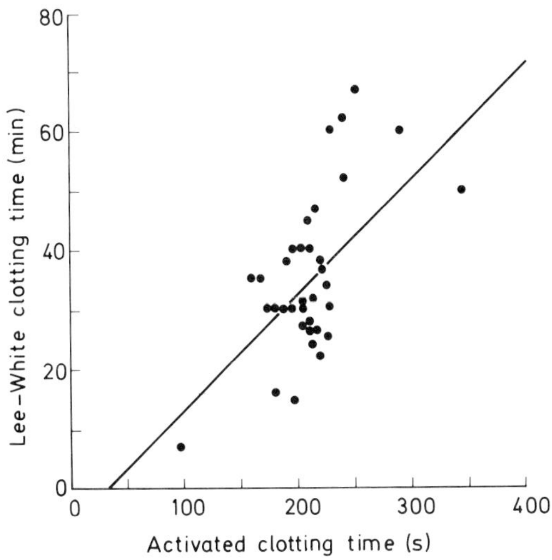

Figure 14.6 Comparison between the ACT and Lee–White clotting time in patients treated by heparin during longterm perfusion. (From de Leval *et al.*[13], by courtesy of *Annales de Chirurgie Thoracique et Cardio-vasculaire*)

and coagulation mechanism by the extracorporeal circuit, and the presence of bleeding tendencies prior to the bypass are the three main factors to be considered[34].

We found that an accurate control of heparin dosage is essential if one is to avoid bleeding complications[13]. We use the activated clotting time (ACT) method[31] to monitor the level of heparin. The ACT is kept basically between 180 and 220 seconds which corresponds to a Lee–White clotting time of 25–40 minutes (*Figure 14.6*). The rapidity, reproducibility and reliability of the ACT test allows for adjustment of the heparin dosage so as to maintain a relatively stable anticoagulation even when the requirements are changing rapidly. *Figure 14.7* shows the rapidly changing heparin requirements in a patient whose urinary output varied sharply. Despite the lability of heparin excretion, we found we could maintain the ACT between 180 and 240 seconds with little difficulty. On the other hand, when factors affecting the metabolism of heparin remain stable, one can maintain a steady state of hypocoagulability with heparin doses varying over a narrow

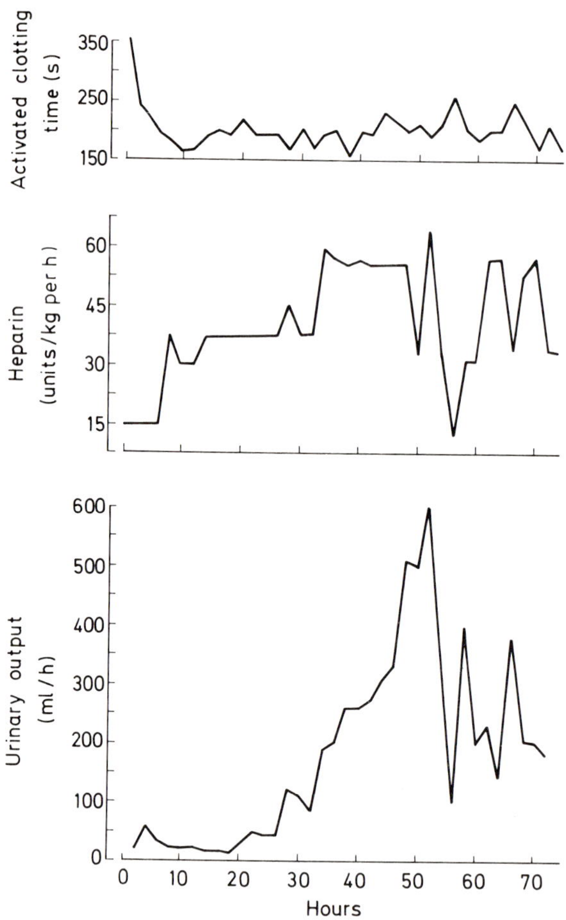

Figure 14.7 Seventy hour bypass for pulmonary insufficiency. Note the rapidly changing heparin requirements in this patient whose urinary output varied sharply. A careful control of the heparinization allowed us to maintain a very stable hypocoagulability. (From de Leval *et al.*[13], by courtesy of *Annales de Chirurgie Thoracique et Cardiovasculaire*)

range. *Figure 14.8* shows a 70-hour bypass in which the heparin requirement ranged between only 10 and 18 units/kg per hour. The average heparin dosage in all our patients was 15–45 units/kg per hour after an initial dose of 100 units/kg of body weight. It is of great importance to administer heparin continuously by an infusion pump in the extracorporeal circuit or in the patient through a catheter which is only used for that purpose.

The level of circulating platelets decreases continuously during the bypass regardless of whether their value was high or low before the perfusion. As indicated by *Figure 14.9*, the number of platelets increases following bypass and there is no appreciable difference in using platelet transfusions. The latter induce at most a short-lived increase in the platelet count.

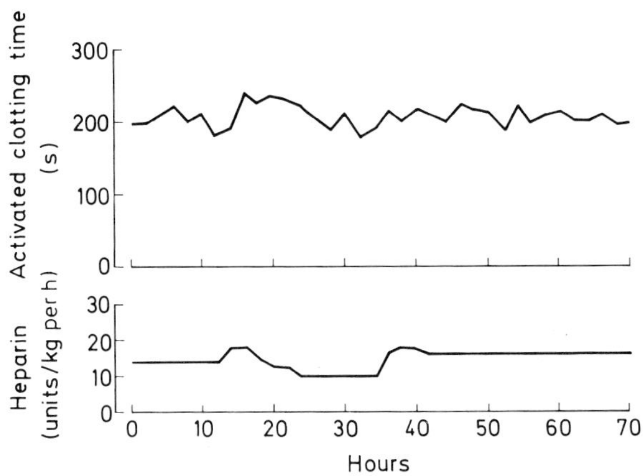

Figure 14.8 Seventy hour bypass where the requirements of heparin were very stable, ranging between only 10 and 18 units/kg per hour

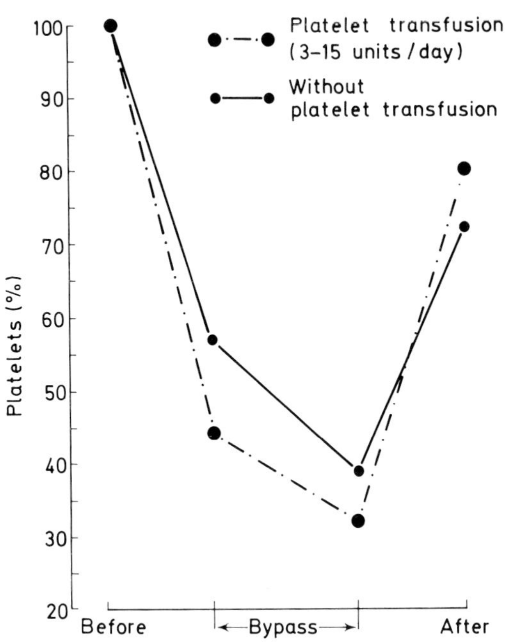

Figure 14.9 Average platelet count changes during longterm perfusion expressed as a percentage of the initial platelet level. There was no sustained or substantial increase in platelet counts obtained by administering platelet transfusion. (From Hill *et al.*[34], by courtesy of *Transactions of the American Society for Artificial Internal Organs*)

The fibrinogen level in the blood remains stable or increases slightly during the perfusion unless a DIC is present.

Prothrombin, partial thromboplastin and thrombin times are affected by heparin and are not reliable indices during bypass. Following bypass, the parameters return to slightly elevated or normal values. The reptilase test, which enables one to measure the thrombin time in the presence of heparin[8], was normal in the patients in whom it was measured.

Of our patients, 4 had laboratory and clinical evidence of disseminated intravascular coagulation before the start of the bypass. In 3 of these, the

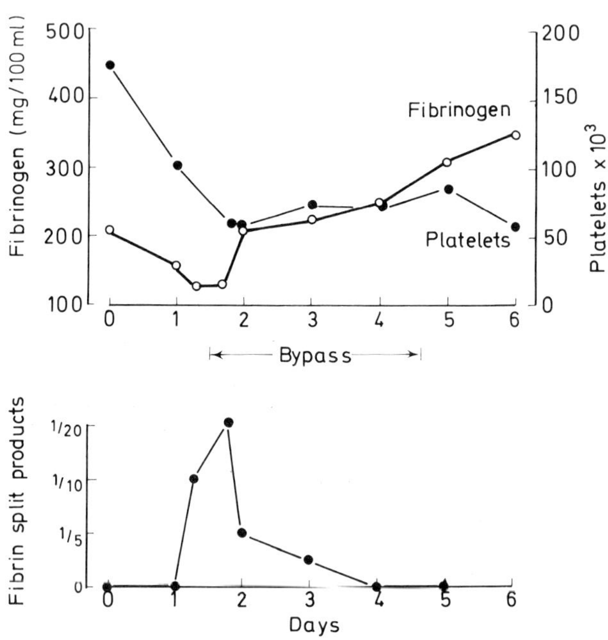

Figure 14.10 Disseminated intravascular coagulation syndrome in a patient undergoing a longterm perfusion for pulmonary insufficiency. DIC had developed before perfusions began. The process was arrested and reversed on bypass. No platelets were given. (From Hill *et al.*[34], by courtesy of *Transactions of the American Society for Artificial Internal Organs*)

process of DIC was stopped and reversed during bypass. This is graphically illustrated in *Figure 14.10*. In this patient, the fibrinogen and platelets were decreasing while the prothrombin time, thrombin time, partial thromboplastin time and fibrin split products were increasing. This trend was accelerating before the beginning of bypass. Following the initiation of bypass and administration of heparin, the consumption coagulopathy was arrested and reversed. In 1 patient who had DIC resulting from amniotic fluid emboli, we were unable to influence the cause of DIC and the patient died while on bypass. These data indicate that a serious consumption coagulopathy is not caused by prolonged extracorporeal circulation.

Microemboli and blood filtration

Microemboli have been implicated as a significant cause of morbidity and mortality following extracorporeal circulation. Pulmonary microemboli have been produced experimentally using pump oxygenators[58, 2]. Hill *et al.*[32] demonstrated the high incidence of cerebral emboli in patients who died after open-heart surgery. Lee *et al.*[45] confirmed the high frequency of neurological deficits and acute psychotic behaviour occurring postoperatively. Approximately one-third of their patients manifested evidence of central nervous system dysfunction after open-heart surgery when careful clinical and objective analysis was carried out.

Aggregated platelets and leukocytes, fat emboli, denatured proteins and air constitute the most usual emboli. The detection of these microemboli has been performed by measuring the screen filtration pressure (SFP), which is the pressure required to pass blood through a micropore filter of known pore size[66], or by a detection chamber employing ultrasound which continuously counts particles in flowing blood[40].

The extracorporeal circuit and the banked blood are the two major sources of these emboli. During storage of the blood, platelets and leukocytes aggregate to form microemboli which are removed from the blood during its passage through the capillary beds of the body. They have been demonstrated by light microscopy[39] and by electron microscopy[12]. These aggregates occur in blood treated with heparin or acid-citrate-dextrose (ACD) but more slowly with the latter. Heparinized blood shows alterations in platelets and leukocytes in a few hours. ACD solution delays the ageing effect from 2 to 10 days[65].

Using a disc oxygenator, it was demonstrated that during extracorporeal oxygenation, platelets and leukocytes developed into aggregates faster than during simple storage[2]. The screen filtration pressure of the preoxygenated blood prior to the institution of bypass is markedly elevated. The direct oxygen-blood interface is responsible for these particular aggregates since the SFP is normal when oxygen is not passed through the oxygenator or when compressed air is used instead of oxygen or when a membrane oxygenator is used[2]. The same investigators found an invariable increase in SFP occurring when the blood from the patient mixes with the blood from the priming volume of the oxygenator. That would suggest the presence of a factor in the priming blood which causes aggregates to form.

The cardiotomy suckers are another cause of emboli, chiefly if the blood from the pericardium is also returned to the pump oxygenator. It is well documented that this blood has sustained the greatest damage of blood anywhere in the extracorporeal circuit[52].

On the basis of these findings, several investigators studied the use of filters in patients undergoing open-heart surgery. Swank and Porter[66] showed that the emboli pass through the stainless steel mesh filters commonly used in pump oxygenators (pore size around 100–150 μm in diameter), but that they can be removed by filtration of the blood through packed fibreglass wool or Dacron wool (pore size 20 μm in diameter). Passing the blood pumped from a bubble oxygenator through a stainless steel mesh which was 6 inches in diameter and contained pores 25 μm in diameter. Patterson, Kessler and Bergland[53] decreased the cerebral damage induced in dogs during extracorporeal circulation. But such stainless steel filters do not have sufficient surface area to pass blood at the flow rates needed for adult humans without causing severe haemolysis[54]. Several disposable blood filters for massive blood transfusions or extracorporeal circulation are currently available for clinical use. The Swank* and the Pall† filters are mostly used in the USA. Swank filters are depth filters made of Dacron wool compressed in a cylindrical package. The model the company designed for blood filtration in the arterial line of the extracorporeal circuit allows a maximum flow of 6000 ml/min and would be effective for retaining and holding adhesive aggregates down to 10 μm in diameter and for removing air bubbles. The Pall filters are constructed of polypropylene except for the filter element which is made of polyester material with a pore size of 40 μm. According to McNamara, Burran and Suchiro[48], the Swank filter has proved to be more effective in removing the debris from banked blood 21 to 23 days old. Solis and Gibbs[63] have also demonstrated the superior effectiveness of the Swank filter as compared to other types of blood filters in removing the microaggregates from the stored blood.

Our own experience is limited to the Swank filters which we have used for open-heart surgery since 1968[16, 35, 52]. With the introduction of the filter, there was a marked improvement in the condition of our patients. They were more alert, more interested in the environment and less confused. The difference was particularly apparent in the first two days after surgery. Our operative mortality in valve replacements has fallen from 19.8 per cent to 6.5 per cent following the utilization of filters. As indicated in Tables 12.1 and 12.2, the operating room death rate was not changed by the filters. This is not unexpected as emboli are more often not fatal when they occur. The incidence of brain fat embolism after open-heart surgery in autopsy specimens decreased from 31 to 4 per cent by the use of filters. However, fat emboli in general were not significantly reduced by filtration.

The possible deleterious effects of filtration were also considered. Haemolysis was found to be lower in patients in whom filtration was used, the number of white cells was unchanged and the platelet count was slightly reduced by passage through the filter. Ashmore *et al.*[3] demonstrated experimentally that platelet counts rapidly increased 30 to 60 minutes after the cessation of bypass when filters were used.

Conclusion

Blood is obviously the first tissue to be considered in extracorporeal circulation and probably the most altered by the passage from normal to artificial maintenance of the circulation and respiration[22]. Its denaturation remains a limiting factor in open-heart surgery and prolonged extracorporeal circulation for respiratory and/or cardiac assistance.

The large blood-gas interface and the suction devices are among the most damaging factors in open-heart surgery. Postoperative bleeding, morbidity and mortality are consequently time-related; the longer the bypass, the more frequently these complications occur.

* Pioneer Filters, Inc., Portland, Oregon, USA
† Pall Corporation, Glen Cove, Long Island, New York, USA

Table 14.1 Mortality following open-heart surgery on patients in whom filter was not used

	Total	*Dead* Operating room	Hospital
Aortic replacement	41	1	10
Mitral replacement	21	5	3
Mitral and aortic non-replacement	33	0	5
Tricuspid replacement	1	0	1
Total	96	6 (6.2%)	19 (19.8%)

Table 14.2 Mortality following open-heart surgery on patients in whom filter was used

	Total	*Dead* Operating room	Hospital
Aortic replacement	50	5	2
Mitral replacement	30	1	5
Mitral and aortic non-replacement	28	0	0
Tricuspid replacement	0	0	0
Total	108	6 (5.5%)	7 (6.5%)

Utilization of a membrane oxygenator without cardiotomy suction has allowed us to perfuse patients with respiratory insufficiency for up to 10 days with a limited alteration of the blood. In these cases, however, we pointed out the importance of a very accurate control of heparinization.

Although little data has been published on the efficiency of the new disposable blood filters, our experience is promising.

Summary

Factors affecting the blood cells and the coagulation system during extracorporeal circulation are considered. Besides the classic aspects of these alterations, we tried to summarize the more recent data.

An experimental study of the platelet kinetics during extracorporeal circulation is reported.

The haematological changes during longterm perfusion with a membrane oxygenator are studied.

The results of disposable filters on the incidence of emboli are discussed.

References

1. Adkins, J. and Hardy, J. 'Sodium heparin neutralization and the anti-coagulant effects of protamine sulphate.' *Archives of Surgery, Chicago*, **94,** 175 (1967)
2. Ashmore, P., Svitek, V. and Ambrose, P. 'The incidence and effects of particulate aggregation and microembolism in pump oxygenator systems.' *Journal of Thoracic and Cardiovascular Surgery*, **55,** 691 (1968)

3. Ashmore, P., Swank, R., Gallery, R., Ambrose, P. and Prichard, K. 'Effect of Dacron wool filtration on the microembolic phenomenon in extracorporeal circulation.' *Journal of Thoracic and Cardiovascular Surgery*, **63,** 240 (1972)
4. Belko, J. and Lerman, F. 'Body response to a second dose of heparin after heparin neutralization by protamine.' *Journal of Cardiovascular Surgery*, **7,** 219 (1966)
5. Bernstein, E. F., Blackshear, P. L. and Keller, K. H. 'Factors influencing erythrocyte destruction in artificial organs.' *American Journal of Surgery*, **114,** 126 (1967)
6. Bernstein, E., Indeglia, R., Shea, M. and Varco, R. 'Sublethal damage to the red blood cell from pumping.' *Circulation*, **45 (Suppl. 1),** 226 (1967)
7. Blackshear, P. L., Dorman, R. and Steinback, J. 'Some mechanical effects that influence haemolysis.' *Transactions of the American Society for Artificial Internal Organs*, **11,** 112 (1965)
8. Britten, A. F. H., Card, R. and Mielke, C. H. 'Reptilase time. Useful monitor of progress in disseminated intravascular coagulation.' *Presented at the International Conference on Haematology*, Munich, Germany (1971)
9. Britten, A. F. H., Salzman, E. W., Grove-Rasmussen, M. and Shaw, R.S. 'Use of ACD bank blood and fresh heparinized blood in open heart surgery.' *Transfusion*, **3,** 368 (1963)
10. Bunn, H. F. and Jandl, J. D. 'Control of haemoglobin function within the red cell.' *New England Journal of Medicine*, **282,** 1414 (1970)
11. Clowes, G. 'Extracorporeal maintenance of circulation and respiration.' *Physiological Reviews*, **40,** 826 (1960)
12. Connell, R. and Swank, R. 'Pulmonary fine structure after haemorrhagic shock and transfusion of aging blood. Microcirculatory approaches to current therapeutic problems.' In *Symposia, 6th European Conference on Microcirculation. Aalborg 1970*, pp. 49–58. Basel: S. Karger (1971)
13. deLeval, M., Hill, J. D., Dontigny, L. and Gerbode, F. 'Controle de l'heparinisation continue par le temps de coagulation active (ACT).' *Annales de Chirurgie Thoracique et Cardiovasculaire*, **11,** 287 (1972)
14. deLeval, M., Hill, J. D., Mielke, C. H., Bramson, M., Smith, C. and Gerbode, F. 'Platelet kinetics during extracorporeal circulation.' *Transactions of the American Society for Artificial Internal Organs*, **18,** 355 (1972)
15. Dieter, R. A., Neville, W. E., Pifarre, R. and Jasuja, M. 'Preoperative coagulation profile and posthaemodilution cardiopulmonary bypass haemorrhage.' *American Journal of Surgery*, **121,** 689 (1971)
16. Egeblad, K., Osborn, J., Burns, W., Hill, J. D. and Gerbode, F. 'Blood filtration during cardiopulmonary bypass.' *Journal of Thoracic and Cardiovascular Surgery*, **63,** 384 (1972)
17. Ekert, H., Friedlander, I. and Hardisty, R. 'Role of platelets in fibrinolysis: studies on the plasminogen activator and antiplasmin activity of platelets.' *British Journal of Haematology*, **18,** 575 (1970)
18. Ekert, H., Gilchrist, G., Stanton, R. and Hammond, D. 'Haemostasis in cyanotic congenital heart disease.' *Journal of Pediatrics*, **76,** 221 (1970)
19. Ekert, H., Montgomery, D. and Aberdeen, E. 'Fibrinolysis during extracorporeal circulation.' *Circulation Research*, **28,** 512 (1971)
20. Friedman, L., Richardson, P. and Galletti, P. 'Observations of acute thrombogenesis in membrane oxygenator.' *Transactions of the American Society for Artificial Internal Organs*, **17,** 369 (1971)
21. Galletti, P. 'Laboratory experience with 24 hour partial heart-lung bypass.' *Journal of Surgical Research*, **5,** 57 (1965)
22. Galletti, P. and Brecher, G. *Heart Lung Bypass*. New York: Grune and Stratton (1962)

23. Gans, H. and Castaneda, A. 'Problems in haemostasis during open-heart surgery: VII. Changes in fibrinogen concentration during and after cardiopulmonary bypass with particular reference to the effect of heparin neutralization and fibrinogen.' *Annals of Surgery*, **165,** 551 (1967)
24. Gans, H., Castaneda, A., Subramanian, V., John, S. and Lillehei, C. 'Problems in haemostasis during open-heart surgery: IX. Changes observed in the plasminogen–plasmin system and their signficance for therapy.' *American Surgeon*, **166,** 980 (1967)
25. Gans, H., Subramanian, V., Lillehei, C. and Castaneda, A. 'Problems in haemostasis during open-heart surgery: VIII. On the *in vivo* turnover rate of plasminogen activator after cardiopulmonary bypass.' *Surgery, St. Louis*, **62,** 292 (1967)
26. Goldman, B., Joison, J. and Austen, G. 'Cardiovascular effects of protamine sulphate.' *Annals of Thoracic Surgery*, **7,** 459 (1969)
27. Gollub, S. and Bailey, C. 'Management of major surgical blood loss without transfusion.' *Journal of the American Medical Association*, **198,** 1171 (1969)
28. Gourin, A., Streisand, R., Greineder, J. and Stuckey, J. 'Protamine sulphate administration and the cardiovascular system.' *Journal of Thoracic and Cardiovascular Surgery*, **62,** 193 (1971)
29. Gralnick, H. and Fischer, D. 'The haemostatic response to open-heart operation.' *Journal of Thoracic and Cardiovascular Surgery*, **61,** 909 (1971)
30. Hara, M., Maris, M., Crumpler, J., Corn, B. and Perkins, W. H. 'Effect of various priming solutions upon red cell mass, plasma volume and extracellular fluid volume of dogs following haemodilution techniques of extracorporeal circulation.' *Journal of Thoracic and Cardiovascular Surgery*, **53,** 354 (1967)
31. Hattersley, P. 'Activated coagulation time of whole blood.' *Journal of the American Medical Association*, **136,** 436 (1966)
32. Hill, J. D., Aguilar, M. J., Baranco, A., de Lanerolle, P. and Gerbode, F. 'Neuropathological manifestations of cardiac surgery.' *Annals of Thoracic Surgery*, **7,** 409 (1969)
33. Hill, J. D., de Leval, M., Fallat, R., Bramson, M., Eberhart, R., Schulte, H., Osborn, J., Barber, R. and Gerbode, F. 'Acute respiratory insufficiency. Treatment with prolonged extracorporeal circulation.' *Journal of Thoracic and Cardiovascular Surgery*, **64,** 551 (1972)
34. Hill, J. D., de Leval, M., Mielke, C. H., Bramson, M. and Gerbode, F. 'Clinical prolonged extracorporeal circulation for respiratory insufficiency: haematological effects.' *Transactions of the American Society for Artificial Internal Organs*, **18,** 546 (1972)
35. Hill, J. D., Osborn, J., Swank, R., Aguilar, M., de Lanerolle, P. and Gerbode, F. 'Experience using a new Dacron wool filter during extracorporeal circulation.' *Archives of Surgery, Chicago*, **101,** 649 (1970)
36. Howland, W. S., Schweizer, O. and Boyan, P. 'The effect of buffering on the mortality of massive blood transfusion.' *Surgery, Gynecology and Obstetrics*, **127,** 777 (1965)
37. Hurt, R., Perkins, H. A., Osborn, J. and Gerbode, F. 'The neutralization of heparin by protamine in extracorporeal circulation.' *Journal of Thoracic and Cardiovascular Surgery*, **32,** 612 (1965)
38. Indeglia, R. A., Dorman, F. D., Castaneda, A. R., Varco, R. and Bernstein, E. F. 'Use of GBH-coated Tygon tubing for experimental prolonged perfusions without systemic heparinization.' *Transactions of the American Society for Artificial Internal Organs*, **12,** 166 (1966)
39. Jenevein, E. and Weiss, D. 'Platelet microemboli associated with massive blood transfusions.' *American Journal of Pathology*, **45,** 313 (1964)
40. Kessler, J. and Patterson, R. 'The production of microemboli by various blood oxygenators.' *Annals of Thoracic Surgery*, **9,** 221 (1970)

41. Kissmeyer-Nielsen, F. and Madsen, C. H. 'Platelets in blood stored in untreated and siliconized glass bottles and plastic bags.' *Journal of Clinical Pathology*, **14,** 626 (1961)
42. Krevans, J. R., Jackson, D. P., Conley, C. L. and Hartmann, R. C. 'Haemorrhagic disorder following massive whole blood transfusions.' *Journal of the American Medical Association*, **159,** 171 (1957)
43. Kusserow, B. K. and Clapp, J. F. 'Red blood cell survival after prolonged perfusion with a blood pump.' *Transactions of the American Society for Artificial Internal Organs*, **12,** 121 (1966)
44. Laufman, H. and Erichson, R. B. *Haematological Problems in Surgery*. Philadelphia: W. B. Saunders (1970)
45. Lee, W. H., Brady, M., Rowe, J. and Miller, W. 'Effects of extracorporeal circulation upon behaviour, personality and brain function. Part II. Haemodynamic metabolic and psychometric correlations.' *Annals of Surgery*, **173,** 1013 (1971)
46. Leveen, H. M., Schatman, B. and Falk, G. 'Cardiac arrest produced by massive transfusions.' *Surgery, Gynecology and Obstetrics*, **109,** 503 (1959)
47. Litwin, M. S., Smith, L. L. and Moore, F. D. 'Metabolic alkalosis following massive transfusion. *Surgery, St. Louis*, **45,** 805, (1959)
48. McNamara, J., Burran, E. and Suchiro, G. 'Effective filtration of banked blood.' *Surgery, St. Louis*, **71,** 594 (1972)
49. Neville, W. E., Faber, L. P. and Peacock, H. 'Total prime of the disc oxygenator with Ringer's and Ringer's lactate solution for cardiopulmonary bypass; clinical and experimental observations.' *Diseases of the Chest*, **45,** 320 (1964)
50. Neville, W. E., Maben, H., Colby, C. and Peacock, H. 'Total prime of the large volume disc oxygenator.' *Annals of Thoracic Surgery*, **1,** 575 (1965)
51. O'Neill, J. A., Ende, N., Collins, J. S. and Collins, H. A. 'A quantitative determination of perfusion fibrinolysis.' *Journal of Thoracic and Cardiovascular Surgery*, **51,** 777 (1966)
52. Osborn, J., Swank, R., Hill, J. D., Aguilar, M. and Gerbode, F. 'Clinical use of a Dacron wool filter during perfusion for open-heart surgery.' *Journal of Thoracic and Cardiovascular Surgery*, **60,** 575 (1970)
53. Patterson, R., Kessler, J. and Bergland, R. 'A filter to prevent cerebral damage during experimental cardiopulmonary bypass.' *Surgery, Gynecology and Obstetrics*, **132,** 71 (1971)
54. Patterson, R. and Twichell, J. 'Disposable filter for microemboli; use in cardipulmonary bypass and massive transfusion,' *Journal of the American Medical Association*, **215,** 76 (1971)
55. Peirce, E. C., II. *Extracorporeal Circulation for Open-Heart Surgery*. Springfield: Thomas (1969)
56. Perkins, H. A., Osborn, J. and Gerbode, F. 'Management of abnormal bleeding following extracorporeal circulation.' *Annals of Internal Medicine*', **51,** 658 (1959)
57. Roe, B. B., Hutchinson, J. C. and Swenson, C. E. 'High flow body perfusion with calculated haemodilution.' *Annals of Thoracic Surgery*, **1,** 581 (1965)
58. Rossi, N., Yu, S., Koepke, J. and Spencer, F. 'Pulmonary injury from prolonged oxygenation with venous blood.' *Surgical Forum*, **15,** 277 (1964)
59. Salzman, E. and Britten, A. F. H. *Hemorrhage and Thrombosis*. Boston: Little, Brown and Co. (1965)
60. Schanberge, J., Barlas, A. and Regan, E. 'Effect of protamine on thromboplastin generation.' *Journal of Laboratory and Clinical Medicine*, **52,** 744 (1958)
61. Smith, R. *Pathologic Physiology for Anesthesiologists*, p. 321. Springfield: Thomas (1956)
62. Smith, R. M. 'Blood replacement in thoracic surgery for children.' *Journal of the American Medical Association*, **161,** 1124 (1956)

63. Solis, R. T. and Gibbs, M. B. 'Filtration of the microaggregates in stored blood.' *Transfusion*, **12,** 245 (1972)
64. Sutera, S., Croce, P. and Mehrjardi, M. 'Hemolysis and subhemolytic alterations of human red blood cells induced by turbulent shear flow.' *Transactions of the American Medical Society for Artificial Internal Organs*, **18,** 335 (1972)
65. Swank, R. 'Alterations of blood on storage: measurement of adhesiveness of "aging" platelets and leucocytes and their removal by filtration.' *New England Journal of Medicine*, **265,** 728 (1961)
66. Swank, R. and Porter, G. 'Disappearance of the microemboli transfused into patients during cardiopulmonary bypass.' *Transfusion*, **3,** 192 (1963)
67. Tarhan, S., Moffit, E., Lundborg, R. and Wallace, R. 'Use of heparinized priming blood after whole body perfusion.' *Surgery, St. Louis*, **67,** 584 (1970)
68. Trimble, A., Herst, R., Grady, M. and Crookston, J. 'Blood loss in open-heart surgery: correlation with laboratory tests for haemostatic function.' *Archives of Surgery, Chicago*, **93,** 323 (1966)
69. Wintrob, M. M. *Clinical Hematology*. (6th edn.). Philadelphia: Lea & Febiger (1967)
70. Woods, J. E., Kirklin, J. W., Owens, C. A., Thompson, J. M. and Taswell, H. F. 'Effects of bypass surgery on coagulation-sensitive clotting factors.' *Mayo Clinic Proceedings*, **42,** 724 (1967)
71. Zucker, M. B., Siegel, M., Cliffton, E. E., Bellville, J. N., Howlands, W. S. and Grossi, C. E. 'Generalized excessive oozing in patients undergoing major surgery and receiving multiple blood transfusions.' *Journal of Laboratory and Clinical Medicine*, **50,** 849 (1957)

15

Microbiological Aspects of Open-Heart Surgery

Roger Freeman

mater artium necessitas

Introduction

In the first edition of this book the opportunity was taken to set out some of the simple principles of microbiology and their application to open-heart surgery. Particular emphasis was placed on the overuse of antibiotics, especially in prophylaxis. Upon reviewing the chapter written at that time it became clear that the lessons of those days have largely been learned, and that microbiological control of open-heart surgery patients has improved markedly. This is partly due to an improvement in clinical microbiology generally, especially in technical fields, and partly due to the maturation of open-heart surgery itself. Better-risks patients are received for operation and the surgical procedure itself is a much smoother and less insulting procedure than before. It would be arrogant to claim that the measures advocated earlier have been in any way responsible for this happy state of affairs, but it may be that they were expressive of a general trend, prevalent at the time, which is now bearing fruit.

Thus, it is not the aim of this new contribution to revise and restate the contents of the first edition. Rather, I have chosen to discuss two topics of some interest, I hope, to those involved in open-heart surgery.

The first topic is hepatitis B, or rather carriage of hepatitis B surface antigen. Few recent discoveries could have galvanized medicine as much as 'Australia antigen' and its associated phenomena. Undoubtedly much unnecessary panic was the result. Fortunately, experience has been accumulated and recent attitudes towards carriers of hepatitis B surface antigen are much more benign, although *acute* hepatitis B is agreed by all to be a highly infective condition. It may, therefore, be timely to give an account of one approach of dealing with this problem.

The second topic is the bane of open-heart surgery – infective endocarditis. I make no excuse for including this disease, since it seems to me that it can never be boring to any surgeon to study the disease which can totally destroy his best work, and even his patient.

Hepatitis B

In recent years the recognition and characterization of infections with the hepatitis B virus (HBV) has become possible due to the development of tests based upon the detection of hepatitis B surface antigen (HBsAg), synonymous with 'Australia antigen' and with hepatitis associated antigen. HBsAg is found in the serum in two conditions, acute hepatitis B and chronic carriers. The former state is an acute illness which would preclude major surgery until well into the convalescent stage and will not enter largely into this discussion for that reason. The latter condition, the chronic carrier state, is relatively common and it is the characterization, management and consequences of this stage which is the problem of relevance to open-heart surgery. First, however, it is important to discuss the diagnosis and epidemiology of HBV infection.

HBV can be transmitted from man to man in several known ways. Parenteral transmission is well known and acute hepatitis B is synonymous with many cases of 'homologous serum jaundice'. Serum of blood containing HBsAg is infective to other human beings when innoculated parenterally in doses as small as 0.5 ml[2]. After an incubation period of several weeks (roughly 40 days) HBsAg appears in the serum, but the patient does not yet fall ill. After a further 40 days, making a total incubation period of approximately 80 days, antibody to the hepatitis B 'core' antigen (HBcAg) appears in addition to HBsAg and an acute hepatitis begins. A short prodromal period often precedes the jaundice and may be characterized by rashes and arthralgia. The clinical illness often lasts only a short while, but both HBsAg and core antibody (anti-HBc) persist in the serum during convalescence. Approximately 3 months after clinical recovery HBsAg disappears from the serum but anti-HBc persists. After several more months antibody to HBsAg (anti-HBs) may appear. This is the normal course of events in an immunologically normal person, and is summarized in

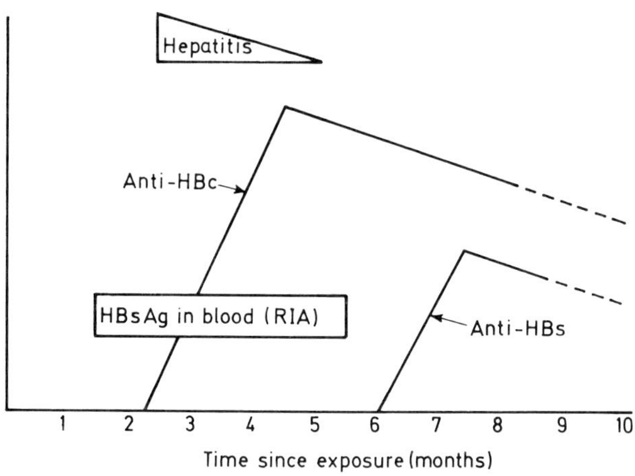

Figure 15.1 Schematic illustration of events following exposure to HBV. RIA = radio-immunoassay

Figure 15.1. Hepatitis BeAg is found in the serum towards the end of the incubation period and the corresponding antibody (anti-HBeAg) usually appears in the serum shortly thereafter, HBeAg having gone. Patients with acute hepatitis B are highly infectious from the first appearance of HBsAg until the end of the clinical illness, and must be barrier-nursed. All the body fluids (blood, faeces, urine etc.) should be regarded as potentially infectious at that time.

HBV can also be transmitted by the oral route, although not as easily as hepatitis A virus ('infective hepatitis'), and transmission from conjunctival contamination by infected material is recognized[5]. Similarly, parenteral transmission need not simply be by transfusion of infected blood or serum, or by 'needle-stick' incidents; acupuncture, intravenous drug abuse and even ear-piercing have all resulted in subsequent cases of hepatitis B[3].

Acute hepatitis B in European races almost always ends in recovery and elimination of HBsAg from the serum, the only residual markers being anti-HBc and anti-HBs. Such persons are of no danger and, indeed, it has been argued that their blood should be accepted for donation. Where, then, do the chronic carriers come from?

A small proportion of those having acute hepatitis B seem unable to eliminate HBsAg from the serum after recovering from the acute illness. The precise reasons are largely unknown, but are supposed to reflect an immunological incompetence. Although rare in Europeans, this tendency is commoner in Asians, and particularly marked in those persons from the Far East. In addition, Europeans with known immunosuppressed states may show the inability to do this. Thus, some carriers may arise from this route. However, the carrier state is much commoner than this group alone would account for.

Asymptomatic HBV infection probably occurs quite commonly in comparison with recognizable cases. It is suspected that asymptomatic HBV infection may also result in the carrier state, possibly more commonly than the symptomatic disease.

Finally, women who are themselves chronic carriers of HBsAg may transmit the virus to their children, resulting in a child which is itself a chronic carrier. Thus, by all these various routes (and possibly by other routes as yet unknown), chronic carriage of HBsAg arises. How, then, may these chronic carriers be recognized?

Carriers of HBsAg fall into two groups. Firstly, a small proportion have progressive liver disease, for instance, chronic aggressive hepatitis. These patients arc usually HBsAg positive, anti-HBc positive and HBeAg positive. It is found that their serum frequently contains the viral DNA-polymerase and it is supposed that replicating HBV is still present within their liver. These patients have a poor outlook, and they are more infectious than the majority of carriers. Liver biopsy will characterize their illness and will help to assess the prognosis.

The second, and major group of carriers are healthy patients, but in whose serum HBsAg can be demonstrated. In addition to HBsAg the serum contains anti-HBc and also (often) anti-HBeAg. These patients have no active liver disease and the serum does not contain the viral DNA-polymerase. They are regarded as patients in whom the virus has probably been eliminated but in whom the liver cells continue to produce one of the components of the virus, namely HBsAg. These carriers have an excellent prognosis and are not as infectious as the first group. However, they are not reliably non-infectious.

Having briefly outlined these various groups of patients, what are the practical implications for open-heart surgery?

Incidence of the carrier state

Carriers of HBsAg occur in the general population at a rate of, roughly, one per thousand. Certain groups have a higher carriage rate, for instance, haemophiliacs, mongols and drug addicts[4]. No actual figure for the incidence of carriage in candidates for open-heart surgery is easily found, but since these patients have often received blood transfusions, injections and other parenteral therapy, the figure may well be above one in a thousand and it is unlikely to be any less.

Detection of the carrier state

Tests for HBsAg exist in varying sensitivity. In acute hepatitis B so much HBsAg is found in the serum that all types of test will usually be positive. Carriers, on the other hand, may well show a disparity between tests of different sensitivity. The most sensitive test is radio-immunoassay (RIA) and all carriers will be positive by this technique. RIA is the usual reference standard for the other tests but it is expensive and therefore unsuitable for mass screening at local level. Passive haemagglutination techniques are relatively inexpensive and rapid tests; their sensitivity, being less than that of RIA, still allows the detection of all but a few carriers. Most centres accept these tests (one commonly used variety is the 'Hepatest') as sufficiently reliable for clinical needs, for instance the decisions necessary for operations and transfusions. Earlier tests, counter-immunoelectrophoresis (CIE) for example, are insufficiently sensitive for this purpose nowadays. Immunoelectronmicroscopy (IEM) is not now used as a primary diagnostic test, but as confirmation of other tests when RIA is not readily available.

Core antibody (anti-HBc) is easily detected by CIE and will normally be found as an accompaniment of HBsAg. Exceptions rarely occur[8].

The presence of anti-HBc and negative Hepatest for HBsAg should lead to the further exclusion of HBsAg by RIA. If RIA is negative, the presence of anti-HBc alone is not a danger, although it does imply HBV infection at some recent time. The findings of anti-HBs along with anti-HBc indicates complete immunological recovery from HBV infection and such patients are safe for operation, and might be usefully guided to show their gratitude by donation of blood for the production of immunoglobulin. (*See later.*)

First steps in the assessment of a positive carrier

As elsewhere in medicine, the first step should be an accurate history, aimed at elucidating the likely source of the infection. The possibility of drug addiction should be borne in mind, and homosexuality is also a possibility. Sexual promiscuity, even if heterosexual, may be important and may have a bearing on other members of the family. Similarly, recent blood transfusions may be important and will lead to tracing the donors who may be HBsAg positive by RIA alone.

Having discharged the obligation to fields other than cardiac surgery, the next step is to determine whether the carrier has serious underlying liver disease. This is probably best done by an experienced gastroenterologist since it will almost certainly include liver biopsy. The time involved in this investigation is not wasted, since it should be a general rule to postpone surgery in all cases for three months on the offchance that HBsAg will disappear from the serum, in case the patient is merely in the early stage of convalescence from an asymptomatic attack of HBV infection. Obviously, postponement of operation is not always feasible but it should be tried wherever possible, especially since the potential rewards are so great.

If the carrier remains positive and is shown to have no serious liver pathology the next step is to attempt to test for the presence of HBeAg or anti-HBe. If the patient is HBeAg positive he should be regarded as highly infectious, whereas the finding of anti-HBe will imply a much lesser (but not absent) degree of infectivity. Unfortunately, the tests for HBeAg and anti-HBe are relatively insensitive and in a large proportion of cases they are negative for both.*

Carriers with proven progressive liver disease have a limited prognosis and their liver disease might well be worsened by operation. The advisability of operation in this group must be the subject of discussion between the surgeon and the gastroenterologist, and many other factors will also need consideration.

Supposing that a patient emerges in whom tests for HBsAg are persistently positive, in whom no serious liver disease is found and whose cardiac lesion is eminently amenable to surgery – in other words a patient in whom operation would readily be offered were he not HBsAg positive. Should surgery be offered, and, if so, can the hazards be contained? The answer to both questions is a cautious 'yes'.

Preoperative precautions

The patient should be admitted to the routine wards, there being no reason at this stage for any elaborate precautions. It is useful to provide a separate room for the patient in order that any blood samples necessary can be taken away from other patients. Similarly, staff taking blood from the patient should wear gloves and take great care. Any accidental inoculation of blood-stained material must be reported. An 'incident book' for the noting of such accidents may be useful if retrospective evidence becomes necessary. Any member of staff having such an accident should be offered specific immunoglobulin (*see later*).

Other than the simple measures outlined above, the patient need not be restricted at this stage. Should he be anticoagulated the possibility of gastrointestinal or renal bleeding ought to be borne in mind and the precautions detailed later may be needed (*see* section on Postoperative care).

Operative precautions

Essentially the aim should be to prevent contact between the infected material from the patient and the susceptible staff. It is reasonable to assume that the following situations constitute 'exposure';

Injection of infected material through intact skin.
Lodgement of infected material in the conjuctiva.
Ingestion of infected material.
Presence of infected material on recent (less than 24-hours'-old) skin cuts or abrasions.
'Massive' contamination of skin, e.g. flooding of large area of skin in blood.

Furthermore, the definition of infected material has to be extended from that used preoperatively. Thus, the patient will be anticoagulated during bypass and so it should be assumed that the gastrointestinal tract and the urinary tract will contain blood, and, therefore, HBsAg. This is especially

*More recently the development of RIA methods for detecting HBeAg and anti-HBe has resulted in very sensitive tests, capable of placing carriers into two categories—viz. HBeAg 'positive' or anti-HBe 'positive'. The precise value of this advance is eagerly awaited

true in the latter case since catheterization of the bladder will be performed and some degree of trauma will necessarily ensue. It should also be realized that all tissue removed at operation will contain HBsAg since it will also contain blood. Finally, suction apparatus will produce aerosols which may (theoretically) contain HBsAg. The following suggestions are put forward to minimize these various risks.

Protection of the staff in the operating theatre

The first essential point is to reduce the staff, and therefore the number of people at risk, to the absolute minimum. It should be clearly understood that surgical operations on HBsAg positive patients are not the occasions on which any gratuitous observations should be undertaken. The staff should consist of the surgeon, his assistant, the theatre sister, her assistant, the anaesthetist, his assistant and one 'runner' nurse. In addition to these, the presence of one, or at the most two, microbiologically expert observers should be allowed. All of the staff operating on the patient (surgeon, surgical assistant and theatre sister) should be protected as follows:–

Goggles should be worn.

An impermeable mask (to prevent ingestion of blood, should blood be sprayed onto the face) should be worn.

An apron of water-resistant material which extends from the neck to the upper surface of the foot wear should be worn.

The arms from elbow to wrist should be covered in water-resistant material (we found that veterinary surgeon's gloves with the hand portion removed served very well).

Rubber boots (autoclavable) should be worn.

Normal theatre clothing is then added (*over* the apron and arm coverings). Double gloving is advised.

(It has been found that the goggles tend to mist over, especially when the impermeable mask – an ordinary mask with cellophane stitched in – is also used. A preferable alternative is a visor, of the welder's type, which serves to protect both eyes and mouth and allows the mask used to be of a normal, i.e. non-impervious, type. The visor can also be hinged-up should misting occur and wiped clean by an assistant.)

The anaesthetist, his assistant and the 'runner' nurse should wear aprons, boots and goggles when attending the bypass machine or closely approaching the patient.

The microbiologist and his assistant are present to observe the operation for any accidental lapses of protocol, to be on hand in order to give advice should some unplanned-for situation arise and to act as a 'fire-brigade' in dealing with spillage of infected material (*see later*).

Preparation of apparatus

The heart-lung machine Modern heart-lung machines are made so that the blood-containing portions are either disposable or capable of being heat-sterilized. However, small modifications are still needed. A membrane oxygenator is preferred since aerosol production is reduced, but in any case the aerosol is ducted out of the operating theatre. We have used the ducts provided for the exhaust of anaesthetic gases for this purpose, having first checked that the ducts opened onto the roof of the building. The ducts are steamed with formaldehyde after use.

All tubing used in the operation is discarded carefully into strong plastic bags for subsequent autoclaving and incineration. The tubing should be removed by placing disposable plastic clamps distal to the steel clamp forceps, usually employed in order that the metal forceps can be saved. The tubing, plus whatever blood remains in it, can then be carefully fed into the plastic sacks. Any spotting of blood which occurs must be dealt with immediately (*see later*).

Suction apparatus Instead of using the modern 'plumbed in' suction system, which may communicate with that of other operating theatres in the same suite, an old-fashioned portable suction machine can be used. The outlet pipe (a theoretical source of aerosol) is connected up to one of the exhaust gas ducts as described above, the duct being steamed with formaldehyde after use. At the end of the operation an equal volume of a strong hypochlorite solution (e.g. 10 mg/100 ml Chloros) containing 10 000 ppm of chlorine is added to the material in the suction jar to inactivate the virus.

Surgical Instruments As the operation progresses, used instruments are discarded into a container filled with 2 mg/100 ml aqueous glutaraldehyde solution (undiluted Cidex). This container should have a lid since the vapour from glutaraldehyde can be troublesome. It should be noted that hypochlorites are unsuitable when dealing with metallic substances since they cause corrosion.

Monitoring equipment As stated earlier, it must be accepted that the less equipment used during the operating the better. However, some monitoring equipment may be indispensable. It should be screened off as far as is practicable and may be covered in plastic sheeting to minimize accidental contamination. Probes and electrodes are often difficult to sterilize. One method is by ethylene oxide, although it should be noted that thorough prior cleaning is advisable with this technique and the cleaning should be done with all necessary precautions against contamination (for instance, the wearing of goggles would probably be necessary).

Cleaning the operating theatre After the conclusion of the operation and the decision that the patient is fit to be transferred to the intensive care unit, the operating theatre must be rendered safe for re-use. All surfaces should be washed in a detergent–hypochlorite mixture (a suitable solution is produced by mixing Lissapol* with Milton). The theatre floor is similarly washed. The exhaust ducts used for the aerosol extraction are fumigated with a 'formalin kettle' for 30 minutes whilst actively extracting. The instruments which have been steeping in glutaraldehyde are cleaned by staff suitably protected with aprons etc. and then packed into a container ready to be autoclaved. All disposable items are double-bagged into plastic bags (forethought is needed to ensure large enough bags of sufficient strength) prior to autoclaving. Having been autoclaved the resultant material is then incinerated. Operating theatre linen is packed into alginate bags and sent for a 'foul linen' wash in which a high temperature is maintained for a long period (and during which the bag dissolves). It should be the duty of a senior member of staff

*Lissapol is now no longer manufactured. Tepol is an acceptable substitute, or Synperonic 'N'.

(preferably the microbiologist) to be present throughout all the above procedures in order to ensure that all the material is safely handled.

After the cleaning of the operating theatre and its thorough cleaning with the detergent–hypochlorite mixture, the theatre ventilation is left full on to promote drying of the cleaned surfaces. The theatre is then ready for re-use.

Duties of the microbiologist during the operation

In addition to carefully observing the operation and being on hand to give advice, the microbiologist and his assistant (both of whom should be wearing aprons, boots and gloves) should furnish themselves with absorbent paper towels and a large container of strong hypochlorite solution. Whenever any drops of blood or other body fluids or any other infected material are spilled they should immediately be mopped up with the absorbent material and discarded into a plastic bag which will subsequently be autoclaved. The area should then be liberally washed with the strong hypochlorite solution. These incidents should be dealt with as they arise, otherwise the material may become transferred onto the footwear of the staff and so become the source of contamination elsewhere in the operating theatre.

Finally, all staff, whether humble or otherwise, MUST be told that any incident should be reported to the microbiologist who should note the incident in order that specific immunoglobulin can be offered if necessary. There is no place in this routine for the 'covering up' of an incident which might be thought to be embarassing to the individual concerned.

Postoperative care

Intensive care unit

As with the operating theatre staff the personnel involved in the intensive care unit (ICU) should be fully protected when closely attending the patient. Because of recent or, in some instances, current, anticoagulation, all the patients' secretions and excretions must be regarded as possibly containing blood, and, therefore, infectious. The operative wounds are a particular risk and staff should understand that serum and other wound exudates are highly infective. Similarly, the intravenous and intra-arterial catheters which are used for pressure monitoring and intravenous therapy should be handled with great care. Urine and faeces may well contain blood and should be treated with strong hypochlorite solution before being discarded. Needles are a particular hazard and suitable receptacles for their safe disposal should be provided. We have found that one simple problem which is easily overlooked is the disposal of excess blood from venepunctures. This should be added to a container in which hypochlorite is already present.

Nurses and doctors attending the patient should be dressed in aprons, gloves and gowns. Goggles should be worn when procedures are to be performed during which aerosols may be generated.

The patient should be nursed in a single room, preferably one with exhaust ventilation. This also allows easier arrangements for controlling the number of staff seeing the patient. These should be reduced to the minimum. For instance, since the nurses attending the patient will necessarily spend much of their time in the room, it is possible for them to perform simple chest physiotherapy. This allows expert physiotherapy to be reserved for complications. In many cases no lung complications will arise and one more person is saved from unnecessary exposure.

Just as the staff should be reduced to the minimum, so the number of intravenous catheters should be curtailed and, if possible, the number of venepunctures. All these measures which may involve much forethought and even some compromise, serve to reduce the chances of exposure to the minimum.

Nursing staff attending the patient should be prevented from attending other patients during the same period. Theoretically, if they were to carefully change out of the protective clothing and carefully wash their hands they would not carry HBsAg elsewhere (they will, after all, go home at the end of their shift) but it cannot be guaranteed in an emergency that care would not be sacrificed for speed. In any case, the benefit of the nurse remaining within the room is that it frees other staff, for instance the physiotherapist, as described above. It should, therefore, be realized that the ICU must be adequately staffed during this period.

Since most patients will initially be intubated and ventilated, it should be assumed that bleeding into the tracheal secretion will occur, and that the sputum or bronchial secretions may be infectious. Gloves should therefore be worn and goggles will be advisable during tracheal suction in case the patient should suddenly cough material into the nurse's face.

A very worrying problem is the procedure to be adopted should the patient develop major complications. Should, for instance, a tracheostomy be required, what then? Most ICUs have the facilities for anaesthesia and minor surgical operations on site and since the isolation room is already contaminated it would be most logical to perform such procedures there. This might also apply to simple measures to secure haemostasis. If, however, a major surgical intervention is necessary the operating theatre protocol will be necessary again. We have adopted the simple measure of retaining the patient in the operating theatre for one hour beyond the normal time before transfer to ICU in the hope that if major local bleeding occurs it will become manifest during that interval. Obviously cleaning and sterilization of the theatre is delayed for that period

Again, an incident book should be kept to record possible cases of exposure in the ICU.

One very useful item on the ICU is the provision of a large window in the isolation room. This allows records of the patient's condition to be kept on the outside and allows visiting staff ready access to the information without any risk at all. Similarly, the nurses inside can easily summon assistance or call for materials without having to go through the tiresome changing and washing necessary on leaving the room. An intercom system would be a bonus.

Laboratory specimens

Blood and its products are highly infectious and the first measure to be adopted regarding the laboratories is the supply of information to the laboratory staff that a patient known to be HBsAg positive is being operated upon. This allows the laboratories to make adequate arrangements for the safe handling of the specimens. The problem of these specimens is familiar to them and no details are required here. The responsibility of informing the laboratories should be given to a senior member of staff, preferably the microbiologist. Specialized laboratories should not be overlooked, for instance those providing blood-gas analysis. Blood specimens should be placed in a screw-cap container and it should be the responsibility of the ward to ensure that the top is secure before the container leaves. The container is then placed inside a stout plastic bag which is then sealed. This ensures that, should the container unexpectedly leak or be dropped and thus broken, any leakage remains confined to the plastic bag. The request form is completed outside the room and is therefore not in any way contaminated and must on no account be placed in the bag with the specimen. All specimens and forms should be clearly marked 'Australia Antigen Positive' or equivalent. Obviously, blood specimens must be kept to the minimum necessary although this must never discourage whatever tests are considered appropriate for the proper management of the patient. Allowing a patient's condition to decline because of reluctance to perform indicated tests probably results in more hazard to more people in the long run.

Investigation of faecal specimens is rarely required during this stage but should it prove necessary a similar procedure can be followed. Likewise for urine specimens. When the patient leaves the ICU the room and equipment are cleaned (*see section on* Cleaning the operating theatre).

Convalescent ward

By this stage the patient will no longer be intubated and will probably have no intravenous or intra-arterial catheters in place. The bladder catheter will similarly have been removed.

The hazards, therefore, have been reduced but NOT eliminated. Thus, taking of blood samples will carry the same risks as before and demands the same precautions. The healing sternotomy wound will remain a possible source of infection until it is soundly healed and completely dry. Thus the patient should be nursed in a single room (preferably with exhaust ventilation) and wound dressings done within the room by staff wearing aprons and gloves.

When do the urine and faeces cease to be a hazard? Since the hazard is due to the admixture of these excreta with blood we have regarded negative tests for the presence of blood in them as indicating that the hazard has passed. Accordingly the nurses test a sample of urine daily until no trace of blood is found, and the laboratory likewise tests the stools for the presence of occult blood.

The patient with a soundly healed wound and no evidence of blood in the faeces and urine thus reverts to his preoperative status.

Management of staff exposed

It has been suggested by well-meaning meddlers that all hospital staff should be screened for HBsAg. It cannot be too strongly emphasized that this is unnecessary, unhelpful and, occasionally, very unfortunate. It is unnecessary because even if a member of the staff were found to be an asymptomatic carrier there is no good evidence that he or she is of any risk to the patients he treats. Indeed, with the exception of haemodialysis units and, possibly, blood transfusion centres, it is widely agreed that no branch of the medical or nursing professions should be barred to such a person. If such a carrier is detected by chance it might be advisable for them to wear gloves when carrying out invasive procedures on patients, but this is all. Since it should always be the aim of the responsible doctor to only perform tests when the result might influence his actions, it can be seen that, with the exception of the specialized groups listed above, the screening of the staff on any routine basis is unhelpful. Such screening of the staff may also be unfortunate since occasionally the finding that an individual is HBsAg positive has resulted in a considerable degree of mental torture for that person. Because of the known association with sexual promiscuity, homosexuality and so on, some individuals have undergone considerable embarrassment (usually with no justification). Since no useful purpose is served, this situation should always be avoided.

Nurses and doctors entering a known 'at risk' situation, i.e. performing major surgery on a known case, however, must be offered the best care possible. Should they be unfortunate enough to acquire HBV infection as a result they will, at least in Great Britain, be eligible for industrial compensation by law. It is, therefore, a useful compromise in these circumstances to take blood from these members of staff at the time of the risk and to store these samples *untested*. Should any person then fall ill and be found to be HBsAg positive the earlier sample can then also be tested and it can be shown that the infection has arisen over the observation period.

Special management of those exposed by accident

Should any nurse or doctor accidentally become exposed to HBsAg-containing material despite the precautions taken, specific protection can be offered. Although no known treatment exists for HBV infection, there is good evidence that the administration of high titre specific immunoglobulin within 10 days of exposure offers substantial protection against the subsequent development of the disease. The immunoglobulin is given at present as a single injection (i.m.) of 500 mg. Although the published trials on the efficacy of this substance are largely encouraging[10] there have been suggestions that in some cases the disease has not been prevented, although the incubation period has been prolonged[1], and it is likely that the dose may be altered in the future or that more than one dose will be given. However, it seems certain that the protection offered is real enough to warrant its use in all genuine cases of exposure. Certain criteria must be met before the immunoglobulin is given:

(1) Exposure must have occurred. This seems obvious but it must be admitted that a certain amount of emotion is generated by hepatitis B infection. It is thought prudent to define exposure as:
  (a) Injection of known positive material.
  (b) Ingestion of known positive material.
  (c) Conjunctival contamination with known positive material.
  (d) Contamination of a recent cut or abrasion with known positive material.
  (e) Gross contamination with known positive material.
(2) The source of the material must be formally shown to be HBsAg positive (in practice within the previous 1 month).
(3) The potential recipient must be shown to be:
  (a) Negative on testing for HBsAg (since if they were positive no action is required).

(b) Negative on testing for anti-HBs (since if they were positive they would be immune to challenge).

The criteria being fulfilled, the immunoglobulin can be given.

In view of the facts mentioned earlier it should be arranged that the recipient of the immunoglobulin be followed up for at least six months, and preferably one year, blood samples being obtained at various intervals and at the onset of any illness, even if not associated with jaundice.

The exposed person should also be advised that even if HBV infection develops it is likely to be a mild self-limiting illness and that subsequent development of the carrier state is unlikely, all things being equal.

Finally, we have taken the view that staff ought to be given the opportunity to decline to be involved in operations performed on HBsAg positive patients if they so desire. Thus, we have used volunteer teams. We do not, however, feel that this practice should be adopted in general and would wish to emphasize that the nursing of carriers of HBsAg on ordinary wards when they have common illnesses is not a hazardous procedure when simple precautions are taken.

Infective endocarditis

Profound changes have occurred in the understanding of the pathogenesis and aetiology of infective endocarditis in recent years. Although some of these changes are not of direct relevance to open-heart surgery, their consequences may be, and many of the other changes have direct implications for the surgeon.

Essentially, the subject of infective endocarditis can be subdivided into:

(1) Studies of the infective agents involved, their modes of access to the circulation and their means of initiating endocarditis.
(2) Studies of the development of the lesions on the endocardium and the changes elsewhere in the body.
(3) Studies of the effects of antibiotic therapy and prophylaxis.

Infective agents involved

Streptococci still account for a predominant amount of cases of subacute bacterial endocarditis (SBE), whilst *Staphylococcus aureus* remains the only common cause of acute bacterial endocarditis. Amongst the streptococci the imprecisely defined '*Streptococcus viridans*' is still commonly found but enterococci (*Streptococcus faecalis*, and similar organisms) account for a larger proportion of streptococcal endocarditis than formerly[2]. Increasing technical ability to identify streptococci has resulted in two separate lines of enquiry of relevance to the study of endocarditis.

Firstly, '*Streptococcus viridans*' is now divisible into many species, for instance *Strep. sanguis*, *Strep. salivarius* and so on. This advance has largely resulted from the work of dental bacteriologists. In the course of their studies on dental caries these dental workers also showed that some of the sub-varieties of '*Strep. viridans*' which they had characterized were more prone to be associated with caries than others. They further suggested that the common link between the caries-associated strains was that of the production of dextrans from a sucrose substrate[9]. This 'bacterial gum', it was suggested, enabled the organisms to stick onto the tooth and initiate dental plaque. Thus, the concept of 'bacterial stickiness' was produced. The relevance of this concept to endocarditis is that it has been a paradox for many years that the α haemolytic streptococci most commonly liberated into the blood at dental extractions etc. are not necessarily the commonest varieties isolated from cases of endocarditis. It may be that this property of 'stickiness' is involved in the ease with which some strains are apparently able to lodge onto the endocardium in comparison with the rest. Indeed, it seems that the dextran-producing strains are more likely to do this. A further extrapolation of this work lies in the observation that postoperative endocarditis is predominantly due to organisms unlike those found in 'classic' SBE. That is, organisms such as *Staphylococcus albus* are found in endocarditis presenting within 6 months of operation, whereas streptococci are less often encountered[11]. Beyond one year after operation, however, the 'classic' organisms reappear. It is known that the surface of a newly replaced heart valve is different from that of a heart valve which has been *in situ* some time, the major change being that of endothelialization which proceeds with time. It may be the case that the recently replaced valve offers a surface more conducive to *Staphylococcus albus* and that this property diminishes as the endothelialization occurs, the end result being a surface which is more conducive to streptococci. Similarly, there may be variations in the susceptibility of different types of artificial valve tissues in this regard. These possibilities deserve further study.

Secondly, it has become apparent that many streptococci which would previously have been placed confidently into either the *Strep. viridans* or enterococci groups, in fact belong to neither. Such organisms as *Streptococcus milleri* might earlier have been wrongly regarded as *Strep. faecalis*. As data builds up concerning these organisms, therapy will doubtless be improved.

From a practical viewpoint the essential initial information with which to guide therapy is not the exact identity of the streptococcus, but its response *in vitro* to sensitivity testing. This point is one which must be stressed to laboratory workers. It is also worth stressing the important fact that simple routine disc-diffusion sensitivity tests are useless in this context. When a streptococcus is isolated which is not of obviously 'faecal' type, the first test performed should be estimation of the minimum inhibitory concentration (MIC) of the organism to penicillin. If the result is very low ($<0.1\ \mu g/ml$) treatment with penicillin alone will probably be sufficient. Should the MIC be high ($>0.1\ \mu g/ml$), penicillin alone will not be sufficient and the laboratory should proceed to test for evidence of synergy between penicillins and aminoglycosides on the organism (*see later*). Several groups of workers have also shown that combinations of penicillin and streptomycin will eradicate *Streptococcus viridans* strains more quickly and completely than penicillin alone, even though that drug is sufficient by itself[17].

Staphylococcal endocarditis presents a much stiffer challenge. It has been shown many times that *Staphylococcus aureus* gains access to the circulation with ease. Although many patients have pre-existing foci of staphylococcal sepsis which serve as the initiating event, a substantial proportion have only a very minor lesion (for instance, a boil) or even no lesion at all. Certain predisposing conditions exist, most commonly diabetes. *Staphylococcus aureus* endocarditis may be a florid disease with rapid progression or it may, much more rarely, pursue a more indolent course. Undoubtedly the commonest variety is the form which accompanies staphylococcal septicaemia and in which the dramatic features of the septicaemia so dominate the clinical picture that the features of endocarditis are masked. It has been estimated that up to 60 per cent of patients with staphylococcal septicaemia suffer acute ulcerative damage to the endocardium during the disease[16]. It should always be remembered that *Staphylococcus aureus* will damage a previously normal endocardium and that a history of previous heart disease is not necessarily found. The only safe course is to treat all genuine cases of *Staphylococcus aureus* septicaemia as cases of acute endocarditis, using prolonged antibiotic therapy which has been carefully selected.

Straphylococcus albus figures largely in the accounts of postoperative endocarditis. The possibility that certain strains of this organism may have a predilection for prosthetic valve materials is referred to above. The source of these organisms is difficult to prove, but it was suggested in the first edition of this book that a large reservoir of intravascular *Staphylococcus albus* was present in the various intravenous and intra-arterial catheters which are used immediately postoperatively in open-heart surgery. This work has been further pursued and the earlier findings confirmed. The next step is the analysis of the many strains of *Staphylococcus albus* isolated from the catheter tips and their comparison with the relatively few strains isolated from endocarditis, in an attempt to find marker characteristics of the 'pathogenic' varieties. Parallels exist in other medical fields, for instance the infection of Spitz-Holter and Pudenz valves in neurosurgery, and it may be that workers in these fields may add to the findings in open-heart surgery. Should it be possible to recognize the 'dangerous' *Staph. albus* among its innocent brothers it may then be possible to eliminate it. Another potent source of *Staph. albus* is the urinary tract where recent reports have incriminated it as a common cause of infection[5]. The strains of *Staph. albus* isolated from urinary tract infection are known to differ in some respects from the commensal types, but in our experience these differences are not found in the endocarditis-causing types.

Diphtheroids are varieties of corynebacteria which are often isolated from blood cultures and which are usually dismissed as 'skin contaminants'. Undoubtedly, in most instances they are contaminants, but it is equally true that in some cases they are not. Again much basic bacteriological work is needed to characterize the truly pathogenic varieties and so allow a more rational diagnosis to follow.

Coxiella burneti is not a common cause of endocarditis, but it is extremely important in that the blood cultures will be 'sterile' since the *Rickettsiae* will not be isolated by ordinary culture. The organism is so infectious and capable of causing laboratory infection that attempts to isolate it should be confined to special laboratories possessing adequate safeguards. Fortunately serological tests suffice to diagnose most cases and they should always be requested in cases of endocarditis with negative cultures. Whereas in acute Q fever the patient will produce only so-called 'phase 2' antibody, in the endocarditis he will produce 'phase 1' antibody as well. The finding of both types of antibody in a single serum specimen makes it a diagnostic feature for all practical purposes.

Lately, *Chlamydia psittaci* (psittacosis) has been claimed to rarely produce a similar clinical syndrome and thus should also be tested for (again serologically) in culture negative endocarditis[13].

Despite the frequency with which Gram-negative bacilli (*E. coli*, pseudomonas, etc.) gain access to the circulation they only rarely cause endocarditis, and this form of the disease is essentially limited to drug addicts and postoperative cases. So unusual is valvular lodgement of these organisms that, save for the special cases just mentioned, it is a relatively safe assumption that 'coliform' bacteraemias can be treated as acute events with a short course of therapy and then the treatment can be withdrawn. Only very rarely is it necessary to recommence treatment for endocarditis. Fungal endocarditis is a specialist subject with its own expertise. Blood cultures are frequently sterile, especially in those cases involving *Aspergillus* species but it is to be welcomed that serological diagnosis of these infections has recently become more precise.

The means whereby organisms gain access to the circulation have been touched upon earlier but it would be unreasonable to conclude without drawing attention to two important, and often overlooked, points. Firstly, it is now realized that virtually any manipulation of the body can induce bacteraemia. Thus rectal biopsies, prostatic massage, enemata and many more 'minor' procedures have joined the obvious instances (delivery, abdominal surgery, prostatic resection, etc.) on the list of circumstances provoking bacteraemia. Even rocking of teeth or eating hard food has been shown to induce bacteraemia, leaving one to conclude that the instances during which antibiotic prophylaxis is offered conventionally are really only the tip of a very big iceberg. Secondly, the neglected phenomenon of 'persorption' which has proved a useful concept in the understanding of the origin of yeasts in patients recovering from open-heart surgery[12] has still to be considered with regard to other organisms, especially bacteria. The evidence from studies on patients suffering from malignant disorders involving neutropaenia has shown that the gut may often be the origin of circulating organisms. The stasis often found in the intestines of open-heart patients may also lead to a build-up of one particular organism and so promote the same phenomenon. This aspect also deserves further study.

Development of the endocardial lesions

The study of endocarditis has been most radically altered by the development of reliable animal models of the disease. Rabbit models have been most widely used, sterile 'endocarditis' being induced by catheters placed across the valve and the resultant lesion being then seeded with organisms given intravenously[6]. The condition produced seems to be acceptably close to the human disease, and has allowed studies of aetiology, pathogenesis and therapy which have a direct bearing on the latter. The conclusions reached are of two groups:

(1) Events on the valvular lesion.
(2) Changes elsewhere in the body.

It has been shown that organisms introduced into the animal's circulation whilst the sterile thrombotic endocarditis remains active will initiate infective endocarditis. If, however, the organisms are introduced sometime after the catheter initiating the thrombotic lesion has been removed, and involution of the thrombotic lesion is occurring, then no infective endocarditis develops. Once infective endocarditis is begun it can be abruptly eliminated by a single dose of a suitable bactericidal drug providing that this drug is given within 24 hours of the introduction of the organism. Once this time interval has elapsed the lesion can only be sterilized by prolonged therapy with the same drug (at least several days in duration). The critical factor, which determines the change of the endocardial infection from one easily treated to one requiring sustained therapy, is the deposition of a layer of fibrin on top of the infected thrombotic lesion. This fibrin layer appears to protect the bacteria from host defences and drugs. Sustained drug treatment will eradicate the infection if two rules are obeyed. Firstly, the oft-repeated clinical observation that only bactericidal drugs are curative has been amply confirmed in the animal model and the prolonged course of therapy found necessary in clinical cases is likewise found in the experimental situation. Durack and Beeson[7] showed that antibiotic therapy would eradicate the vast majority of the bacteria within a few dose intervals, but that a small subgroup of the bacteria appeared capable of remaining alive, albeit in a low state of metabolism and not dividing in any way, in the presence of the antibiotics. Finally these few remaining organisms would divide and become susceptible to the drug and the infection would be cured. This whole process took approximately two weeks—a time interval remarkably similar to clinical events. These findings raise some very interesting points regarding the merits of anticoagulation and antifibrin drugs in patients having prosthetic valves. Whilst it is undoubtedly true that 'endocarditis' occurs in patients receiving anticoagulation for their prosthetic valves it has been my clinical impression on more than one occasion that such cases have responded dramatically well to antibiotics, and in two such patients, both of whom had 'endocarditis' proven by blood culture, reoperation disclosed only very small vegetations. One would not want to rush into fibrinolytic therapy but further experimental work will be awaited with great interest and might provide the first addition to the armamentarium against endocarditis in many years. Finally, the proof of the fibrin layer's importance in the establishment of endocarditis provides firm evidence of the need for the high antibiotic concentration in the serum during treatment. This allows a diffusion gradient to develop between the serum and the interior of the lesion and thus ensures the production of an adequate amount of the drug in the area of the organisms.

If the bacteria-laden vegetation is also regarded as a large mass of bacterial antigen floating in a sea of antibody, it can be seen that the stage is set for circulating immune complexes to be formed as minute amounts of antigen are released from the valve. It seems that the body has three responses to bacterial invasion. The commonest is the production of pus. In endocarditis, however, the organisms are immured from the body's cellular attack and polymorphs cannot kill them. How well the body could cope with these organisms if given the opportunity is seen in the situation occurring whem emboli from the valve lodge in normal tissue. The septic embolus usually results in a sterile infarct since the bacteria cease to be protected and the normal cellular mechanisms rapidly kill them. The body's second line of defence is used against those bacteria which can survive the polymorph attack, e.g. tubercle bacilli, *Listeria* and *Brucella*. All these infections are characterized by a granulomatous reaction. Since this, too, requires access of cells it cannot be used by the body to heal endocarditis. The third, and only remaining response is that of humoral antibody production. This occurs in BE to a massive degree. Thus, antigen–antibody complexes are formed in the circulation and may be deposited in many distant parts of the body. If they lodge in the kidney, immune complex nephritis may result; if in the skin, an 'allergic vasculitis', and so on. Many of the inexplicable manifestations of BE have now been elucidated on this basis. This revolutionary concept has two important consequences. Firstly, it is very likely that in cases of established endocarditis immune disturbances will be well advanced. Thus, in a personal series of over 20 proven cases of endocarditis no case was found in which the immunoglobulin concentrations (IgG, IgM and IgA) in the serum were all normal. (Two further cases were found with normal levels but both had been treated with antibiotics for several days, having been referred for surgery on haemodynamic grounds). The disturbance of immunoglobulins found was not always the same. A raised IgG was the most common, occasionally together with a raised IgM, and sometimes a raised IgG and IgA were found. A rare pattern was a single raised IgM and this was found in a case of Q fever endocarditis. This association has been described before. One pattern not seen was a single raised IgA. Disturbances of the immunoglobulins is not specific to BE but such a finding may help in suspected cases in which blood cultures are negative. More importantly, it has proved a remarkably useful rule that if blood cultures are negative and the immunoglobulins are normal then BE is extremely unlikely to be the cause of the patient's illness. Some claims have been made that the serum complement (usually measured as 'C3') is equally useful, in that a depressed level is typical of BE and that normal level excludes the disease. This is a dangerous fallacy. While in cases of BE with advanced immune complex deposition a low C3 will be found, particularly in those with nephritis, a substantial number of cases have a normal, or even elevated level, but nonetheless have disturbed immunoglobulin levels. The second consequence of the immune complex 'theory' of endocarditis has been dubbed 'immune complacency'. It must be stressed that immunology does not explain everything and that emboli have not been explained away; they still occur and it would be a foolish man who opined from the bottom of the bed that all the patients' ills were due to immune complexes. Unfortunately, patients are occasionally denied treatment, especially surgical operation, because it has been assumed that what would have previously been thought to be recurrent emboli was really an immune phenomenon. Finally, it is not thought necessary to treat the immune complex disease specifically, e.g. with steroids, if the primary disease has been well controlled. Indeed they may be contraindicated because of the infection.

Therapy of endocarditis

The treatment of endocarditis has undergone four important changes. Firstly, our understanding of the pathogenesis of the disease, due in large part to the experimental models, has allowed a better insight into the principles underlying therapy. Secondly, better laboratory testing has allowed rational choice of antibiotics and more complete laboratory control.

Thirdly, new drugs have entered the lists as contenders for use in therapy, and fourthly, surgery has ceased to be a desperate measure invoked as a last throw, and has advanced to become a valuable adjunct to medical treatment.

The rabbit models have confirmed the basic principles in therapy which had been arrived at by careful clinical observation in the past. Thus, the essential use of bactericidal as opposed to bacteriostatic agents has been confirmed. Similarly, the need for therapy to be prolonged and a rational basis for this has also been shown. These observations have been alluded to earlier.

Laboratory testing has improved in two ways. Firstly, it is to be welcomed that many more laboratories are now providing MIC values on organisms isolated from BE and that many are also doing tests of possible synergy and antagonism. Thus, good practice is spreading from a few centres to much larger numbers. Similarly, the range of useful tests to be applied to isolated organisms has largely increased. Since, broadly speaking, organisms (bacteria in this context) fall into two categories, that is, those capable of being killed by a single drug and those requiring a combination of drugs, the following is a general guide to the information needed by the clinician.

Streptococci

(a) MIC to penicillin less than 0.1 μg/ml These organisms can be treated with penicillin alone, or by penicillin combined with streptomycin. In the former case, penicillin should be given parenterally for four weeks, usually at a dose of 2 megaunits, 6 hourly. Check assays in the serum should show a level of at least four times the MIC or, better, a result in the back-titration method of greater than 1 in 4 (*see later*). If a combination of penicillin and streptomycin is used it has been claimed that only 2 weeks' therapy is necessary but similar results in the back-titration must be shown. Some therapists use 4 weeks' penicillin but include streptomycin for the first 2 weeks. Our practice has been to use penicillin alone, adding streptomycin if relapse occurs (this latter possibility is rare if back-titration results have been adequate). If the patient is said to be allergic to penicillin the procedure described below should be adopted. If treatment with an alternative drug becomes necessary, cephalosporins or clindamycin may be used, but in all cases back-titration assays are advised.

(b) MIC to penicillin greater than 0.1 μg/ml A synergic combination of antibiotics will be needed. Usually this will consist of a penicillin (penicillin, ampicillin or amoxycillin) and an aminoglycoside (streptomycin, kanamycin or gentamicin). The laboratory should arrange the appropriate tests for these organisms (enterococci, group D streptococci, *Streptococcus milleri* and so on) and it has to be stressed that these tests must be done for the safe treatment of the patient. Assays of the aminoglycoside component of the combination should be performed to control the risk of toxicity, and back-titrations should be done to determine the efficacy of therapy. In very rare instances the organism cannot be shown to be sensitive to the usual combinations. In such cases vancomycin in combination with aminoglycosides, usually streptomycin, has been used. The use of two nephrotoxic and ototoxic drugs in combination is not a happy prospect but has proved useful on occasion. Back-titration must be done, since to persist with a very dangerous therapy if it is shown to be ineffective would be contraindicated.

Staphylococci

(a) Coagulase positive As mentioned earlier, *Staphylococcus aureus* endocarditis can be relatively easy to treat, or it can be one of the worst clinical problems imaginable. There seems no easy prediction, and often the problems emerge on testing. If the strain is sensitive to penicillin and does not, on formal testing, produce penicillinase, the drug of choice is penicillin and, as the sole therapy, will usually succeed. Back-titrations should demonstrate a level of 1 in 4 or greater. Unfortunately, resistance to penicillin is the rule rather than the exception these days. If the strain is sensitive to most other drugs, the laboratory should test combinations of them, especially cloxacillin and Fucidin, cloxacillin and clindamycin and clindamycin and Fucidin. Any combination showing synergy is then selected and given. Back-titrations are needed to assess the therapy. When cloxacillin is used in endocarditis it may be useful to employ the closely related drug methicillin since it is much less protein-bound in the serum. Strains showing resistance to cloxacillin often show synergy to a combination of methicillin and gentamicin. If all the above combinations fail it becomes necessary to consider combinations involving rifampicin and erythromycin. Finally, vancomycin remains a potent antistaphylococcal drug, alone or in combination with others. In all cases back-titrations must be done to monitor therapy.

(b) Coagulase negative staphylococci The sensitivity pattern of coagulase negative staphylococci is very unpredictable. For instance, unlike their coagulase positive relatives they may often be sensitive to cephalosporins whilst being resistant to cloxacillin. In general, if sensitive to cloxacillin this drug should form the backbone of therapy. If resistant, but shown to be sensitive to the cephalosporins, these agents should be used. Failing these two drugs, vancomycin should be considered, and in all instances back-titrations are necessary.

Diphtheroids

Most patients documented in the literature with diphtheroid endocarditis have been treated with either penicillin alone or in combination with streptomycin. However, many strains are resistant to penicillin and the cephalosporins. It should be remembered that the most active drug against these organisms, erythromycin, may not be useful in BE because of its bacteriostatic nature. Vancomycin has great activity and Fucidin has also been used. Again it must be emphasized that MIC estimations in sensitivity tests are mandatory and the slow-growing nature of these organisms makes such tests technically difficult on occasions. Finally, back-titrations are advised.

Other organisms

It has been emphasized that organisms other than those listed above are rare, but many species such as haemophili, actinobacilli, coliform bacilli and fungi are encountered from time to time. The reader is advised to consult more comprehensive accounts for details.

Back-titrations

This test has gained more acceptance in recent years. It is still undoubtedly underused. The principle is simple, namely the assessment of the ability of the patient's serum, containing the antibiotics he is receiving plus whatever natural defences he has, to extinguish the organism isolated from his blood. If the serum is shown to be cidal to the organism at a dilution of 1 in 4, or greater, therapy is adjudged to be adequate. It is important to realize the advantages and limitations of this method. Regarding its limitations, the test has two categories of fault. Firstly, it is essential that serum sample is taken at the correct time. Thus, if the patient is receiving a combination of drugs, samples should be taken at various times in order that the effects of differing ratios of the mixture can be assessed. Similarly, even when a single drug is used, samples should be taken at times when the drug is likely to be present in maximal amounts.

The second category of fault with the test is that of technical error. The test involves doubling dilutions and it is widely accepted that a technical limit of one dilution is the best that can be expected. Thus, a result of at least 1 in 8 may be a prudent level to be taken, ensuring, as it does, a level of 1 in 4. The test also involves subculture of the organism from the dilutions tested in order to demonstrate the cidal effect. This involves obtaining a sample of the liquid culture, and it cannot be certain that a fully representative subsample is always obtained.

These limitations apart, the test has many advantages. Firstly, it overcomes the problems inherent in monitoring the progress of patients receiving a synergic combination of drugs, in whom mere estimations of drugs levels would fail to assess the possible effects of the synergy. Although it would be possible to devise other means of measuring these effects, the back-titration test provides a simple and quick answer to the problem. Secondly, the test includes all elements present in the serum in its assessment. In addition to the drugs there may be antibodies and further synergy may be possible between these factors and the drugs.

The back-titration test does not provide a complete answer to monitoring the patient's progress, many patients having recovered from the disease with levels which have been inadequate in the test, although some of these results may have reflected the technical limitations referred to earlier. The test probably finds its greatest use in the patient whose progress is worrying. In such a patient an adequate level in the test implies that inadequate antibiotic therapy is not the cause of the problem. Probably the commonest example is the patient with a drug fever, usually due to penicillin. The wellbeing of the patient, combined with the adequate bactericidal level demonstrated by the test, allows the decision to continue with therapy to be made with confidence and the defervescence which occurs when drugs are eventually withdrawn provides gratifying confirmation. Drug fever is much commoner than realized.

Much more serious is the problem of continuing cardiac deterioration in the face of demonstrably adequate back-titration results. In our experience the explanations fall into two groups. Firstly, there may be a complication of the endocarditis which has resulted in a metastatic lesion which the drugs are unable to cure. One example is a splenic abscess. Another situation occurs in patients with prosthetic heart valve replacement due to the presence of local suppuration, classically an annular abscess located at the sewing rim of the valve. Thus, this combination of findings (deterioration plus adequate bactericidal levels) should lead to early consideration of surgical intervention. Finally, a patient occasionally presents in whom bacteraemia persists despite adequate back-titration results. This should lead to a full reappraisal of all the tests, in case the organism had been incorrectly identified or tested. Failing this, there may be a source of bacteraemia outside the circulation, for instance a renal stone, which will require further treatment. In the last patient we had with such a problem surgery was performed and an undiagnosed patent ductus arteriosus was discovered. In conclusion, therefore, the back-titration test is not a magic talisman. It has limitations, but as experience accrues it seems to be emerging as a simple guide to rational decision-making in the management of BE. The last point which should always be remembered is that patients with BE may develop intercurrent infection, for instance urinary tract infection, during their treatment. Here again the back-titration test will read out as satisfactory and should therefore lead to appropriate investigation of the other infection.

Finally, one is left with the two infective forms of endocarditis which have unsatisfactory treatment at present. Endocarditis due to *Coxiella burneti* (Q fever) is an infection with an organism which is only regularly susceptible to tetracyclines, drugs which are bacteriostatic. It is, therefore, not surprising that treatment is not usually successful with antibiotics alone. Two avenues have been explored. Firstly, the surgical removal of the valve under tetracycline cover. The results of this method are difficult to evaluate, but are not uniformly curative. Secondly, the addition of co-trimoxazole to tetracycline has been shown to produce a clinical cure in at least one case, and the progress of several others has seemed to be satisfactory to date. On the other hand, at least one patient has been treated with this combination, has been subjected to reoperation (for haemodynamic reasons) and the organism was isolated from the excised valve tissue. More experience is needed with both these approaches before any firm conclusions can be reached. Similar, but even more cautious, comments apply to the endocarditis associated with psittacosis, in which co-trimoxazole would not in any case be appropriate. More recently rifampicin has been shown to act on Q fever and psittacosis. It is, of course, a highly potent bactericidal drug and may thus transform the treatment of these two forms of BE if initial promise is fulfilled.

The role of surgery

With modern antibiotic therapy it should be possible in most cases to present a patient for surgical operation on purely haemodynamic grounds. Operation to control the infection may still occasionally be necessary, especially when the infected valve is a prosthesis, because of abscess formation etc., but in most instances it will only be indicated because of valve disintegration despite adequate antibacterial therapy (as shown by back-titrations). There is no doubt that operative intervention in such cases, especially when the aortic valve is the one affected, is life-saving and it cannot be stressed too often that the adequately controlled infection is no contraindication. The patients respond so well under these circumstances that my personal hope is that all cases of endocarditis, particularly those of the aortic valve, will be treated in a hospital having facilities for emergency open-heart surgery. It is our normal practice to give a complete course of therapy after valve replacement to ensure that the new tissue is unaffected by the infection. Obviously, if valve replacement is undertaken electively many weeks or months after an adequate course of therapy, when observations in the intervening period indicate cure of the infection, we treat the patient in the same way as any other patient subjected to valve replacement and do not re-treat his endocarditis.

References

1. Alter, H. J., Holland, P. V. and Schmidt, P. J. 'Gamma-globulin and hepatitis B: prevention or extension?' *Lancet*, **1,** 1110 (1972)
2. Cherubin, C. E. and Neu, H. C. 'Infective endocarditis at the Presbyterian Hospital in New York City, 1938–1967 ' *American Journal of Medicine*, **51,** 83 (1971)
3. Cossart, Y. E. *Virus Hepatitis and its Control.* p. 132. London: Bailliere-Tindall (1977)
4. Cossart, Y. E. *Virus Hepatitis and its Control.* p. 133. London: Bailliere-Tindall (1977)
5. Cossart, Y. E. *Virus Hepatitis and its Control.* p. 220. London: Bailliere-Tindall (1977)
6. Durack, D. T. and Beeson, P. B. 'Experimental endocarditis. I. Colonization of a sterile vegetation.' *British Journal of Experimental Pathology*, **53,** 44 (1972)
7. Durack, D. T. and Beeson, P. B. 'Experimental endocarditis. II. Survival of bacteria in endocardial vegetations.' *British Journal of Experimental Pathology*, **53,** 50 (1972)
8. Freeman, R. and Hambling, M. H. 'Routine use of counterimmuno-electrophoresis for detecting antibody to hepatitis B virus core antigen.' *Journal of Clinical Pathology*, **31,** 832 (1978)
9. Gibbons, R. J., Van Houte, J. and Liljemark, W. F. 'Parameters that affect the adherence of *Streptococcus salivarius* to oral epithelial surfaces.' *Journal of Dental Research*, **51,** 424 (1972)
10. Grady, G. F. and Lee, V. A. 'Hepatitis B virus immune globulin: prevention of hepatitis following accidental exposure among medical personnel.' *New England Journal of Medicine*, **293,** 1067 (1975)
11. Johnson, W. D., Jr. 'Prosthetic valve endocarditis.' In *Infective Endocarditis*. Ed. D. Kayc, Ch. 9. Baltimore: University Park Press (1976)
12. Krause, W., Matheis, H. and Wulf, K. 'Fungaemia and funguria after oral administration of *Candida albicans.*' *Lancet*, **1,** 598 (1969)
13. Levison, D. A., Guthrie, N., Ward, C., Green, D. M. and Robertson, P. G. C. 'Infective endocarditis as part of psittacosis.' *Lancet*, **2,** 844 (1971)
14. MacCallum, F. O. and Bauer, J. D. 'Homologous serum jaundice. Transmission experiments with human volunteers.' *Lancet*, **1,** 622 (1944)
15. Maskell, R. 'Importance of coagulase-negative staphylococci as pathogens in the urinary tract.' *Lancet*, **1,** 1155 (1974)
16. Rogers, D. E. 'Staphylococcal infections.' *Disease-a-month*, April, 23 (1958)
17. Wolfe, J. C. and Johnson, W. D. 'Penicillin-sensitive streptococcal endocarditis. *In vitro* and clinical observations on penicillin–streptomycin therapy.' *Annals of Internal Medicine*, **81,** 178 (1974)

Suggested references

Cossart, Y. E. *Virus Hepatitis and its Control.* London: Bailliere-Tindall (1977)
Kaye, D. (Ed.) *Infective Endocarditis*. Baltimore: University Park Press (1976)

16

Mycological Aspects of Open-Heart Surgery

E. G. V. Evans

ex umbra in solem

Introduction

The most serious mycological complication following open-heart surgery is fungal endocarditis which affects valvar prostheses and grafts. Less serious fungal infections, such as superficial yeast infections at drip and catheter sites and yeast cystitis, also occur but are relatively easily dealt with and it is not proposed to discuss them here.

The diagnosis and management of all forms of infective endocarditis presents difficulties and this is particularly true for fungal endocarditis. This infection was regarded as uniformly fatal[2] and although the prognosis has improved in recent years the outlook is still poor, particularly if dissemination to other organs occurs.

Occurrence and types

Fungal endocarditis is not as common as its bacterial counterpart but it has gained notoriety because of the difficulties associated with its management and its often fatal outcome. Relatively, it accounts for a high proportion of fatal postoperative infections.

The occurrence of opportunistic fungal endocarditis after cardiac surgery is extensively documented[45, 57, 58, 70, 71, 92, 93] and these review articles which deal with aspects of diagnosis and therapy are recommended.

The most frequent type is a yeast endocarditis[2, 3, 11, 17, 28, 43, 44, 56, 65, 69, 81, 84, 90, 92, 93, 112], usually caused by a *Candida* species, the most commonly involved being *Candida albicans* and *Candida parapsilosis*. Endocarditis caused by *Aspergillus* species also occurs[5, 10, 13, 14, 24, 42, 45, 48, 53, 68, 76, 113], and occasionally fungi less well known as the cause of endocarditis are implicated[9, 33, 34, 55, 82, 97, 104].

Source of the infection

In the case of yeast endocarditis (*Candida* endocarditis) the source of the yeast is usually the patient himself, although the organisms also abound in the hospital environment. A large proportion of open-heart surgery patients have yeasts in the mouth and/or gut on admission to hospital and, of those who do not, many rapidly acquire them. In the immediate postoperative period there is a marked increase in the patients' yeast population providing a significant reservoir for potential endogenous infection[20]. There are several possible routes of entry for yeasts into the bloodstream. The introduction of yeasts through a contaminated intravenous (IV) catheter line is thought to be a common route of infection[83, 93] and patients receiving IV hyperalimentation appear worst affected[99]. Other possibilities are colonization of the surgical wound with subsequent bloodstream invasion or direct contamination of the operative site, but these are thought to occur relatively infrequently[99]. What is now emerging as probably the most important route of entry for yeasts into the bloodstream is the persorption mechanism of the gut[110] which allows paracellular passage of particles across intestinal mucosa. Persorption of *Candida albicans* occurs quite readily from the jejunum of experimental animals[99] and there is one account of such an event in man when ingestion of 10^{12} *Candida albicans* cells resulted in candidaemia and candiduria[51]. If transient candidaemias due to persorption are common, then it is likely that IV catheters become contaminated by the bloodstream rather than vice versa. However, contaminated catheters will act as a secondary reservoir of yeasts and reseed the bloodstream, and so their early removal remains good practice.

The rate of persorption is enhanced by increases in the quantity of yeasts present[99] and so yeast levels in the small intestine should be kept low to minimize the risks of bloodstream invasion. Yeasts do not proliferate at this site or in the stomach and so the number of yeasts present depends on seeding from above. It seems likely, therefore, that the mouth will emerge as the most important reservoir of yeasts for potential systemic infection and the presence of large quantities of yeasts in the mouth of 'special risk' patients, such as open-heart surgery patients, assumes a new importance. Whatever the route of infection, the build-up of potentially pathogenic yeasts in the immediate postoperative period is undesirable and should be suppressed.

The postoperative yeast overgrowth in our patients could be successfully suppressed by simple antifungal prophylaxis with polyene antifungals[20] and the routine use of this procedure over the last 5 years has virtually eliminated yeast sepsis among our patients. Antifungal prophylaxis, at least with polyene antifungals, does not appear to have the attendant problems of antibacterial prophylaxis, namely development of resistant strains and replacement of the existing flora with other potentially more hazardous organisms. Prophylactic pre- and postoperative antifungal therapy should therefore receive serious consideration as a routine procedure in cardiac surgery patients.

The source of *Aspergillus* species is less clear. Unlike yeasts they are not present as commensals in normal individuals. They are, however, present as airborne contaminants and it is likely that contamination takes place during the surgical procedure[24, 76].

In our experience, based on cultural studies, the actual valve graft material used during surgery for heart valve replacement has never been contaminated with either *Candida* or *Aspergillus*. This was also the experience of others[14].

Clinical picture

Clinically *Candida* and *Aspergillus* infections resemble bacterial endocarditis but there is a higher frequency of large vegetations on the valves and consequently of emboli in the large arteries.

Candida endocarditis, as with bacterial infections, occurs in two distinct situations. It may become apparent in the immediate postoperative period accompanied by a septicaemia, or it appears several weeks or even months postoperatively. *Aspergillus* endocarditis usually takes the latter form.

Diagnosis

Early diagnosis of these infections is essential. Probably the most important single point that can be made concerning diagnosis is that clinicians should be aware of the possibility of fungal endocarditis from the outset so that specific requests for mycological investigations can be made along with those for bacteriological investigations. For too long the possibility of a fungal infection has been considered only after failure to implicate any other organism.

Clinical

Clinical criteria can only be used to make a presumptive diagnosis of fungal infection. However, recent observations that endophthalmitis is a common complication in patients with systemic forms of candidiasis, especially in those with candidaemia, has provided the clinician with a most useful diagnostic sign[18, 32, 63]. Endogenous endophthalmitis can also occur in patients with invasive aspergillosis[23, 66]. Furthermore, echocardiography has recently been used to demonstrate fungal vegetations on heart valves in *Candida* endocarditis of the aortic valves[4, 29, 31] and mitral valve[75] and also in *Aspergillus* endocarditis of a Starr–Edwards mitral prosthesis[87].

Laboratory

The laboratory procedures most useful for diagnosis are blood culture and serology.

Blood culture

In the case of *Candida* endocarditis blood cultures are frequently negative although they tend to become positive in the later stages of infection[92]. A series of blood cultures may therefore be necessary before the organism is grown. In one study, cultures of arterial rather than venous blood were found to be more reliable for recovery of *Candida* from the bloodstream[99]. Arterial blood cultures may therefore be indicated when venous blood cultures have failed in a patient with an infection of unknown aetiology.

Unfortunately, the isolation of a yeast from a blood culture is not absolute proof of systemic infection as reports of transient candidaemias of no clinical significance are common. These are often related to IV catheterization and usually disappear after removal of the catheter or, alternatively, they may result from persorption of yeasts from the gut. Repeated isolation of *Candida* from the bloodstream distinguishes between transient candidaemia and true infection. The possibility that a blood culture isolate is a contaminant, for example from the patient's skin, is remote. Specific mention of the possibility of yeast infection by the clinician should help suppress the tendency of a few microbiologists to look upon all fungi, in the first instance, as being contaminants. All fungi isolated from blood cultures should be identified fully and regarded as significant until proved otherwise. It is important to remember that species other than *Candida albicans* may cause an infection; indeed, members of other genera such as *Torulopsis glabrata* have been implicated on rare occasions[96]. This latter organism was, in fact, responsible for a fatal infection in one of our patients who developed a massive septicaemia in the immediate postoperative period and died within 48 hours.

Some patients may have a concomitant bacterial and yeast endocarditis[7, 37, 92]. It should, therefore, be borne in mind that yeasts are slower growing than bacteria and that the presence of both in blood cultures may be a source of error; once a bacterial cause has been isolated the cultures may be discarded[73].

Recovery of *Candida* from clinical material such as urine, faeces, sputum or bronchial secretions is of relatively little diagnostic significance as the numbers isolated may be considerable in the absence of systemic infection. However, it has been said that patients with negative urine cultures are unlikely to have systemic yeast infection[99].

In the case of *Aspergillus* infections blood cultures are usually completely negative[24, 76, 116].

Serology

Serological tests for both *Candida* and *Aspergillus* should be carried out when fungal endocarditis or septicaemia is suspected.

Tests for the estimation of agglutinins and precipitins to *Candida* are recommended[21, 93, 102]. The patient's serum should be tested against antigens from more than one *Candida* species. Other serological tests for the detection of antibodies to *Candida* such as haemagglutination, latex particle agglutination and fluorescent antibody are also available but have been less widely evaluated.

The problem with available serological tests for *Candida* is that they lack specificity and results must be interpreted with care[21, 30]. Antibodies to *Candida* have, for example, been found postoperatively among open-heart surgery patients who had no demonstrable systemic *Candida* infection[22, 65, 74] and often at titres previously regarded as indicative of invasive disease[22]. It has been shown that the appearance of these antibodies is related to the commensal yeast overgrowth seen postoperatively in open-heart surgery patients and that when this yeast multiplication is suppressed by antifungal prophylaxis the antibody response is reduced[22].

Serological tests for candidiasis are likely to be more useful when performed regularly over a period of time[21, 27]; a high or rapidly rising antibody titre suggests infection and, conversely, a reduction in antibody titre is associated with recovery from infection[93]. In open-heart surgery patients the antibodies that develop in response to yeast overgrowth in the immediate postoperative period disappear as the commensal yeast flora returns to normal levels[22]. Conversely, one would expect that in patients with *Candida* endocarditis the antibody titre would either continue to rise or be maintained at a high level.

There have been attempts to increase the specificity of the precipitin test in candidiasis and some of the results are encouraging[26, 101]; developments in this area and the current status of serological tests in the diagnosis of systemic candidiasis have recently been reviewed[19].

The appropriate test for *Aspergillus* infection is the precipitin test. Again it is important that the serum is tested against a range of antigens from several *Aspergillus* species. The test should be positive in those with *Aspergillus* endocarditis but it is also positive in patients with pulmonary forms of aspergillosis and these should be excluded. However, in one series of 7 patients with fatal prosthetic valve endocarditis due to *Aspergillus* the precipitin test was not found to be diagnostically helpful[76].

Despite the difficulties, serological tests are a useful *aid* to diagnosis but their results must be interpreted with care and considered along with the other findings.

Prognosis and therapy

Without treatment fungal endocarditis is uniformly fatal and prompt therapy is vital[92, 93, 103]. There are isolated reports of the successful medical treatment of endocarditis but it is unlikely, judging from the general results in the literature, that any available antifungal therapy, when used alone, will cure fungal endocarditis, particularly when the infection follows open-heart surgery. A combination of chemotherapy and surgical procedures such as replacement of infected valves, removal of infected tissues or repair of an aneurysm offers the best chance of success[47, 65, 92, 93, 103, 105]. This is particularly so when, as is usually the case, the condition is not diagnosed until the infection is well advanced. In a review of 107 patients with yeast endocarditis[103] the mortality for surgical therapy or antifungal therapy alone was 82 per cent whereas mortality was reduced to 20 per cent among 20 patients for whom these treatments were combined. Early surgical treatment is indicated[103] and antifungal therapy can be started preoperatively to reduce infection to a level which permits surgical intervention and to prevent dissemination.

Most of the information in the literature relates to the therapy of yeast endocarditis—the treatment of *Aspergillus* endocarditis is less well documented. It is clear, however, that the prognosis for *Aspergillus* endocarditis is poor[24, 76]. Experience with other forms of invasive aspergillosis underlines the fact that early diagnosis and treatment is essential[1] and that, generally, therapeutic results are disappointing[1, 79].

The most widely used antifungal for treatment of fungal endocarditis is amphotericin B but more recently flucytosine has also been used either alone or in combination with amphotericin B. Several imidazole antifungals have become available but the role of these in the treatment of endocarditis has yet to be fully assessed.

Amphotericin B

The polyene antifungal amphotericin B is still regarded by many as the drug of choice for the treatment of fungal endocarditis or septicaemia, despite its well known side-effects and renal toxicity[38, 107], as it has a proven antifungal effect *in vivo*. Amphotericin B is not absorbed from the gut and is administered IV as an infusion in dextrose. There are several schemes in the literature for administration of amphotericin B and most contain hints on how to reduce toxic and side-effects to a minimum[15, 16, 38, 50, 91, 106, 114]. Practice varies widely but therapy is usually started with a 1 mg test dose or a dose of 0.1–0.25 mg/kg per day and is gradually increased, as tolerance permits, to a maximum of 1.0 or 1.5 mg/kg per day. More aggressive dosage schedules are used in critically ill patients[117, 118]. Peak serum levels are usually attained on a dose of 0.5 mg/kg per day. Satisfactory blood levels are maintained when a higher dose is given on alternate days[6]. If toxic effects necessitate interruption of therapy for more than a few days then treatment is normally resumed with the low initial dose and then increased gradually again[50]. In one scheme[16] the dose of amphotericin B is increased until a daily peak serum level is achieved which is 2 or 3 times the minimum concentration of the drug that inhibits growth of the patient's organism *in vitro*. Although this allows the administration of considerably less amphotericin B it is not clear whether these lower doses are suitable for the treatment of fungal endocarditis[85]; other low dosage schemes[60, 61] are acknowledged to be unsuitable for therapy of this condition.

It has been suggested that the concomitant administration of IV mannitol may protect against the nephrotoxic effects of amphotericin B[36, 72] but a later study has failed to confirm the protective effect of mannitol[8].

Blood cultures rapidly become negative on commencement of amphotericin B therapy but the patient should not be regarded as clear of infection even after several weeks of negative cultures. There is a temptation in these circumstances to discontinue therapy but experience has shown that a relapse is inevitable unless an adequate total dose of amphotericin B has been administered. The difficulty lies in deciding what constitutes an adequate dose. One would expect this to vary from patient to patient and there are few guidelines to be found in the literature. As an empirical guide, it has been suggested that therapy should continue for a minimum of 10–12 weeks after surgical intervention[16, 47], and that the patient should receive a total of 2 500 mg of amphotericin B[103]; cultural monitoring of the patient should always continue following discontinuation of therapy. A decision to stop therapy must be made in individual cases on the basis of the clinical and mycological findings. It has been suggested that treatment should continue either until the patient's precipitins disappear or until titres are clearly falling; regular monitoring of fungal precipitins is recommended during and after cessation of therapy[93]. Complete recovery can normally be assumed when the patient's precipitins disappear and the patient has remained asymptomatic, with negative blood cultures, for a minimum of 1 year[47, 50].

It is advisable, because of the hazards of amphotericin B therapy, that anyone contemplating its use should first consult detailed literature on the subject.

Flucytosine (5-fluorocytosine)

Flucytosine, a fluorinated pyrimidine, is well absorbed from the gut and can reach blood levels of up to 100 μg/ml after oral administration without toxic effects[95]. Most yeasts are sensitive to the drug at this concentration *in vitro* but some 12 per cent of strains show primary resistance to flucytosine at concentrations of 25 μg/ml or more[35, 71, 88]. It is useful for treating yeast infections caused by sensitive strains but it should be added that these may lose a degree of sensitivity during therapy. Repeat determinations of sensitivity should therefore be carried out on any fresh isolates obtained during the course of treatment with flucytosine[39, 41, 111].

The current recommended dose of flucytosine is 150 mg/kg per day in 4 equal parts. Peak serum levels are attained 4–6 hours after the dose. Initially there were signs of potentially serious toxic effects in some patients treated with flucytosine[80]. However, in most instances, the early problems with toxicity were due to accumulation of the drug in patients with renal impairment which led to excessively high blood levels[46]. Patients with poor renal function and those on renal dialysis should be given a much reduced dose of flucytosine[12, 89]; their flucytosine serum level should be monitored at regular intervals and the dosage adjusted as necessary. Dosage can also be adjusted according to creatinine clearance rates[106]. It is preferable that the serum level of flucytosine should not be allowed to rise above 80 μg/ml.

The use of flucytosine for the treatment of systemic yeast infections is well documented[106]. It has been used with varying success for the treatment of yeast endocarditis[67, 80, 96] and has also been used successfully in combination with surgical treatment[62].

Amphotericin B + flucytosine

Combined therapy with amphotericin B and flucytosine has been used for treatment of fungal endocarditis following reports that these antifungals have a synergistic activity against yeasts *in vitro*[59, 64]. This combination enables administration of lower doses of both drugs, thereby reducing the risks both of toxicity and development of resistance but at the same time achieving therapeutically useful results[108].

There are instances where combined flucytosine and amphotericin B therapy has resulted in a medical cure of *Candida* endocarditis[17, 54] but in most instances successful therapy has been achieved by the use of these two antifungals in conjunction with surgical treatment[25, 28, 29, 84, 98]. There is also one instance of this combination being used to cure a patient with *Aspergillus* endocarditis of a prosthetic valve[10].

Imidazole antifungals

Clotrimazole was the first imidazole antifungal to be extensively studied[40]. Like amphotericin B, it has a broader spectrum of activity than flucytosine[77, 94] and there are no reported cases of primary resistance. However, the drug is poorly absorbed after oral administration, with serum levels often below the minimum inhibitory concentration (MIC) of many pathogenic fungi *in vitro*[35]. Furthermore, in some patients, clotrimazole induces liver enzymes that break down the active drug[106]. Evidence of transitory liver toxicity[52] and side-effects such as nausea, vomiting, anorexia and fatigue have been noted in some patients[106]. Although clotrimazole has been used successfully to treat systemic candidiasis after cardiac surgery[49], its use for the treatment of systemic mycoses has been discontinued because of its poor tolerance in some patients, but mainly because of its inconsistent therapeutic results.

Several other imidazole derivatives including miconazole, econazole and ketoconazole have more recently become available but they are still under evaluation. Miconazole has been the most extensively documented so far[78, 86, 109]. It is poorly absorbed from the gut and is given IV to achieve satisfactory blood levels[100]. Miconazole has been used on a limited scale for the treatment of systemic fungal infections, including systemic candidiasis[115], and there is one instance of its use as part treatment of *Candida* endocarditis[28]. It is too early, however, to assess the eventual role of miconazole in the therapy of the systemic mycoses.

Whatever the antifungal drug used, it is important that an accurate test of the fungus' sensitivity (MIC/MCC value) is carried out and also that the patient's serum levels be monitored during therapy.

Systemic antifungal therapy, because of its hazards, should never be lightly undertaken but done only after careful clinical appraisal and discussion of the laboratory data with an experienced mycologist/microbiologist.

References

1. Aisner, J., Schimpff, S. C. and Wiernik, P. H. 'Treatment of invasive aspergillosis: relation of early diagnosis and treatment to response.' *Annals of Internal Medicine*, **86**, 539 (1977)
2. Andriole, V. T., Kravetz, H. M., Roberts, W. C. and Utz, J. P. '*Candida* endocarditis. Clinical and pathological studies.' *American Journal of Medicine*, **32**, 251 (1962)
3. Arnon, R. G. and Ehrlich, R. 'Systemic candidiasis following cardiac surgery: an improved outlook.' *Southern Medical Journal*, **70**, 585 (1977)
4. Arvan, S., Cagin, N., Levitt, B. and Kleid, J. J. 'Echocardiographic findings in a patient with *Candida* endocarditis of the aortic valve.' *Chest*, **70**, 300 (1976)
5. Aslam, P. A., Gourley, R., Eastridge, C. E. and Pate, J. W. '*Aspergillus* endocarditis after aortic valve replacement.' *International Surgical Digest*, **53**, 91 (1970)
6. Bindschadler, D. D. and Bennett, J. E. 'A pharmacologic guide to the clinical use of amphotericin B.' *Journal of Infectious Diseases*, **120**, 427 (1969)
7. Boyce, J. M. H. 'A case of prosthetic valve endocarditis caused by *Corynebacterium hofmanni* and *Candida albicans*.' *British Heart Journal*, **37**, 1195 (1975)
8. Bullock, W. E., Luke, R. G., Nuttall, C. E. and Bhathena, D. 'Can mannitol reduce amphotericin B nephrotoxicity? Double blind study and description of a new vascular lesion in kidneys.' *Antimicrobial Agents and Chemotherapy*, **10**, 555 (1976)
9. Canlas, M. S. and Dillon, M. L. Jr. '*Histoplasma capsulatum* endocarditis: report of a case following heart surgery.' *Angiology*, **28**, 454 (1977)
10. Carrizosa, J., Levison, M. E., Laurence, T. and Kaye, D. 'Cure of *Aspergillus ustus* endocarditis on a prosthetic valve.' *Archives of Internal Medicine*, **133**, 486 (1974)
11. Climie, A. R. W. and Rachmaninoff, N. 'Fungal (*Candida*) endocarditis following open-heart surgery.' *Journal of Thoracic and Cardiovascular Surgery*, **50**, 431 (1965)
12. Dawborn, J. K., Page, M. D. and Schiavone, D. J. 'Use of 5-fluorocytosine in patients with impaired renal function.' *British Medical Journal*, **4**, 382 (1973)
13. Dayal, Y., Weindling, H. K. and Price, D. L. 'Cerebral infarction due to fungal embolus. A complication of *Aspergillus* infection on an aortic valve prosthesis.' *Neurology*, **24**, 76 (1974)
14. Doshi, R. '*Aspergillus fumigatus* endocarditis of an aortic homograft with aneurysm of the ascending aorta.' *Journal of Pathology*, **103**, 263 (1971)

15. Drutz, D. J. 'Antibiotic therapy in compromised hosts.' *California Medicine*, **119,** 49 (1973)
16. Drutz, D. J., Spickard, A., Rogers, D. E. and Koenig, M. G. 'Treatment of disseminated mycotic infections. A new approach to amphotericin B therapy.' *American Journal of Medicine*, **45,** 405 (1968)
17. Dupont, B., Drouhet, E. and Lapresle, C. 'Première guérison médical d'une endocardite à *Candida* sur prosthèse valvulaire.' *Annales de Médecine Interne*, **128,** 699 (1977)
18. Edwards, J. E., Jr., Foos, R. Y., Montgomerie, J. Z. and Guze, L. B. 'Ocular manifestations of *Candida* septicaemia: review of seventy-six cases of hematogenous *Candida* endophthalmitis.' *Medicine*, **53,** 47 (1974)
19. Evans, E. G. V. 'Diagnosis of systemic fungal infections.' In *Recent Advances in Infection*. Eds D. Reeves and A. Geddes. p. 55. Edinburgh: Churchill Livingstone (1979)
20. Evans, E. G. V. 'The incidence of pathogenic yeasts among open-heart surgery patients – the value of prophylaxis.' *Journal of Thoracic and Cardiovascular Surgery*, **70,** 466 (1975)
21. Evans, E. G. V. (Ed.) *Serology of Fungal Infection and Farmer's Lung Disease. A Laboratory Manual*. Leeds: British Society for Mycopathology (1976)
22. Evans, E. G. V. and Forster, R. A. 'Antibodies to *Candida* after operations on the heart.' *Journal of Medical Microbiology*, **9,** 303 (1976)
23. Friedman, A. H., Chishti, M. I. and Henkind, P. 'Endogenous ocular aspergillosis.' *Ophthalmologica*, **168,** 197 (1974)
24. Gage, A. A., Dean, D. C., Schimert, G. and Minsley, N. '*Aspergillus* infection after cardiac surgery.' *Archives of Surgery, Chicago*, **101,** 384 (1970)
25. Gladstone, J. L., Friedman, S. A., Cerruti, M. M. and Jomain, S. L. 'Treatment of *Candida* endocarditis and arteritis.' *Journal of Thoracic and Cardiovascular Surgery*, **71,** 835 (1976)
26. Glew, R. H., Buckley, H. R., Rosen, H. M., Moellering, R. C., Jr. and Fischer, J. E. 'Serologic tests in the diagnosis of systemic candidiasis. Enhanced diagnostic accuracy with crossed immunoelectrophoresis.' *American Journal of Medicine*, **64,** 586 (1978)
27. Glew, R. H., Buckley, H. R., Rosen, H. M., Moellering, R. C., Jr. and Fischer, J. E. 'Value of prospective *Candida* precipitins in fungemia in patients with hyperalimentation.' *Surgical Forum*, **26,** 113 (1975)
28. Goenen, M., Reynaert, M., Jaumin, P., Chalant, C. H. and Tremouroux, J. 'A case of *Candida albicans* endocarditis 3 years after an aortic valve replacement. Successful combined medical and surgical therapy.' *Journal of Cardiovascular Surgery*, **18,** 391 (1977)
29. Gomes, J. A. C., Calderon, J., Lajans, F., Sakurai, H., Friedman, H. S. and Tatz, J. S. 'Echocardiographic detection of fungal vegetations in *Candida parapsilosis* endocarditis.' *American Journal of Medicine*, **61,** 273 (1976)
30. Gordon, M. A. 'Serodiagnosis of opportunistic mycoses.' In *Opportunistic Pathogens*. Eds J. E. Prier and H. Friedman. p. 147. London: Macmillan (1974)
31. Gottlieb, S., Khuddus, S. A., Balooki, H., Dominguez, A. E. and Myerburg, R. J. 'Echocardiographic diagnosis of aortic valve vegetations in *Candida* endocarditis.' *Circulation*, **50,** 826 (1974)
32. Griffin, J. R., Pettit, T. H., Fishman, L. S. and Foos, R. Y. 'Blood-borne *Candida* endophthalmitis. A clinical and pathologic study of 21 cases.' *Archives of Ophthalmology, N. Y.*, **89,** 450 (1973)
33. Haldane, E. V., MacDonald, J. L., Gittens, W. O., Yuce, K. and Rooyen, C. E. Van. 'Prosthetic valvular endocarditis due to the fungus *Paecilomyces*.' *Canadian Medical Association Journal*, **111,** 963 (1974)

34. Hall, W. J., III. '*Penicillium* endocarditis following open-heart surgery and prosthetic valve insertion.' *American Heart Journal*, **87,** 501 (1974)
35. Hamilton-Miller, J. M. T. 'A comparative *in vitro* study of amphotericin B, clotrimazole and 5-fluorocytosine against clinically isolated yeasts.' *Sabouraudia*, **10,** 276 (1972)
36. Hellebush, A. A., Salama, F. and Eadie, E. 'The use of mannitol to reduce the nephrotoxicity of amphotericin B.' *Surgery, Gynecology and Obstetrics*, **134,** 241 (1972)
37. Henderson, J. and Nickerson, J. F. 'Bacterial endocarditis with *Candida albicans* superinfection.' *Canadian Medical Association Journal*, **90,** 452 (1964)
38. Hildick-Smith, G., Blank, H. and Sarkany, I. *Fungous Diseases and their Treatment*. London: Churchill (1964)
39. Hoeprich, P. D., Ingraham, J. L., Kleker, E. and Winship, M. J. 'Development of resistance to 5-fluorocytosine in *Candida parapsilosis* during therapy.' *Journal of Infectious Diseases*, **130,** 112 (1974)
40. Hoffbrand, B. I., Allen, H. B. and Good, C. S. (Eds) '*Clotrimazole*.' *Postgraduate Medical Journal*, **50 (Suppl. 1)**, (1974)
41. Holt, R. J. and Newman, R. L. 'The antimycotic activity of 5-fluorocytosine.' *Journal of Clinical Pathology*, **26,** 167 (1973)
42. Horten, B. C., Abbott, G. F. and Porro, R. S. 'Fungal aneurysms of intracranial vessels.' *Archives of Neurology*, **33,** 577 (1976)
43. Jamshidi, A., Pope, R. H. and Friedman, N. H. 'Fungal endocarditis complicating cardiac surgery.' *Archives of Internal Medicine*, **112,** 370 (1963)
44. Juffe, A., Miranda, A. L., Rufilanchas, J. J., Maronas, J. M. and Figuero, D. 'Prosthetic valve endocarditis by opportunistic pathogens.' *Archives of Surgery*, **112,** 151 (1977)
45. Kammer, R. B. and Utz, J. P. '*Aspergillus* species endocarditis. The face of a not so rare disease.' *American Journal of Medicine*, **56,** 506 (1974)
46. Kauffman, C. A. and Frame, P. T. 'Bone marrow toxicity associated with 5-fluorocytosine therapy.' *Antimicrobial Agents and Chemotherapy*, **11,** 244 (1977)
47. Kay, J. H., Bernstein, S., Tsuji, H. K., Redington, J. V., Milgram, M. and Brem, T. 'Surgical treatment of *Candida* endocarditis.' *Journal of the American Medical Association*, **203,** 621 (1968)
48. Khan, H. T., Kane, E. G. and Dean, C. '*Aspergillus* endocarditis of mitral prosthesis.' *American Journal of Cardiology*, **22,** 227 (1968)
49. Kozinn, P. J., Lynfield, J. and Seelig, M. S. 'Successful treatment of systemic candidiasis following cardiac surgery.' *American Journal of Diseases of Children*, **128,** 106 (1974)
50. Kozinn, P. J., Taschdjian, C. L., Seelig, M. S., Caroline, L. and Teitler, A. 'Diagnosis and therapy of systemic candidasis.' *Sabouraudia*, **7,** 98 (1969)
51. Krause, W., Matheis, H. and Wulf, K. 'Fungaemia and funguria after oral administration of *Candida albicans*.' *Lancet*, **1,** 598 (1969)
52. Mahgoub, E. S. 'Laboratory and clinical experience with clotrimazole (BAYb5097).' *Sabouraudia*, **10,** 210 (1972)
53. Mahvi, T. A., Webb, H. M., Dixon, C. D. and Boone, J. A. 'Systemic aspergillosis caused by *Aspergillus niger* after open-heart surgery.' *Journal of the American Medical Association*, **203,** 520 (1968)
54. Mayrer, A. R., Brown, A., Weintraub, R. A., Ragni, M. and Postic, B. 'Successful medical therapy for endocarditis due to *Candida parapsilosis*. A clinical and epidemologic study.' *Chest*, **73,** 546 (1978)

55. McClellan, J. R., Hamilton, J. D., Alexander, J. A., Wolfe, W. G. and Reed, J. B. '*Paecilomyces varioti* endocarditis on a prosthetic aortic valve.' *Journal of Thoracic and Cardiovascular Surgery*, **71,** 472 (1976)
56. McConnell, E. M. and Roberts, C. 'Pathological findings in three cases of fungal endocarditis complicating open-heart surgery.' *Journal of Clinical Pathology*, **20,** 555 (1967)
57. McLeod, R. and Remington, J. S. 'Fungal endocarditis.' In *Infective Endocarditis*. Ed. S. H. Rahimtoola. p. 211. New York: Grune and Stratton (1978)
58. McLeod, R. and Remington, J. S. 'Postoperative fungal endocarditis.' In *Infections of Prosthetic Heart Valves and Vascular Grafts*. Ed. R. J. Duma. p. 163. Baltimore: University Park Press (1977)
59. Medoff, G., Comfort, M. and Kobayashi, G. S. 'Synergistic action of amphotericin B and 5-fluorocytosine against yeast-like organisms.' *Proceedings of the Society for Experimental Biology and Medicine*, **138,** 571 (1971)
60. Medoff, G., Dismukes, W. E., Meade, R. H., III and Moses, J. M. 'A new therapeutic approach to *Candida* infections. A preliminary report.' *Archives of Internal Medicine*, **130,** 241 (1972)
61. Medoff, G., Dismukes, W. E., Meade, R. H., III and Moses, J. M. 'Therapeutic program for *Candida* infection.' *Antimicrobial Agents and Chemotherapy*, **–1970,** 286 (1971)
62. Montague, N. T. and Sugg, W. L. '*Candida* endocarditis with femoral emboli. Treatment with surgery and 5-fluorocytosine.' *Journal of Thoracic and Cardiovascular Surgery*, **67,** 322 (1974)
63. Montgomerie, J. Z. and Edwards, J. E., Jr. 'Association of infection due to *Candida albicans* with intravenous hyperalimentation.' *Journal of Infectious Diseases*, **137,** 197 (1978)
64. Montgomerie, J. Z., Edwards, J. E., Jr and Guze, L. B. 'Synergism of amphotericin B and 5-fluorocytosine for *Candida* species.' *Journal of Infectious Diseases*, **132,** 82 (1975)
65. Murray, I. G., Buckley, H. R. and Turner, G. C. 'Serological evidence of *Candida* infection after open-heart surgery.' *Journal of Medical Microbiology*, **2,** 463 (1969)
66. Naidoff, M. A. and Green, W. R. 'Endogenous *Aspergillus* endophthalmitis occurring after kidney transplant.' *American Journal of Ophthalmology*, **79,** 502 (1975)
67. Naveh, Y., Friedman, A., Merzbach, D. and Hashman, N. 'Endocarditis caused by *Rhodotorula* successfully treated with 5-fluorocytosine.' *British Heart Journal*, **37,** 101 (1975)
68. Newman, W. H. and Cordell, A. R. '*Aspergillus* endocarditis after open-heart surgery. Report of a case and review of literature.' *Journal of Thoracic and Cardiovascular Surgery*, **48,** 652 (1964)
69. Newsom, S. W. B., Lee, W. R. and Rees, J. R. 'Fatal fungal infection following open-heart surgery.' *British Heart Journal*, **29,** 457 (1967)
70. Norenberg, R. G., Sethi, G. K., Scott, S. M. and Takaro, T. 'Opportunistic endocarditis following open-heart surgery.' *Annals of Thoracic Surgery*, **19,** 592 (1975)
71. Odds, F. C. *Candida and Candidosis*. Leicester: Leicester University Press (1979)
72. Olivero, J. J., Lozano-Mendez, J., Ghafary, E. M., Eknoyan, G. and Suki, W. N. 'Mitigation of amphotericin B nephrotoxicity by mannitol.' *British Medical Journal*, **1,** 550 (1975)

73. Paisley, J. W., Todd, J. K. and Roe, M. H. 'Early detection and preliminary susceptibility testing of positive blood cultures with the steers replicator.' *Journal of Clinical Microbiology*, **6,** 367 (1977)
74. Parsons, E. R. and Nassau, E. '*Candida* serology in open-heart surgery.' *Journal of Medical Microbiology*, **7,** 415 (1974)
75. Pasternak, R. C., Cannom, D. S. and Cohen, L. S. 'Echocardiographic diagnosis of large fungal verruca attached to mitral valve.' *British Heart Journal*, **38,** 1209 (1976)
76. Petheram, I. S. and Seal, R. M. E. '*Aspergillus* prosthetic valve endocarditis.' *Thorax*, **31,** 380 (1976)
77. Plempel, M., Bartmann, K., Buchel, K. H. and Regel, E. 'Experimental study of a new orally effective broad-spectrum antimycotic agent.' *German Medical Monthly*, **14,** 532 (1969)
78. Proceedings International Symposium, Antwerp. 'New possibilities in the treatment of systemic mycoses. Reports on the experimental and clinical evaluation of miconazole.' *Proceedings of the Royal Society of Medicine, London*, **70, (Suppl. 1**), (1977)
79. Prystowsky, S. D., Vogelstein, B., Ettinger, D. S., Merz, W. G., Kaizer, H., Sulica, V. I., Zinkham, W. H. 'Invasive aspergillosis.' *New England Journal of Medicine*, **295**, 655 (1976)
80. Record, C. O., Skinner, J. M., Sleight, P. and Speller, D. C. E. '*Candida* endocarditis treated with 5-fluorocytosine.' *British Medical Journal*, **1,** 262 (1971)
81. Robboy, S. J. and Kaiser, J. 'Pathogenesis of fungal infection on heart valve prostheses.' *Human Pathology*, **6,** 711 (1975)
82. Roberts, F. J., Allen, P. and Maybee, T. K. '*Petriellidium boydii (Allescheria boydii*) endocarditis associated with porcine valve replacement.' *Canadian Medical Association Journal*, **117,** 1250 (1977)
83. Rose, H. D. 'Venous catheter-associated candidemia.' *American Journal of Medical Science*, **275,** 265 (1978)
84. Rotheram, E. B., Jr. and Magovern, G. J. 'Two-year cure of *Candida* infection of prosthetic mitral valve.' *Postgraduate Medicine*, **61,** 237 (1977)
85. Rubinstein, E., Noriega, E. R., Simberkoff, M. S. and Rahal, J. J., Jr. 'Tissue penetration of amphotericin B in *Candida* endocarditis.' *Chest*, **66,** 376 (1974)
86. Schär, G., Kayser, F. H. and Dupont, M. C. 'Antimicrobial activity of econazole and miconazole *in vitro* and in experimental candidiasis and aspergillosis.' *Chemotherapy*, **22,** 211 (1976)
87. Schelbert, H. R. and Muller, O. F. 'Detection of fungal vegetations involving a Starr–Edwards mitral prosthesis by means of ultrasound.' *Vascular Surgery*, **6,** 20 (1972)
88. Schönebeck, J. and Ånsehn, S. '5-fluorocytosine resistance in *Candida* spp. and *Torulopsis glabrata*.' *Sabouraudia,* **11,** 10 (1973)
89. Schönebeck, J., Polak, A., Fernex, M. and Scholer, H. J. 'Pharmacokinetic studies on the oral antimycotic agent 5-fluorocytosine in individuals with normal and impaired kidney function.' *Chemotherapy*, **18,** 321 (1973)
90. Scully, R. E. and McNeely, B. U. '*Candida* septicaemia after double valve replacements.' *New England Journal of Medicine*, **291,** 1021 (1974)
91. Seabury, J. H. and Dascomb, H. E. 'Experience with amphotericin B for the treatment of systemic mycoses.' *Annals of the New York Academy of Science*, **89,** 202 (1960)
92. Seelig, M. S., Speth, C. P., Kozinn, P. J., Taschdjian, C. L., Toni, E. F. and Goldberg, P. 'Patterns of *Candida* endocarditis following cardiac surgery: importance of early diagnosis and therapy (an analysis of 91 cases).' *Progress in Cardiovascular Diseases*, **17,** 125 (1974)

93. Seelig, M. S., Speth, C. P., Kozinn, P. J., Toni, E. F. and Taschdjian, C. L. 'Candida endocarditis after cardiac surgery: clues to earlier detection.' *Journal of Thoracic and Cardiovascular Surgery*, **65**, 583 (1973)
94. Shadomy, S. '*In vitro* antifungal activity of clotrimazole (BAYb5097).' *Infection and Immunity*, **4**, 143 (1971)
95. Shadomy, S. '*In vitro* studies with 5-fluorocytosine.' *Applied Microbiology*, **17**, 871 (1969)
96. Sharpe, D. N., Singh, B. N., Cornere, B. M. and Allwood, G. K. '*Torulopsis glabrata* endocarditis complicating aortic homograft valve treated with 5-fluorocytosine: case report with discussion of antifungal chemotherapy.' *New Zealand Medical Journal*, **81**, 294 (1975)
97. Slifkin, M. and Bowers, H. M. Jr. '*Phialophora mutabilis* endocarditis.' *American Journal of Clinical Pathology*, **63**, 120 (1975)
98. Stone, D. L. '*Candida* endocarditis treated with a combination of antifungal chemotherapy and aortic valve replacement.' *British Heart Journal*, **37**, 1191 (1975)
99. Stone, H. H., Kolb, L. D., Currie, C. A., Geheber, C. E. and Cuzzell, J. Z. 'Candida sepsis: pathogenesis and principles of treatment.' *Annals of Surgery*, **179**, 697 (1974)
100. Sung, J. P., Grendahl, J. G. and Levine, H. B. 'Intravenous and intrathecal miconazole therapy for systemic mycoses.' *Western Journal of Medicine*, **126**, 5 (1977)
101. Syverson, R. E., Buckley, H. R. and Gibian, J. R. 'Increasing the predictive value positive of the precipitin test for the diagnosis of deep-seated candidiasis.' *American Journal of Clinical Pathology*, **70**, 826 (1978)
102. Taschdjian, C. L., Seelig, M. S. and Kozinn, P. J. 'Serological diagnosis of candidal infections.' *CRC Critical Reviews in Clinical Laboratory Sciences*, **4**, 19 (1973)
103. Turnier, E., Kay, J. H., Bernstein, S., Mendez, A. M. and Zubiate, P. 'Surgical treatment of *Candida* endocarditis.' *Chest*, **67**, 262 (1975)
104. Upshaw, C. B., Jr. '*Penicillium* endocarditis of aortic valve prosthesis.' *Journal of Thoracic and Cardiovascular Surgery*, **68**, 428 (1974)
105. Utley, J. R., Mills, J. and Roe, B. B. 'The role of valve replacement in the treatment of fungal endocarditis.' *Journal of Thoracic and Cardiovascular Surgery*, **69**, 255 (1975)
106. Utz, J. P. 'Chemotherapy for the systemic mycoses.' *British Journal of Hospital Medicine*, **15**, 112 (1976)
107. Utz, J. P., Bennett, J. E., Brandriss, M. W., Butler, W. and Hill, G. J. 'Amphotericin B toxicity. Combined clinical staff conference at the National Institutes of Health.' *Annals of Internal Medicine*, **61**, 334 (1964)
108. Utz, J. P., Garriques, I. L., Sande, M. A., Warner, J. F., Mandell, G. L., McGehee, R. F., Duma, R. J. and Shadomy, S. 'Therapy of cryptococcosis with a combination of flucytosine and amphotericin B.' *Journal of Infectious Diseases*, **132**, 368 (1975)
109. Van Cutsem, J. M. and Thienpont, D. 'Miconazole, a broad-spectrum antimycotic agent with antibacterial activity. *Chemotherapy*, **17**, 392 (1972)
110. Volkheimer, G. and Schulz, F. H. 'The phenomenon of persorption.' *Digest*, **1**, 213 (1968)
111. Warner, J. F., Duma, R. J., McGehee, R. F., Shadomy, S. and Utz, J. P. '5-fluorocytosine in human candidiasis.' *Antimicrobial Agents and Chemotherapy*, **–1970**, 473 (1971)
112. Watanakunakorn, C., Carleton, J., Goldberg, L. M. and Hamburger, M. '*Candida* endocarditis surrounding a Starr–Edwards prosthetic valve. Recovery of *Candida* in hypertonic medium during treatment.' *Archives of Internal Medicine*, **121**, 243 (1968)

113. Wheeler, E. O. and Robboy, S. J. 'Fever, cardiac arrhythmias and pericarditis after aortic-valve replacement.' *New England Journal of Medicine*, **295,** 718 (1976)
114. Winn, W. A. 'Coccidioidomycosis and amphotericin B.' *Medical Clinics of North America*, **47,** 1131 (1963)
115. Wust, H. J. and Lennartz, H. 'Miconazole in systemic candidiasis.' *Proceedings of the Royal Society of Medicine, London*, **70** (**Suppl. 1**), 18 (1977)
116. Young, R. C., Bennett, J. E., Vogel, C. L., Carbone, P. P. and De Vita, V. T. 'Aspergillosis. The spectrum of the disease in 98 patients.' *Medicine*, **49,** 148 (1970)

Recommended recent comprehensive reviews on antifungal chemotherapy

117. Medoff, G. and Kobayashi, G. S. 'Strategies in the treatment of systemic fungal infections'. *New England Journal of Medicine*, **302,** 145 (1980)
118. Speller, D. C. E. (Ed.) *Antifungal Chemotherapy*. Chichester: Wiley (1980)

17

Extracorporeal Circulation, Anaesthesia and Postoperative Management for Surgery of Myocardial Ischaemia

Lawrence H. Cohn, Anna Mae Fosberg, Stanley Lee-Son and John J. Collins, Jr.

sapiens qui prospicit

Introduction

Aortocoronary bypass on a large scale was begun by Favaloro and associates at the Cleveland Clinical Foundation in 1967[24] following the introduction of selective coronary arteriography by Sones in 1962[44]. In the ensuing twelve years, the coronary artery bypass operation (CABG) has become the most common cardiovascular operation in the world. In the United States alone more than 75 000 CABG operations are performed each year. Angina is relieved, exercise capability improved and the quality of life enhanced after such operations[4, 5, 8, 35, 42]. With increasing follow-up direct myocardial revascularization also appears to have a significant positive effect on longevity[14, 34, 40, 46, 47]. Thus, until the basic aetiology of arteriosclerosis is determined, this operation will continue to be an important and effective treatment for coronary arteriosclerosis.

In recent years there has been an increasingly aggressive operative approach for patients with extensive coronary artery disease as well as for those with left ischaemic ventricular dysfunction. More grafts per patient and more complete revascularization are now accomplished with low mortality rates due to improved methods of coronary artery grafting, safer extracorporeal circulation, pharmacological and mechanical modification of acute myocardial ischaemia, improved myocardial protection, and increased awareness that the time prior to cardiopulmonary bypass is the most critical period for patients undergoing CABG.

This chapter will review the preoperative care, intraoperative myocardial protection, management of both anaesthesia and extracorporeal circulation, and essentials of postoperative care for patients undergoing coronary artery bypass grafting for acute and chronic myocardial ischaemia.

Preoperative preparation

Patients undergoing elective coronary bypass surgery with previous coronary angiography detailing the coronary lesions enter the hospital two days prior to operation to familiarize themselves with the hospital surroundings and to become orientated to the Intensive Care Unit and postoperative procedures. Chest radiographs, electrocardiograms (ECG) and SMA-12 are done and medical conditions commonly present such as diabetes and systemic hypertension, and other manifestations of arteriosclerosis are evaluated at this time. For example, systemic hypertension is a significant factor which should be controlled prior to surgery as it may increase myocardial oxygen consumption by increasing left ventricular wall tension which may result in myocardial ischaemia[19].

In general, cardiotonic agents and diuretics are discontinued to help restore body potassium and to decrease serum digoxin levels. Anticoagulation is stopped two days prior to surgery. Fresh frozen plasma is prepared for the post-bypass period in these patients. Propranolol is not discontinued in any patient who is to undergo coronary bypass operation. If a patient is continuing to have angina, however mild, the dosage remains the same; if the patient is pain-free, the dose is halved. At the inception of CABG surgery in the early 1970s, it was suggested that propranolol be discontinued three weeks prior to operation because of its myocardial depressant effects in the immediate postcardiopulmonary bypass period[22, 50]. This has not been our experience or that of others[6, 11, 20, 21, 29, 30, 43]; in fact, there has been considerably more difficulty when beta blockers have been discontinued in patients prior to CABG who require the depression of myocardial oxygen requirements until new myocardial blood flow can be established by coronary bypass grafting. There have been few instances of depressed postcardiopulmonary bypass ventricular function with such agents. However, if post-bypass myocardial depression is encountered, it can be alleviated by inotropic drugs such as dopamine and/or by electrical pacing. In patients with unstable angina, it is even more important to maintain therapeutic levels of propranolol prior to surgical treatment because of the depressive effect on myocardial oxygen consumption which favourably influences the balance of oxygen supply and demand to jeopardized myocardial function[11, 19].

Cigarette smoking is discontinued two weeks in advance of surgery. Detailed pulmonary function tests are not routinely ordered but bedside spirometry and respiratory therapy evaluation are carried out prior to surgery for a baseline estimation of pulmonary function.

In the preparation of the patient with unstable angina refractory to medical therapy and for which operation is required on an emergency or urgent basis, intra-aortic balloon counterpulsation is occasionally indicated to stabilize the patient and protect him during the critical bypass period[10, 51]. It is particularly indicated in those patients with a tight left main coronary occlusion and unstable angina with continuing pain, arrhythmias and hypo- or hypertension[14]. We do not routinely use this device in patients with left main stem coronary stenosis unless the patient is in an unstable haemodynamic condition. This device is also of importance if the anaesthesia service is inexperienced in handling patients with unstable angina or if operating room logistics are uncertain.

Anaesthetic management

Until myocardial revascularization is accomplished by coronary artery bypass grafts, coronary blood flow cannot increase to meet an increased myocardial oxygen demand. Appropriate control of the determinants of myocardial oxygen consumption should allow the myocardium to work within the physiological constraints set by the obstructive lesions. Ideal anaesthetic management of patients undergoing CABG should avoid interference with the limited oxygen supply and avoid factors which might increase myocardial oxygen demand.

Preoperative preparation

At the preoperative visit the anaesthesiologist acquaints himself with the patient's history, physical findings and results of investigations including cardiac catheterization and coronary angiography. At this time a rapport is established with the patient and the findings are reviewed with particular attention paid to his drug history. The anaesthetic plan is explained to the patient, thus keeping the patient informed and reassuring him. This has been shown to be a useful non-pharmacological antidote to anxiety.

Examination of the haemodynamic parameters provides an indication of the contractility of the myocardium. With the catecholamine release in response to stress, a myocardium with increasing contractile performance may increase its oxygen demand beyond the limits of its blood supply resulting in ischaemia. An anaesthetic technique which decreases this contractility may be needed. On the other hand, a myocardium with poor contractility may be unable to maintain an adequate cardiac output if the anaesthetic agents depress contractility.

The patient for coronary artery surgery may be receiving many medications and interaction of these drugs with the anaesthetic agents is very possible. Beta adrenergic blockade with propranolol is frequently used in the medical management of the patient with angina. As noted above, continuation of this drug up to the time of surgery has not caused any major adverse reactions during surgery, while abrupt withdrawal of propranolol may increase the risk of myocardial infarction[6, 21]. Drugs used in the treatment of hypertension may act at various sites in the autonomic nervous system and control of hypertension should be maintained until the time of surgery. The reactivity of the sympathetic nervous system may be obtunded and therefore the circulatory depressant action of anaesthetic agents might be aggravated. If the mechanism of action of the antihypertensive agents is known, appropriate counter-measures may be instituted should marked hypotension occur. Diuretics may be used in the management of hypertension and congestive heart failure. There may be a decreased extracellular volume[13] which may only become manifest when vasodilatation occurs under anaesthesia. Diuretics may also lead to a loss of potassium which may be masked by an accompanying metabolic alkalosis and aggravated by dilution during cardiopulmonary bypass and urinary loss.

The preoperative visit includes examination of sites for placement of intravenous infusions, and performance of Allen's test to check the patency of the radial and ulnar arteries. Note is also made of the patient's airway and any feature which might make endotracheal intubation difficult.

Preoperative orders include sedatives to ensure a good night's sleep. The aim of preanaesthetic medication is to have a calm and sedated patient on arrival in the operating room. One hour before surgery the patient receives pentobarbital 1–2 mg/kg body weight intramuscularly, morphine sulphate 0.1 mg/kg body weight intramuscularly and scopolamine 0.4 mg intramuscularly. Diazepam 5–10 mg orally is added if the patient is very anxious and is scheduled for surgery later in the day. At the time of premedication the patient also receives oxygen by mask and a supply of nitroglycerin tablets.

Before the arrival of the patient in the operating room, the anaesthetic drugs and equipment and monitors are prepared and checked. In addition, infusions of vasoactive drugs are prepared such as:

(1) neosynephrine (alpha adrenergic agonist) : 2 mg in 500 ml solution;
(2) isoproterenol (beta adrenergic agonist) : 2 mg in 500 ml solution;
(3) dopamine (beta adrenergic agonist) : 800 mg in 500 ml solution of 5 mg/100ml dextrose in water.

Other cardioactive drugs that should be readily available include lidocaine and sodium nitroprusside.

On arrival in the operating room, the patient is identified and his records and vital signs are checked. An electrocardiogram (ECG) monitor is attached to the patient. Under local anaesthesia, two large bore intravenous infusion catheters are placed, the usual sites being the dorsum of the right hand and the left external jugular vein. An 18-gauge arterial catheter is inserted percutaneously into the left radial artery for continuous monitoring of arterial pressure and for withdrawal of samples for arterial blood gases and acid–base balance estimation. Central venous pressure is monitored by either a catheter introduced via the right external jugular vein using a J-wire to facilitate passage of the catheter centrally or via an internal jugular puncture.

Induction of anaesthesia

Preoxygenation is carried out during the preparatory stages of anaesthesia which is induced using morphine in incremental doses until the patient is no longer responsive to command. This usually occurs after about 1–2 mg/kg body weight have been administered. If the patient is still alert, diazepam 5–10 mg is used to provide additional sedation. Succinylcholine is used to facilitate endotracheal intubation. Nitrous oxide 50–70 per cent in oxygen is added to maintain anaesthesia and ventilation is controlled using a mechanical ventilator set to deliver a tidal volume of 10 ml/kg body weight at 10 times per minute. Ventilation is adjusted to maintain the arterial $P\text{CO}_2$ in the range of 30–35 mmHg depending on the arterial blood-gas analysis. Muscle relaxation is maintained with tubocurarine administered in increments to avoid hypotension. An oesophageal temperature probe is placed to monitor central body temperature. Two units of compatible blood are checked and made readily available and appropriate prophylactic antibiotics are administered. A bladder catheter is passed and urine output measured every 30 minutes.

Anaesthesia is maintained with nitrous oxide and oxygen. Further doses of morphine and neuromuscular blocking agents are used as needed. Bradycardia below 50 beats per minute is sometimes seen and this usually responds to administration of atropine 0.4 mg intravenously or isoproterenol infusion. It is important to treat this aggressively since venous pooling and decreased venous return with morphine anaesthesia plus bradycardia may depress the cardiac output. Hypotension may occur with induction of anaesthesia and the response to fluid administration is first determined. If hypotension below 100 mmHg occurs, a neosynephrine infusion is begun.

Hypotension may also occur following surgical preparation of the lower limbs when these are lowered and pooling of blood in the legs occurs. This can be minimized by lowering the legs gradually. Hypotension may occur during cardiac cannulation, caused by blood loss or obstruction of venous return which is corrected by altering the position of the cannula or by starting the heart-lung bypass as soon as possible.

Hypertension may also occur in response to incision and to sternotomy. Sodium nitroprusside is occasionally needed to reduce the blood pressure. The 'Double Product'[2] is conveniently used as a practical guide to myocardial oxygen consumption. If the product of heart rate multipled by systolic blood pressure is 12 000, measures are instituted to reduce this product. Usually introduction of halothane in a concentration of 0.5 to 1 per cent will suffice.

Because of the dilutional effect of cardiopulmonary bypass, further doses of morphine and neuromuscular blocking agents are given. Ventilation is maintained during partial heart-lung bypass but discontinued during total bypass.

During cardiopulmonary bypass, preparations are made for the post-bypass period. A dose of neuromuscular blocking agent is added prior to electrical defibrillation of the heart to minimize muscular response by the electrical stimulus. Blood transfusions are prepared for the post-bypass period as well as the protamine infusion. The dose of protamine is estimated by titration of the heparin levels or from the activated clotting time and the protamine is administered when decannulation has been accomplished (*see below*).

After the heart is defibrillated a return is made to partial bypass and ventilation is begun. The blood pressure is maintained at 90–100 mmHg systolic and the central venous and left atrial pressures are kept at levels that give an optimal systemic arterial pressure—usually about 15 cmH_2O.

Extracorporeal circulation and operative techniques

The extracorporeal system

We currently utilize a Cobe Optiflo-II bubble oxygenator mounted on an Olson console with DeBakey roller pumps. The oxygenator used is designed for a low gas flow/blood flow ratio, continuous monitoring of arterial and venous blood temperatures and easy and safe access to blood sampling ports. Its design also incorporates an integral gas filter, scavenger vent, heat exchanger, and stopcocks, all of which, in conjunction with the sterile precut tubing set, makes for the fastest and safest assembly of an extracorporeal system possible.

Arterial line filters*, cardiotomy reservoir† and an integral in-depth filter are used to remove particular microemboli up to 20 microns in size which are

*Johnson and Johnson Intercept filter
†Cobe reservoir

a cause of postoperative cerebral dysfunction[1] and to serve as potential fail-safe mechanism to prevent gross air embolization.

A Sarnes Heater-Cooler unit is the source of a constant, dependable flow of water for the heat exchanger. The patients are routinely cooled to 28°C and the central body temperature is monitored with an oesophageal probe. The oxygenator non-blood prime consists of 1600 ml of lactated Ringer's solution, 25 g of dextrose, antibiotics and 2000 units of heparin, a solution simulating human plasma. This prime will generally lower the patient's haematocrit to the range of 20–25. If the patient is markedly anaemic, a unit of blood will be substituted for the lactated Ringer's solution. The arterial perfusion rate is 1.5–2.0 ℓ/min per m^2 to obtain a perfusion pressure of approximately 70–90 mmHg.

Blood gases are monitored when the patient's temperature has reached 28–30°C. Thereafter, samples are taken every 60 minutes unless the clinical situation warrants more frequent determinations.

The initial dose of heparin for cardiopulmonary bypass is 300 units/kg body weight, injected directly into the right atrium by the surgeon. The anticoagulation level is measured by the whole-blood activated clotting time as described by Hattersley[27]. Additional heparin and protamine dosage is calculated from the dose-response curves prepared by Bull *et al.*[7]. We also use the Hepcon System A/10R, an automatic heparin–protamine titration device which will calculate the heparin dose based on the patient's sex, height, weight and pump prime according to a formula devised by Allen[2]. The system will precisely detect the heparin level at any concentrations by a protamine titration cartridge; the protamine neutralizing dose can also be determined.

Cannulation technique

The cannulation technique for extracorporeal circulation is illustrated in *Figure 17.1*. We use a single large right atrial cannula (size 38 French) which is placed through the right atrial appendage and secured by a simple pursestring. The tube is introduced so that it lies just at the mouth of the inferior vena cava. We have found this single tube cannulation to be satisfactory for the vast majority of patients undergoing coronary bypass surgery. If coronary bypass is combined with mitral valve replacement double caval cannulation is carried out. The arterial perfusion cannula is placed into the ascending aorta at the pericardial reflection except in those patients with ascending aortic aneurysms or with excessively short aortas. In these cases the femoral artery is used for arterial inflow. The size 20 or 22 French arterial cannula* is trimmed appropriately so that a black marker line is at the level of the aortic adventitia. The cannula is secured in place by a pursestring suture to the aorta and to the chest retractor by a heavy black silk ligature.

Following insertion of cannulae, the air is evacuated from the cardiopulmonary bypass circuit and the patient is connected to the heart-lung machine. Bypass tubing clamps are removed only by the surgeon and bypass is established. When the systemic (oesophageal) temperature reaches 28°C the heart is fibrillated and the aorta cross-clamped.

*United States Catheter and Instruments

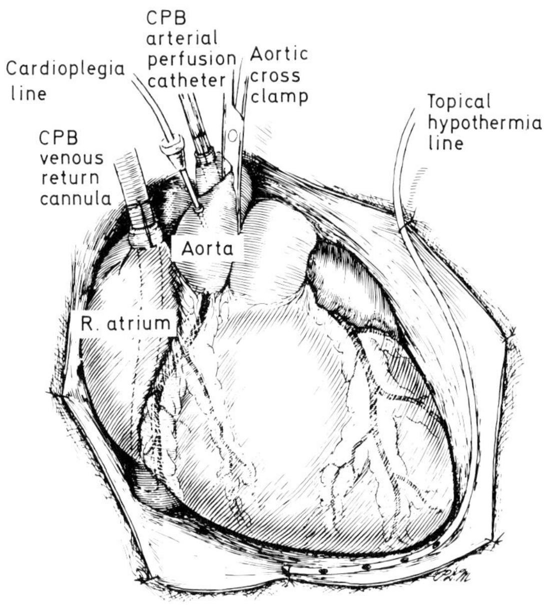

Figure 17.1 Cardiopulmonary bypass technique and one of the current methods of myocardial protection during coronary bypass surgery. A single right atrial cannula and distal ascending aortic cannula without left ventricular vent is used for most patients. Topical hypothermia is maintained by perfusion of 4°C lactated Ringer's solution throughout the pericardium while the cardioplegic solution is perfused into the aortic root. (Reproduction by permission from *Treatment of Acute Myocardial Ischemia: An Integrated Medical Surgical Approach*. Ed L. H. Cohn. (1979). New York: Futura Publishing Co. Inc.)

Myocardial protection

The ascending aorta proximal to the cross-clamp is cannulated by a size 14 Medicut cannula for perfusion of a hyperkalaemic (30 mmol/ℓ) basic (pH 7.5) hypermolar (330 mmol/ℓ) cardioplegic solution while local cardiac hypothermia is simultaneously instituted by cold perfusing (4°C) lactated Ringer's solution into the pericardial cavity through a nasogastric tube[15]. During cardiopulmonary bypass, 300–500 ml of cardioplegic solution are administered every 30 minutes by the perfusionist through a haemacoil unit submerged in ice slush and using an inflated cuff with a pressure of 300 mmHg. This method of myocardial protection produces a flaccid cold heart within a short time of aortic flow interruption, lowering the interventricular septal temperature to 12–15°C[25, 32]. With these protection methods the perioperative infarction rate following CABG (new Q wave, loss of R wave) is less than 5 per cent[9, 31].

In most cases, left ventricular venting is not used. Following cross-clamping of the aorta the heart is flaccid and the left ventricle rarely becomes distended. If the left ventricle should distend because of an unusually large bronchial return, a left ventricular vent is placed in the apex of this cavity. In patients with left ventricular aneurysms, with severely depressed left ventricular function, or in those subjected to concomitant valve replacement operations, an apical ventricular vent is routinely used.

Grafting technique

After the aorta is cross-clamped and hyperkalaemic cardioplegia is instituted, all distal venocoronary anastomoses are made using a single period of cardiac ischaemia. The anastomoses are made each with a single running 6-0 monofilament polypropylene (Prolene) suture in order to reduce the duration of the operating time. After all the distal anastomoses are completed, the aortic cross-clamp is removed and the heart reperfused. The patient's body temperature is progressively returned to 37°C during the last anastomosis and the heart is defibrillated as soon as possible following the removal of the aortic cross-clamp. After cardioplegia, defibrillation occurs spontaneously in about half the patients who have this form of myocardial protection. The proximal anastomoses to the ascending aorta are then made using a tangential, partially-occluding aortic clamp while the heart is recovering from the period of ischaemia.

Air is evacuated from the grafts by inserting a 25-gauge needle in the apex of the graft and milking them prior to removing a black Fogarty® bulldog clip which has occluded the graft just proximal to the anastomotic site of the coronary artery in order to prevent ingress of air through the vein graft and into the coronary bed. If a vent has been used, air is expressed through the left ventricular apex and through an ascending aorta air vent. The patient is then weaned off heart-lung bypass by reducing the cardiopulmonary bypass flow to 1 litre/min and transfusing the patient until adequate ventricular filling pressures are reached. A temporary pacemaker wire is placed on the epicardial surface of the right ventricle in all patients. A right atrial pacing wire is inserted in those patients in whom left ventricular compliance is reduced and it is considered that atrial contraction would be helpful in increasing the cardiac output. Chest tubes are placed in the mediastinum. Both pleural cavities are kept intact in order to minimize the possibility of trauma to the lungs or the transpleural migration of microorganisms which may contaminate the mediastinum. The drainage tubes are connected to a disposable three-bottle suction apparatus and are vigorously milked and stripped for several hours following the return of the patient to the intensive care unit.

Blood conservation

In 1971, Roche and Stengle[38] reported that, on average, 8 units of whole blood were used for each patient undergoing CABG in the United States. Had that rate of blood utilization continued to the present, blood supplies would have been severely depleted solely by CABG operations[39–41, 53]. We use a blood conservation programme consisting of oxygenator haemodilution, pre-bypass phlebotomy with autotransfusion and the judicious use of plasma and blood to maintain the patient's haematocrit in the low range of

®Edwards Laboratory

30 per cent. Phlebotomy is not performed in any patient with acute myocardial ischaemia or in those with left main coronary stenosis. Recently, the Haemonetics Cell Saver system has been used to rescue autologous red cells from the heart-lung machine and to transfuse the packed cells from the pump oxygenator back to the patient beginning at the time of closure of the sternum and continuing in the postoperative period. This is done in order to elevate the patient's haematocrit by using his own red cells[12, 18, 49].

Postoperative management

The postoperative care of the patients following CABG does not differ greatly from the routine postoperative care of any patient undergoing open-heart surgery. In fact, because of the excellent state of the patient's myocardium, in most instances, the postoperative care is straightforward and less complicated than in patients with intracardiac correction of complex congenital anomalies or in those with cardiac valve operations.

Control of haemorrhage

Most patients will have blood loss from the mediastinal drainage tubes that ceases almost completely within the first three to five hours following return to the intensive care unit. Any bleeding, i.e. 100–200 ml/h, that continues beyond this point is considered to be surgical bleeding which will necessitate return of the patient to the operating room. Should a mediastinal chest tube clot and the patient exhibit evidence of continued loss of blood, two manoeuvres may be done to declot the tube: gentle irrigation under sterile conditions with warm saline or the use of a Fogarty arterial embolectomy catheter which can be introduced through the tube to extract the clot by the embolectomy principle. A bedside check of the clotting time and a laboratory evaluation of prothrombin, partial thromboplastin and platelet count should be done early and clotting factor deficiency corrected. Platelet counts after haemodilution and extracorporeal circulation average approximately 90 000[18] and will occasionally need replenishment if this level falls below 50 000. In our experience, bleeding from cut blood vessels are the rule rather than the exception in cases of postoperative haemorrhage.

Leg compression is accomplished by rubber bandages to the leg from which the vein has been removed to prevent postoperative haematomata. Ambulation is begun on the first postoperative day and prolonged sitting is avoided to prevent phlebitis and pulmonary embolism.

Postoperative respiratory care

Respiratory care is tailored to the type of anaesthetic agent used during the operation. Since morphine is the predominant anaesthetic agent used at our hospital for CABG, overnight endotracheal intubation and positive pressure respiration is required. In the occasional patient who has had a relatively short operation and who exhibits normal respiratory mechanics, extubation is performed after return to the intensive care unit. An Emerson volume respirator is used. At the end of the operation, the patient is transferred to the intensive care unit until the patient gradually regains consciousness over a period of hours. Blood gases are checked at regular intervals and adjustments of oxygen concentration and minute ventilation made as needed. When the patient is fully conscious and is haemodynamically stable, weaning from controlled ventilation is begun. The patient should be able to achieve a vital capacity greater than 10 ml/kg body weight, or generate an inspiratory force of at least 30 cm water. The patient is then allowed to breathe spontaneously from a T-piece circuit using a Brigg's adaptor so that oxygen enriched air can be delivered to the patient. At the end of one hour, artrial blood gases and respiratory mechanics are evaluated and if they are satisfactory, the patient is extubated. During this period, the patient's general condition, respiration and cardiac function are also monitored. Following extubation, the patients are maintained on an ultrasonic nebulized oxygen source through a face mask. Postural drainage, cupping, deep breathing exercises and coughing are carried out by respiratory therapists. It is rare in our experience with a programme of intensive pulmonary physical therapy, for patients to require endotracheal suctioning or the use of intratracheal 'cough' catheters.

Renal function

Renal impairment is rare after cardiopulmonary bypass operations of moderate length in patients with normal preoperative renal function (<1 per cent). (The average time for a triple CABG is about 70 minutes). Modern pump oxygenator systems and haemodilution are relatively atraumatic to red cells so that haemoglobinuria is uncommon. Though flow in most extracorporeal systems is non-pulsatile and renal failure unusual (<1 per cent), urine flow may decrease somewhat during heart-lung bypass due to systemic hypothermia and reduction in mean perfusion pressure. If there is haemoglobinuria, osmotic diuretics such as mannitol, which increase renal blood flow, are effective in washing out the haemoglobin.

Postoperatively, volume replacement will usually ensure adequate urine flow but furosemide (Lasix) is often given to stimulate urine flow if cardiac volumes are adequate. The spontaneous or Lasix-induced diuresis causes significant potassium loss requiring aggressive supplementation. Patients with chronic renal failure commonly sustain a worsening of their renal function postoperatively and occasionally require temporary peritoneal-or haemodialysis.

Fluid and electrolytes

This area of management is slightly different from that of the adult patient with surgical treatment for valvular or congenital heart disease. The amount of exogenous fluid and colloid that these patients require may be considerably more than expected and above the actual losses sustained during the first 24 hours following the operation. This is due, in part, to the chronically contracted plasma volume in patients with coronary artery disease prior to surgery[13]. Thus, what was once termed 'stress' polycythaemia' in many patients with coronary artery disease[33] is, in fact, intrinsic plasma oligaemia. Once the patient undergoes coronary bypass surgery and has returned to an asymptomatic status, the plasma oligaemia is still present when measured six months postoperatively[16]. In addition, these patients do not have a similar expansive response of the extracellular fluid space after cardiopulmonary bypass as do patients who have been in chronic congestive failure with valvular heart disease[33]. Hypokalaemia is a constant finding in patients undergoing cardiac surgery with extracorporeal circulation, particularly when associated with haemodilution[13]. The serum potassium may, of course, not reflect intracellular potassium levels, the largest ion in the intracellular space. Therefore, we routinely replenish potassium both intraoperatively and postoperatively until the serum K+ is 4.5–5.0 mmol/litre.

Maintenance of normal postoperative cardiac output

Following CABG operations there is a normal rewarming period that occurs with vasodilation which produces a mild 'physiological' hypotension[36]. This rewarming vasodilation without other significant haemodynamic abnormalities is a very consistent finding in patients treated with a haemodilution prime and moderate systemic hypothermia during perfusion. The mild hypotension is accompanied by increased body temperature, improved peripheral perfusion and decreased cardiac filling pressures. Volume infusion is the treatment of choice and within a short period of time the cardiac and systemic volumes are replenished and the patient's blood pressure returns to normal. Though appearing well perfused with adequate cardiac volumes, the cardiac index may still be somewhat depressed[36].

An obvious cause of decreased cardiac output after CABG is haemorrhage and cardiac tamponade. This will be noted by the marked elevation of both left and right atrial pressures, a decrease in cardiac output, tachycardia, and decreased peripheral perfusion. Mediastinal drainage tubes which have probably ceased draining should be stripped and the tubes irrigated and/or thromboectomized. If this does not result in immediate relief, the patient should be returned to the operating room immediately. If the patient's condition deteriorates significantly and rapidly, thoracotomy should be performed in the intensive care unit and the tamponade relieved. Following this, the patient is taken back to the operating room for surgical closure of the sternotomy.

A significant cause of hypotension and decreased cardiac output is cardiac arrhythmia. Space does not permit a detailed description of the variety of arrhythmias that may occur in the recovery phase of patients undergoing coronary bypass surgery but the general treatment of arrhythmias depends on the patient's haemodynamic condition. With all arrhythmias serum potassium should be checked and replenished by urgent intravenous bolus infusion. If a patient has a supraventricular tachycardia (which in 10 per cent of cases is atrial fibrillation) and is hypotensive despite adequate filling pressures, DC electrocardioversion should be carried out urgently. If, however, the patient is not hypotensive and peripheral perfusion is relatively good, the ventricular rate may successfully be reduced by intravenous digoxin therapy and therefore emergency cardioversion may not be required. Regardless of the perfusion status, atrial fibrillation should be aggressively treated so that the ventricular rate is controlled and kept below 100 beats/minute. Our patients are not digitalized preoperatively and if they are on digitalis when admitted for the operation, this drug is discontinued. This is done so that if a patient does develop an arrhythmia postoperatively, it is almost invariably due to inadequate digitalization rather than too much digitalis. Maintenance digoxin therapy, 0.125–0.25 mg/day postoperatively is begun so that if rapid atrial fibrillation does develop the amount of digoxin required to control the ventricular rate will be considerably less than if no digoxin had been given. If a patient has recurrent bouts of ventricular tachycardia and/or persistent ventricular irritability (VEA), aggressive potassium replenishment and intravenous lidocaine infusion are concomitantly carried out. The minimum lidocaine dose which generally suffices to control VEA is usually 2–4 mg/minute. Repeated boluses of 100–150 mg lidocaine may be given in addition to the continuous intravenous infusions to control VEA and occasionally, in refractory cases, intravenous administration of pronestyl, either in combination or in addition to lidocaine, is necessary[52]. These drugs in high doses may cause myocardial depression so that dopamine may be required to counteract the hypotensive effects of these agents. If bradycardia develops, the temporary pacing wire sutured to every patient's right ventricle is used to pace the heart rate at 80–90 beats/minute which appears to be the optimum rate for most patients following cardiac surgery, as determined by cardiac output measurements[32]. Electrical pacing also minimizes the occurrence of irritable foci (VEA).

Depression of intrinsic myocardial contractility may cause postoperative hypotension. This is uncommon in patients having coronary bypass operations with a normal left ventricular ejection fraction and with adequate myocardial protection during the operation but may be relatively common in those patients who have severely depressed preoperative ejection fractions. If the decreased ejection fraction is due to ventricular scarification rather than ischaemia these patients may have postoperative hypotension even if the afterload is reduced and the preload is adequate. If the intrinsic myocardial contractility is depressed, continuous dopamine infusion is the treatment of choice in most instances although a judicious mixture of different catecholamine agents may sometimes be necessary in extreme situations. If dopamine or other catecholamines do not improve the cardiac output, then an intra-aortic balloon counterpulsation device should be inserted to further reduce the afterload as well as the preload. Dobutamine, a new sympathetic amine, has been recently introduced which may have an improved inotropic response without increasing the heart rate[45].

The most ominous cause of postoperative hypotension is acute myocardial ischaemia. In this situation, patients who are experiencing graft failure or have suffered a major perioperative myocardial infarction due to inadequate myocardial protection or inadequate revascularization may become hypotensive, have poor systemic perfusion, elevation of the ST segments on the precordial ECG leads, a significant (>200 mg/100ml rise in the SGOT and a positive MB–CPK band. If the patient does not quickly stabilize with conventional methods of management, an intra-aortic balloon counterpulsation device should be inserted to prevent further myocardial necrosis and to increase coronary blood flow. In certain selected instances, reoperation for aortocoronary graft failure and thrombectomy may be indicated.

Systemic hypertension is a relatively common complication in patients following coronary bypass surgery and its occurrence in the postoperative period is reported to be between 20 and 30 per cent[28, 37]. The aetiology of post-CABG hypertension seems to be an increased plasma catecholamine level and activation of the angiotensin–renin system with increased sympathetic vascular tone and systemic blood pressure[48]. The treatment of hypertension is accomplished by vasodilation therapy with intravenous infusion of sodium nitroprusside (0.1 mg/ml) to titrate the blood pressure below 150 mmHg. It is important to treat the hypertension aggressively in order to prevent suture line bleeding which may occur despite normal blood clotting status if there is a sudden increase in pulse pressure and also to prevent sudden increases in myocardial oxygen consumption associated with increased left ventricular wall tension which may precipitate or worsen myocardial ischaemia.

Conclusions

The course of a patient after a coronary bypass grafting for chronic or acute myocardial ischaemia depends primarily on a complete and accurate coronary revascularization, expeditiously carried out under ideal conditions of perfusion and myocardial protection. This includes the preoperative preparation, anaesthetic management, myocardial protection and atraumatic extracorporeal circulation. Technical excellence is the *sine qua non* of uncomplicated patient care. No amount of postoperative treatment can ever compensate for an operation inadequately or inaccurately performed. Patients who have had properly performed operations, efficiently done, with the elements of care that we have outlined being observed, will have an uncomplicated early and late postoperative course. Simplification of preoperative, intraoperative, and postoperative techniques, and the performance of these techniques by a small, close-knit, experienced staff will lead to uniform and meticulous patient care which in turn will lead to increased safety and longevity for patients undergoing coronary bypass grafting.

References

1. Aguilar, M. J., Gerbode, F. and Hill, J. D. 'Neuropathologic complications of cardiac surgery.' *Journal of Thoracic and Cardiovascular Surgery*, **61**, 676 (1971)
2. Allen, T. H., Peng, M. T., Chen, K. P., Huang, T. F., Chang, C. and Fang, H. S. 'Prediction of blood volume and adiposity in man from body weight and cube height.' *Metabolism*, **5**, 328 (1956)

3. Amsterdam, E. A., Hughes, J. L., DeMaria, A. N., Zelis, R. and Mason, D. T. 'Indirect assessment of myocardial oxygen consumption in the evaluation of mechanisms and therapy of angina pectoris.' *American Journal of Cardiology*, **33,** 737 (1974)
4. Barbovak, J. J., Hughes, C. V., Anderson, A. J., Rimm, A. A. 'Effect of aortocoronary bypass operation on factors precipitating angina.' *Journal of Thoracic and Cardiovascular Surgery*, **75,** 47 (1978)
5. Barry, W. H., Pfeifer, J. F., Lipton, M. J., Tilkian, A. G. and Hultgren, H. N. 'Effects of coronary artery bypass grafting on resting and exercise haemodynamics in patients with stable angina pectoris: A prospective randomized study.' *American Journal of Cardiology*, **37,** 823 (1976)
6. Boudoulas, H., Snyder, G. L., Lewis, R. P., Kates, R. E., Karayannacos, P. E. and Vasko, J. S. 'Safety and rationale for continuation of propranolol therapy during coronary bypass operation.' *Annals of Thoracic Surgery*, **26,** 222 (1978)
7. Bull, B. S., Huse, W. M., Brauer, F. S. and Korpman, R. 'Heparin therapy during extracorporeal circulation. II. The use of a dose-response curve to individualize heparin and protamine dosage.' *Journal of Thoracic and Cardiovascular Surgery*, **69,** 685 (1975)
8. Chatterjee, K., Matloff, J. M. and Swan, H. J. C. 'Improved angina threshold and coronary reserve following direct myocardial revascularization.' *Circulation*, **51 (Suppl. I)** 81 (1975)
9. Cohn, L. H. 'Myocardial preservation: local hypothermia plus cardioplegia.' *Panel presentation, Pan-Pacific Surgical Association*, **April** (1978)
10. Cohn, L. H. 'Physiologic basis and clinical application of intra-aortic balloon counterpulsation in low cardiac output states.' *Surgical Clinics of North America*, **55,** 545 (1975)
11. Cohn, L. H., Alpert, J., Koster, J. K., Mee, R. B. B. and Collins, J. J., Jr. 'Changing indications for the surgical treatment of unstable angina.' *Archives of Surgery*, **113,** 1312 (1978)
12. Cohn, L. H., Anderson, W., Fosberg, A. and Collins, J. J., Jr. 'The effects of phlebotomy, haemodilution and autologous transfusion on blood utilization in open-heart surgery.' *Chest*, **68,** 283 (1975)
13. Cohn, L. H., Angell, W. W. and Shumway, N. E. 'Body fluid spaces following cardiopulmonary bypass. I. Effects of cardiac failure and haemodilution.' *Journal of Thoracic and Cardiovascular Surgery*, **62,** 423 (1971)
14. Cohn, L. H., Boyden, C. M. and Collins, J. J., Jr. 'Improved long-term survival after aorto-coronary bypass for advanced coronary artery disease.' *American Journal of Surgery*, **129,** 380 (1975)
15. Cohn, L. H. and Collins, J. J., Jr. 'Local cardiac hypothermia by myocardial protection.' *Annals of Thoracic Surgery*, **17,** 135 (1974)
16. Cohn, L. H., Klovekorn, P., Moore, F. D. and Collins, J. J., Jr. 'Intrinsic plasma volume deficits in patients with coronary artery disease: effects of myocardial revascularization.' *Archives of Surgery*, **108,** 57 (1974)
17. Cohn, L. H., Koster, J. K., Mee, R. B. B. and Collins, J. J., Jr. 'Surgical treatment of left main coronary artery stenosis.' *World Journal of Surgery*, **2,** 701 (1978)
18. Cohn, L. H., Solomon, S., Lee-Son, S., Sandberg, G. and Collins, J. J., Jr. 'Sequestration of platelet-rich plasma for patients undergoing coronary bypass operations.' *Proceedings, Haemonetics Blood Conservation Institute*, **11,** 20 (1978)
19. Cohn, P. F., and Cohn, L. H. 'Medical/surgical treatment of unstable angina.' In *Treatment of Acute Myocardial Ischemia: An Integrated Medical/Surgical Approach*. Ed. L. H. Cohn. p. 240. New York: Futura Publishing Company (1979)

20. Coltart, D. J., Dayen, M. N., Stinson, E. B., Goldman, R. H., Davies, R. O. and Harrison, D. C. 'Investigation of the safe withdrawal period for propranolol in patients scheduled for open-heart surgery.' *British Heart Journal*, **37,** 1228 (1975)
21. Diaz, R. G., Freeman, E. and Levitt, B. 'Myocardial infarction after propranolol withdrawal.' *American Heart Journal*, **88,** 257 (1974)
22. Effler, D. B. and Vilkoen, J. F. 'Extracorporeal circulation, anaesthesia and immediate postoperative management for coronary artery disease surgery.' In *Current Techniques in Extracorporeal Circulation*. Ed. M. I. Ionescu. p. 183. London: Butterworths (1976)
23. Ellis, R. J., Pryor, W. and Ebert, P. A. 'Advantages of hypothermia and potassium cardioplegia in left ventricular hypertrophy.' *Annals of Thoracic Surgery*, **24,** 229 (1977)
24. Favaloro, R. G. 'Saphenous vein graft in the surgical treatment of coronary artery disease. Operative technique.' *Journal of Thoracic and Cardiovascular Surgery*, **58,** 178 (1969)
25. Gay, W. A., Jr. and Ebert, P. A. 'Functional, metabolic, and morphologic effects of potassium-induced cardioplegia.' *Surgery*, **74,** 284 (1973)
26. Gregg, D. E. and Green, H. O. 'Effects of viscosity, ischaemia, cardiac output and aortic pressure on coronary blood flow measured under a constant perfusion pressure.' *American Journal of Physiology*, **130,** 108 (1940)
27. Hattersley, P. C. 'Activated coagulation time of whole blood.' *Journal of the American Medical Association*, **196,** 436 (1966)
28. Hoar, P. F., Hickey, R. F. and Ullyott, D. J. 'Systemic hypertension following myocardial revascularization.' *Journal of Thoracic and Cardiovascular Surgery*, **71,** 859 (1976)
29. Jones, E. L., Kaplan, J. A., Dorney, E. R., King, S. B., III, Douglas, J. S., Jr. and Hatcher, C. R., Jr. 'Propranolol therapy in patients undergoing myocardial revascularization.' *American Journal of Cardiology*, **38,** 696 (1976)
30. Kirsh, M. M., Behrendt, D. M., Jackson, A. P., Dhadphale, P., Alseri, S., Brymer, J., Orringer, M. B. and Sloan, H. 'Myocardial revascularization in patients receiving longterm propranolol therapy.' *Annals of Thoracic Surgery*, **25,** 117 (1978)
31. Koster, J. K., Cohn, L. H., Collins, J. J., Jr. Sanders, J. H., Muller, J. E. and Young, E. 'Continuous hypothermia arrest versus intermittent ischaemia for myocardial protection during coronary revascularization.' *Annals of Thoracic Surgery*, **24,** 330 (1977)
32. Kouchoukos, N. T. and Karp, R. B. 'Management of the postoperative cardiovascular surgical patient.' *American Heart Journal*, **92,** 513 (1976)
33. Lawrence, J. H. and Berlin, N. I. 'Relative polycythemia: the polycythemia of stress.' *Yale Journal of Biology and Medicine*, **24,** 498 (1951)
34. Lawrie, G. M., Morris, G. C., Jr., Chapman, D. W., Winters, W. L. and Lie, J. T. 'Patterns of patency of 596 vein grafts up to seven years after aorto-coronary bypass.' *Journal of Thoracic and Cardiovascular Surgery*, **73,** 443 (1977)
35. McIntosh, H. D. and Garvia, J. A. 'The first decade of aorto-coronary bypass grafting, 1967–1977.' *Circulation*, **75,** 405 (1978)
36. Morgan, A. P., Anderson, W., Bevilacqua, R., Cohn, L. H., Moore, F. D. and Collins, J. J., Jr. 'Effects of computer controlled transfusion on recovery from cardiac surgery.' *Annals of Surgery*, **178,** 391 (1973)
37. Roberts, A. J., Niarchos, A. P., Subramanian, V. A., Abel, R. M., Herman, S. D., Sealey, J. F., Case, D. B., White, R. P., Johnson, G. A., Laragh, J. H. and Gay, W. A., Jr. 'Systemic hypertension associated with coronary bypass.' *Journal of Thoracic and Cardiovascular Surgery*, **74,** 846 (1977)

38. Roche, J. K. and Stengle, J. M. 'Open-heart surgery and the demand for blood.' *Journal of the American Medical Association*, **225,** 1516 (1973)
39. Sandiford, F. M., Chiariello, L., Hallman, G. L. and Cooley, D. A. 'Aorto-coronary bypass in Jehovah's Witnesses.' *Journal of Thoracic and Cardiovascular Surgery*, **68,** 1 (1974)
40. Sheldon, W. C., Rincon, G., Pichard, A. D., Razavi, M., Cheanvechai, C. and Loop, F. D. 'Surgical treatment of coronary artery disease: pure graft operations with study of 741 patients followed 3–7 years.' *Progress in Cardiovascular Diseases*, **18,** 237 (1975)
41. Sherman, M. M., Dobnik, D. B., Dennis, R. C. and Berger, R. L. 'Autologous blood transfusions during cardiopulmonary bypass.' *Chest*, **70,** 592 (1976)
42. Siegel, W., Lim, J. S., Proudfit, W. L., Sheldon, W. C. and Loop, F. D. 'The spectrum of exercise test and angiographic correlations in myocardial revascularization surgery.' *Circulation*, **51 (Suppl. I)**, 156 (1975)
43. Slogoff, S., Keats, A. S. and Ott, E. 'Preoperative propranolol therapy and aorto-coronary bypass operation.' *Journal of the American Medical Association*, **240,** 1487 (1978)
44. Sones, F. M., Jr. and Shirey, E. K. 'Cine coronary arteriography.' *Modern Concepts in Cardiovascular Disease*, **31,** 735 (1962)
45. Sonnenblick, E. H., Frishman, W. H. and LeJemtel, T. H. 'Dobutamine: a new synthetic cardioactive sympathetic amine.' *New England Journal of Medicine*, **300,** 17 (1979)
46. Stiles, Q. R., Lindesmith, G. G., Tucker, W. L., Hughes, R. K. and Meyer, B. W. 'Long-term follow-up of patients with coronary artery bypass grafts.' *Circulation*, **54 (Suppl. III)**, 32 (1976)
47. Takaro, T., Hultgren, H. N., Lipton, M. and Detre, K. M. 'The VA cooperative randomized study of surgery for coronary arterial occlusive disease. II. Subgroup with significant left main lesions.' *Circulation*, **54 (Suppl. III)**, 107 (1976)
48. Taylor, K. M., Morton, I. J., Brown, J. J., Bain, W. H. and Caves, P. K. 'Hypertension and the renin–angiotensin system following open-heart surgery.' *Journal of Thoracic and Cardiovascular Surgery*, **74,** 840 (1977)
49. Tucker, W. Y. and Cohn, L. H. 'Intraoperative use of the Haemonetics Cell Saver in open-heart surgery.' *Proceedings, Haemonetics Seminar*, **7,** 25 (1976)
50. Viljoen, J. F., Estafanous, G. and Kellner, G. A. 'Propranolol and cardiac surgery.' *Journal of Thoracic and Cardiovascular Surgery*, **64,** 826 (1972)
51. Weintraub, R. M., Voukydis, P. C., Arvesty, J. M., Cohen, S. I., Ford, P., Kurland, G. S., LaRaia, P. J., Morkin, E. and Paulin, S. 'Treatment of pre-infarction angina with intra-aortic balloon counterpulsation and surgery.' *American Journal of Cardiology*, **34,** 809 (1974)
52. Wynne, J., Alpert, J. S. and Koster, J. K., Jr. 'Medical/surgical treatment of arrhythmias of myocardial ischaemia.' In *The Treatment of Acute Myocardial Ischemia: An Integrated Medical/Surgical Approach*. Ed. L. H. Cohn. p. 240. New York: Futura Publishing Company (1979)
53. Yeh, T., Shelton, L. and Yeh, T., Jr. 'Blood loss and bank blood requirement in coronary bypass surgery.' *Annals of Thoracic Surgery*, **26,** 11 (1978)

18

The Place of Extracorporeal Circulation in Operations upon the Thoracic Aorta

Harris B. Shumacker, Jr.

hoc opus, hic labor es

Introduction

Many of the operations performed upon the thoracic aorta require total or partial cardiopulmonary bypass. Some surgical procedures are best carried out with a heart-lung machine on standby while others can be accomplished without such assistance. Certain lesions of the thoracic aorta have been treated over a sufficiently long period of time and in large enough numbers to permit firm conclusions regarding their management. Some of the necessary operative procedures are well enough established so that there is general agreement regarding most phases of their accomplishment, but not all. Some other conditions and their treatment are still in such an unsettled state that comments concerning them are on very insecure grounds; indeed, some of these comments must be considered quite speculative. As a consequence, it is not possible to include in this discussion only factual material concerning procedures universally utilized and results which are clear and satisfactory. Instead, what is written must be necessarily regarded only as the author's views of the current status of the art and his conjectures about future developments in this field.

When total cardiopulmonary bypass is necessary, the operator naturally should utilize the apparatus and the methods he finds work best in his hands. My associates and I generally induce moderate body hypothermia and on rare occasions profound hypothermia. When it is necessary to stop the natural coronary circulation by ascending aortic cross-clamping, for all but the briefest periods, we keep the heart chilled and arrested by periodic coronary perfusion with cold balanced electrolyte potassium-containing solution. In addition, we place electrolyte ice slush in the pericardial sac after positioning a pack along the left lateral side to offer some protection against cold injury to the adjacent phrenic nerve. If the operation does not

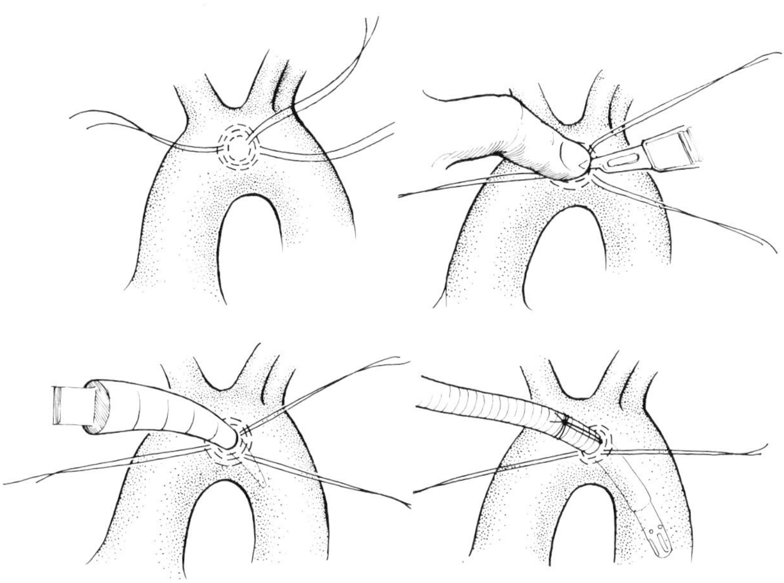

Figure 18.1 Method of introducing arterial inflow catheter into aortic arch

involve the distal ascending aorta and this segment is in reasonably good condition, the arterial inflow cannula is placed in this location. If the entire ascending aorta must of necessity be involved in the operative procedure, the inflow can often be safely placed in the aortic arch (*Figure 18.1*). It is not advisable, however, to insert an arterial inflow cannula into the ascending aorta or arch if the patient is known to have cystic medial disease, because of the danger of inducing dissection. When these sites are unsuitable, the inflow cannula can be passed upward through the exposed femoral or iliac artery, and there may be rare occasions when the left subclavian artery is preferred for cannulation.

The ascending aorta

In general, all lesions of the ascending aorta and aortic root requiring operative treatment necessitate the use of total cardiopulmonary bypass. An extraordinarily rare case is that of the well defined and delimited saccular aneurysm which can be excised by excluding the mouth of the aneurysm and the sac from the main aortic pathway with a clamp placed tangentially across its 'neck'. Even under these circumstances it is imperative to have a heart-lung apparatus on standby. Before attempting such excision by clamp exclusion, one should be certain that the instrument can be positioned in such a way that it will permit an adequate outflow tract through the aorta during the operation, that it will leave an aorta of suitable size in place after the repair is completed, and that the required manipulations can be performed without hazard of dislodgement of any mural thrombus within the sac. Far more commonly it is advisable to place such patients on total cardiopulmonary bypass, excise the aneurysm completely, and repair the resultant defect by suturing in position a patch of woven Dacron or Teflon graft material. Whenever such patches are used additional assurance against blood ooze penetration can be secured by suturing to the inner surface of the prosthetic material a properly fashioned portion of the patient's own pericardium.

In very few situations do stenotic lesions of the ascending aorta require surgical correction. One of these is the congenital supravalvular aortic stenosis. In such cases it is important to open the aorta through the involved area well beyond the limits of the stenosis, to excise any intraluminal obstructing ridge and to place a patch of proper size and shape in order to restore as nearly normal aortic dimension and configuration as is possible. Though the aortic valve is often deformed, it can ordinarily be left intact although careful incision of one or two fused commissures may be required at times. If the patient is old enough, the aortic annulus of adequate size, and the valve function sufficiently bad, the valve should be replaced. Aortic valve substitution may also become necessary later in life in those patients operated upon when young if valvular malfunction becomes great enough to justify replacement. Another type of stenotic lesion is that produced by acute or subacute dissection resulting from cystic medial disease. Such stenosis may be of extreme degree. In one personal instance, the aortic lumen visualized angiographically had a pathway hardly larger than that of one of the main coronary arteries. Management of constrictions of this sort is an essential part of the treatment of dissections of the ascending aorta.

A third extremely rare stenotic lesion may occur acutely with circumferential disruption of the aorta as a consequence of deceleration trauma. These injuries occur far more commonly in the proximal part of the descending thoracic aorta distal to the origin of the left subclavian artery, but those in the supravalvular area, though second in incidence, are very uncommon. They should be borne in mind, however, as should all such disruptions, whenever a patient has had a chest injury, particularly one occurring as the result of rapid deceleration and especially when there is any indication of widening of the mediastinal shadow on a plain chest radiograph. Their presence or absence should be confirmed or ruled out by an immediate arteriographic study. Generally the aorta is simply torn and only rarely is the inner flap of the injured portion so dislocated that it produces a significant outflow stenosis. This condition is corrected, as are the more simple circumferential tears, by proper debridement of the damaged ends of the disrupted vessel and resuture, either directly or by the interposition of an appropriate prosthetic tube as the situation demands.

Aneurysms of the ascending aorta due to syphilis, once seen commonly, are now encountered exceedingly rarely. Whenever they are dealt with surgically, one should always keep in mind the fact that the aortic wall disease may involve the ostia of the coronary arteries in such a way as to leave only pinpoint openings into them. In such cases it may be necessary to improve the coronary circulation by aortic-coronary grafting procedures if the orifice cannot be adequately opened.

Far more common are arteriosclerotic aneurysms of the ascending aorta. When they involve the aortic root they are frequently associated with annular dilatation and significant aortic valve insufficiency so that the valve requires replacement. The surgeon naturally selects the valve of his choice (*Figure 18.2*). For some years my associates and I have been using by preference glutaraldehyde-preserved, mounted porcine aortic valve substitutes unless the annulus is unusually small or the patient not beyond middle age in which case we have utilized the Björk–Shiley prosthesis. When the latter valves have been employed, we have advised continuous anticoagulation with Coumadin.

There is general agreement about the management of chronic aneurysms of the ascending aorta due to cystic medial disease with or without an old dissection. They are frequently well delimited to the ascending aorta and the terminal portion of the ascending aorta is quite suitable for attachment of a prosthetic tube. In the majority of cases, the annulus has undergone dilatation with the creation of wide-open aortic regurgitation and left ventricular failure. Physicians as well as surgeons concur that surgical intervention is mandatory. The entire aneurysm should be removed, the aortic valve replaced, and an ascending aortic prosthetic tube inserted. Though not all surgeons hold the same view, I feel strongly that additional security of the anastomosis between the prosthetic tube and the aorta is achieved by suturing a cuff of Teflon felt around both the aortic root and the distal cut end of the aorta so that when the prosthesis is united with the host tissues, they are buttressed on the one side by the Dacron tube and on the

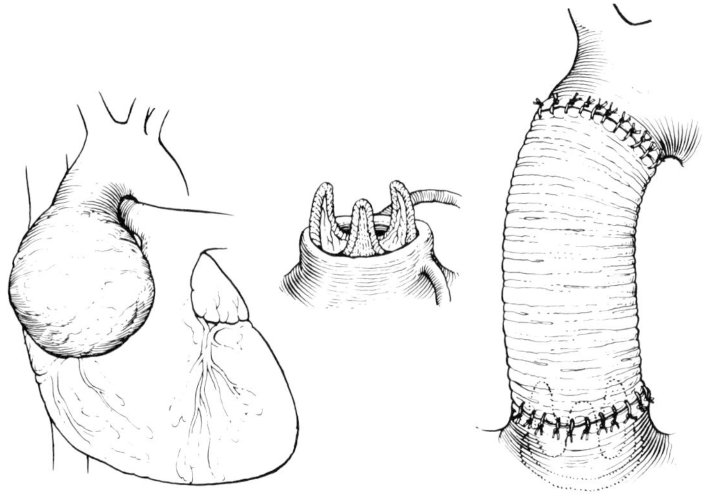

Figure 18.2 Drawing illustrating graft and valve insertion in case of ascending aortic aneurysm with aortic insufficiency

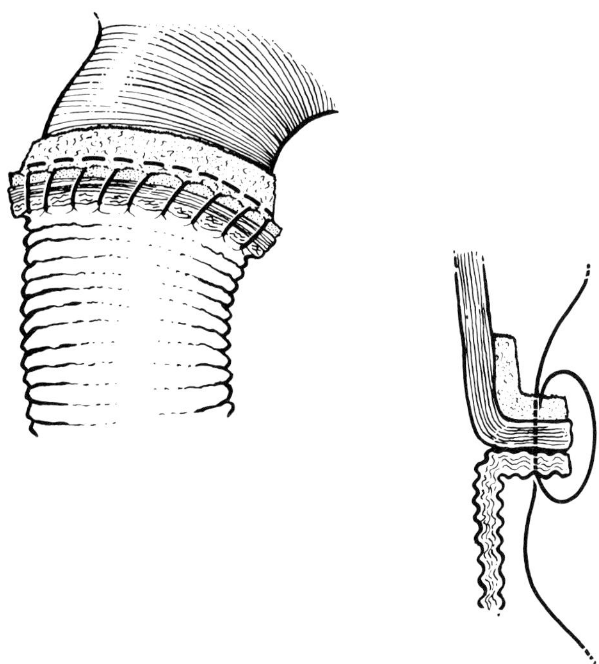

Figure 18.3 Use of a strip of Teflon felt to repair the split aorta and reinforce the approximation of aorta and graft. (Reproduced from Shumacker, H. B. (1978) by courtesy of *Journal of Cardiovascular Surgery*)

other by the felt material (*Figure 18.3*). Suturing pericardium as a cover over prosthetic grafts is very useful in controlling any tendency for blood to ooze through the interstices of the material. The results are generally quite good and the operative mortality low.

There are wider differences of opinion concerning the management of acute and subacute dissecting aneurysms beginning from a tear in the supravalvular aortic area. The principal point of disagreement concerns what is to be done in the case of the acutely insufficient aortic valve, so frequently produced by dissection in the regions of the commissural attachments in such a way as to make the valve leaflets flail. Some hold the view that all such cases should be managed by valve replacement. Others have pointed out that a number of the valves can safely be left in place and rendered competent by making the affected leaflets bicuspid. All too often in my experience, however, the dissection involves too many commissures to make this plan feasible. I have found that careful reapproximation of the split aortic wall in the region of the commissures with properly buttressed sutures has restored valvular competence (*Figure 18.4*) and that good function has been maintained over long periods of time. Hence, it is my feeling that the valve should not be replaced unless the valve leaflets themselves are obviously diseased as well as flailing. Another point of debate concerns whether one should remove the entire sinuses of Valsalva along with the rest of the aorta and restore coronary blood flow by

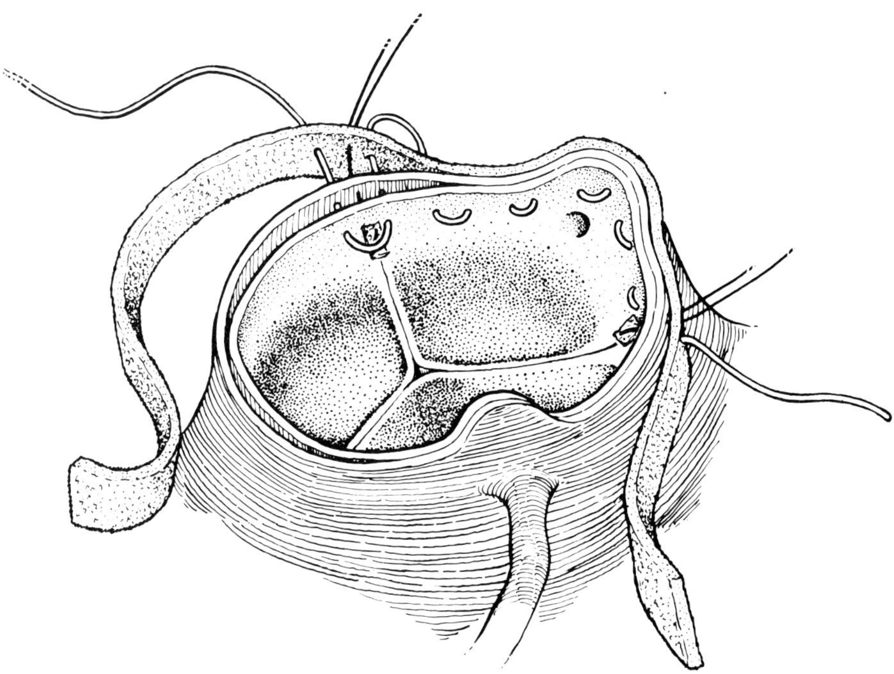

Figure 18.4 Drawing illustrating repair of split aortic root, suspension of flail valve leaflets by buttress suture approximation of separated commissures and excision of sinuses of Valsalva leaving only oval lips containing the coronary orifices. (Reproduced from Shumacker, H. B. (1978) by courtesy of *Journal of Cardiovascular Surgery*)

reattaching the coronary ostia directly to the prosthetic tube (making the procedure more easy, if feasible, by leaving a cuff of the original aortic wall about the coronary orifice), or place autogenous vein grafts between the aortic prosthetic tube and the coronary arteries at more distal sites. The latter procedure naturally must be utilized in those cases where the dissection extends directly into the coronary artery itself and interferes with blood flow into it. It is my opinion that in most instances the major portion of the sinuses of Valsalva area can be excised almost *in toto* leaving only enough wall tissue to obviate the necessity of coronary artery transplantation and I have not seen untoward events consequent upon the use of this method afterwards (*Figure 18.4*). This technique should not, however, be employed if the coronary ostia are a considerable distance from the aortic root, a situation which is much more likely to prevail with respect to the right than the left coronary orifice. Instead, transplantation of the coronary ostia or saphenous vein bypass grafting should be performed in such cases. Once again, it is my conviction that a more secure union between the prosthetic tube and aorta in cases of this sort is achieved by attaching a cuff of Teflon felt both about the aortic root and the more distal aortic end prior to insertion of the prosthesis.

Two difficult problems associated with acute and subacute dissection will be dealt with when considering the management of arch lesions. One is the rare case in which adequate arteriograms fail to disclose the point of aortic rupture and none is found in the opened aorta. The other is the uncommon instance of the tear beginning not in the supravalvular area but in the distal ascending aorta near the origin of the innominate artery.

The aortic arch

The management of aneurysms of the aortic arch remains in a very unsettled state. Fortunately, such lesions are not common. The fact that they are rarely encountered and therefore seldom operated upon, however, explains in no small measure the high mortality which has generally prevailed during and after their resection and the differing methods which have been utilized for repair and graft replacement. In the very uncommon instance in which the proximal portion of the ascending aorta is in a relatively normal state, one might consider utilizing the original methods used in their early cases by Cooley, DeBakey, and their associates (*Figure 18.5*). A Dacron bypass prosthetic tube is placed between the proximal ascending aorta and the descending thoracic aorta beyond the aneurysm. This bypass tube is employed either as a temporary measure or as a permanent replacement of the arch. Smaller Dacron grafts attached to the main bypass tube are successively united as rapidly as possible to the divided ends of the innominate, left carotid, and subclavian branches. If the ascending aorta and arch are involved, total bypass is utilized and catheter perfusion is employed while the innominate and carotid artery reconstruction is being

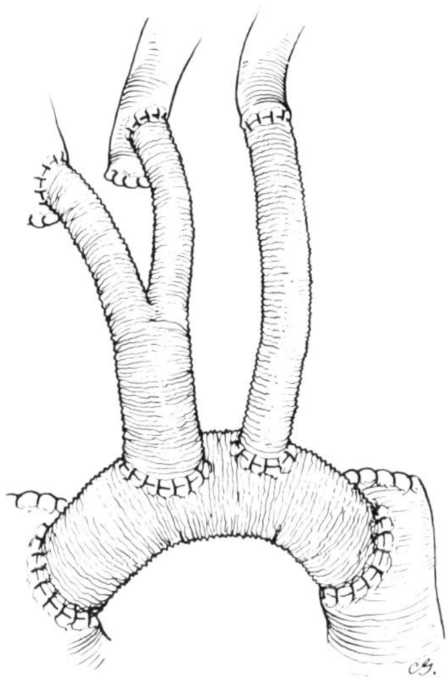

Figure 18.5 Temporary–permanent graft for aortic arch resection

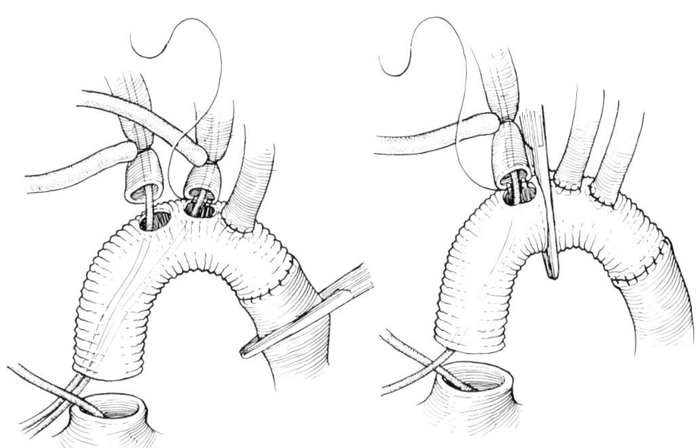

Figure 18.6 Method of aortic resection utilizing total cardiopulmonary bypass and catheter perfusion of innominate and carotid arteries

performed (*Figure 18.6*). Waldhausen has suggested a modification applicable when the ascending aorta is extensively involved as well as the arch (*Figure 18.7*). The aortic prosthetic graft is first attached to the uninvolved segment of the descending thoracic aorta and then, in succession, union is made with the left subclavian, the carotid, and the innominate arteries, the clamp being moved proximal to each branch once the anastomosis is completed, thus allowing retrograde perfusion of these vessels. Finally, the

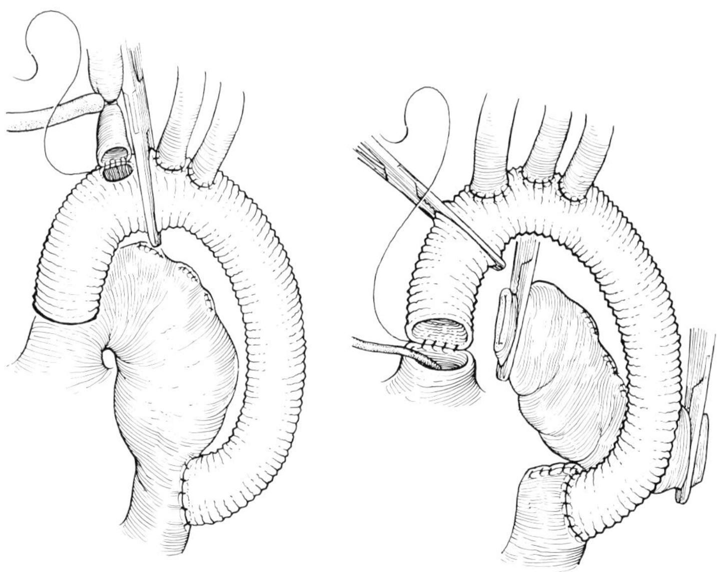

Figure 18.7 Method for aortic replacement utilizing, first, retrograde aortic perfusion and, later, total cardiopulmonary bypass

patient is placed on total cardiopulmonary bypass for completion of the operation by resecting the ascending aortic portion of the aneurysm and attaching the graft to the aortic root. Some success has been achieved with each of these procedures but altogether they have proved generally difficult and associated with too high a risk.

Judging from the four cases reported by Griepp and his colleagues and the experience of my associates, Isch, Jolly and others with two such cases, it would be my conjecture that the use of total cardiopulmonary bypass and profound hypothermia will replace other methods for dealing with aortic arch aneurysms. A median sternotomy approach alone or one extended by a left intercostal incision as necessary is employed. The body temperature is lowered as far as possible. As much dissection is carried out as can be accomplished with safety before beginning the cardiopulmonary bypass. The aneurysm is opened and partially unroofed, the clot and intimal debris removed, and the graft inserted first to the uninvolved distal end of the aorta, next to an oval segment of the wall from which the three branch vessels arise, and then to the proximal aorta. While the aneurysm is open and the distal anastomosis has begun a very small pump flow is maintained in order to keep the thoracic and abdominal aorta and their branches filled and free of air. During the period of rewarming and restoration of normal cardiac function, time is available for taking care of any remaining bleeding points. The aneurysmal wall may then be sutured over the graft to aid in haemostasis. In general, we always leave the aneurysm in place in all operations upon the arch, descending thoracic and abdominal aorta, and carry out an intrasaccular suture, a technique which saves time and blood loss and provides a useful cover for the graft. It is not unlikely that this method of profound hypothermia will prove better in the long run than the others currently being utilized.

Should this method prove as successful as I believe it will, it may be applicable in other situations now managed in a somewhat unsatisfactory way. These include cases in which not only the arch but all, or portions, of the ascending or descending thoracic aorta are involved as well. They embrace the unusual instances of dissecting aneurysms previously mentioned, those in which the site of the tear cannot be identified by arteriographic study and is not present in the opened portion of the aorta, and those in which the tear occurs so far distally in the ascending aorta that it is difficult to approximate securely its split end before attaching the prosthetic graft. In two instances of the first sort of difficulty, the ascending aorta was opened, the haemopericardium evacuated, the flail valve suspended, and a graft tube inserted in such a way that its distal end was sutured to a fenestrated aorta. Though both did well, one does not feel confident about this method. In a third case, the opened descending aorta did not exhibit the expected tear and though the patient survived graft replacement, death occurred later at home from rupture of the ascending aorta. With respect to the second problem, I have successfully replaced the ascending aorta, but only with an insecure approximation of the split distal end. One of my colleagues, however, seeking to place the clamp farther and farther across the proximal arch in an effort to unite more accurately the split wall before attaching the graft, finally was left with an unstable cuff and the patient did not survive. If deep hypothermia proves effective for arch aneurysms, it might, in both types of these cases of dissection, permit the surgeon to deal better with the ascending aorta or, if it seems preferable, to resect partially or totally the affected arch as well.

The descending thoracic aorta

The operative management of certain lesions of the descending thoracic aorta, or of this segment and the distal portion of the arch, frequently does not require bypass support or shunt. Coarctation of the aorta, for example, can almost always be so repaired. The occasional case in which the constricted area lies proximal to the take-off of the left subclavian artery can generally be treated in the same manner as the more common variety. However, when the arch is involved, it is a wise precaution to have a heart-lung machine on standby in case its use may facilitate better reconstruction. Furthermore, some type of bypass is necessary in cases of coarctation with unusually poor collateral circulation, when reoperation is required for bleeding after some time has elapsed and the previously existent collateral circulation is no longer functional, and in instances when expansion of a previously implanted aortic prosthetic graft makes replacement necessary. Though almost all cases of patent ductus arteriosus also are divided and closed well without bypass support, some are best performed with a standby apparatus. These exceptional cases include those with extensive calcification of the ductus or of the adjacent aorta, and those with a large aneurysm of the ductus or of the nearby aorta below an associated coarctation. Total bypass is also naturally required if the division accompanies an intracardiac surgical procedure.

Most of the other disorders involving the descending aorta have been accomplished with some sort of bypass. This measure has been used with the hope that it would minimize the risk of ischaemic spinal cord damage, avoid excessive hypertension in the cephalad portion of the body during aortic cross-clamping, and ensure adequate blood flow to the abdominal viscera. This brings us into an area of conflicting views, for some surgeons prefer one type of shunting mechanism, some another, and some feel that no shunt at all is needed.

One of the most widely utilized methods involves withdrawing blood from the left atrium and delivering it into a femoral or external iliac artery by means of a roller pump. Though 15 to 30 ml/kg per minute have been thought adequate, most surgeons have tried to maintain a flow of 30 ml/kg per minute or more. The radial or brachial pressure should be monitored and the flow adjusted, if possible, to avoid excessive hypertension proximally and reasonably good pressure distally. In general, this method has proved relatively satisfactory. It has, however, several potential or real disadvantages. In rare instances, especially when the left auricular appendage is small and the heart enlarged, the atrium may be torn during placement of the cannula. In other unusual cases, an inadequate flow is obtained despite repeated adjustments of the position of the left atrial cannula. In still other cases, fortunately encountered uncommonly, and principally in patients with arteriosclerotic heart disease, the manoeuvres associated with the insertion of the cannula or the blood loss related to the manipulation may precipitate life-threatening disturbances in cardiac function. These difficulties are avoided if blood is withdrawn from the right brachial artery, a method which has worked well in the few cases in which it has been utilized. More experience with this technique is, however, needed. It has been wisely suggested that the proximal left subclavian artery should not be used for any sort of bypass because of its importance in collateral circulation to the dorsal spinal cord. Regardless of the source of the oxygenated blood withdrawn, the closed mechanical bypass method has the distinct disadvantage of potentially increasing blood loss during the surgical procedure because of the necessary heparinization without providing any good mechanism for recovering and reinfusing the blood immediately. If a bypass of this type is used, it may be preferable to alter the usual closed arrangement in order to permit suction withdrawal of blood lost into the thorax and its prompt return to the patient or to employ an autotransfusion device.

The speedy recovery and return of any blood lost is one of the real advantages of another widely used method – that of utilizing a peripheral pump oxygenator system. Venous blood is generally withdrawn from a cannula placed in a femoral or iliac vein and often advanced into the inferior vena cava, though the cannula may sometimes be introduced directly into the distal thoracic vena cava if the location of the lesion to be treated makes this feasible. Femoral or iliac arterial inflow has usually been employed. I have preferred the external iliac vessels which are easily exposed through a small extraperitoneal incision. Fairly large cannulae can be used and they can ordinarily be passed without difficulty as far proximally as is desired. There is much to commend the method; the heart is not manipulated; there are no tubes in the operative field, the blood flow can usually be maintained at any level considered ideal and the blood lost during the operation, as mentioned previously, can be salvaged and reintroduced into the patient with no time lag.

Other methods which require neither pump nor oxygenator can be employed. One method involves the intraluminal intubation of the affected segment of the aorta while another one utilizes temporary non-pump bypass from a proximal arterial source or from the left ventricle to the aorta distal to the lesion or into a femoral or iliac artery. As early as 1910 Alexis Carrel mentioned the applicability of these methods and described experiments both with direct aortic intubation and with left ventricular-aortic shunts.

Temporary intraluminal shunts have been studied experimentally, and some of the early resections of aneurysms of the descending thoracic aorta were accomplished with this aid. This method has, however, never gained wide usage. It can be employed only in cases in which there is a length of uninvolved aorta proximal and distal to the lesion adequate for circumferential fixation of the tube. Safe introduction of the tube may require longer aortic cross-clamping than desirable when mural thrombus and diseased intima must be removed beforehand. The excision of the aneurysm and the interpolation of the graft may prove more difficult than they would otherwise be because of the presence of the rigid or semi-rigid tube. The aorta must be occluded and the tube removed before completion of the final graft-aortic anastomosis.

Left ventricular-aortic bypass has been utilized successfully in a small number of patients. The reported experiences, however, deal largely with traumatic rupture of the aorta and do not include instances of arteriosclerotic aneurysms with their greater likelihood of being associated with intrinsic heart disease, nor the more difficult instances of cystic medial disease. The method, however, does provide another means of bypass and may prove useful on occasions.

Experimental and clinical experiences with temporary non-pump arterial–arterial bypass have been largely with aorta-to-aorta shunts. They have the advantage of permitting utilization of grafts or tubes of large calibre. They can be inserted with ease in instances of relatively small midthoracic aneurysms or more proximal ones, especially those of traumatic origin. Unfortunately, such lesions are encountered rather infrequently. All too often the lesions to be bypassed involve the first part of the descending thoracic aorta or the distal arch and when this is the situation the more proximal arch may be relatively inaccessible through the incision utilized to permit safe and easy introduction of the tube proximally. Furthermore, the ascending aorta may also be difficult to use safely through the posterolateral incision so advantageously employed for lesions of the descending aorta. At times it is also impossible to place the other end of the shunt in the distal thoracic aorta with ease and security either because there is not a sufficient length of it uninvolved or because a very large aneurysm makes its adequate exposure difficult or unsafe. The tube or graft can, of course, be implanted in a femoral or iliac artery. Aortic bypass shunts may be hazardous in the presence of severe disease at the available site of insertion, whether this is due to arteriosclerosis, syphilis, or cystic medial disease, and should, I feel, never be used in the latter disorder because of fear of producing dissection.

The proximal portion of the left subclavian artery is often readily accessible but, as has been previously mentioned, its use may be ill-advised because of interference with collateral flow to the spinal cord. Recent studies indicate that non-pump shunts from the distal right brachial to the femoral artery provide good protection in dogs. This was also true of early experiments with left subclavian-aortic bypass. I know of no clinical experiences with non-pump direct distal right brachial to femoral or external iliac shunts. If they should prove as effective as they are in animals, they would be most useful. The vessels are quickly and easily exposed and either tube or graft bypass readily established. The arm can be positioned so that the antecubital area is quite close to the femoral or iliac artery and hence short segments of grafts or tubes can be employed. It would seem advisable, in suitable cases, to establish such shunts, measure flow with the aorta occluded, and either utilize them or convert to another bypass method according to the adequacy of the measured flow. In this way, this method of bypass could be safely evaluated in man.

Regardless of the arterial source or site of return, one can shunt by intubation with cannulae and non-pervious tubes or by woven prosthetic grafts sutured to incisions in the arteries. The first method has the advantage that it can be instituted and terminated a little more rapidly than the second. It has the disadvantage that the intraluminal cross-sectional area of the ends to be introduced cannot be as great as that of the main portion of the tube itself, nor as large as that of the artery into which the tube or cannula is introduced. In contrast, the graft sutured in place can be larger than the artery. The prosthetic graft has the added benefit of greater flexibility. I have been inclined to favour the graft, therefore, when it can be utilized with reasonable ease.

Although flow through such shunts can be measured, the magnitude of flow is dependent upon intrinsic haemodynamic factors and cannot be controlled externally. All the methods which employ pump-determined flow allow some variation, within limits—an advantage under certain circumstances. The experiments performed by Austen and Shaw indicate that blood can be withdrawn by pump from an artery more rapidly than it would be shed from the open artery bleeding freely against no resistance.

The management of traumatic disruptions of the first portion of the descending thoracic aorta is in a very satisfactory state and this is also true of traumatic aneurysms, and, in general, of all types of aneurysms that are reasonably small and situated in the proximal or mid-portion of the thoracic aorta, regardless of the type of shunt protection which is utilized.

The operative treatment of acute and subacute dissections of the descending thoracic aorta is not as satisfactory as is that of those present in the ascending aorta. For one thing, those in the latter situation are treated with total cardiopulmonary bypass and any blood lost is immediately returned to the pump oxygenator system and to the patient. The methods of bypass used in general for the treatment of dissection of the descending thoracic aorta have not included this protection of immediate recovery and replacement of blood lost. Almost all the dissections in the descending thoracic aorta are very extensive and involve the abdominal aorta and often the iliac and femoral arteries as well. It is not ordinarily difficult to free the distal end of the arch and obtain a suitable segment of aorta to which a graft can be attached proximal to the site where the dissection begins. In dealing with the distal segment, however, one is frequently confronted with a large dissection involving the very distal portion of the thoracic aorta often extending beyond the diaphragm. Despite the utilization of a circumferential cuff of Teflon felt to approximate the dissected aortic wall prior to attachment of the graft, the large size of the split wall itself presents a problem. In addition, in ligating the intercostal, oesophageal, and bronchial vessels one must isolate them individually outside the aneurysm or transfix them from within it one at a time, and even if one attempts to minimize blood lost from them by placing the distal clamp successively farther down the aorta as the operation proceeds, blood loss is frequently substantial and replacement sometimes falls behind loss. The infradiaphragmatic dissection not uncommonly detaches from the main lumen important branches to the abdominal viscera and sometimes causes obstruction to the flow of blood through the iliac-femoral system into the lower extremity with resultant ischaemia. These problems generally cause no difficulty and any persistent lower extremity ischaemia, which is rare, can almost invariably be eliminated by the simple manoeuvre of balloon dilatation through the exposed femoral artery. It is possible that all these factors may contribute to the somewhat higher risk associated with operating upon descending thoracic dissections as compared with that of treating similar lesions in the ascending portion of the aorta. Certainly, it is hoped that the techniques utilized and the results of treatment can be improved.

The same difficulties are associated with the treatment of very large extensive aneurysms involving the entire thoracic aorta or a major portion of it regardless of aetiology. Indeed, the problems are somewhat similar to those encountered in operating upon aneurysms involving the thoracic and the upper abdominal aorta or the entire abdominal aorta.

The thoracoabdominal aorta

The management of thoracoabdominal aneurysms, though reasonably satisfactory, has been far from ideal. The most widely employed method is that described by DeBakey and his colleagues. This entails the insertion of a prosthetic graft end-to-side into the thoracic aorta above the aneurysm and into the abdominal aorta or iliac arteries below it. The renal and the superior mesenteric arteries as well as the coeliac trunk are divided one at a time and

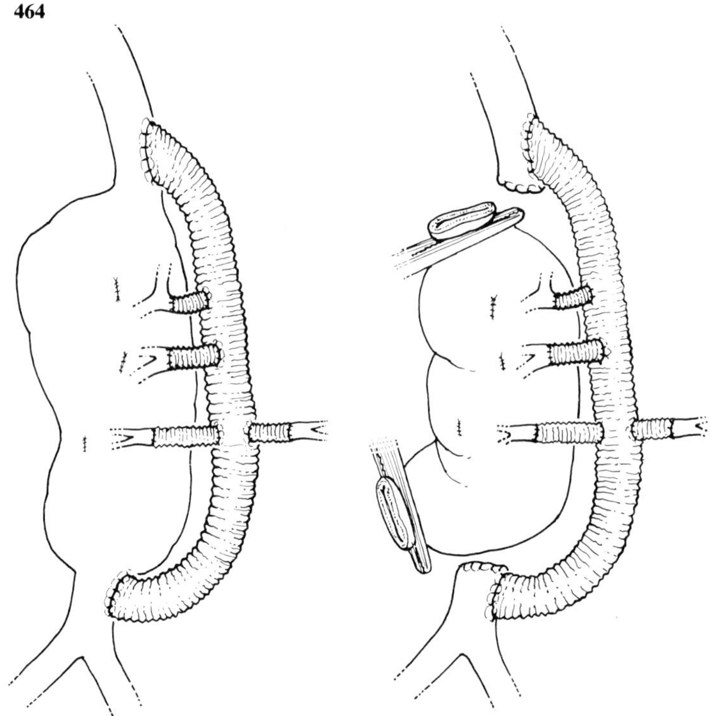

Figure 18.8 Method of resecting thoracoabdominal aneurysm using a permanent bypass graft

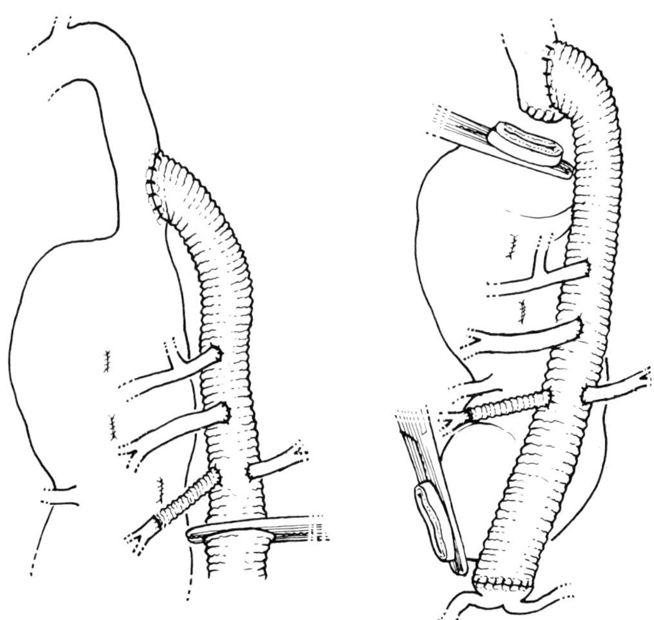

Figure 18.9 Alternative method of repairing thoracoabdominal aneurysm using a permanent bypass graft

anastomosed directly to the parent graft or to branch grafts attached to it (*Figure 18.8*). The aneurysm is then resected or obliterated. For the rare circumstances in which the aneurysm involves the entire abdominal aorta and the iliac arteries are too severely diseased, other methods of treatment are available. A graft is similarly attached to the thoracic aorta. The abdominal visceral branches are stepwise divided and sutured to the graft, and as each anastomosis is accomplished flow is established by repositioning of the occluding clamp (*Figure 18.9*). Finally, the aorta is cross-clamped above the iliacs and the distal end of the graft is sutured to the orifices of the iliac arteries or the terminal portion of the aorta if it is usable. Unfortunately, the results of these operations are not entirely gratifying as the mortality is still too high.

Most surgeons have felt it too hazardous from the standpoint of the likelihood of inducing paraplegia to remove aneurysms which involve practically the entire thoracic and the upper abdominal aorta. These dangerous lesions have thus been generally considered inoperable.

The recent publication of Crawford and his associates may significantly modify the future operative approach to pathological conditions of the entire thoracic aorta or most of it, to thoracoabdominal aortic aneurysms, and to abdominal aneurysms of the aorta involving the principal visceral branches. They have demonstrated in over eighty cases that extensive thoracoabdominal and upper abdominal aortic aneurysms, some involving the entire thoracic and abdominal aorta, can be removed completely with a much lower fatality rate than has previously been achieved.

The operative techniques which Crawford and his colleagues have followed in obtaining such excellent results do not include the utilization of any bypass support whatsoever for protecting the spinal cord and viscera. Heparinization is not required and the aneurysm is not excised but rather an intrasaccular implantation of the graft is made. Following this, oval segments of the aortic wall giving rise to important visceral branches, including the larger intercostal and spinal arteries, are attached to appropriate defects cut in the graft tube. These authors have certainly had an eminently satisfactory survival rate and they encountered very few cases of paraplegia. Their experiences during the more recent years would indicate, however, that the incidence of paraplegia can be reduced at least to half and perhaps can be practically eradicated by salvaging the larger intercostal and spinal arteries. Furthermore, paraplegia was encountered only in their patients with the most extensive aneurysms. Elimination of the excision of the aneurysm and intrasaccular insertion of the graft tube has been employed with satisfactory results by others and, as has been mentioned, I have long used this method by choice. The salvage of a segment of aortic wall containing more than one branch has also been utilized on occasions, as has been the retroperitoneal exposure of the abdominal aorta and its principal branches from the left side. Crawford's colleagues at Baylor University, DeBakey, McCollum and Graham, have just reported upon 117 cases of descending thoracic aortic aneurysms treated without shunt but with one dose of heparin at the time of cross-clamping and with ligation of the intercostal arteries. The previous mortality was lowered by half to 9.4 per cent and no increase in paraparesis (2.5 per cent) occurred—an excellent achievement, indeed. The combination of measures suggested by Crawford's group has certainly worked beautifully in their hands.

Since I have some fear that surgeons, without the very large background experience of the Crawford group and the capability of operating as rapidly as they in performing such sizable operative procedures, might not be able to achieve such success, there has occurred to me a modification of their method which possibly would prove safer in the hands of most surgeons. It might make possible the avoidance of errors which could result as a consequence of their feeling forced to get the procedure completed hastily. The suggestion involves the utilization of cardiopulmonary bypass and as low a body temperature as can be induced by it. One would make a large thoracoabdominal incision and carry out as much of the preliminary dissection as can be accomplished safely before institution of cardiopulmonary bypass. There is every likelihood that this could be done with very little blood loss. The cardiopulmonary bypass could be quickly and safely instituted through such an incision by placing the outflow venous drainage cannula through the main pulmonary artery or the right ventricular wall and the arterial inflow cannula through the uninvolved portion of the left subclavian artery (*Figure 18.10*). Ordinarily, one would anticipate that this

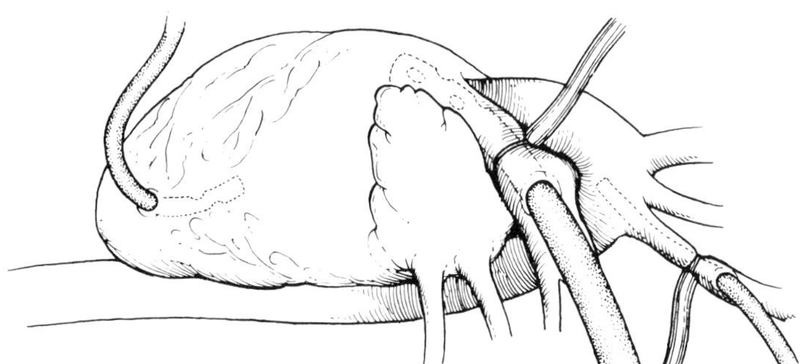

Figure 18.10 Method of establishing cardiopulmonary bypass and left ventricular decompression through left thoracotomy incision

inflow cannula could be advanced into the arch of the aorta safely. Once partial heart-lung bypass were started, it could be made complete by occluding the pulmonary artery around the drainage cannula or distal to it. Certainly, repair of the subclavian itself should present no problem since there has been essentially none with the utilization of femoral or iliac arteries for this purpose. As soon as cardiopulmonary bypass was instituted, one would cool the patient just as quickly and as profoundly as possible, isolate the lesion between clamps, and then proceed with the remainder of the operation according to Crawford's technique. The aneurysm would be opened but not resected and one would salvage the branch arteries and the principal spinal and intercostal vessels in the manner he has suggested. The proposed method has, of course, the theoretical disadvantage of requiring a little additional time to institute heart-lung bypass and to discontinue it and of having to heparinize the patient with the potentiality of more blood loss than would otherwise occur. Since the aorta and its branches would be occluded until the grafting procedure were completed, one would not, however, anticipate much loss of blood and what was lost could be quickly recovered and returned to the extracorporeal unit. The proposed method has the advantage of permitting cooling of the body with its additional safety margin from the standpoint of ischaemic damage to the spinal cord and viscera as well as the advantage of making it possible to perfuse the head and the proximal portion of the body.

It is reasonable to suspect that the less than ideal mortality which has accompanied the currently used methods is caused in great part by the inadequate exposure of the distal portion of the involved aorta, the frequency with which the affected segment is not entirely removed and therefore the graft tube has to be united with a diseased and dilated aortic segment. Furthermore, the tedious and exacting necessity of isolating, clamping, dividing, and attaching to the graft tube the important visceral arteries involved, and the failure to preserve blood flow into the large patent intercostal and spinal arteries, have contributed to suboptimal results and to the high mortality reported. The wide exposure, the leaving in place of the aneurysm itself, the preservation of all the important branches, the technique of using oval segments of the aorta so that the branches can be united with the graft tube more expeditiously, should save time, make the operation more complete, and, in general, add safety. Only further experience with Crawford's technique or with the proposal which I have made, will determine, however, their applicability and safety. Only then will it be clearly established that patients with aneurysms involving practically the entire thoracic and abdominal aorta are, as a matter of fact, suitable candidates for operative treatment, and whether in dealing with acute and subacute dissections of the thoracic aorta the operation will be made better by extending it to include the involved abdominal segment as well. Should all of this prove to be true, patients with large aneurysms affecting the major portion of the thoracic and abdominal aorta, up to the present ordinarily abandoned to a policy of watchful waiting, will be salvaged. Equally, patients with extensive dissections of the aorta will not be left with large uninvolved segments of the aorta—segments which so frequently dilate with the passage of time and sometimes require secondary operative manipulations or are considered so extensive as not to be amenable to operative treatment. One feels a certain hesitation in making these suggestions without adequate background experience, but I have seen no reasonable alternative. It is my feeling that Crawford's technique, or the proposed alternative method, will prove in the long run to be the treatment of choice in cases such as those described and discussed in this chapter.

Suggested Bibliography

Alley, R. D., Sewell, W. H., Formel, P. F., Stanahan, A., Kausel, H. and Koth, D. R. 'Experimental evolution of external shunts for by-passing the thoracic aorta.' *Surgical Forum*, **5**, 85 (1954)

Austen, W. G. and Shaw, R. S. 'Experimental studies with extracorporeal circuits as a method to enable surgical thoracic aneurysms.' *Journal of Thoracic and Cardiovascular Surgery*, **39,** 337 (1960)
Bahnson, H. T. 'Definitive treatment of saccular aneurysms of the aorta with excision of sac and aortic suture.' *Surgery, Gynecology and Obstetrics*, **96,** 382 (1953)
Bloodwell, R. D., Hallman, G. L. and Cooley, D. A. 'Partial cardiopulmonary bypass for pericardiectomy and resection of descending thoracic aortic aneurysms.' *Annals of Thoracic Surgery*, **6,** 46 (1968)
Carrell, A. 'On the experimental surgery of the thoracic aorta and the heart.' *Annals of Surgery*, **52,** 83 (1910)
Clatworthy, H. W. and Varco, R. L. 'A small bore polythene shunt to prevent mechanical shock after prolonged cross-clamping of the thoracic aorta.' *Proceedings of the Society for Experimental Biological Medicine*, **74,** 434 (1950)
Cole, P. T. and Gutelius, J. R. 'Paraplegia resulting from use of subclavian artery as a shunt source during resection of the descending thoracic aorta.' *Annals of Surgery*, **169,** 293 (1969)
Cooley, D. A. and DeBakey, M. E. 'Resection of entire ascending aorta in fusiform aneurysm using cardiac bypass.' *Journal of the American Medical Association*, **162,** 1150 (1956)
Cooley, D. A. and DeBakey, M. E. 'Surgical considerations of intrathoracic aneurysms of aorta and great vessels.' *Annals of Surgery*, **135,** 660 (1952)
Cooley, D. A., DeBakey, M. E. and Morris, G. C., Jr. 'Controlled extracorporeal circulation in surgical treatment of aortic aneurysm.' *Annals of Surgery*, **146,** 475 (1957)
Cooley, D. A., Mahaffey, D. E. and DeBakey, M. E. 'Total excision of the aortic arch for aneurysm.' *Surgery, Gynecology and Obstetrics*, **101,** 667 (1955)
Crawford, E. S., Snyder, D. M., Cho, G. C. and Roehm, J. O. F., Jr. 'Progress in treatment of the thoracoabdominal and abdominal aortic aneurysms involving celiac, superior mesenteric, and renal arteries.' *Annals of Surgery*, **188,** 404 (1978)
Cross, F. S., Hirose, Y., Jones, R. D., Hudack, S. S. and Kay, E. B. 'Evaluation of a mechanical shunt to bypass segments of the thoracic aorta including the arch.' *Surgical Forum*, **6,** 166 (1955)
DeBakey, M. E., Crawford, E. S., Cooley, D. A. and Morris, G. C., Jr. 'Successful resection of fusiform aneurysm of aortic arch with replacement by homograft.' *Surgery, Gynecology and Obstetrics*, **105,** 657 (1957)
DeBakey, M. E., Crawford, E. S., Garrett, C. H., Beall, A. C., Jr. and Howell, J. F. 'Surgical considerations in the treatment of aneurysms of the thoraco-abdominal aorta.' *Annals of Surgery*, **162,** 650 (1965)
DeBakey, M. E., Crawford, E. S. and Morris, G. C., Jr. 'Aneurysms of the thoracic aorta: analysis of 179 patients treated by resection.' *Journal of Thoracic Surgery*, **36,** 393 (1958)
DeBakey, M. E., Creech, O. and Morris, G. C. 'Aneurysm of thoraco-abdominal aorta involving the celiac, superior mesenteric and renal arteries. Report of four cases treated by resection and homograft replacement.' *Annals of Surgery*, **144,** 549 (1956)
DeBakey, M. E., McCollum, C. H. and Graham, J. M. 'Surgical treatment of the descending thoracic aorta.' *Journal of Cardiovascular Surgery*, **19,** 571 (1978)
DeCamp, P. T., Spencer, R. and Overstreet, J. W. 'Experimental studies in delayed homologous arterial grafting utilizing an intra-arterial shunt.' *Surgical Forum*, **1,** 282 (1951)
Diloon, M. L., Young, W. G. and Sealy, W. C. 'Aneurysms of the descending thoracic aorta.' *Annals of Thoracic Surgery*, **3,** 430 (1967)

English, T. A. H. 'Direct left ventriculofemoral bypass during resection of coarctation of the aorta with anomalous subclavian arteries.' *Thorax*, **20,** 36 (1965)
Gerbode, F., Baimbridge, M., Osborn, J. J., Hood, M. and French, S. 'Traumatic thoracic aneurysms: treatment by resection and grafting with the use of an extra-corporeal bypass.' *Surgery*, **42,** 975 (1957)
Griepp, R. B., Stinson, E. B., Hollingsworth, J. F. and Buehler, D. 'Prosthetic replacement of the aortic arch.' *Journal of Thoracic and Cardiovascular Surgery*, **70,** 1051 (1975)
Gunning, A. J. 'A disposable one-piece left ventriculo-aortic bypass cannula.' *Thorax*, **27,** 371 (1972)
Izant, R. J., Hubay, C. A. and Holden, W. D. 'A nonsuture aortic shunt—an experimental study.' *Surgery*, **33,** 233 (1953)
Johnson, J., Kirby, C. K. and Lehr, H. B. 'A method of maintaining adequate blood flow through the thoracic aorta while inserting an aorta graft to replace an aortic aneurysm.' *Surgery*, **37,** 54 (1955)
Kahn, D. R., Valhayanon, S. and Sloan, H. 'Resection of descending thoracic aneurysms without left heart bypass.' *Archives of Surgery, Chicago*, **97,** 336 (1968)
King, H. and Shumacker, H. B., Jr. 'Mechanical by-pass during thoracic aortic cross-clamping.' *Journal of Thoracic Surgery*, **34,** 485 (1957)
Kirsh, M. M., Kahn, D. R., Crane, J. D., Anastasia, L. F., Lui, A. H., Moores, W. Y., Valhayanon, S., Bookstein, J. J. and Sloan, H. 'Repair of acute traumatic rupture of the aorta without extracorporeal circulation.' *Annals of Thoracic Surgery*, **10,** 227 (1970)
Lam, C. R. and Aram, H. H. 'Resection of the descending thoracic aorta for aneurysm: a report of the use of a homograft in a case and an experimental study.' *Annals of Surgery*, **134,** 743 (1951)
Leshnower, A. C. and Shumacker, H. B., Jr. 'Experimental unassisted right brachial-to-femoral bypass.' *Archives of Surgery, Chicago*, **109,** 542 (1974)
Mahorner, H. and Spencer, R. 'Shunt grafts.' *Annals of Surgery*, **139,** 439 (1954)
Mallory, P. J. 'Repair of the ruptured aorta using left 'ventriculo-aortic support.' *Thorax*, **25,** 213 (1970)
Neville, W. E., Thomason, R. D., Peacock, H. and Colby, C. 'Cardiopulmonary bypass during noncardiac surgery.' *Archives of Surgery, Chicago*, **92,** 576 (1966)
Powley, P. H. 'Traumatic rupture of the aorta: repair using ventriculo-aortic bypass.' *Proceedings of the Royal Society of Medicine*, **64,** 1085 (1971)
Shafer, P. W. and Hardin, C. A. 'The use of temporary polythene shunts to permit occlusion, resection, and frozen homologous graft replacement of vital vessel segments. A laboratory and clinical study.' *Surgery*, **31,** 186 (1952)
Shumacker, H. B., Jr. 'Cystic medial necrosis.' *Journal of Cardiovascular Surgery*, **19,** 639 (1978)
Shumacker, H. B., Jr. 'Innovation in operative management of thoraco-abdominal aortic aneurysms.' *Surgery, Gynecology and Obstetrics*, **136,** 793 (1973)
Stanahan, A., Alley, R. D., Sewell, W. H. and Kausel, H. W. 'Aortic arch resection and grafting for aneurysm employing an external shunt.' *Journal of Thoracic Surgery*, **29,** 54 (1955)
Waldhausen, J. A. 'Excision and replacement of the entire thoracic aorta for aneurysm.' *Journal of Thoracic and Cardiovascular Surgery*, **48,** 78 (1964)

19

The Technique of Intracardiac Repair in Infancy using Deep Hypothermia with Circulatory Arrest and Limited Cardiopulmonary Bypass

Brian G. Barratt-Boyes

clavam extorquere Herculi

Introduction

For many years the surgical management of symptomatic congenital heart disease presenting in infancy has consisted, where possible, of palliation and later second stage intracardiac repair. This management has been accepted in most clinics and for the majority of correctable forms of congenital heart disease until recently because, with few exceptions, the results of primary repair had been unsatisfactory.

In an attempt to improve the results of primary repair in infancy, a number of cardiac surgical groups have adopted profound hypothermia techniques in order to provide a sufficient period of circulatory arrest during which to perform an accurate and rapid repair of even complex defects within a totally relaxed and bloodless heart. While the provision of ideal operating conditions is a most important feature of profound hypothermia techniques, a second major advantage is that it reduces the duration of cardiopulmonary bypass regardless of the complexity of the lesion. There is ample evidence that conventional cardiopulmonary bypass has many deleterious effects and that these are related to the duration of perfusion and are less well tolerated in infants and neonates than in older patients. It is theoretically an advantage, therefore, when operating upon infants, to limit the duration of perfusion if this can be done safely. Circulatory arrest techniques at low body temperatures appear to make this possible.

The principles involved in the use of hypothermia and circulatory arrest were established by Bigelow, Callaghan and Hepps[10] and later practised by Lewis and Taufic[30] and Swan *et al.*[37], while profound hypothermia with longer periods of arrest was used by Drew and Anderson[22] chiefly in adult patients. The advantages of profound hypothermia in infancy were recognized early by the Japanese surgeons, who used various methods of cooling and rewarming, and the technique described in detail here is similar to that recommended by the Kyoto group (Hikasa *et al.*[25]).

There are a number of ways in which the body temperature can be manipulated to provide an adequate period of circulatory arrest.

Entirely by surface means (surface cooling and surface rewarming)

This technique has been used by the Seattle group since 1967[19]. Ether anaesthesia is considered important and a respiratory alkalosis is induced. Surface cooling and rewarming are provided by a water bath. Heparinization is not required but low molecular weight dextran is used to reduce blood viscosity. Results using this technique have been good[20], although the numbers reported are insufficient to establish a clear superiority over conventional extracorporeal circulation.

The technique has significant disadvantages, which include a prolonged anaesthetic time, mainly due to the slowness of surface rewarming, and the necessity for manual cardiac massage during the early stages of surface rewarming. More importantly, in the absence of cardiopulmonary bypass, there is no way, in cyanotic patients, to oxygenate the tissues fully prior to the circulatory arrest period, or to support the circulation in the post-arrest period when arrhythmias occur.

Metabolic data using this technique have been collected by Baum *et al.*[8]. Infants who survived had peak lactate concentrations from 10.4 to 16.7 mmol/ℓ and those who died reached levels of 10.6 to 23.8 mmol/ℓ. There is thus a considerably greater lactacidosis with this technique than with either of the subsequent methods.

Entirely by cardiopulmonary bypass (core cooling and core rewarming)

This is similar to the technique introduced by Drew and Anderson in 1959[22], except that a mechanical oxygenator is used rather than the patient's own lungs. Its main attraction is a saving in anaesthetic time, although this varies with the flow rate and the temperature gradient between machine blood and patient, and the optimum for these two variables is by no means established. It is known that core cooling produces wide temperature gradients within the body because of altered distribution of blood flow[32]. The skeletal muscle mass is poorly perfused and remains at a relatively high temperature while the liver and heart cool rapidly and cease to function early. This technique was discredited when some groups reported a significant incidence of neurological complications in adult patients, partly related to wide variations in details of technique[11].

When core cooling is used, steps must be taken to protect the lungs when there is direct run-off from the aorta into the pulmonary artery (patent ductus arteriosus, truncus arteriosus etc.), and to protect the ventricles when there is direct run-off into either of these chambers (aortic incompetence, ruptured sinus of Valsalva aneurysm, etc.).

Metabolic data have been collected with this technique in infants at Green Lane Hospital for comparison with surface cooling and core rewarming[23]. The studies were not, however, contemporaneous nor were the infants matched as regards weight so that a meaningful comparison with the latter technique is difficult. The results are also dependent on perfusion flow rates (which varied in this instance from 100 to 150 ml/kg per min) and the temperature gradients between the perfusate and the nasopharynx. The study suggested, however, that while lactic acid production may be different with these two techniques, variations in P_{CO_2}, pH and base deficit were roughly comparable. The main difference was in oxygen uptake. Thus, at the same pre-arrest temperature of 22°C and the same blood flow, the oxygen uptake following cooling entirely by bypass was twice that obtained when cooling was largely by surface means. This presumably results from uneven body cooling with core cooling techniques and suggests that the safe circulatory arrest time following core cooling is less at any given temperature than with surface cooling.

Surfacing cooling and bypass rewarming

This technique, which combines cooling with core rewarming[25], has been in use at Green Lane Hospital since July 1969[7]. Surface cooling is provided by a water bed and ice bags, but a 5 minute period of core cooling is often required to complete the cooling process or, in the cyanotic group, to oxygenate fully the tissues prior to circulatory arrest. Core rewarming requires a 20–30 minute period of heart-lung bypass and is assisted by circulating water at 40°C through the water bed. On theoretical grounds this method is superior to other techniques[40] because surface cooling is more even than core cooling, the liver functions for a longer time and the heart continues to beat and to provide a pulsatile flow. Core rewarming rapidly increases the temperature of these central organs so that the heart can eject and again provide pulsatile flow and the liver can begin to metabolize lactate[1]. The period of cardiopulmonary bypass is also reduced to a minimum.

Metabolic data

Changes in arterial blood P_{CO_2}, base deficit, pH and lactate are depicted in *Figure 19.1* in relation to the nasopharyngeal temperature and the periods of bypass and circulatory arrest[33]. A number of postoperative measurements are also included.

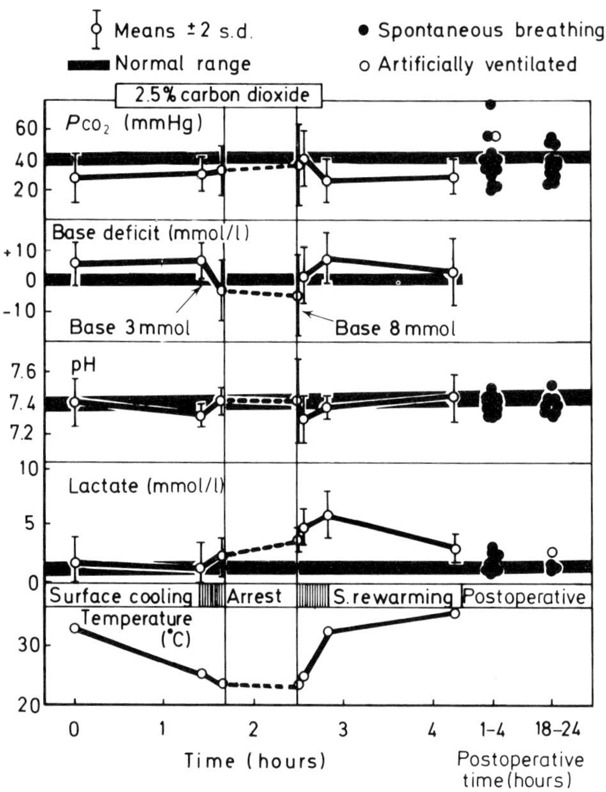

Figure 19.1 Metabolic changes during profound hypothermia in infancy using surface cooling (followed by a short period of core cooling) and core rewarming (followed by surface rewarming). The temperature changes and sampling times relative to these events are depicted in the lower panel. In this series of 10 infants[33] circulatory arrest was established at an average of 22°C and core rewarming discontinued at 32°C. This should be compared with *Figure 19.4*. The amounts shown for added base are the resultants of machine blood plus bicarbonate solution with which each period of perfusion began

The P_{CO_2} level is altered by the rate of ventilation and the addition of 2.5 per cent CO_2 at temperatures below 30°C. The mean level varies between 28 and 40 mmHg and approximates 34 mmHg at the time of circulatory arrest.

The base deficit represents the metabolic component of the acid–base change, consisting of lactic acid, hydrogen ion from other sources and administered bicarbonate. It does not change during surface cooling but falls significantly (alkaline shift) with the short terminal period of core cooling, this change being only partly due to the addition of bicarbonate. After arrest and during the rewarming phase there is a significant rise (acid shift), despite the addition of bicarbonate, which reaches its peak at the end of rewarming perfusion and then returns to normal.

The pH is the resultant of the above two factors and, when measured at the temperature of the blood, there is only minor variation from 7.40.

Arterial blood lactate remains unchanged during surface cooling, rises slightly during bypass cooling and then increases sharply to a mean maximum of 5.5 mmol/ℓ during rewarming perfusion as a result of washout of ischaemic tissues. This significant lactacidosis corrects itself when natural circulation is re-established. It is not much greater than that occurring after conventional bypass in adults at 30°C where the mean level rises to 3.2 mmol/ℓ[24].

It is usually assumed that lactate changes are the prime cause of the variation in base deficit, or, expressed differently, that in hypoxic situations the metabolic acidosis results purely from the release of lactic acid. That this is not so, is shown in *Figure 19.2* where the lactate concentration

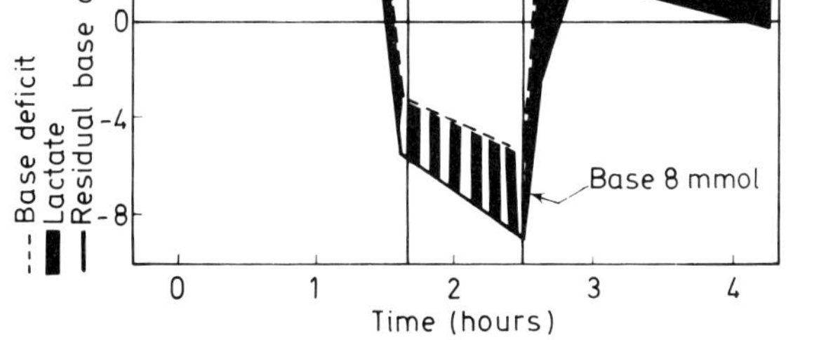

Figure 19.2 Mean variation in residual base deficit in the same 10 infants as in *Figure 19.1*

is subtracted from the base deficit to give the non-lactic (or residual) base deficit. The non-lactic base deficit shows a swing to the alkaline side during the initial short cooling perfusion (from + 5 to − 6) only partly accounted for by the addition of bicarbonate, and an acid shift (− 9 to + 2) during rewarming perfusion despite the addition of further base.

Similar changes occur during conventional bypass at 30°C without circulatory arrest, but they do not occur during profound hypothermia when the terminal short period of cooling bypass is omitted[33]. They appear, therefore, to be the result of cooling plus bypass and not cooling alone. They are presumed to result from massive hydrogen ion shifts and do not appear to be harmful.

Total body oxygen uptake falls during cooling to an average of 1.26 ml/kg per min just before circulatory arrest at 22°C. Within two minutes of starting rewarming perfusion, uptake trebles due to rapid repayment of oxygen debt and remains near this level throughout the rewarming period.

Biochemical changes have been studied by Brown *et al.*[12] and by others. During cooling there is a fall in serum potassium and plasma insulin and a rise in plasma glucose. The changes in serum sodium and magnesium are insignificant.

Disadvantages of this technique

(1) It is more time-consuming and complex than conventional extracorporeal circulation. The increase in total operating (anaesthetic) time in infants weighing five kilograms or less is minimal using current methods of surface cooling and even in heavier infants seldom exceeds one hour[2]. The need for some additional equipment and expertise is, however, undeniable.

(2) There is a possibility of brain damage. Reported experience from numerous centres using this technique in infants[2,35,36] makes it clear that brain damage is rarely recognized during hospital convalescence. It should not occur if recommended arrest times are strictly adhered to and cerebral air embolism is avoided. Later psychometric testing of infants operated upon at Green Lane Hospital using surface cooling and core rewarming techniques has been completed recently[16]. This confirms earlier impressions that these children show no significant deviation from normal. It requires re-emphasis that previous reports of brain damage following circulatory arrest at low temperatures have occurred when core cooling techniques, not surface cooling techniques, have been used.

(3) Perhaps the major disadvantage is the strict limit placed on intracardiac repair time. Some surgeons find this intolerable and it may make repair of more complex lesions impractical for some operators. It is vital not only that the surgeon should be expert and expeditious but also that the details of intracardiac pathology are available preoperatively. Only in this way can the procedure be fully planned before the arrest period, rather than during it.

An alternative technique which overcomes this disadvantage and combines deep hypothermia with low flow perfusion has been described by Kirklin *et al.*[27]. Its safety has still to be established.

(4) Subcutaneous fat necrosis does occur in about 20 per cent of infants. Painful subcutaneous nodules appear and make the infant feverish and irritable. In our experience resolution has been complete in all instances, although involvement of the sternotomy wound with delayed healing has been reported[36]. Methods to prevent it are under study—probably the most important is the avoidance of prolonged contact with ice chips or ice-cold water.

Comparison with cardiopulmonary bypass

Conventional cardiopulmonary bypass at euthermia or mild hypothermia has been applied to infants with success in the repair of ventricular septal defects and, more recently, in some other conditions. In comparing the two techniques the age of the infant and the complexity of the lesion repaired must be documented for these become most important in the neonatal period. Circulatory arrest techniques are probably greatly superior in the first few months of life when the heart is very small, although the experience with cardiopulmonary bypass in this age group still remains insufficient to allow a valid comparison.

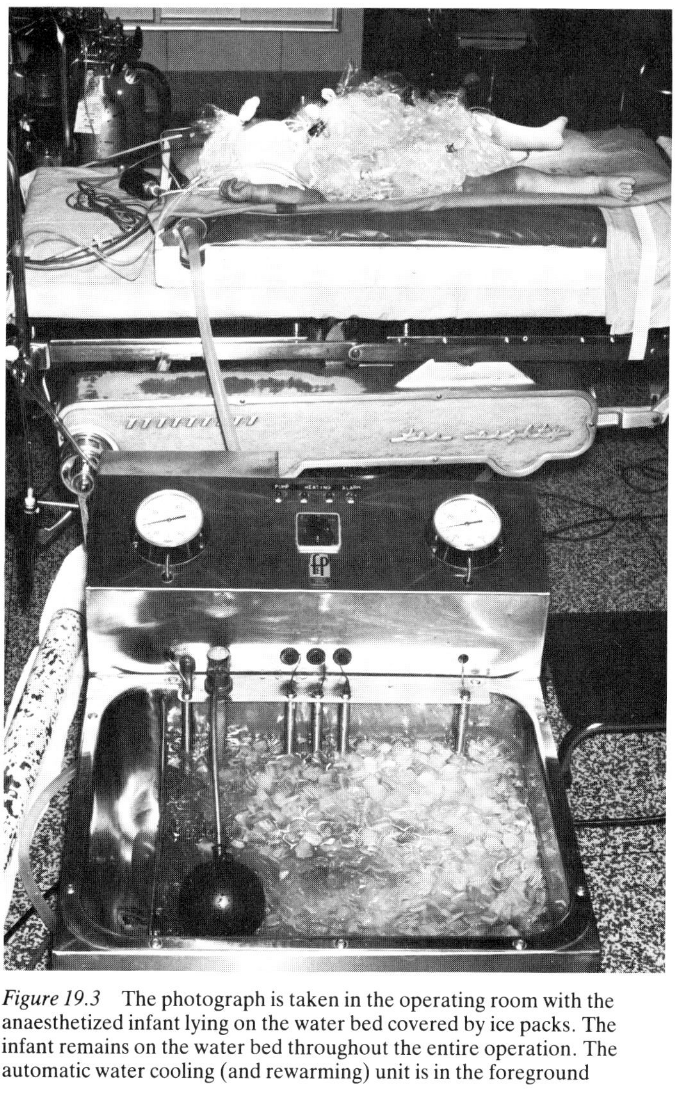

Figure 19.3 The photograph is taken in the operating room with the anaesthetized infant lying on the water bed covered by ice packs. The infant remains on the water bed throughout the entire operation. The automatic water cooling (and rewarming) unit is in the foreground

Technique of profound hypothermia (surface cooling and core rewarming)

Equipment

Water bed and ice bags

The water bed is constructed of heavyweight plastic, supported in a low-profile wooden frame which fits the table top. Water at 1°C is rapidly circulated through the bed using a specially designed circuit (*Figure 19.3*). To allow as much as possible of the infant to come into direct contact with the bed, it is not permitted to overfill.

The rate of cooling with this system is depicted in *Figure 19.4* for a 4 kg subject. For this weight of infant the nasopharyngeal temperature falls 1°C in 5 minutes. The rate is slowed by approximately 1 minute per degree for each additional kilogram of body weight.

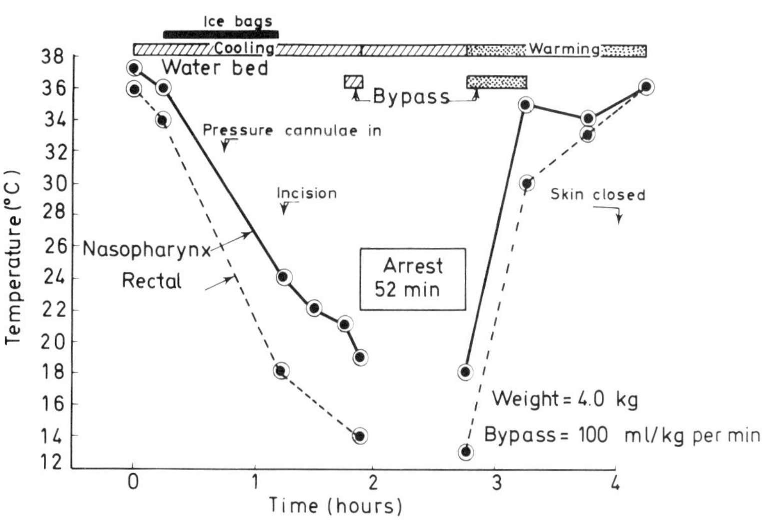

Figure 19.4 Graphic representation of events during profound hypothermia and circulatory arrest in a 4 kg infant. Note the slight fall in temperature during the circulatory arrest period

The water bed is also used to aid rewarming. Its temperature is altered more rapidly by emptying out the cold water before refilling it with warm. When the bed is empty the infant sinks towards the table top, and the zero level of the pressure transducers must be adjusted accordingly.

Operating on a water bed has the theoretical disadvantage that the infant is not completely stable. In practice, the surgeon is unaware of this and is not inconvenienced.

Bypass circuit

Components These have been reduced to a minimum to limit priming volume (*Figure 19.5*). (1) A 5 inch diameter double-roller pump head is used for arterial return. When fitted with ⅜ inch internal diameter Mayon tubing the maximum output is 1100 ml/min and with 5⁄16 inch internal

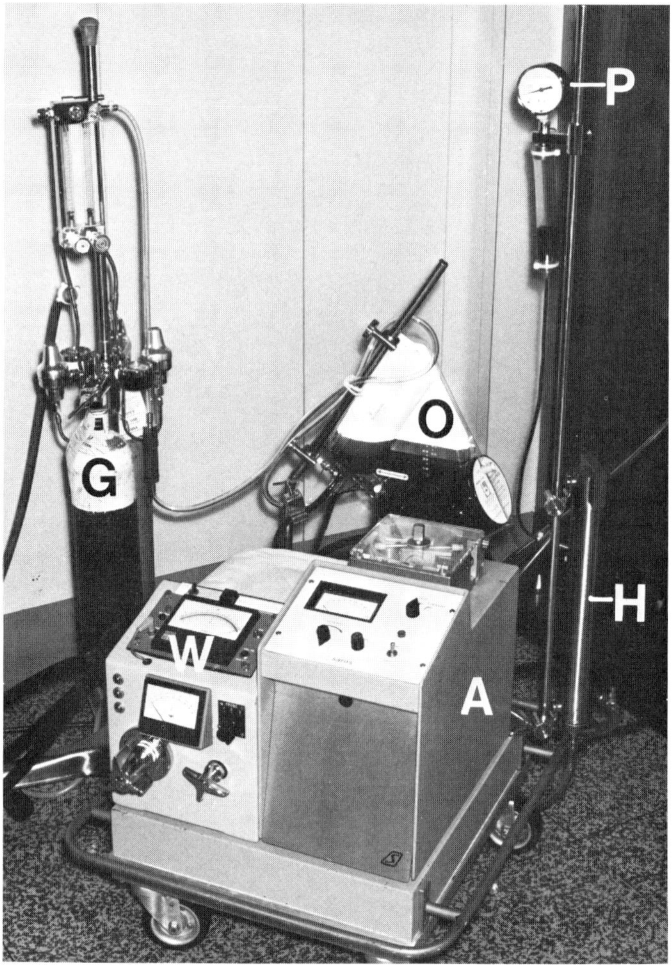

Figure 19.5 The infant heart-lung bypass circuit. A = arterial pump unit; G = carbon dioxide gas cylinder with flow meter and mixing valve; H = infant heat exchanger; O = infant 'Temptrol' oxygenator; P = pressure gauge on arterial line; W = water mixing valve unit and temperature gauge

diameter tubing, it is 800 ml/min. Open-heart pumps are not required. (2) An infant Temptrol oxygenator receives blood directly from the single venous line. (3) An infant heat exchanger is mounted between the oxygenator and the arterial filter and has a 60 ml priming volume. The temperature of the blood leaving it is identical to the circulating water temperature at the flow rates and temperature gradients used and only the water temperature is therefore monitored. The water temperature is adjusted by a thermostatically controlled water-mixing valve. (4) The arterial line pressure is monitored from a side arm in the line beyond the heat exchanger. (5) The line tubing is ¼ inch internal diameter Mayon throughout.

Prime This consists of two units of heparinized blood collected on the morning of the operation (within two to three hours of use). Each unit contains 50 ml of 5 mg/100 ml glucose as diluent for the heparin (20 mg/500 ml). Further dilution is not practised unless the infant's haematocrit level is in excess of 35 per cent, when an appropriate amount of N/5 saline plus 4.2 mg/100 ml glucose solution and 4 mg/100 ml serum albumin is added to reduce it to this level.

Protocol

(1) The infant is premedicated 45 minutes before the operation with 0.1 ml/kg body weight of a mixture of pethidine 25 mg, chlorpromazine 6.25 mg and promethazine 6.25 mg/ml.
(2) The naked infant is placed supine on the cold water bed (*Figure 19.3*) from which he is partly insulated at this stage by a dry towel. Limb leads for the electrocardiogram are positioned and anaesthesia is induced by mask using equal parts of nitrous oxide and oxygen plus 0.5 per cent to 1 per cent halothane. Intravenous pancuronium bromide (0.2 mg/kg) is given and followed by insertion of an orotracheal airway and accurately positioned nasopharyngeal and rectal temperature probes. The dry towel is removed and replaced by a single layer of linen cloth to ensure more direct cold transference. Ventilation is continued with humidified nitrous oxide and oxygen and 0.5 per cent halothane, using a modified Ayr's T-piece technique. Hyperventilation is avoided as far as possible.
(3) Water at 1°C is rapidly recirculated through the water bed throughout the cooling phase and ice bags are placed over the chest and flanks (*Figure 19.3*).
(4) An intravenous cannula is inserted percutaneously in the left wrist or forearm and infusion with N/5 saline with 4.2 mg/100 ml glucose at 3 ml/kg per hour begun. In infants under six months of age the pressure monitoring lines are inserted by cutdown via the left femoral artery and long saphenous vein and advanced into the abdominal aorta and inferior vena cava. A size 18 gauge arterial cannula is preferred as this does not usually obstruct forward arterial flow. In infants over six months of age the arterial line is often inserted percutaneously into the left radial artery. Induction of anaesthesia and cannulation usually take 40–45 minutes, by which time the nasopharyngeal temperature has already fallen significantly (*Figure 19.4*).
(5) Further ice bags are positioned to cover the abdomen, protecting the genital area and avoiding contact with peripheral parts (*Figure 19.3*).
(6) At 30°C and below, 2.5 per cent CO_2 is added to the anaesthetic gas mixture.
(7) Surface cooling is continued until the nasopharyngeal temperature reaches 24°C. Halothane inhalation is stopped at lower temperatures if the arterial blood pressure falls consistently below 30 mmHg, but sinus bradycardia is not corrected. In complex defects which require an arrest temperature of 18°C, surface cooling is continued until 22°C is reached, provided the blood pressure remains above 25 mmHg.

(8) The ice bags are removed and the skin painted and draped. A median sternotomy is made with a vibrating saw and the pericardium opened vertically. When needed for the intracardiac repair, an appropriate piece of pericardium is removed. The patient is heparinized (300 units/kg body weight).

(9) The venae cavae are encircled with tapes, including a left superior vena cava when present, using an aneurysm needle for the inferior vena cava tape, as this avoids any manipulation of the heart which can induce ventricular fibrillation. If the latter occurs, the heart is electrically defibrillated. If defibrillation is not achieved (and this is rare,) cannulation is completed without undue haste with the heart arrested.

(10) A single right atrial cannula (4–6 mm internal diameter) is inserted through the appendage and the arterial return line is placed in the ascending aorta close to the valve, using a size 14F nasal suction catheter (*Figure 19.6*). Each of these structures is excluded in a

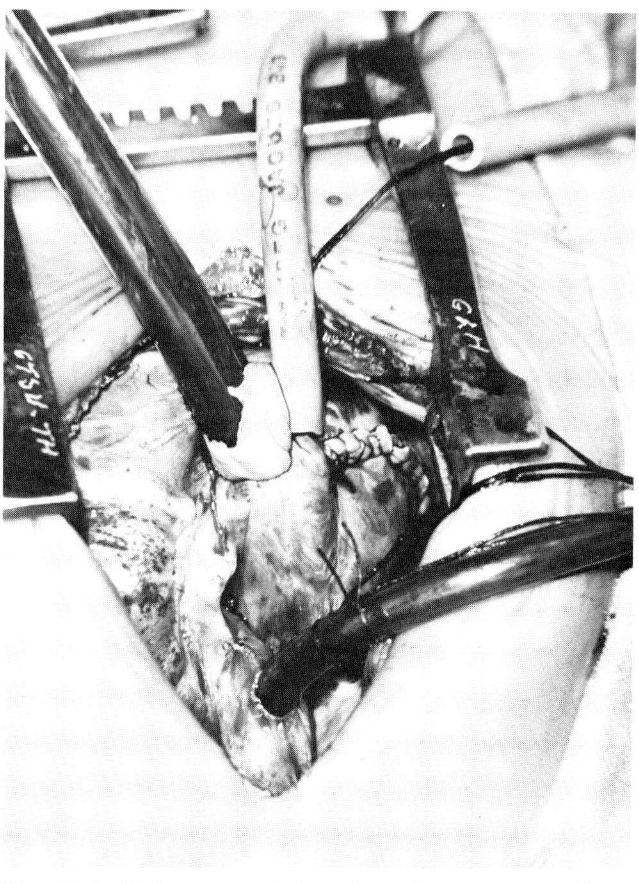

Figure 19.6 The heart exposed through a median sternotomy with arterial and venous cannulae in position. (From Barratt-Boyes *et al.*[5] by courtesy of *Progress in Cardiovascular Diseases*)

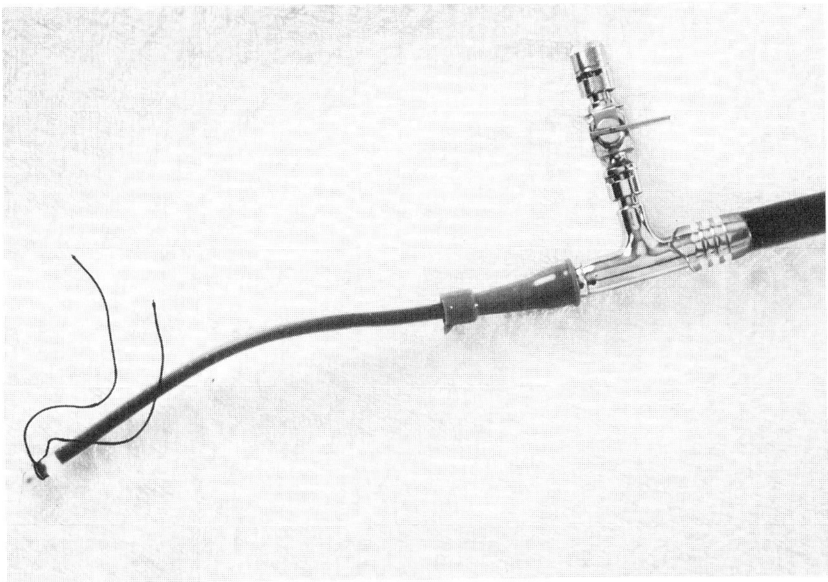

Figure 19.7 The arterial cannula with the silk tie in position near its obliquely cut tip. It is connected to the arterial line with a metal connector containing a Luer lock side arm which is used for aspiration of air and for injection of the cardioplegic solution. (Most of the assembly has been filled with blood)

curved clamp and opened before the pursestrings are placed. The tip of the arterial catheter is cut obliquely and a silk ligature tied 3 mm from its end to mark and limit the depth of insertion of the catheter into the ascending aorta (*Figure 19.7*).

(11) The venous and arterial lines are connected to the primed perfusion circuit, incorporating a two-way tap in the arterial connector, partly for use later to aspirate air from the ventricle. The arterial line is clamped on the heart-lung machine side of the connector. Two mmol of potassium chloride, 5 mmol of sodium bicarbonate and 500 mg of ascorbic acid are added to the machine prime, the latter for its effect in lowering blood viscosity[38].

(12) Iced water has continued to circulate through the water bed during these manoeuvres and the temperature will have dropped a further 2 to 3°C.

(a) In patients with acyanotic conditions, where an arrest time of 30 to 45 minutes is expected and the temperature has already reached 20°C, the gas mixture is changed to 97.5 per cent oxygen and 2.5 per cent CO_2 for 5 minutes and blood then drained through the venous line into the oxygenator to empty the heart and lungs of most of their contained blood. The aorta is then cross-clamped downstream of the arterial line cannulation site, the caval tapes snared down and the venous line clamped.

(b) In all patients having cyanotic cardiac anomalies and whenever the repair time is expected to approach or exceed 60 minutes, cooling perfusion is started at a flow rate of 100 ml/kg per min. The temperature of the blood leaving the heat exchanger is maintained at 10°C lower than the nasopharyngeal temperature. A minimum 3 minute perfusion time is allowed to oxygenate the tissues as fully as possible. At the desired temperature of 18°C the perfusion is stopped, blood drained from the venous line, the aorta and cavae occluded and both lines clamped.

(13) A single injection of cold cardioplegic solution (15 ml/kg body weight of St. Thomas's solution)[26] is made into the aortic root by means of a syringe connected to the Luer tap in the arterial line (*Figure 19.7*). Care is taken not to overpressurize the coronary artery bed. The solution is allowed to escape from the right atrium by removing the venous line from the appendage. The heart immediately becomes completely flaccid and the operating field still and blood-free. The heart is opened where appropriate and any fluid sucked away and discarded.

(14) During circulatory arrest the water bed temperature is raised to 15°C and an oxygen flow of 1.5 ℓ/min is maintained through the Temptrol oxygenator to ensure that the gas-vent holes are not occluded by dried blood. The lungs are kept slightly inflated but are not ventilated.

(15) With the intracardiac repair completed the cardiotomy is closed. The right atrium is always opened to close any atrial communication, including a patent foramen ovale, and blood is injected by syringe through any atrial defect to flush air from the atrium into the ventricle.

(16) To expel air from the heart the usual procedure is as follows:

(a) A small catheter is introduced through a stab wound in the apex of the left ventricle and controlled with a pursestring stitch. Blood, which has been aspirated from the oxygenator into two or three 50 ml syringes via the Luer tap on the arterial line connector during the arrest period, is syringed through the left ventricular catheter and aspirated into a dry syringe connected to the Luer tap, gently massaging the heart and ventilating the lungs. The solution passes through any Teflon patch used for ventricular septal defect repair into the right ventricle. Air in the right heart is therefore readily evacuated by inserting a fine forceps between the right ventriculotomy closure sutures and passing these also upwards through the pulmonary valve to render it temporarily incompetent. The catheter is not removed from the ventricle until a later stage (*see* Protocol (17)).

(b) Following atrial baffle repair for transposition of the great arteries, the catheter is introduced through the right atrial appendage pursestring and air flushed from the right heart (the left heart has been filled with blood before completing the baffle suture line).

(17) Rewarming bypass is commenced, adding 2 mmol of potassium chloride, 10 mmol of sodium bicarbonate and a further 500 mg of ascorbic acid to the perfusate. The first return from the arterial line is allowed to distend the ascending aorta momentarily and flush the coronary arteries before the aortic cross-clamp is released. The perfusion flow is kept at 100 ml/kg per min and the mean right atrial pressure at 5 to 10 mmHg. The heart usually returns to a co-ordinated beat spon-

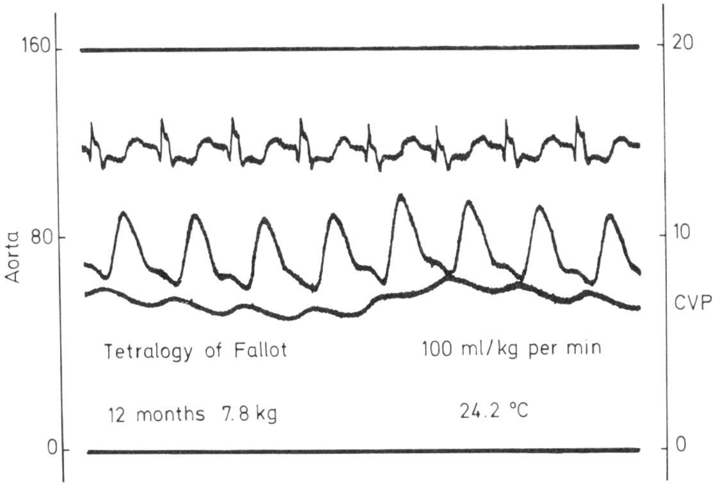

Figure 19.8 Aortic pulse contour recorded 4 minutes after commencing rewarming bypass at a flow rate of 100 ml/kg per min. The central venous pressure (CVP) at this time was 8 mmHg. (From Barratt-Boyes *et al.*[5] by courtesy of *Progress in Cardiovascular Diseases*)

taneously within minutes of commencing perfusion, but if not it is electrically fibrillated. The raised filling pressure allows it to eject and contribute a normal arterial pulse contour (*Figure 19.8*)). In case air should remain inside the ventricle, the ascending aorta is needled proximal to the arterial cannula and allowed to bleed. The left ventricle is also dislocated and suction applied to the catheter in the apex of the ventricle with the syringe, following which the catheter is removed and the stab wound closed.

As the heart is contributing to the circulation, the lungs are ventilated. If the heart rate is slow due to heart block, and this is common early in the rewarming phase, the heart is electrically paced at an adequate rate.

(18) The temperature of the blood leaving the heat exchanger is initially 10°C above the arrest temperature and is raised to 37°C within 5 minutes. At the start of the rewarming period the water bed is recirculated with water at 40°C and this is continued until the chest is closed.

(19) During rewarming, a left atrial pressure line is inserted either through the base of the right superior pulmonary vein or through the left atrial appendage. If pacemaker wires are not already in position they are now inserted.

(20) Rewarming perfusion is stopped after 20 to 30 minutes when the nasopharyngeal temperature reaches 35°C and the rectal temperature 28°C or more (*Figure 19.4*). Should the arterial pressure be inadequate, isoprenaline is given intermittently or continuously and this is occasionally substituted with adrenaline. The heart is decannulated. Heparin is reversed with protamine sulphate (6 mg/kg) given slowly

intravenously over a period of 5 minutes. The sternum is closed over two drainage catheters.

(21) The effects of pancuronium bromide are reversed with an appropriate dose of neostigmine and atropine, and further blood samples are taken. If the infant is awake and breathing well with a stable circulation, the tracheal tube is removed[34]. A chest x-ray is taken before extubation to confirm that both lungs are fully expanded. Blood loss is replaced to maintain a mean left atrial pressure of 10 to 15 mmHg using reconstituted fresh lyophilized plasma or whole blood, depending on the haematocrit. Calcium chloride 100 mg is given after the first 100 ml of blood replacement and a further 50 mg after the second 100 ml.

Special situations

Complex situations requiring excessive circulatory arrest time

These are rare, the most frequent being complex transpositions or malpositions with an associated large ventricular septal defect. The ventricular septal defect is closed first and if there is insufficient time remaining for the atrial baffle insertion, the right ventriculotomy is closed and air flushed from the heart (in case it should eject with the aortic clamp released, although at these low temperatures this is unlikely). A second period of

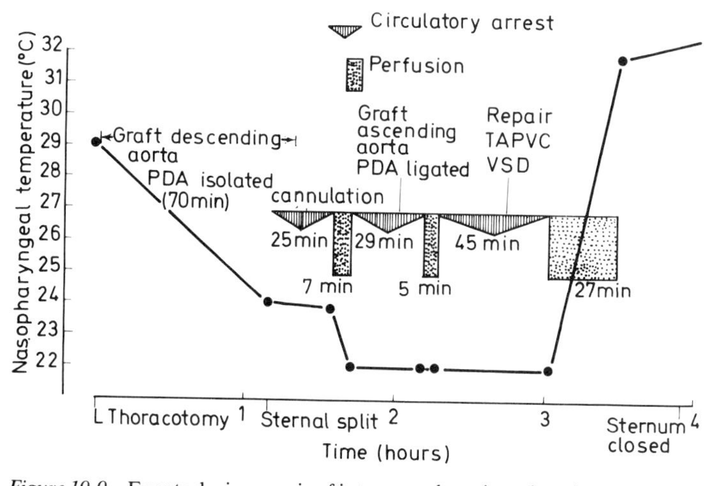

Figure 19.9 Events during repair of interrupted aortic arch and associated defects using several periods of circulatory arrest and cold perfusion. (From Barratt-Boyes *et al*,[6] by courtesy of *Journal of Thoracic and Cardiovascular Surgery*)

perfusion is begun at the arrest temperature and continued for 15 to 20 minutes. This is followed by a second circulatory arrest period for the insertion of the atrial baffle.

A further example, where three arrest periods were used, is shown in *Figure 19.9*. This infant had interrupted aortic arch, large ventricular septal defect (VSD) and total anomalous pulmonary venous connection (TAPVC) to the coronary sinus[6].

Associated aortic coarctation
In two instances repair of coarctation of the aorta has been combined with ventricular septal defect closure. The coarctation has been repaired first through a left thoracotomy during surface cooling, the chest then closed, and the infant placed supine for further core cooling, circulatory arrest and repair of the ventricular septal defect. As it is likely that this technique is associated with an increase in risk when performed in neonates, we now prefer to repair the coarctation (and band the pulmonary artery) as a first stage. Ventricular septal defect closure and debanding is performed between three and six months of age.

Associated patent ductus arteriosus (PDA)
This has been closed without difficulty from the anterior approach regardless of its size. The low blood pressure at the end of the period of surface cooling makes exposure simple and, if necessary, the caval snares can be tightened to empty the heart completely while the ductus is dissected and ligated. Ligation only has been practised in these infants using the anterior approach, but two ligatures are required when the duct is large.

Reoperations
The heart is more irritable at low temperatures and, while no important arrhythmia has occurred prior to opening the chest even at temperatures as low as 22°C, ventricular fibrillation has occurred occasionally with manipulation of the heart. Accordingly, when pericardial adhesions are expected, the chest is opened at about 27°C rather than 24°C and cooling subsequently completed by a rather longer period of cooling bypass.

Comments on protocol

Anaesthetic management
The premedication is designed to promote drowsiness and vasodilatation and to limit the maintenance anaesthetic dose required in infants. Halothane induction and maintenance also serves to prevent vasoconstriction and, in practice, there has been no obvious disadvantage from its known myocardial depressant effect. An adequate dose of relaxant is considered important to prevent subclinical shivering and pancuronium bromide is now preferred to *d*-tubocurarine for this purpose as it avoids the hypotensive effect of the latter drug.

Temperature
Monitoring While the Kyoto[31] and Seattle[20] groups have both relied on rectal temperature, we prefer the nasopharyngeal one because our experimental studies and those of many others show a closer correlation between this and brain temperature. Using surface cooling, the rectal temperature falls faster than the nasopharyngeal and at the time of circulatory arrest it is between 2°C and 6°C (lower than the nasopharyngeal temperature (*Figure 19.3*).

Gradients
The optimum temperature gradient between arterial pump blood and the nasopharynx remains speculative. During core cooling the gradient is

limited to 10°C chiefly because a wider gradient (with very cold blood) will produce more rapid capillary shutdown and more uneven body cooling. During rewarming it is theoretically possible for oxygen bubbles to form in the plasma if the temperature gradient is too wide[21]. This is less likely to occur if the Po_2 in the oxygenator is kept below 150 mmHg, and if the heart is ejecting vigorously into the ascending aorta thereby diluting the flow from the arterial pump line.

Pressure monitoring

In order to monitor arterial pressures postoperatively in tiny infants for several days, rather than hours, either the femoral or brachial arteries must be cannulated. We prefer the femoral artery route particularly as this has not resulted in infection or impaired limb viability.

The central venous pressure is monitored during and after operation usually with a catheter introduced through the saphenous vein into the inferior vena cava, or alternatively, with a 3F catheter introduced directly into the right atrium during the operation. The left atrial pressure is also always monitored postoperatively using a similar catheter introduced into the left atrium during the rewarming phase of the operation. The left atrial pressure must not be allowed to remain above 20 mmHg at any time during the operation, otherwise pulmonary oedema may occur. During surface cooling this will rarely occur if the heart rhythm remains normal, but in the terminal stages of core cooling there is a possibility if ventricular fibrillation occurs or if there is run-off from the aorta. At this time a needle may be introduced into the left atrium to monitor the pressure. During core rewarming an excessive rise in left atrial pressure is also possible but it is unlikely if the heart is ejecting vigorously (*Figure 19.8*).

Cardiopulmonary bypass

Prime The fresh heparinized blood prime has not been diluted routinely because of the increase in interstitial fluid and total body water that occurs in the postperfusion period under these circumstances[18]. Citrated blood is also avoided, in part because it increases the sodium load (both from the citrate itself and the additional bicarbonate necessary to reconstitute the blood and return the pH to near normal). These factors may be unimportant in 'good-risk' patients but could be detrimental in neonates, many of whom present for surgery with severe congestive heart failure.

It is relevant to note that each unit of heparinized blood contains 50 ml of 5 mg/100 ml glucose as diluent. There is thus some haemodilution and there is also a considerable glucose load. The added ascorbic acid has been shown experimentally to lower blood viscosity at low temperatures[38].

Potassium and base The amounts of potassium chloride and sodium bicarbonate added to the heart-lung machine prime before cooling perfusion and again prior to rewarming perfusion are empirical and should, strictly speaking, be varied depending on the infant's weight. The metabolic data would also suggest that rather more base could be added during rewarming (*Figure 19.1*) to correct the acid shift. However, the rapid correction of acidosis with resumption of a natural circulation at the end of the rewarming perfusion (*Figure 19.1*) indicates that additional base is seldom necessary and it is deliberately kept to a minimum in order to reduce the sodium load.

Flow rates Rates of 100 ml/kg per min are used during both cooling and rewarming perfusion. At the low temperatures already prevailing when the short period of cooling perfusion is begun, this flow is considered adequate; and during rewarming perfusion the pump flow is deliberately kept below the expected cardiac output to allow the contracting heart to contribute a pulsatile arterial flow. Pulsatile flow is probably important in providing better capillary perfusion. Should the heart rate be inadequate during rewarming it is paced at 120 beats/minute.

The CO_2 gas concentration. This is increased to 2.5 per cent at temperatures below 30°C to keep the $P\text{CO}_2$ reasonably close to 40 mmHg. It could be argued that higher levels are desirable to raise the $P\text{CO}_2$ towards 70 mmHg, a level which has been shown to improve cerebral blood flow[29]. Others have maintained the $P\text{CO}_2$ at 40 mmHg by varying the CO_2 concentration[27]. We have not further increased the CO_2 concentration however, because with surface cooling the brain appears to have been adequately protected during the circulatory arrest period, and it is postulated that the lower pH which would result might not be an advantage at low temperatures[23].

Cooling and rewarming techniques and duration of bypass A water bed, when compared with the less efficient water blanket used previously[5], has almost doubled the rate of surface cooling. It is possible with this technique to surface cool rapidly to low temperatures, particularly as efficient cooling continues after the ice bags have been removed and the heart is being exposed. In contrast to earlier reports[6,7] ice bags are not now removed and the thoracotomy begun until a temperature of at least 24°C is reached. With this system there is often no need to add a period of cooling perfusion to lower the temperature further as it will have reached the pre-arrest level by the time the heart has been cannulated. Similarly, the rewarming period is more efficient as the water bed contributes during core rewarming and after perfusion has been stopped, until the skin incision is closed. For these reasons rewarming perfusion is now continued only until the temperature has reached 35°C.

These factors have reduced the total operating time to approximately 4 hours in 4 kg infants (*Figure 19.4*). They have also reduced cardiopulmonary bypass time to a minimum, namely no more than 5 minutes for cooling perfusion and 30 minutes for rewarming perfusion.

Prevention of air embolism The danger of entrapment of air in the left heart, after the repair has been completed and as the bypass is being continued, is well recognized. It is not so apparent that air may enter the ascending aorta through the arterial cannulation site during circulatory arrest. This is apt to occur because the vascular bed is largely exsanguinated and the pursestring stitch may not be airtight. Positioning of the aortic cross-clamp distal (downstream) to the arterial cannulation site throughout the arrest period prevents air from reaching the cerebral vessels and also allows easy aspiration, through the arterial line connector, of the blood used to flush out the left ventricle.

Circulatory arrest times The 'safe' circulatory arrest time in infants at a given temperature can be established only by trial and error for any particular technique. Figures given by others may not be relevant if, for example, core cooling is used or rectal temperature is relied upon or adults are opeated upon. Our experience indicates that with surface cooling to at least 25°C and terminal core cooling (and following the details of the protocol outlined), one hour of circulatory arrest is safe (will not produce brain damage) at 20°C nasopharyngeal (16–18°C rectal) and 70 minutes is safe at 18°C nasopharyngeal (12–14°C rectal) temperature. Nasopharyngeal temperature has not been reduced below 18°C as there may be deleterious effects on the brain at temperature much below this level.

Patient selection and results of intracardiac repair

Up to the end of 1973 it was our policy to attempt one-stage repair using profound hypothermic techniques in all severely symptomatic infants with potentially correctable varieties of congenital heart disease regardless of age or weight[5]. This approach was then modified however, because analysis of results indicated an excessive mortality in most neonates (30 days of age or less) particularly when the lesion was complex or the repair was incomplete. The hospital (30 day) mortality over the period July 1969 (when the profound hypothermia technique was introduced) to December 1976 is listed in *Table 19.1* It was highest in neonates (63 per cent) and fell progressively thereafter to 11 per cent between the ages of 6 and 23 months. As 3 of the 10 deaths in the 6–11 month group occurred in totally uncorrectable lesions, the mortality with correctable lesions in this age range was 8 per cent.

This mortality is related to the type of congenital heart disease in *Table 19.2* and to the year of operation in *Table 19.3*. In both tables the neonates operated upon are also specified. Changes in patient selection were introduced in 1974 to reduce the number of neonates from 15.6 per cent (1969–1973) to 4.4 per cent (1974–1976). This was the main factor associated with the reduction in mortality from 23.4 per cent to 16.2 per cent, respectively.

Examination of the neonatal mortality indicated that (1) The result was reasonable when the lesion was not complex and the repair was complete (ventricular septal defect without coarctation of the aorta, tetralogy of Fallot, total anomalous pulmonary venous connection, simple transposition of the great arteries). (2) The result was often disappointing when correction was incomplete, for example, in *congenital aortic stenosis* when there is often associated fibroelastosis of the left ventricle, and in *pulmonary atresia* when the right ventricle is often small. In this latter condition we have returned to the use of palliative procedures (blind valvotomy with or without a shunt) even when the right ventricular cavity is of reasonable or good size. (3) The most disappointing results occurred in neonates with complex conditions, namely transposition plus large ventricular septal defect with or without coarctation of the aorta or pulmonary atresia with a large ventricular septal defect. There was only one survivor (who died later) in these two groups (*Table 19.2*). Accordingly, in *transposition associated with large VSD* which cannot be controlled medically in very early life, pulmonary artery banding has replaced the intracardiac repair.

Table 19.1 The relationship between age at operation and hospital mortality (1969–1976)

Age (months)	*Number of patients*	*Hospital deaths*	
		Number	*%*
< 1	38	24	63.2
1–2	58	14	24.1
3–5	82	14	17.1
6–11	92	10	10.9
12–23	72	8	11.1
Totals	342	70	20.4

Table 19.2 The relationship between type of congenital heart disease and hospital mortality (1969–1976). Included are 10 infants in whom cooling was entirely by cardiopulmonary bypass and a further 10 infants aged 18–23 months with a body weight over 10 kg operated upon with conventional bypass without circulatory arrest

Diagnosis	*Total*	*Hospital deaths*		*Neonates*	*Hospital deaths*	
		Number	*%*		*Number*	*%*
VSD	71	4	5.6	3	1	33
Tetralogy of Fallot	65	7*	10.8	3	1	33
Simple TGA	70	9	12.8	4	2	50
Complex TGA	39	21	53.8	9	8	89
TAPVC	23	3	13	8	2	25
DOV ± PS	11	1	9			
Pulmonary atresia + VSD	16	7	44	3	3	100
Pulmonary atresia (IVS)	5	4**	80	4	3	75
PS + underdeveloped RV	2	2	100	1	1	100
Truncus arteriosus	8	2	25			
ASD***	9					
Total AV canal	3	2	66			
AP window	1					
Aortic stenosis	7	5	71	3	3	100
Pulmonary stenosis	6					
Mitral stenosis	2					
Tricuspid atresia	2	1	50			
Anomalous coronary	2	2	100			
Total	342	70	20.4	38	24	63.2

* Includes 3 deaths in tetralogy of Fallot variants
** Includes 1 with Ebstein's anomaly
*** Includes 1 with Ebstein's anomaly and 6 with partial AV canal
AP = aortopulmonary; ASD = atrial septal defect; DOV = double outlet ventricle; IVS = intact ventricular septum; PS = pulmonary stenosis; RV = right ventricle; TAPVC = total anomalous pulmonary venous connection; TGA = transposition of the great arteries; VSD =ventricular septal defect

Table 19.3 The relationship between year of operation and hospital mortality

Year of operation	*Total*	*Hospital deaths* *Number*	*%*	*Neonates* *Number*	*%*
1969 (July–Dec)	16	5	31	3	19
1970	52	9	17	7	13
1971	49	11	22	9	18
1972	38	10	26	5	13
1973	50	13	26	8	16
1974	43	8	19	1	2
1975	50	8	16	3	6
1976	44	6	14	2	4
Totals	342	70	20.4	38	11

Table 19.4 Palliative cardiac operations in early infancy (1974–1976)

Type of palliation and age	*Age at hypothermia repair (months)*	*Outcome*
Complex TGA		
Coarctation repair + banding: 2 days	5	Late death
Coarctation repair + banding: 2 days	3	Hospital death
Blalock: 7 days	No	Satisfactory
Banding + PDA division: 18 days	3	Satisfactory
Pulmonary atresia + VSD		
Waterston: 1 day	No	Satisfactory
Waterston: 2 days	No	Satisfactory
Waterston: 3 days	13	Satisfactory

Second stage intracardiac repair is carried out at approximately 6 months of age (or earlier if symptoms demand it). Similarly, in pulmonary atresia associated with large ventricular septal defect presenting in the neonatal period with increasing cyanosis, a shunt procedure is performed. The use of E-type prostaglandins to maintain ductus patency has made this operation safer. Currently, a Blalock shunt is preferred to a Waterston shunt. As *Table 19.4* shows, the results in the 7 neonates treated in this fashion have been better than with primary repair.

Current management is clarified further by an analysis of all 44 infants who had undergone corrective operation during 1976 (*Table 19.5*). Only two were neonates (one with Ebstein's anomaly with pulmonary atresia who died following tricuspid valve replacement and pulmonary valvotomy; and one with simple transposition who survived.) There were 4 other hospital deaths, all occurred in patients with complex lesions and none was related to technical errors.

Table 19.5 Experience with corrective surgery in infancy during 1976

Diagnosis	*Number of patients*	*Hospital deaths*
VSD	10	
Tetralogy of Fallot	11	
Simple TGA	9	1 (I-L-D heart)
Complex TGA	3	1
TAPVC	1	
DORV + PS	1	
Pulmonary atresia + VSD	2	2
Truncus arteriosus	1	
AP window	1	
Aortic stenosis	1	
Pulmonary stenosis	1	
Tricuspid atresia	2	1
Ebstein's anomaly*	1	1
Total	44	6 (14%)

* With pulmonary atresia
DORV = double outlet right ventricle

Table 19.6 Ventricular septal defect repair (1969–1976)

Age (months)	*Number of patients*	*Hospital deaths*	*Late deaths*
< 1	3	1*	
1–2	12	1*	
3–5	20		
6–11	18	1	
12–23	18	1	1
Totals	71	4 (5.6%)	1

* Coarctation of the aorta also present

The higher mortality in neonates and in the rarer complex conditions should not be permitted to overshadow the good results achieved in the less complex correctable lesions. Thus in those with left-to-right shunts and in the commoner cyanotic conditions, the combined mortality was 8.8 per cent (23 hospital deaths in 261 infants). It should also be emphasized that these lesions were present in by far the majority (77 per cent).

Management and results in some of these lesions are as follows:

Ventricular septal defect

In the absence of moderate or severe coarctation of the aorta the mortality following ventricular septal defect (VSD) closure was 3.3 per cent (*Table 19.6*). Many of the younger infants had associated shunts at atrial or ductal level which were corrected without influencing the mortality. When coarctation was also present however, there were 2 deaths in 11 patients. One of these deaths occurred in a neonate (*Table 19.2*) in whom both lesions were corrected during the course of a one-stage operation. This is no longer advocated. Instead, in neonates and in the second month of life, the coarctation is repaired and the pulmonary artery banded. Reoperation is performed electively at 6 months of age (or earlier if persistent heart failure demands it).

The results using this management which was introduced in 1974, are given in *Table 19.7*. It will be noted that one of these infants had multiple

Table 19.7 Coarctectomy and pulmonary artery banding in early infancy

Age of patients	*Age at hypothermia repair (months)*	*Outcome*
2 days	4	Satisfactory
3 weeks	3	"
6 weeks	15	"
7 weeks	10	"
8 weeks	7	"
9 weeks*		"

* Multiple Swiss cheese defects

(Swiss-cheese) ventricular septal defects. This lesion, whether or not it is combined with coarctation of the aorta, is also managed by preliminary pulmonary artery banding rather than primary repair. All other symptomatic VSDs are managed by primary repair.

The only morbidity in this series was one reoperation of a large midmuscular defect and two instances of cerebral damage which followed postoperative cardiac arrest.

Eleven of the surviving patients with residual systolic murmurs were recatheterized and none had left-to-right shunts detectable on oxygen saturation data[4].

Tetralogy of Fallot

The results of repair of cyanotic tetralogy of Fallot are listed in *Table 19.8*. As in VSD the mortality was highest when operation was required under the age of three months. The neonatal death occurred in association with a high preoperative dose of propranolol (10 mg/kg per day) with high blood levels persisting postoperatively. High dose propranolol therapy is now avoided; a dose of 5 mg/kg is probably safe although it should be discontinued 24 hours preoperatively. The only death in an older infant (aged 21 months) occurred because of severe obstructive pulmonary vascular disease from cyanosis and polycythaemia. There has been one late death and one reoperation for recurrent VSD. Recatheterization of the first 22 of these infants[13] revealed one tiny residual VSD and one instance

Table 19.8 Tetralogy of Fallot repair (1969–1976)

Age (months)	*Number of patients*	*Hospital deaths*	*Late deaths*	*Outflow patch*
< 1	3	1		2
1–2	6	2		5
3–5	7			3
6–11	25		1	6
12–22	21	1		11
Totals	62	4 (6.4%)	1	27 (43%)

of moderate outflow tract obstruction (right ventricular/aortic systolic pressure ratio of 0.88)

Because of these results primary repair is preferred to palliative aorto-pulmonary shunts except in those rare instances where there is marked underdevelopment of the pulmonary arteries (right and left proximal pulmonary arteries smaller than 2 mm in diameter). An open pulmonary valvotomy is an alternative and possibly preferable form of palliation in such instances.

Simple transposition of the great arteries (TGA)

This group (*Table 19.9*) includes a number of infants with small and moderate-sized VSDs which required closure and six infants with pulmonary stenosis which required valvotomy or excision of tissue from the left

Table 19.9 Baffle repair for simple transposition of the great arteries (1969 – June 1978)

Age (months)	*Number of patients*	*Hospital deaths Number*	*%*	*Late deaths*
< 1	4	2	50	
1–2	14	2	14	2
3–5	25			3
6–11	33	3	9	
12–23	12	2	17	
Totals	88	9	10.2	5

ventricular outflow tract. Four also had a moderate or large patent ductus arteriosus which was ligated at the time of atrial baffle repair. One of the two neonatal deaths occurred in association with a large ductus and severe heart failure. This combination is now managed by ductus division via a left thoracotomy with postponement of baffle repair until the time of elective operation (3–6 months of age).

The results in *Table 19.9* have been extended into 1978 because recent alterations in the surgical technique of baffle placement have improved the results. Thus, in the last two years, using a V-Y atrioplasty to enlarge the newly created pulmonary venous atrium, the hospital mortality has fallen to 4 per cent (1 death in 25 infants). Moreover, all these infants were under 12 months of age and 16 were under 6 months of age and there was no mortality in this latter group.

There have been only five late deaths, three due to baffle obstruction, and only three reoperations for baffle complications. Many of the surviving infants have been recatheterized and show satisfactory haemodynamics[17]. Thus the incidence of baffle obstruction has been low and with current techniques should be insignificant. Disabling arrhythmias are also rare[14]. We recommend atrial baffle repair electively before the infant reaches 6 months of age and at an earlier age, no matter how young, in those instances where progress is unsatisfactory following the initial balloon septostomy. A Blalock–Hanlon atrial septectomy is not recommended.

Total anomalous pulmonary venous connection

Profound hypothermia-circulatory arrest techniques have been largely responsible for the marked improvement in the hospital mortality following repair of this lesion (*Table 19.10*), despite the fact that many are neonates. When these babies are critically ill very early in life with obstruction to pulmonary venous return there is no alternative to early corrective surgery. Mortality is unrelated to the type of anomalous drainage or to the degree of right ventricular hypertension, although babies who are referred for surgical treatment late, in a moribund state, are less likely to survive.

Table 19.10 Repair of total anomalous pulmonary venous connection (1969–1976)

Age (months)	*Type of anomalous drainage* *Infracardiac*	*Cardiac*	*Supracardiac*	*Hospital deaths*	*Late deaths*
< 1	5	2	1	2	2
1–2		1*	1		
3–5	1	6	2	1	2
6–10		3	1		
Totals	6	12	5	3 (13%)	4

* Mixed drainage to coronary sinus and left vertical vein

Late postoperative cardiac catheterization has not revealed any instances of obstruction at the surgical anastomosis[39]. Two of the four late deaths in the series were due to stenosis of the terminal portions of the pulmonary veins, a rare and uncorrectable form of pulmonary venous obstruction[39].

Double outlet ventricle

Double outlet right or left ventricle is prone to present in infancy (though rarely in the neonatal period) either with signs of heart failure from a large left-to-right shunt or with severe cyanosis due to tight pulmonary stenosis. On the basis of exact preoperative assessment of the morphology[3], it is possible usually to proceed with repair using indications similar to those for large VSD or, when there is pulmonary stenosis, for tetralogy of Fallot. As shown in *Table 19.2* the hospital mortality in these cases is low. Palliation is preferred to repair in tiny infants where a conduit would be essential to relieve the pulmonary stenosis or in infants with associated complete atrioventricular canal defect.

Truncus arteriosus

Primary repair is preferred to pulmonary artery banding in this condition despite the need for a conduit. In the absence of important malfunction of the truncal valve the hospital mortality should be low. Both deaths in this series were due to technical error (damage to the left anterior descending coronary artery in one patient and the use of a non-valved pericardial conduit in the other). An antibiotic-treated valved aortic homograft conduit is used with a diameter of 18–20 mm which is large enough to allow for considerable growth. It has not yet been necessary to replace such a conduit.

Atrial septal defect and atrioventricular canal defects

Occasionally an atrial septal defect presents with severe heart failure in infancy, usually in association with partial anomalous pulmonary venous connection. Repair is indicated forthwith. A partial atrioventricular canal defect may also present in infancy particularly when there is important mitral incompetence. Six such infants have had a very satisfactory repair. Complete AV canal classically presents in early life and is now also amenable to repair with a relatively low risk[9]. The total Green Lane Hospital experience now includes eight infants with two deaths.

Miscellaneous conditions

Tricuspid atresia with normally related great arteries may be amenable to a Kreutzer operation[28] (a direct anastomosis between the right atrial appendage and the dislocated pulmonary artery) provided the pulmonary valve is normal. The procedure is attractive because the anastomosis should grow with the child.

Ebstein's anomaly frequently presents in infancy and may be corrected by tricuspid valve repair or replacement (as the 'ring' is large).

Anomalous origin of the left coronary artery from the pulmonary artery is theoretically correctable by transposing the anomalous origin with a button of pulmonary artery wall to the aorta, or to the subclavian artery. Our two such operations appeared to be technically satisfactory but were unsuccessful due primarily, we believe, to the extensive left ventricular infarction which accompanied early presentation of this defect. For this reason we have now returned to ligation of the anomalous coronary artery.

Summary of results

The hospital mortality in this series of 342 infants was 20 per cent and varied from 63 per cent in the neonatal period to 11 per cent in the age group 6–23 months. The high neonatal mortality has led to a reappraisal of the indications for primary repair in neonates and the reintroduction of palliative procedures for VSD associated with severe coarctation, complex TGA, and pulmonary atresia plus large VSD. Intracardiac repair then follows at about six months of age. These modifications in management have improved significantly the mortality in these specific lesions.

Age limits of technique

We continue to use this technique for all infants less than 10 kg in weight. Most children over 10 kg in weight, even when under 2 years of age, have the operation performed using conventional cardiopulmonary bypass, although 6 additional children over 2 years of age and over 10 kg in weight have had operations under profound hypothermia. Four of these had transposition of the great arteries, one an isolated atrial inversion[15] and one a total atrioventricular canal. The technique was used in each instance because of the ideal operating conditions it provides in these complex atrial repairs.

Summary

A technique of profound hypothermia with circulatory arrest and limited cardiopulmonary bypass is described in detail and advocated for use in infants under 10 kg in weight and particularly in the first six months of life.

Cooling is provided largely or entirely by surface means using a water bed and rewarming largely by cardiopulmonary bypass. The total operating time averages 4 hours for a 5 kg infant and the total duration of bypass 35 minutes regardless of the complexity of the lesion. The technique provides ideal operating conditions and avoids complications related to prolonged cardiopulmonary bypass. It is associated with a moderate lactacidosis and a wide variation in the non-lactic base deficit. These changes are not much greater than those which occur following conventional cardiopulmonary bypass and are rapidly corrected once the natural circulation is re-established.

The results of a programme of primary intracardiac repair rather than palliation indicate that the risks are significant only in complex lesions particularly in the neonatal period. Appropriate modifications in the indications for primary repair have led to a reduction in hospital mortality from 23 per cent in the years 1969–73 to 16 per cent in the years 1974–1976. In the commoner, less complex conditions which comprised almost four-fifths of the total, the mortality is 8.8 per cent.

The morbidity of corrective surgery under profound hypothermia has been low and has not been associated with cerebral damage. The recommended maximal circulatory arrest time following surface cooling is 60 minutes at 20°C and 70 minutes at 18°C (nasopharyngeal temperature).

Success in infant surgery depends upon attention to detail both in the preoperative diagnosis, which must be complete, and in the intraoperative and postoperative management, both of which must be free of errors.

Acknowledgements

This work is the result of a combined effort from many people trained in this discipline. I would particularly like to thank Drs J. B. Lowe, J. M. Neutze and P. W. T. Brandt for their help in diagnosis and Drs E. R. Seelye and Marie Simpson for their skilled anaesthetic and intensive care management.

References

1. Ballinger, W. F., II, Vollenweider, H., Templeton, J. Y., III and Pierucci, L., Jr. 'Acidosis of hypothermia.' *Annals of Surgery*, **154,** 517 (1961)
2. Barratt-Boyes, B. G. 'Complete correction of cardiovascular malformations in the first two years of life using profound hypothermia.' In *Heart Disease in Infancy: Diagnosis and Surgical Treatment.* Eds B. G. Barratt-Boyes, J. M. Neutze and E. A. Harris. p. 25. Edinburgh: Churchill Livingstone (1973)
3. Barratt-Boyes, B. G. and Calder, A. L. 'Double outlet ventricle: Classification and surgical management.' In *Second Henry Ford Hospital International Symposium on Cardiac Surgery*. Ed. J. C. Davila. p. 283. New York: Appleton-Century-Crofts (1977)
4. Barratt-Boyes, B. G. Neutze, J. M., Clarkson, P., Shardey, G. C. and Brandt, P. W. T. 'Repair of ventricular septal defect in the first two years of life using profound hypothermia-circulatory arrest techniques.' *Annals of Surgery*, **184,** 376 (1976)
5. Barratt-Boyes, B. G., Neutze, J. M., Seelye, E. R. and Simpson, M. 'Complete correction of cardiovascular malformations in the first year of life.' *Progress in Cardiovascular Diseases*, **15,** 229 (1972)
6. Barratt-Boyes, B. G., Nicholls, T. T., Brandt, P. W. T. and Neutze, J. M. 'Aortic arch interruption associated with patent ductus arteriosus, ventricular septal defect and total anomalous pulmonary venous connection. Total correction in an eight-day-old infant using profound hypothermia and limited cardiopulmonary bypass.' *Journal of Thoracic and Cardiovascular Surgery*, **63,** 367 (1972)
7. Barratt-Boyes, B. G., Simpson, M. and Neutze, J. M. 'Intracardiac surgery in neonates and infants using deep hypothermia with surface cooling and limited cardiopulmonary bypass.' *Circulation*, **43,** 25 (1971)
8. Baum, D., Dillard, D. H., Mohri, H. and Crawford, E. W. 'Metabolic aspects of deep surgical hypothermia in infancy.' *Pediatrics*, **42,** 93 (1968)
9. Berger, T. J., Kirklin, J. W., Blackstone, E. H., Pacifico, A. D. and Kouchoukos, N. T. 'Primary repair of complete atrioventricular canal in patients less than two years old.' *American Journal of Cardiology*, **41,** 906 (1978)
10. Bigelow, W. G., Callaghan, J. C. and Hepps, J. D. 'General hypothermia for experimental cardiac surgery.' *Annals of Surgery*, **132,** 531 (1950)
11. Björk, V. O. and Holmdahl, M. H. 'The oxygen consumption in man under deep hypothermia and the safe period of circulatory arrest.' *Journal of Thoracic and Cardiovascular Surgery*, **42,** 392 (1961)
12. Brown, T. C. K., Dunlop, M. E., Stevens, B. J., Clarke, C. P. and Shanahan, E. A. 'Biochemical changes during surface cooling for deep hypothermia in open-heart surgery.' *Journal of Thoracic and Cardiovascular Surgery*, **65,** 402 (1973)

13. Calder, A.L., Barratt-Boyes, B. G., Brandt, P. W. T. and Neutze, J. M. 'Postoperative evaluation of patients with tetralogy of Fallot repaired in infancy: including criteria for the use of outflow patching and a radiological assessment of pulmonary regurgitation.' *Journal of Thoracic and Cardiovascular Surgery*, **77 No. 5,** 704 (1979)
14. Clarkson, P. M., Barratt-Boyes, B. G. and Neutze, J. M. 'Late dysrhythmias and disturbances of conduction following Mustard operation for complete transposition of the great arteries.' *Circulation*, **53,** 519 (1976)
15. Clarkson, P. M., Barratt-Boyes, B. G. and Neutze, J. M. '"Isolated atrial inversion". Visceral situs solitus, visceroatrial discordance, discordant ventricular d-loop without transposition, dextrocardia: diagnosis and surgical correction.' *American Journal of Cardiology*, **29,** 877 (1972)
16. Clarkson, P. M., MacArthur, B. A., Barratt-Boyes, B. G., Whitlock, R. M. and Neutze, J. M. 'Developmental progress following cardiac surgery in infancy using profound hypothermia and circulatory arrest.' *Circulation*, **62 No. 4,** 855 (1980)
17. Clarkson, P. M., Neutze, J. M., Barratt-Boyes, B. G. and Brandt, P. W. T. 'Late postoperative haemodynamic results and cineangiocardiographic findings after Mustard atrial baffle repair for transposition of the great arteries.' *Circulation*, **53,** 525 (1976)
18. Cohn, L. H., Angell, W. W. and Shumway, N. E. 'Body fluid shifts after cardiopulmonary bypass. 1. Effects of congestive heart failure and haemodilution.' *Journal of Thoracic and Cardiovascular Surgery*, **62,** 423 (1971)
19. Dillard, D. H., Mohri, H., Hessell, E. A., II, Anderson, H. N., Nelson, R. J., Crawford, E. W., Morgan, B. C., Winterscheid, L. C. and Merendino, K. A. 'Correction of total anomalous pulmonary venous drainage in infants utilizing deep hypothermia with total circulatory arrest.' *Circulation*, **35 (Suppl. I),** 105 (1967)
20. Dillard, D. H., Mohri, H. and Merendino, K. A. 'Correction of heart disease in infancy utilising dep hypothermia and total circulatory arrest.' *Journal of Thoracic and Cardiovascular Surgery*, **61,** 64 (1971)
21. Donald, D. E. and Fellows, J. L. 'Relation of temperature, gas tension and hydrostatic pressure to the formation of gas bubbles in extracorporeally oxygenated blood.' *Surgical Forum*, **10,** 589 (1959)
22. Drew, C. E. and Anderson, I. M. 'Profound hypothermia in cardiac surgery: report of three cases.' *Lancet*, **1,** 748 (1959)
23. Harris, E. A. 'Metabolic aspects of profound hypothermia.' In *Heart Disease in Infancy: Diagnosis and Surgical Treatment.* Eds B. G. Barratt-Boyes, J. M. Neutze and E. A. Harris. p. 65. Edinburgh: Churchill Livingstone (1973)
24. Harris, E. A., Seelye, E. R. and Barratt-Boyes, B.G. 'Respiratory and metabolic acid–base changes during cardiopulmonary bypass in man.' *British Journal of Anaesthesia*, **42,** 912 (1970)
25. Hikasa, Y., Shirotani, H., Satomura, K., Huraoka, R., Abe, K., Tsushial, K., Yokota, Y., Mikis, S., Kawai, J., Mori, A., Okamoto, Y., Kolo, H., San, Y., Kanzaki, Y. and Yokota, M. 'Open-heart surgery in infants with an aid of hypothermic anaesthesia.' *Archiv fur Japanische Chirurgie*, **36,** 495 (1967)
26. Jynge, P., Hearse, D. J., Baimbridge, M. V. 'Myocardial protection during ischaemic cardiac arrest.' *Journal of Thoracic and Cardiovascular Surgery*, **73,** 848 (1977)
27. Kirklin, J. W., Pacifico, A. D., Hannah, H. and Allarde, R. R. 'Primary definitive intracardiac operations in infants: intraoperative support techniques.' In *Advances in Cardiovascular Surgery*. Ed. J. W. Kirklin. Ch. 9, p. 85. New York: Grune and Stratton (1973)

28. Kreutzer, G., Galindez, E., Bono, H., De Palma, C. and Laura, J. P. 'An operation for the correction of tricuspid atresia.' *Journal of Thoracic and Cardiovascular Surgery*', **66,** 613 (1973)
29. Larson, C. P., Jr. 'Anaesthesia and control of the cerebral circulation.' In *Extracranial Occlusive Cerebrovascular Disease, Diagnosis and Management.* Eds E. J. Wylie and W. K. Ehrenfeld. Ch. 8. Philadelphia: W. B. Saunders Co. (1970)
30. Lewis, F. J. and Taufic, M. 'Closure of atrial septal defects with aid of hypothermia: experimental accomplishments and report of one successful case.' *Surgery*, **33,** 52 (1953)
31. Okamoto, Y. 'Clinical studies for open-heart surgery in infants with profound hypothermia.' *Archiv fur Japanische Chirurgie*, **38,** 188 (1969)
32. Rudy, L. W., Boucher, J. K. and Edmunds, L. K., Jr. 'The effect of deep hypothermia and circulatory arrest on the distribution of systemic blood flow in rhesus monkeys.' *Journal of Thoracic and Cardiovascular Surgery*, **64,** 706 (1972)
33. Seelye, E. R., Harris, E. A., Squire, A. W. and Barratt-Boyes, B. G. 'Metabolic effects of deep hypothermia and circulatory arrest in infants during cardiac surgery.' *British Journal of Anaesthesia*, **43,** 449 (1971)
34. Simpson, M. M. and Seelye, E. R. 'Postoperative care of infants in the first year of life.' In *Heart Disease in Infancy: Diagnosis and Surgical Treatment.* Eds B. G. Barratt-Boyes, J. M. Neutze and E. A. Harris. p. 316. Edinburgh: Churchill Livingstone (1973)
35. Stewart, S., III, Edmunds, L. H., Jr., Kirklin, J. W. and Allarde, R. R. 'Spontaneous breathing with continuous positive airway pressure after open intracardiac operations in infants.' *Journal of Thoracic and Cardiovascular Surgery*, **37,** 65 (1973)
36. Subramanian, S., Wagner, H. R., Vlad, P. and Lambert, E. C. 'Experiences with deep hypothermia in infancy using surface cooling.' In *Heart Disease in Infancy: Diagnosis and Surgical Treatment.* Eds B. G. Barratt-Boyes, J. M. Neutze and E. A. Harris. p. 37. Edinburgh: Churchill Livingstone (1973)
37. Swan, H., Virtue, R. W., Blount, S. G. and Kircher, L. T. 'Hypothermia in surgery: analysis of 100 clinical cases.' *Annals of Surgery*, **142,** 382 (1955)
38. Tanaka, T., Bennett, L. R., Maloney, J. V., Jr. 'Ascorbic acid as an antisludging agent in extracorporeal circulation.' *Surgical Forum*, **14,** 275 (1963)
39. Whight, C. M., Barratt-Boyes, B. G., Calder, A. L., Neutze, J. M., Brandt, P. W. T. 'Total anomalous pulmonary venous connection: long-term results following repair in infancy.' *Journal of Thoracic and Cardiovascular Surgery*, **75,** 52 (1978)
40. Wolfson, S. K., Jr., Yalav, E. H. and Eisenstat, S. 'An isothermic technique for profound hypothermia and its effect on metabolic acidosis.' *Journal of Thoracic and Cardiovascular Surgery*, **45,** 466 (1963)

20

Intracardiac Surgery in Infants with Conventional Cardiopulmonary Bypass

Lawrence I. Bonchek and Albert Starr

This chapter has been reprinted without alteration from the first edition of this book, which was published originally in 1976.

dignus vindice nodus

Introduction

The use of conventional cardiopulmonary bypass for intracardiac surgery in infants has been reported for well over a decade. Early reports dealt primarily with lesions for which effective palliative operations were unavailable, such as total anomalous pulmonary venous return[7], or with lesions in which the results of early palliation and late correction were not wholly satisfactory, such as ventricular septal defect[14,24]. Cumulative experience with miniaturized equipment has now significantly extended the applicability of cardiopulmonary bypass[16,21]. At the University of Oregon Medical School, cardiopulmonary bypass has been used for the correction of virtually all types of cardiac anomalies in 100 infants under 2 years of age[5,26] The success of the operations has depended invariably upon the nature of the defects, rather than upon the use of the cardiopulmonary bypass technique (*Table 10.1*).

Methods

Preoperative preparation and anaesthesia

In general, nutritional deficits respond poorly to intensive management until the cardiac abnormality is corrected, and they should not delay surgery. Deficits in serum electrolytes are corrected meticulously, however. In emergency cases, such management proceeds simultaneously with cardiac catheterization, and corrective surgery follows promptly thereafter. Preoperative digitalization with digoxin is carried out according to standard paediatric dosage tables, but all digoxin is withheld beginning 24 hours prior to operation. Prophylactic antibiotics are begun the evening before surgery.

Premedication consists of atropine (0.1–0.15 mg) and morphine (0.2 mg/kg). Anaesthesia is induced with intramuscular ketamine (8–9 mg/kg) and is maintained with nitrous oxide (50–60 per cent) and supplemental intravenous ketamine (1 mg/kg). Halothane was used earlier in our experience, but ketamine is now preferred because it is not a myocardial depressant and it is anti-arrhythmic. Morphine is no longer used extensively in infants because it is slowly metabolized, and recovery is prolonged after high doses. Muscle relaxation for intubation is obtained with succinylcholine (2 mg/kg), but it is subsequently maintained with curare (0.1–0.3 mg/kg). Following the induction of anaesthesia, an uncuffed nasotracheal tube* is inserted in all cases and is retained for postoperative respiratory support. Orotracheal tubes are tolerated poorly, increase pharyngeal secretions and are more difficult to maintain in a stable position. The smallest acceptable nasotracheal tube is 3.5 mm external diameter, to permit the introduction of at least a No. 8 Fr suction catheter for postoperative bronchial toilet. Even the smallest infants will ordinarily accept a 3.5 mm external diameter tube, and we do not hesitate to employ larger tubes if the larynx can accommodate them, as laryngeal and subglottic stenosis have not been a problem.

* Portex Ltd., Hythe, Kent, England

In every infant, a central venous pressure catheter is inserted through the external or internal jugular vein. A Doppler ultrasonic transcutaneous flow probe* is placed over the brachial or radial artery, and in conjunction with a standard manometer cuff, accurate blood pressures are readily obtained with pulsatile or non-pulsatile flow. Elimination of arterial catheters saves time, presents catheter occlusion at inconvenient moments and avoids problems with flush solutions that increase the fluid load in small infants.

Operative techniques

Median sternotomy incisions are employed almost exclusively, to facilitate adaptation of the operative approach should unexpected abnormalities be encountered. Aortic cannulation is performed first through a single pursestring suture in the ascending aorta. A 14 to 18 Fr short Bardic catheter is inserted 1–1.5 cm through a stab wound, with the aid of a partial exclusion clamp. The catheter should be as short as is convenient, since resistance to flow is proportional to length. The catheter is sewn securely to

* Parks Laboratories Inc., Beaverton, Oregon, USA

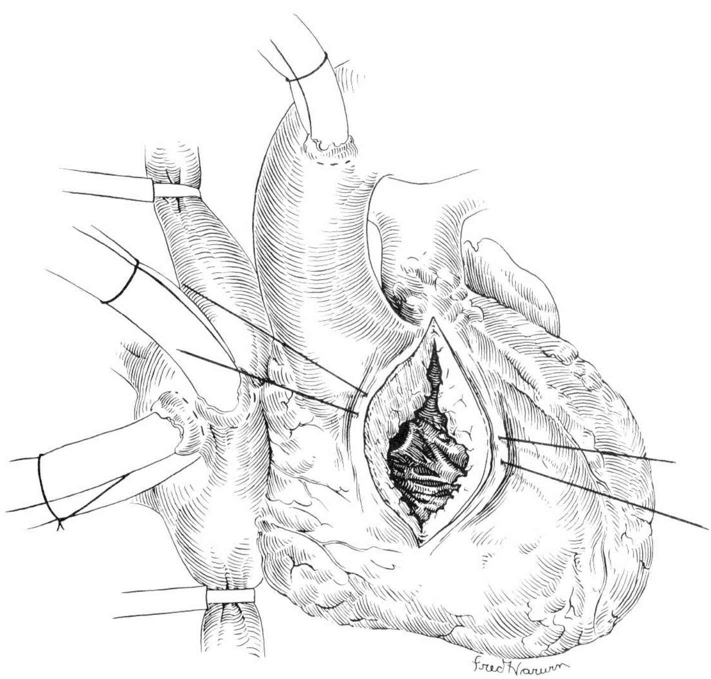

Figure 20.1 Routine cannulation technique for intracardiac operations. Ascending aorta cannulated through a single pursestring suture; caval catheters inserted through separate sutures and crossed within the atrium. All catheters are secured with single ligatures that bind the catheter to the tourniquet. (From Starr, Bonchek and Sunderland[26], by courtesy of *Journal of Thoracic and Cardiovascular Surgery*)

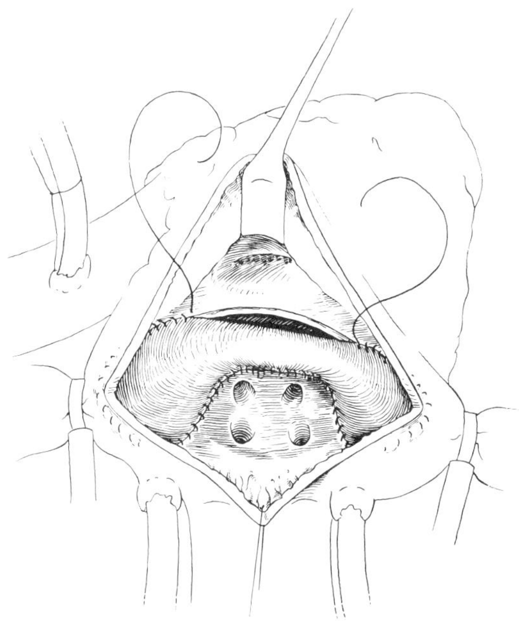

Figure 20.2 Cannulation technique used for Mustard procedure. The atrial appendage is not cannulated, and catheters are placed to the patient's right, to facilitate exposure. Right-angle catheters are particularly convenient. For closure of atrial septal defects, the superior caval catheter is inserted through the atrial appendage, the inferior caval catheter is the same as illustrated, and the atriotomy is between the two catheters. (From Bonchek and Starr[5], by courtesy of *Annals of Thoracic Surgery*)

the drapes. The intracardiac anatomy should then be assessed through an atrial appendage pursestring suture, if the size of the appendage and the infant's condition permit. Caval cannulae (size 16 to 22 Fr) are introduced through separate pursestring sutures. Catheters with tapered basket-type tips* simplify cannulation. Ordinarily the inferior caval catheter is inserted through the atrial appendage, and the superior caval catheter is introduced through a separate pursestring suture so that the catheters cross within the atrium (*Figure 20.1*). For exposure of atrial septal defects, or for the Mustard procedure, the technique is reversed and the catheters are not crossed (*Figure 20.2*). In the latter instance, right-angle catheters are often useful.* Insertion of catheters into the cavae prior to the institution of bypass may impair venous return and result in hypotension; catheters must therefore occasionally remain in the atrium until bypass is instituted. To provide optimal drainage, separate caval cannulation is employed even for operations limited to the left side of the heart, such as aortic commissurotomy.

If a concomitant patent ductus arteriosus is present or suspected, exposure is carried out through the median sternotomy incision by

* Polystan (Canada) Ltd., Scarborough, Ontario, Canada

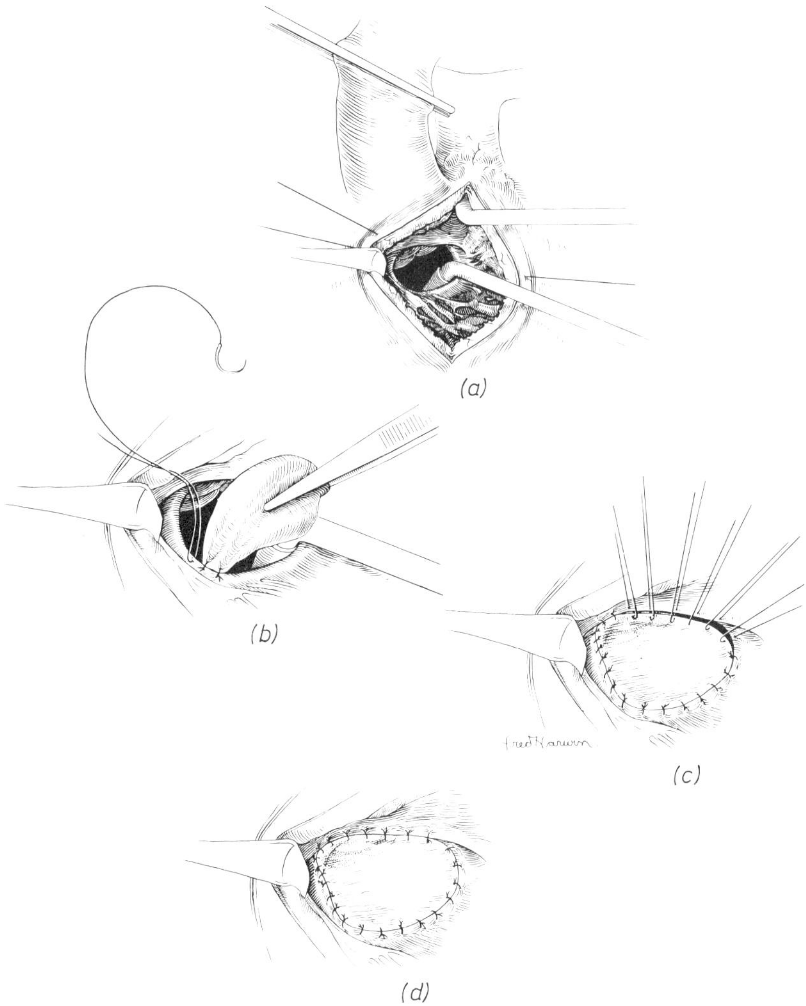

Figure 20.3 Closure of a ventricular septal defect. (*a*) Aortic cross-clamping is used for exposure of the ventricular septal defect. An intracardiac sucker is inserted through the defect and retracted to the left to remove left ventricular blood and enhance exposure. (*b*) Suturing proceeds clockwise from the midportion of the caudal rim of the defect. Each suture is tied immediately after placement. (*c*) Sutures are then placed counter-clockwise beginning again at the caudal margin. The last few sutures are left untied and the aortic clamp is removed. Air is evacuated through the defect as the heart resumes beating. (*d*) The last few sutures are tied in the beating heart. A left ventricular vent is unnecessary

downward traction on the main pulmonary artery and the right ventricular outflow tract. The ductus is surrounded with a heavy silk ligature or braided tape. If immediate ligation is considered unwise, it is ligated upon institution of bypass while aortic pressure is low. A left superior vena cava returning to the coronary sinus may be present and will not be diagnosed in cases that have not had catheterization through the left brachial vein. If one is found by intrapericardial inspection, and the right atrium or ventricle is to be opened, the accessory cava is surrounded with a braided tape and occluded with a tourniquet during perfusion.

Aortic cross-clamping for as much as 20 consecutive minutes is employed to provide myocardial relaxation and a quiet, bloodless field during exposure of ventricular septal defects, or during suturing in the vicinity of the coronary sinus. A left ventricular vent is required only for operations on the left ventricular outflow tract. A vent is unnecessary whenever the right heart is opened and there is an interatrial or interventricular communication as in tetralogy of Fallot, transposition of the great arteries or ventricular septal defect (*Figure 20.3*). During closure of a ventricular septal defect the last few sutures at the cephalic edge of the patch are left untied. The aortic cross-clamp is removed and the aortic valve is momentarily held open with a clamp to prevent coronary air embolism. Air in the left ventricle is evacuated through the defect as the heart resumes beating, and the remaining sutures are tied in the beating heart. When the Mustard procedure is carried out the heart is electrically fibrillated prior to opening the atrium and is defibrillated as the suture line in the new left atrium is completed. Before defibrillation, the operating table is positioned so that the apex of the heart is depressed, the anatomic tricuspid valve is tripped with a clamp inserted through the atrial suture line, and a needle vent is inserted in the ascending aorta.

A wire of Teflon-coated, braided stainless steel is attached directly to the ventricle for electrical fibrillation, and it is retained for postoperative pacing. At the conclusion of the operation, similar wires are attached to the atrium as well.

Techniques of cardiopulmonary bypass

The venous and arterial catheters are connected to a disposable Temptrol infant oxygenator (Model Q-130) with 0.25 inch internal diameter tubing. With this tubing the standard roller-pump head delivers a stroke volume of 15 ml. For more precise control of perfusion rate in infants with pump flows below 800–900 ml/min, the coronary perfusion-pump head is used. This smaller pump head delivers 10 ml per revolution with 0.25 inch internal diameter tubing. High flow cardiopulmonary bypass at 2.4 ℓ/min per m^2 is instituted gradually. The infant Temptrol oxygenator with integral heat exchanger and a priming volume of only 500 ml is employed for all infants with body surface area (BSA) 0.54 m^2 or less (approximately 10–12 kg). Larger children (BSA > 0.54 m^2) are not considered within this discussion as they ordinarily require the paediatric Temptrol oxygenator (Model Q-110). Cardiopulmonary bypass technique in these larger children does not differ appreciably from that used with the adult oxygenator.

Initial prime with the infant oxygenator consists of 1 unit whole blood and 7.5 ml/kg of 10 mg/100 ml mannitol. This avoids the excessive haemodilution that can result when a non-blood prime combines with the small intravascular volume of infants. The routine use of mannitol has virtually eliminated postoperative renal failure[22]. If the anticipated length of bypass is less than 20–30 minutes, the mannitol dose is reduced to 5 ml/kg. Until recently, heparinized blood drawn within 24–48 hours of operation was used for priming, but we currently use fresh ACD blood buffered to pH 7.25–7.35 with 22.3 mmol (½ ampule) $NaHCO_3$[4]. If additional blood is required during bypass, unbuffered ACD blood is added, and the acid load is metabolized without difficulty during perfusion. Each unit of ACD blood is heparinized with 2500 units sodium heparin, after which 800 mg calcium chloride and 300 mg magnesium sulphate are added. If the infant's haematocrit is high, lactated Ringer's solution is partially substituted for blood in the prime, to yield an haematocrit of 40–42 during perfusion. Priming blood is passed through a commercial filter to eliminate microaggregates that can increase pulmonary vascular resistance[17]. A commercial Dacron wool filter has recently been used in the cardiotomy suction circuit also, but its effect on platelets in infants has not yet been adequately elucidated and is the subject of current investigation.

It is clearly established that in bubble oxygenators at low blood flow rates, high oxygen flow rates can result in foaming and transmission of bubbles to the arterial line[11]. Oxygen flow is therefore maintained at less than 3 × blood flow, and 2–2.5 × blood flow is usually adequate.

Blood gases and serum electrolytes are determined every 20 to 30 minutes during bypass. Hypokalaemia is corrected promptly with potassium chloride. Metabolic acidosis is not encountered with this perfusion routine, and bicarbonate or THAM are not administered as they obscure an assessment of the adequacy of perfusion. Arterial oxygen saturation is always > 95 per cent (with P_{O_2} often > 200mmHg) and P_{CO_2} is < 40 mmHg once pump flow is maximal and all desaturated blood has passed through the oxygenator.

As a result of the open chest in an air-conditioned operating room, an infant's temperature at the beginning of bypass is ordinarily approximately 35 to 36°C. More profound hypothermia is not commonly employed, but in the repair of tetralogy of Fallot, if bronchial collateral flow is disturbing, hypothermia to 30 or 32°C will often diminish the volume of blood returning through the pulmonary veins. Rewarming is carried out prior to termination of bypass. The water to blood temperature gradient is always kept below 10°C during rewarming to prevent bubble formation in the blood or damage to the formed elements.

Bypass is terminated slowly by progressive occlusion of the venous drainage lines with simultaneous diminution in arterial return. Cardiac volume is monitored visually and pulmonary artery pressure by digital palpation: direct monitoring of left or right atrial pressures is not ordinarily required. A left atrial catheter is often inserted before chest closure, however, for postoperative monitoring and for withdrawal of arterial blood samples. Protamine sulphate is used to neutralize the heparin in a dose 1.5 × the amount of heparin administered. If inadequate clotting results, an additional 25 per cent of the protamine dose is administered slowly.

Postoperative management

The nasotracheal tube is retained initially in all patients. Respiratory assistance is provided with a Bourns respirator* which provides a maximum tidal volume of 150 ml. High tidal volumes are essential to prevent

* Model LS104–150, Bourns Life Systems Inc., Riverside, California 92506, USA

diffuse atelectasis. Regardless of theoretical calculations, we routinely employ a tidal volume of 15 ml/kg with a respiratory rate of 20–30/minute in small infants. The respiratory alkalosis that could result from such a high minute volume is avoided by adding 5 to 20 ml of dead space between the respirator circuit and the nasotracheal tube. The initial inspired oxygen concentration of 100 per cent is rapidly decreased to 40 per cent to minimize oxygen injury to the lungs. Ultrasonic humidification is provided routinely, and should hyponatraemia develop, the volume of fluid absorbed by the lungs should be considered in the daily fluid allowance. Complete respiratory control is ordinarily provided for the first 24 hours using morphine, and occasionally curare, for sedation, except for simple lesions such as aortic stenosis or atrial septal defects. When an emergency operation has been carried out in moribund infant, postoperative cardiac function may be so severely compromised by the preoperative situation that the mere transition from controlled to assisted ventilation can result in metabolic acidosis in a previously compensated infant. The Bourns respirator is a volume-cycled respirator which lends itself readily to assisted as well as controlled ventilation in infants because of its extreme sensitivity to negative airway pressures (0.5 cmH_2O), and its relatively short and non-compliant tubing. The compression factor for this respirator is only 0.6 ml/cmH_2O airway pressure with the usual length of tubing. After the infant has demonstrated satisfactory respiratory function in the assist mode, as determined by frequent blood-gas determinations, a trial of spontaneous respiration is provided with the nasotracheal tube in place. Extubation is then accomplished within 1 to 5 days after operation. Endotracheal tubes have occasionally been left in place up to 2 weeks, and tracheostomy has been necessary only 3 times in our entire series of infants. Spontaneous respiration with the nasotracheal tube in place is occasionally impractical in very small infants, as the smaller nasotracheal tubes can increase the work of spontaneous breathing. If this is suspected, the infant is extubated, but is reintubated promptly if hypoxaemia, bradycardia, laboured respirations or respiratory acidosis develop. Following extubation, frequent tracheal suction under direct vision with a laryngoscope is essential and will obviate most tracheostomies. Positive end-expiratory pressure during mechanical respiratory support or spontaneous breathing have been employed infrequently. However, they are valuable in certain patients with particular respiratory problems, and the Bourns respirator lends itself readily to positive end-expiratory pressure in the control mode.

The intial fluid allowance is 50 ml/kg per 24 hours of 10 mg/100 ml glucose in water. A high central venous pressure (13–18 cmH_2O) and/or left atrial pressure is advantageous in most cases to exploit fully the Frank–Starling mechanism, except when the left ventricle has had diminished volume-loading preoperatively, as in total anomalous pulmonary venous return. Whole blood, fresh frozen plasma and Plasmanate are used for volume expansion; selection is guided by the infant's haematocrit. Potassium and sodium replacement are governed by frequent determinations of serum levels; 2.5 mmol/kg of potassium and 2 mmol/kg of sodium are usually given daily. Neonates and infants can develop hypocalcaemia

Table 20.1 Intracardiac surgery in infants with cardiopulmonary bypass

Cardiac anomaly	*No.*	*Deaths*	*%*	*Causes of death (no.)*
Fallot's tetralogy				
Intracardiac correction	30	3	10	Error in case selection (2); technical error (1)
Infundibulectomy	2	0	0	
Transposition of the great arteries (simple and complex)	20	6	30	Arrhythmia (2); anaesthesia (1); bleeding (1); respiratory (1); technical error (1)
Total anomalous pulmonary venous return	7	3	43	High pulmonary vascular resistance (1); arrhythmia (1); left ventricular failure (1)
Ventricular septal defect (simple)	8	1	12.5	Respiratory (1)
Ventricular septal defect (complex)	8	5	63	Uncorrectable (2); high pulmonary vascular resistance (2); arrhythmia (1)
Single ventricle (pulmonary artery banding)	2	1	50	Uncorrectable
Atrial septal defect (secundum)	5	0	0	
Atrial septal defect (primum)	1	0	0	
Persistent common atrioventricular canal	1	1	100	Left ventricular failure
Cor triatriatum	1	0	0	
Aortic stenosis	5	1	20	Technical error
Hypoplastic left ventricle	3	3	100	Uncorrectable
Pulmonic stenosis	5	1	20	Arrhythmia
Double outlet right ventricle	2	2	100	Arrhythmia (1); anaesthesia (1)
Total cases	100	27	27	
Total correctable cases	94	21	22	

or hypoglycaemia when given routine intravenous fluids, and these possibilities must also be considered in all cases. The mannitol diuresis induced by the priming fluid persists noticeably for only 1–2 hours postoperatively. Thereafter, urine output of 1 ml/kg per hour is considered quite adequate and less than 0.5 ml/kg per hour is inadequate in virtually all infants. Between these extremes, urine output is assessed in conjunction with the usual clinical parameters, and additional doses of mannitol or diuretic agents are occasionally indicated. Urine specific gravity is assessed with a refractometer.*

Management of arrhythmias is facilitated by the atrial and ventricular pacing wires inserted routinely at surgery. Permanent surgical heart block has not occurred in our experience.

Surgical results

The results with these techniques are summarized in *Table 20.1* and will be briefly discussed only as they pertain to this chapter[5,26]. Correction of a large number of complicated lesions has been carried out. Twenty-seven infants were less than 3 months old, 20 were 3 to 6 months, 15 were 6 to 12 months and 38 were 1 to 2 years old.

Causes of death

There were 27 deaths (27 per cent). Six cases were considered uncorrectable. In 2 infants, peculiarities of papillary muscle attachment prevented closure of complicated ventricular septal defects. In 3 others, the preoperative diagnoses were mitral stenosis, ventricular septal defect and double outlet right ventricle, respectively, but a rudimentary left ventricle was found at operation. In one other, a hypoplastic aorta complicated closure of a ventricular septal defect. If these 6 uncorrectable cases are excluded, the overall mortality was 22 per cent (21/94).

Two deaths attributed to anaesthetic complications resulted from unrecognized traumatic intubations. The infants died in the operating room before the heparin was neutralized with protamine. Clotted blood was found in the trachea or endotracheal tube at necropsy and must have been present before bypass. Sixteen other deaths were due to the usual variety of causes: arrhythmias (6); cardiac failure (2); high pulmonary vascular resistance (3) (2 infants with ventricular septal defects had preoperative right-to-left shunts on room air); technical error (3); and error in case selection (2). No deaths were directly related to the use of cardiopulmonary bypass, and only 3 (3 per cent) could have been indirectly related. One death resulted from postoperative bleeding and tamponade and could have been prevented by an earlier diagnosis of the cause of clinical deterioration. Only 2 deaths were due primarily to respiratory failure, and the ultimate causes of such problems are always complex[10].

* TS meter model 10400, American Optical Corp. Buffalo, New York 14214., USA

Selection of oxygenator system for cardiopulmonary bypass

A 6 inch disc oxygenator was used for infant cases before 1968, but this has been completely discarded. The Temptrol bubble oxygenator is now employed routinely because of its convenience and ease of assembly, disposability, small priming volume, integral heat exchanger and effective bubble dissipation. A separate bubble trap has not been employed, and central nervous system complications have not been observed. Although the bubble oxygenator has been considered 'a second class ticket' by Shumway[23] and 'properly relegated to museums' by Peirce[20], we have found it as effective in small infants as in adults. High blood flow rates are sustained with no accompanying difficulty in complete oxygenation or dissipation of carbon dioxide. Metabolic acidosis does not occur and buffers are not required. Membrane oxygenators, on the other hand, are still in a developmental stage. The limited gas exchange capacity of many current membrane oxygenators[6] could be a particular disadvantage in infants. Urgent operations are commonly performed on cyanotic infants with profound respiratory and metabolic acidosis. An oxygenator system with abundant reserve is able to restore normal blood-gas concentrations and to correct metabolic acidosis during the bypass period. Adequate gas exchange in the larger membrane units is achieved at the expense of a high priming volume[15]. In certain recently available smaller units with low priming volumes, gas exchange is adequate at low flow rates. In experimental studies by Housman and Braunwald[13], however, the addition of THAM or bicarbonate was routinely required, and this suggests that high flow rates could not be maintained.

At a flow rate of 2.4 ℓ/min per m^2 tissue O_2 consumption is determined by O_2 needs and is not limited by O_2 supply[25]. This flow rate corresponds to over 100 ml/kg in infants. A normal buffer base concentration was present at the conclusion of bypass in all of our cases, despite the fact that bicarbonate or THAM were not added to the pump. Ten infants were overtly acidotic at the beginning of bypass (mean pH 7.24, range 7.13–7.32), and even in these cases, a substantial rise in pH occurred by the end of bypass (mean pH 7.40, range 7.30–7.54).

Although it has been clearly demonstrated that membrane oxygenators lack the deleterious effect on pulmonary function shared by all oxygenator systems with an air–blood interface, this advantage is apparent primarily during long perfusions. Following the usual clinical perfusions, pulmonary function has not differed measurably between patients perfused with a bubble oxygenator and those perfused with a membrane oxygenator[15]. Respiratory failure resulted in 2 deaths (2 per cent) in our entire series and has been encountered with similar frequency by others in infants operated upon with the use of a membrane oxygenator or with profound hypothermia[1]. In most such cases, the cardiac lesion was clearly responsible (total anomalous pulmonary venous return, high flow ventricular septal defect, etc.). The major advantages of the membrane oxygenator with regard to protein denaturation and destruction of formed elements in the blood are thus not as apparent in infants, since the length of perfusion is relatively short.

Haemolysis during cardiac surgery is primarily related to cardiotomy suction with its obligatory air–blood interface and mechanical trauma to blood[19]. The use of a membrane oxygenator thus cannot prevent haemolysis when cardiotomy suction is required. Renal failure as a result of haemoglobinuria has not been seen in our series. Plasma haemoglobin at the conclusion of bypass ranged from 13 to 238 mg/100 ml with a mean of 78 mg/100 ml. These values were related to the amount of suction used.

Rationale for the use of cardiopulmonary bypass or circulatory arrest

The feasibility of intracardiac surgery in small infants with cardiopulmonary bypass or with profound hypothermia and circulatory arrest – with or withot partial circulatory support – has now been amply demonstrated in many large centres. The use of cardiopulmonary bypass avoids the profound and incompletely understood metabolic abnormalities and the potential for cerebral injury associated with circulatory arrest[3, 2]. The technique of deep hypothermia without cardiopulmonary bypass, as advocated by the University of Washington group[9], has not met with widespread acceptance. On the other hand, the technique initiated in Kyoto by Hikasa *et al.*[12] and Mori *et al.*[18], and applied extensively by Barratt-Boyes, Simpson and Neutze[2], not only requires a time-consuming period of cooling, but exposure to a pump oxygenator system with its attendant theoretical disadvantages is required for rewarming in any event. In Barratt-Boyes's reports, pump times have averaged one-half hour. Many intracardiac operations can be carried out in 30 to 40 minutes of routine bypass. The range of bypass times in our series has been 18 to 145 minutes, with a mean of 69 minutes. This reflects the preponderance of complex repairs (e.g. tetralogy and transposition) in our series.

Many infants have severe metabolic acidosis prior to bypass as a result of congestive heart failure, profound cyanosis and low cardiac output. High flow cardiopulmonary bypass corrects these abnormalities simply by restoring normal systemic blood flow, as discussed earlier[25]. Hypothermia may be induced during cardiopulmonary bypass when brief circulatory arrest is essential, as for closure of a Potts shunt. Intermittent aortic cross-clamping is available to provide a quiet field and myocardial relaxation. Bronchial collateral return can be minimized by mild hypothermia and temporary reduction in the perfusion rate.

There is no question that prolonged cardiopulmonary bypass disturbs coagulation mechanisms, particularly in cyanotic infants, and unusually meticulous and often time-consuming attention to haemostasis after bypass has been necessary in many of our cases. One death resulted from postoperative bleeding and cardiac tamponade. We currently perform a preoperative coagulation screening test in all infants, and the same tests are repeated following the termination of cardiopulmonary bypass and 24 hours later. Results thus far indicate a significant fall in platelet count, but similar findings have been reported with the use of the membrane oxygenator[8, 15] and are probably related to cardiotomy suction. This can be treated with platelet transfusions. Abnormalities in other clotting factors are variable and are controlled by the administration of readily available fresh-frozen plasma immediately following termination of bypass. The administration of freshly drawn whole blood corrects virtually all clotting abnormalities and is usually readily obtainable since the quantities required in infants are small.

Psychological and social development testing in 19 of our patients who have undergone correction of tetralogy of Fallot with high flow cardiopulmonary bypass has revealed normal or above-normal intellectual and social development[26]. Similar studies after longterm follow-up are not yet available in infants who have had total circulatory arrest.

It has been our feeling that circulatory support should be maintained during intracardiac surgery if the anatomic result is not compromised. From a technical standpoint, the caval catheters rarely interfere with operative exposure, and aortic cannulation is required by the Hikasa–Barratt-Boyes technique as well. Our experience has been almost exclusively with infants over the age of 6 weeks, however. In neonates, particularly with lesions that require intra-atrial correction such as transposition of the great arteries and total anomalous pulmonary venous return, the caval catheters are inconvenient. If longterm follow-up of these neonates proves that cerebral function is unaffected by circulatory arrest under deep hypothermia for prolonged periods, the technique may prove particularly applicable in such cases.

Summary

Successful intracardiac repair of congenital heart defects in infants can be carried out with conventional cardiopulmonary bypass and normothermia using miniaturized equipment and a disposable bubble oxygenator. The system employed has important advantages: an extremely small priming volume, excellent gas exchange at the highest flows employed, an integral heat exchanger, ease of assembly and operation, and disposability. At high flow (2.4 ℓ/min per m^2) oxygen supply is adequate for tissue oxygen needs. At present, in the current state of their development, the practical disadvantages of membrane oxygenators appear to outweigh their theoretical advantages.

The need for atrial catheters has not prevented intra-atrial repairs such as those of total anomalous pulmonary venous return or transposition of the great arteries. In the smallest neonates, however, the technique of profound hypothermia with circulatory arrest and limited heart-lung bypass may prove useful if longterm follow-up demonstrates the absence of cerebral injury following its use. In infants subjected to intracardiac operations with conventional cardiopulmonary bypass, late follow-up has documented normal intellectual and social development.

References

1. Barratt-Boyes, B. G., Neutze, J. M., Seelye, E. R. and Simpson, M. 'Complete correction of cardiovascular malformations in the first year of life.' *Progress in Cardiovascular Diseases*, **15,** 229 (1972)
2. Barratt-Boyes, B. G., Simpson, M. and Neutze, J. M. 'Intracardiac surgery in neonates and infants using deep hypothermia with surface cooling and limited cardiopulmonary bypass.' *Circulation*, **43** and **44 (Suppl. I),** 25 (1971)

3. Baum, D., Dillard, D. H., Mohri, H. and Crawford, E. W. 'Metabolic aspects of deep surgical hypothermia in infancy.' *Pediatrics*, **42,** 93 (1968)
4. Bigelow, J. C., Dobbs, H. L. and Fogdahl, R. P. 'Acid-citrate-dextrose vs. heparinized whole blood prime.' *Archives of Surgery, Chicago*, **96,** 65 (1968)
5. Bonchek, L. I. and Starr, A. 'Total correction of transposition of the great arteries in infancy as initial surgical management.' *Annals of Thoracic Surgery*, **14,** 376 (1972)
6. Carlson, R. G., Landé, A. J., Ivey, L. W., Starek, P. J., Rees, J. R., Subramanian, V. A., Twichell, J., Baxter, J., Bloch, J. H. and Lillehei, C. W. 'Total cardiopulmonary support with disposable membrane oxygenator during aortocoronary artery vein-graft operations.' *Chest*, **62,** 424 (1972)
7. Cooley, D. A. and Ochsner, A., Jr. 'Correction of total anomalous pulmonary venous drainage.' *Surgery, St. Louis*, **42,** 1014 (1957)
8. deLeval, M., Hill, J. D., Mielke, H., Bramson, M. L., Smith, C. and Gerbode, F. 'Platelet kinetics during extracorporeal circulation.' *Transactions of the American Society for Artificial Internal Organs*, **18,** 355 (1972)
9. Dillard, D. H. Mohri, H. and Merendino, K. 'Correction of heart disease in infancy utilizing deep hypothermia and total circulatory arrest.' *Journal of Thoracic and Cardiovascular Surgery*, **61,** 64 (1971)
10. Downes, J. J., Nicodemus, H., Peirce, W. S. and Waldhausen, J. A. 'Acute respiratory failure in infants following cardiovascular surgery.' *Journal of Thoracic and Cardiovascular Surgery*, **59,** 21 (1970)
11. Fisk, G. D., Stacey, R. B. and Horton, D. A. 'Bubbles in an infant oxygenator at very low flow rates.' *Journal of Thoracic and Cardiovascular Surgery*, **64,** 98 (1972)
12. Hikasa, Y., Shirotani, H., Satomura, K., Muraoka, R., Abe, K., Tsushimi, K., Yokota, Y., Miki, S., Kawai, J., Mori, A., Okamoto, Y., Koie, H., Ban, T., Kanzaki, Y., Yokota, M., Mori, C., Kamiya, T., Tamura, T., Nishii, A. and Asawa, Y. 'Open-heart surgery in infants with an aid of hypothermic anaesthesia.' *Archiv fur Japanische Chirurgie*, **36,** 495 (1967)
13. Housman, L. B. and Braunwald, N. S. 'Experimental evaluation of the Travenol and Landé–Edwards membrane oxygenator for use in neonate perfusions.' *Annals of Thoracic Surgery*, **14,** 150 (1972)
14. Kirklin, J. W. and DuShane, J. W. 'Repair of ventricular septal defect in infancy.' *Pediatrics*, **27,** 961 (1961)
15. Kirsh, M. M., Peirce, E. C., Gago, O., Dufek, J., Lee, R., Jordan, F., Reinisch, J., Straker, J., Poloff, D., Rhodes, L. and Sloan, H. 'Clinical use of Peirce–General Electric membrane oxygenator.' *Annals of Thoracic Surgery*, **14,** 140 (1972)
16. Malm, J. R., Bowman, F. O., Jesse, M. J. and Blumenthal, S. 'Open-heart surgery in the infant.' *American Journal of Surgery*, **119,** 63 (1970)
17. McNamara, J. J., Burran, E. L., Larson, E., Omiya, G., Suchiro, G. and Yamose, H. 'Effect of debris in stored blood on pulmonary microvasculature.' *Annals of Thoracic Surgery*, **14,** 133 (1972)
18. Mori, A., Muraoka, R., Yokota, Y., Okamoto, Y., Ando, F., Fukemasu, H., Oku, H., Ikeda, M., Shirotani, H. and Hikasa, Y. 'Deep hypothermia combined with cardiopulmonary bypass for cardiac surgery in neonates and infants.' *Journal of Thoracic and Cardiovascular Surgery*, **64,** 442 (1972)
19. Osborn, J. J., Cohn, K., Hait, M., Russi, M., Salel, A., Harkins, G. and Gerbode, F. 'Haemolysis during perfusion: sources and means of reduction.' *Journal of Thoracic and Cardiovascular Surgery*, **43,** 459 (1962)
20. Peirce, E. C. *Extracorporeal Circulation for Open Heart Surgery*, p. 27. Springfield: Charles C. Thomas (1969)
21. Pierce, W. S., Raphaely, R. C., Downes, J. J. and Waldhausen, J. 'Cardiopulmonary bypass in infants: indications, methods and results in 32 patients.' *Surgery, St. Louis*, **70,** 839 (1971)

22. Porter, G. A., Starr, A., Kimsey, J. and Lenertz, H. 'Mannitol haemodilution–perfusion: the kinetics of mannitol distribution and excretion during cardiopulmonary bypass.' *Journal of Surgical Research*, **7,** 447 (1967)
23. Shumway, N. In *A Technic for Extracorporeal Circulation* by R. C. Stofer, p. VII. Springfield: Charles C. Thomas (1968)
24. Sloan, H., Mackenzie, J., Morris, J. D., Stern, A. and Sigman, J. 'Open-heart surgery in infancy.' *Journal of Thoracic and Cardiovascular Surgery*, **44,** 459 (1962)
25. Starr, A. 'Oxygen consumption during cardiopulmonary bypass.' *Journal of Thoracic and Cardiovascular Surgery*, **38,** 46 (1959)
26. Starr, A., Bonchek, L. I. and Sunderland, C. O. 'Total correction of tetralogy of Fallot in infancy.' *Journal of Thoracic and Cardiovascular Surgery*, **65,** 45 (1973)

21

Intra-Aortic Balloon Counterpulsation

David Bregman

at spes non fracta

Introduction

It has been calculated that more than 40 million Americans are afflicted by heart and blood vessel diseases, with more than 4.3 million people involved with coronary artery disease. Myocardial infarction is the single greatest killer, having claimed 650 000 lives in 1978[2].

While the overall mortality rate from myocardial infarction has greatly improved with the development of coronary care and shock units and with the expeditious treatment of conduction disturbances, nevertheless, once patients develop cardiogenic shock and are refractory to medical therapy, the mortality rate is 85–100 per cent, death ensuing from progressive pump failure[39–43, 92, 188]. It has been estimated that in approximately 15–20 per cent of patients who are hospitalized for myocardial infarction, the clinical picture is complicated by an acute perfusion failure. Since it has not been possible to salvage these patients with medical therapy alone, the magnitude and pathological extent[1, 62, 165] mandates that a more aggressive mechanical means of assisting or relieving the pump be utilized in treating their disease.

Many cardiac assist devices have been suggested for the treatment of refractory left ventricular power failure, but the most effective clinical devices to date have been those which employ the principle of counterpulsation[30, 32, 36–43, 47–49, 62, 68, 72, 74, 75, 84, 86, 88, 89, 94, 95, 100–102, 106–113, 120, 127, 128, 130, 132–137, 140, 142–147, 151–156, 161, 165–169, 174, 177, 179–182, 184, 188, 189, 194–196, 199, 203–207, 209]. The single most effective device utilizing this concept is the intra-aortic balloon[30, 32, 36–43, 86] whose versatility has been widely demonstrated both in the laboratory[50, 56, 72, 74, 84, 110, 120, 133, 137, 142, 143, 168, 169, 174, 194, 195, 206, 207, 209, 217] and clinically[30, 32, 36–43, 57–59, 75, 86, 95, 106, 113, 127, 132, 135, 144–147, 151–156, 161, 172, 184, 196, 205].

The concept of counterpulsation, which is the basis of intra-aortic balloon pumping (IABP), was first described by Harken in 1958[94] and, as originally proposed, involved the removal of blood via the femoral route from the arterial tree during ventricular systole and the rapid reinfusion of the same blood during diastole to increase coronary perfusion pressure. By this method, in the normotensive preparation, one could decrease left ventricular work and increase coronary blood flow, thereby improving the balance between myocardial oxygen supply and oxygen demand[25]. This concept was initially received with great enthusiasm and several investigators have reported some success with its clinical application[101, 102, 179, 203]. However, the method as described has several drawbacks: (1) The excessive turbulence caused by the rapid withdrawal and reinfusion of the blood causes appreciable haemolysis and therefore limits the duration of clinical applicability; (2) Either bilateral femoral arteriotomies or a subclavian arteriotomy is required for this procedure; (3) It has been shown by Dormandy, Goetz and Kripke[74] that counterpulsation via the femoral route in the hypotensive state does not increase the coronary blood flow. Because of these drawbacks to the potential requirement for prolonged circulatory support, other investigators chose to apply the principle of counterpulsation in another, unique, fashion.

In 1962, Moulopoulos, Topaz and Kolff[142, 143] suggested the use of a single-chambered intra-aortic balloon positioned in the descending thoracic aorta to accomplish the same purpose of counterpulsation, but without its drawbacks. The balloon is inflated in diastole beginning with closure of the aortic valve and is held in inflation until the onset of ventricular systole, when the balloon is rapidly deflated. The inflation of the balloon displaces intra-aortic blood towards the coronary tree, thereby augmenting coronary perfusion pressure and blood flow. The collapse of the balloon creates a 'sink' which decreases the impedance to left ventricular ejection or left ventricular afterload, and consequently reduces left ventricular work[68]. After a hiatus of 7 years, Kantrowitz *et al.*[109] reported the first successful clinical application of single-chambered IABP.

The main advantages of IABP over conventional arterio-arterial counterpulsation are: (1) Circulatory assistance is possible for extended periods of time since there is minimal haemolysis; (2) A single femoral arteriotomy is required; (3) Coronary blood flow is augmented even in the hypotensive state[206].

Two additional significant advantages result from the use of either counterpulsation or IABP: (1) It has been demonstrated by Jacobey *et al.*[101] that after a short period of counterpulsation, dormant intercoronary collateral beds are opened and these channels remain open after the procedure is terminated; (2) It has been demonstrated by Nachlas and Sieband[157], Cox *et al.*[69], Sugg, Webb and Ecker[204] and Maroko *et al.*[133] that early institution of IABP or counterpulsation decreases the size of the potential myocardial infarction after coronary occlusion. Thus intra-aortic balloon pumping has emerged as the single most important mechanical support adjunct in the treatment of refractory left ventricular power failure[30, 32, 36–43].

This technique appears to be at present the most promising method of assisting the failing heart, both through its ease of application and through its effectiveness in decreasing left ventricular work and in increasing coronary blood flow while causing minimal haemolysis[30, 32, 36, 39–43, 86, 206, 207].

Recent reports[30, 32, 36, 39–43, 57–61, 75, 86, 128, 151–156, 184, 196, 213] indicate that patients with cardiogenic shock refractory to conventional therapy can now be supported by an intra-aortic balloon device, can safely undergo ventriculography or selective cinecoronary angiography, and can survive until they are placed on cardiopulmonary bypass for open-heart surgery or myocardial revascularization. A survival rate of 50 per cent has now been reported by McEnany *et al.*[139].

There is clinical and experimental evidence to demonstrate that the critical factor which improves the performance of a heart suffering from an acute myocardial infarction and power failure is an increase in coronary blood flow[63, 115, 117, 118, 177]. It has also been shown that a major determinant of improved retrograde coronary flow is an elevation in the mean aortic diastolic pressure[51, 85, 211, 214, 216]. Under conditions of hypoxaemia, cardiac performance is coronary-flow dependent, and unloading of the left ventricle does not improve myocardial efficiency by itself. Therefore, any method of mechanical assistance should aim at maximally increasing coronary blood flow.

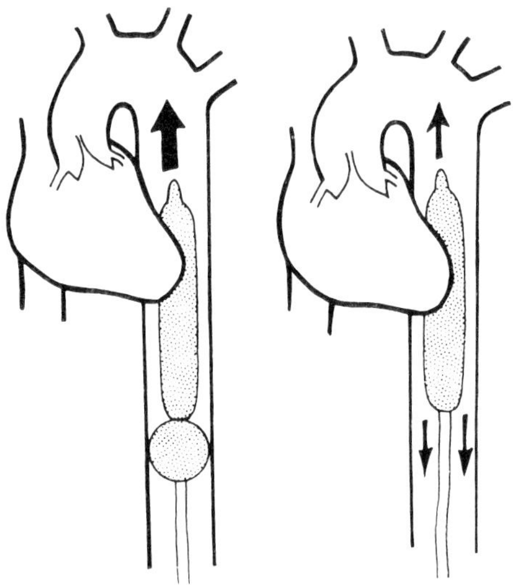

Figure 21.1 Intra-aortic pumping action of single-chambered (omnidirectional) versus dual-chambered (unidirectional) balloons. (Reproduced from Bregman, Kripke and Goetz[43] by courtesy of *Transactions of the American Society for Artificial Internal Organs*)

The cylindrically shaped, omnidirectional, single-chambered intra-aortic balloon that is at present in use,[106, 107, 109] or its modifications[56, 57, 127, 132, 151–156, 184, 218], displaces blood both cranially and caudally in diastole, thereby dissipating much of its effectiveness in augmenting coronary blood flow[30, 32, 36–43, 86] (*Figure 21.1*). It is the purpose of this chapter to describe laboratory and clinical experience with the dual-chambered intra-aortic balloon* which pumps intra-aortic blood unidirectionally towards the coronary and cerebral circulation[30, 32, 36–43, 86] resulting in a 66–100 per cent greater increment in coronary blood flow over that obtained with a single-chambered balloon of equal volume displacement[206, 207]. In addition, initial clinical experience with percutaneous IABP will also be discussed.

The dual-chambered intra-aortic balloon

Experimental rationale

In studies designed to compare the single-chambered omnidirectional balloon with the unidirectional dual-chambered intra-aortic balloon, all parameters of left ventricular work were diminished in both (*Figure 21.2*). Using the single-chambered balloon, left ventricular work (gram-metres/min) fell 28.8 per cent and the tension–time index fell 35.4 per cent. In the

* Developed at the Albert Einstein College of Medicine, Bronx Municipal Hospital Center, Bronx, New York, USA

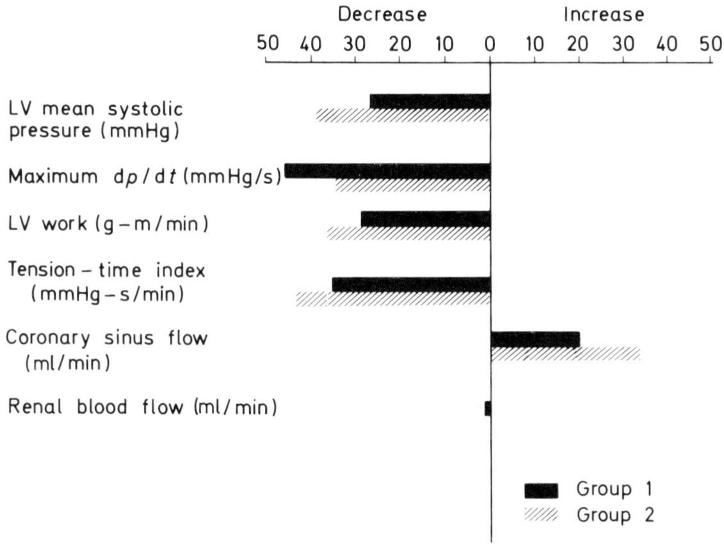

Figure 21.2 Effects of IABP on central and peripheral canine haemodynamics. All parameters of left ventricular work are diminished while coronary sinus flow is increased. A 66 to 100 per cent increase in coronary blood flow is obtained using a dual-chambered balloon without impairing distal perfusion. Group 1 = single-chambered balloon; group 2 = dual-chambered balloon. (Reproduced from Talpins *et al.*[207] by courtesy of *Surgical Forum*)

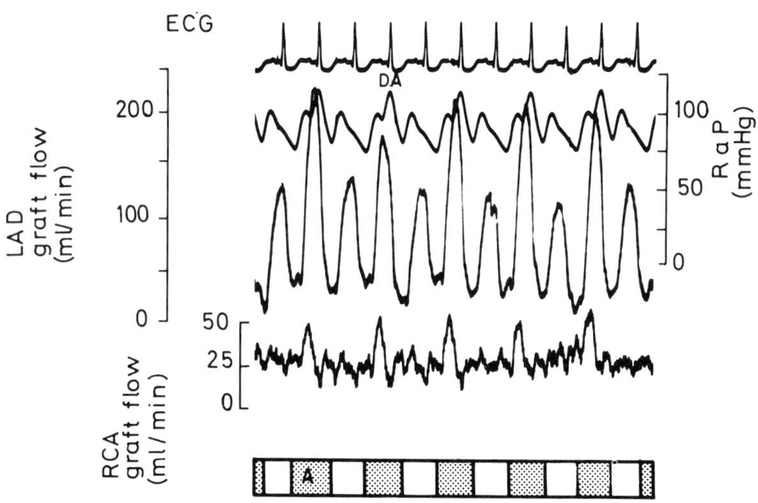

Figure 21.3 Dual-chambered IABP in a patient assisted after aortocoronary bypass graft surgery. RaP = radial artery pressure; DA = diastolic augmentation; LAD = left anterior descending coronary artery; RCA = right coronary artery; A = assist (IABP) periods. Flows were measured with a square-wave electromagnetic flowmeter. With patient assisted every other beat, note the 100 per cent increase in LAD and RCA graft flows during diastole. Tracing speed: 25 mm/s

dual-chambered group, these parameters decreased by 37.2 per cent and 43.1 per cent, respectively ($P < 0.001$). However, of greater significance is the fact that the dual-chambered balloon increased coronary sinus blood flow an average of 66–100 per cent over and above that obtained with a single-chambered balloon[206, 207]. These observations have been confirmed experimentally with electromagnetic flowmeters and, more recently, in the operating room in patients assisted after coronary reconstructive surgery where increases averaging 83 per cent (range 50–100 per cent) were recorded[48] (*Figures 21.3* and *21.4*).

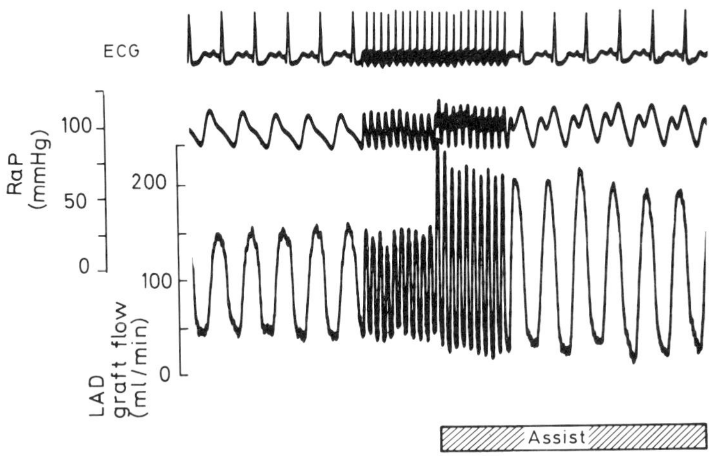

Figure 21.4 *See* legend to *Figure 21.3*. Note doubling of LAD graft flow during the assist (IABP). Tracing speeds: 25 and 10 mm/s

The beneficial haemodynamic effects of unidirectional intra-aortic balloon pumping have been confirmed by Furman *et al.*[84].

Experimentally, free plasma haemoglobin determinations never rose above 5.2 mg/100 ml during one hour of IABP[206, 207]. Clinically, the values obtained have been negligible[30, 32, 36–43, 86], and therefore haemolysis does not pose a time limitation on IABP as it does on arterio-arterial counterpulsation[74].

Mechanism of balloon action

Our clinical experience has been with the unidirectional dual-chambered intra-aortic balloon (*Figure 21.5*). The balloon has a spherical distal chamber which inflates early in diastole and occludes the aorta. This is sequentially followed by the inflation of a narrower cylindrical proximal pumping chamber, in the same diastolic interval, which displaces intra-aortic blood entirely (unidirectionally) towards the aortic root. Both chambers are completely deflated by an active vacuum just prior to ventricular ejection. Two human balloon configurations are available. For the average size adult patient with a normal-calibre common femoral

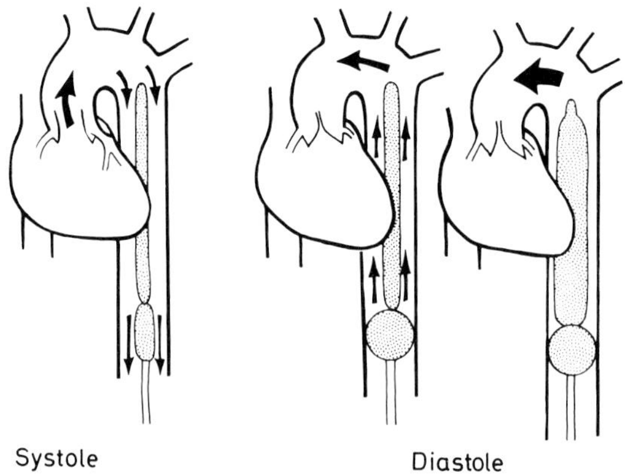

Figure 21.5 Mechanism of action of the dual-chambered intra-aortic balloon. The distal spherical balloon inflates slightly earlier in diastole and phasically obstructs aortic flow. The larger cylindrical proximal balloon then pumps the blood unidirectionally towards the aortic root. Both balloons are then completely deflated by an active vacuum just prior to ventricular ejection. (Reproduced from Bregman and Goetz[40] by courtesy of *Journal of Thoracic and Cardiovascular Surgery*)

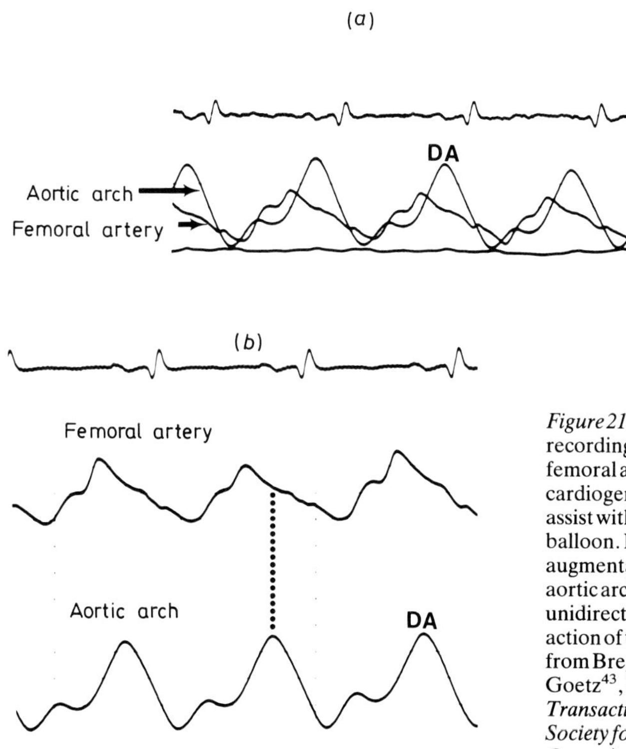

Figure 21.6 Simultaneous recordings of aortic arch and femoral artery pressure tracings in a cardiogenic shock patient during assist with the dual-chambered balloon. Note large diastolic augmentation (DA) obtained in the aortic arch pressure tracing due to unidirectional intra-aortic pumping action of the balloon. (Reproduced from Bregman, Kripke and Goetz[43], by courtesy of *Transactions of the American Society for Artificial Internal Organs*)

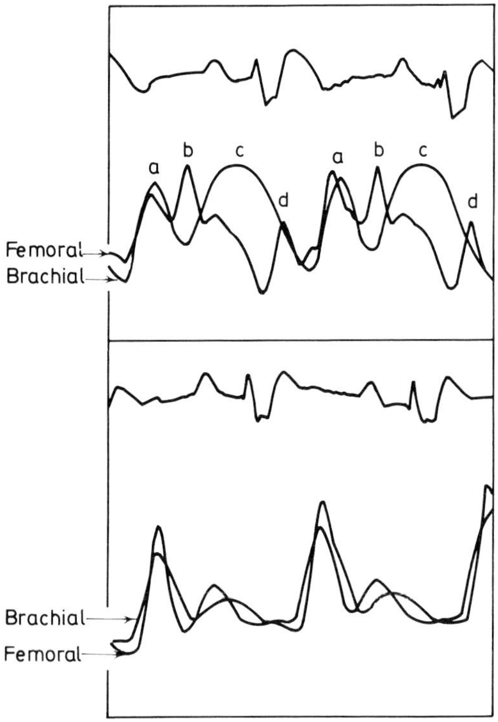

Figure 21.7 Simultaneous recordings of pressures proximal (brachial artery) and distal (femoral artery) to a dual-chambered intra-aortic balloon in an assisted patient. *Top panel*: assist off. *Bottom panel*: assist on. a = ventricular systole; b = deflection resulting from inflation of occluding balloon in femoral artery trace – note its absence in brachial artery trace; c = diastolic augmentation produced by pumping balloon – observe its absence in femoral artery trace; d = equilibration of brachial and femoral artery pressures with deflation of balloons

artery, a 30 ml dual-chambered balloon is utilized with an 18 mm outer diameter distal occluding balloon and a 14 mm proximal pumping balloon. For a patient with a larger vascular tree, a 40 ml dual-chambered balloon is available with a 20 mm occluding balloon and a 16 mm proximal pumping balloon. Both are mounted on a 12F catheter.

The action of the dual-chambered balloon in a patient is illustrated in *Figure 21.6*. With the onset of inflation of the occluding balloon, a small pressure wave is transmitted to the femoral artery. However, when the occluding balloon is maximally inflated, pumping is entirely unidirectional towards the aortic root, and the diastolic augmentation is seen only in the aortic arch tracing and not in the femoral artery tracing. *Figure 21.7* illustrates the same physiology in another patient.

Balloon construction and safety

Balloon membrane

The basic dual-chambered balloon is a single-cast tubular membrane of a specially formulated polyurethane polymer[38]. Wall thickness is generally 4 to 5 mils* and, for a given balloon, is consistent within ½ mil over the major wall section. Tapered end sections are slightly thicker to counter additional end stresses. The polyurethane formula utilized has a very non-linear stress characteristic peculiar to the needs of the intra-aortic balloon. *Figure 21.8* shows the behaviour of a 4 ml cast of this polyurethane film subjected to increasing stress. In region 1, length changes very little

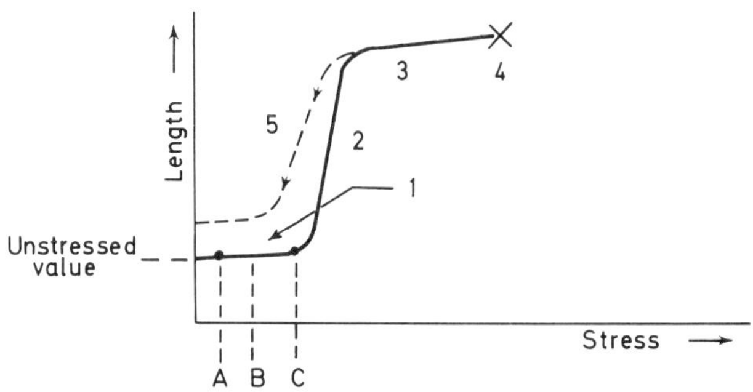

Figure 21.8 Stress/strain characteristics of polyurethane formula in dual-chambered intra-aortic balloon (*see* text). (Reproduced from Bregman, D and Goetz, R. H.[38] by courtesy of *Transactions of the American Society for Artificial Internal Organs*)

with stress. Region 2 is an elastic zone; the molecular chains, normally folded and entangled, begin to straighten after the stress reaches the threshold value and the material stretches similar to a rubber band. When the chains are fully straightened, the curve then enters a saturation region, 3, and 'locks' at its ultimate length. Sufficient force, at region 4, will break the chain and then cause rupture. The dual-chambered balloon is operated totally within region 1 for several reasons. The obvious reason is that we make use of a safety chamber (*Figures 21.9* and *21.12*) and utilize only enough gas to 'fill', but not to 'distend', the intra-aortic balloon. Since work equals force times distance, one can see that cyclic forces within region 1 cause very little distance change and, consequently, very little work is expended on the balloon material, resulting in minimal fatigue. Balloons operated in region 2 will exhibit fatigue as evidenced by the fact that once stretched, the material takes a different return path (as indicated by Number 5, *Figure 21.8*). In physics, this can be recognized as a rudimentary hysteresis loop in which the energy dissipated is proportional to the loop area. The minor loop in region 1 is virtually non-measurable.

The stretched molecular chains do not fully return to their folded state. The linkages are weakened, and ultimately they will fail. The stress required to reach point C (all other factors remaining equal) will depend

* 1 mil = 10^{-3} inches (25.4 μm)

upon the thickness of the polyurethane. The film thickness used, therefore, is determined by the size of the folded balloon, when inserted, and by the stress range, to keep it within region 1. With a 4 ml film in a typical human dual-chambered balloon, point C is reached at 8 to 12 psi (400–600 mmHg) of differential pressure. Each balloon manufactured is statically and dynamically tested to point B, and the exact value is marked on a quality control sheet accompanying the balloon. For example, a typical value might be 4 psi (200 mmHg). When the balloon is used with a safety chamber, the peak pressure only reaches point A, usually 1 to 2 psi or 50 to 100 mmHg. The polyurethane formula chosen is a prudent compromise between good folding properties and a low degree of initial distensibility. Over the test range (region B), this formula stretches about 1 per cent. Since balloon volume varies with the square of the radius (axial stress being less significant in an elongated balloon than radial stress), this is equivalent to a 2 per cent variation in volume.

Balloon catheter

A one-piece polyurethane catheter is utilized with a 10 per cent radio-opaque filler. Hence the entire catheter is radio-opaque, which aids proper intra-aortic balloon positioning. In addition, a flexible stainless steel strut has been built into the proximal balloon section to facilitate insertion and to prevent a balloon from folding over upon itself after it has been inserted into the aorta. The basic stiffness of the catheter is such that a stylet is not required for insertion, but the balloon cannot be forced so as to initiate an aortic dissection as has been reported with a more rigid balloon catheter design[62].

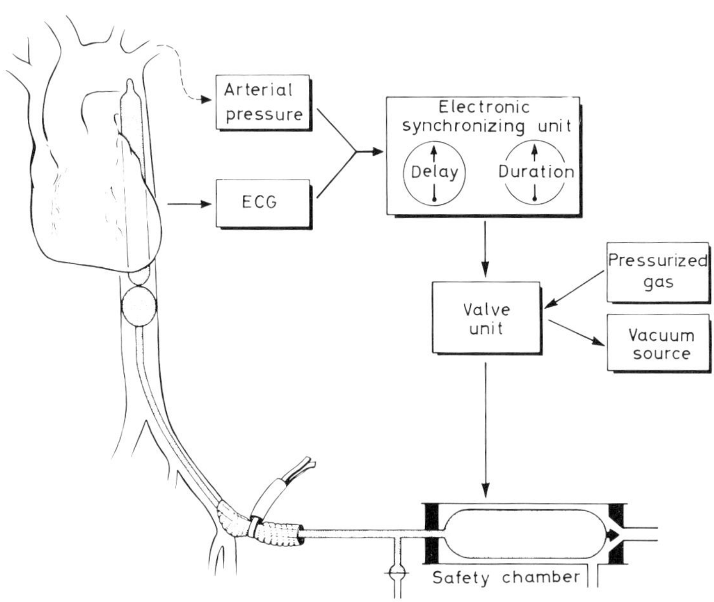

Figure 21.9 Schematic representation of clinical dual-chambered IABP. (Reproduced from Bregman, Kripke and Goetz[43], by courtesy of *Transactions of the American Society for Artificial Internal Organs*)

In the new percutaneous balloon (PERCOR TM Balloon, Datascope Corporation, Paramus, New Jersey), the catheter section is replaced by a straight wire that swivels inside the balloon catheter and balloon membrane. The balloon membrane may be compactly wrapped around the wire enabling easy insertion through a No. 12F sheath (*Figure 21.9A*). The driving gas enters the balloon at the junction of the catheter and the balloon membrane through a port of entry that is slightly less than No. 12F in size. The balloon membrane is constructed of polyurethrane similar to that used in the standard single-and dual-chambered Datascope intra-aortic balloons. The new balloon is currently available in a 40 ml size mounted on a 12F catheter.

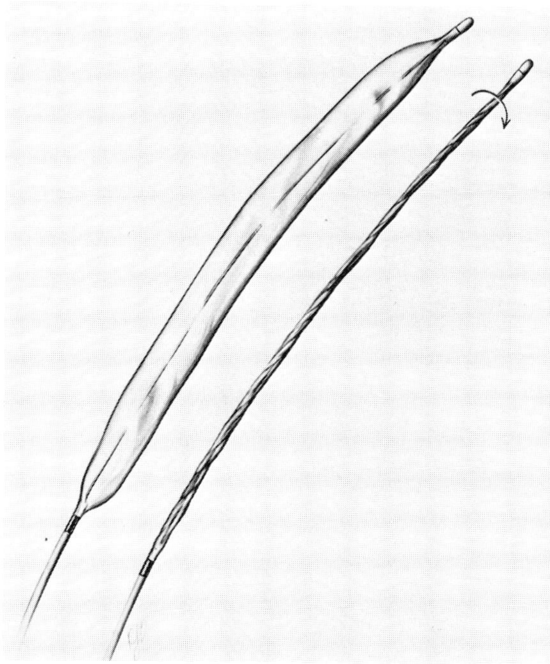

Figure 21.9A Percutaneous balloon (PERCOR TM) wrapped and unwrapped

Seals

The dual-chambered balloon is chemically welded onto the polyurethane catheter so that a polyurethane seal is obtained. In addition, the proximal and distal ends of the balloon are overcoated with additional polyurethane layers to complete the seal.

Arterial grafts

As will be described subsequently, a Dacron graft is sutured onto the common femoral artery and the dual-chambered balloon is inserted through the graft and is then positioned just distal to the left subclavian artery in the descending thoracic aorta. When the graft and catheter are snared, this allows distal perfusion of the extremity during the period of cardiac assist (*Figure 21.9*).

The clinical system for intra-aortic balloon pumping

Our clinical experience most recently has been with the Datascope System 82* (*Figures 21.10* and *21.11*). The System 82 has incorporated several significant improvements over its predecessor, the Datascope System 80, which was described in detail in the previous edition of this chapter.

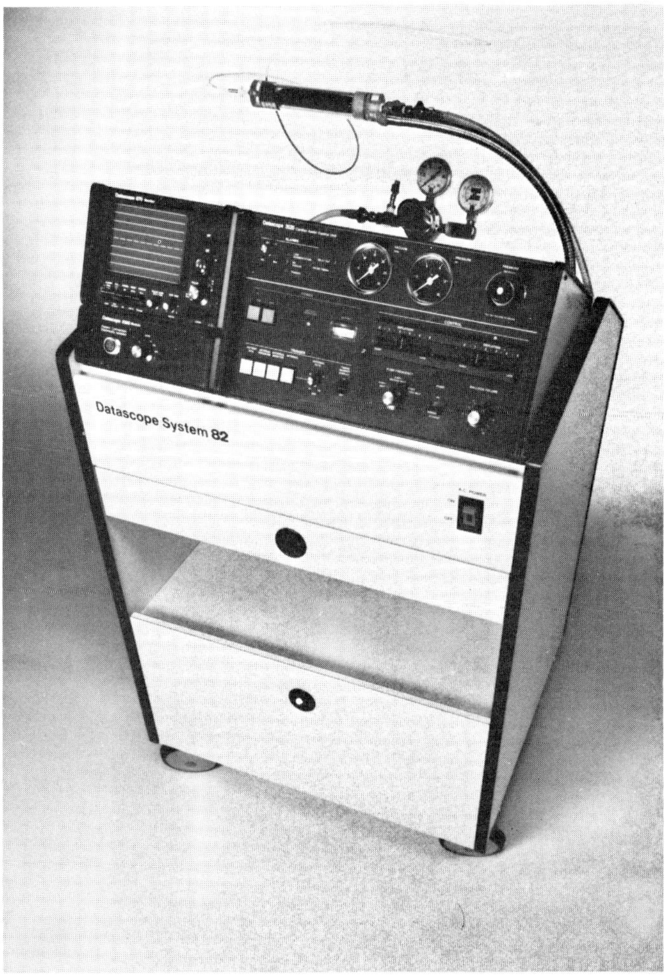

Figure 21.10 System 82 – improved, simplified, failsafe, mobile cardiac assist console

Particular attention has now been devoted to redesigning and simplifying the operating controls, since, with greater frequency, nursing staff and other paramedical personnel are in actual fact running the balloon pump console. As a result, the setting of two prominent slide controls is essentially all that is needed for proper operation of the balloon pump. The

* Manufactured by the Datascope Corporation, Paramus, New Jersey, USA

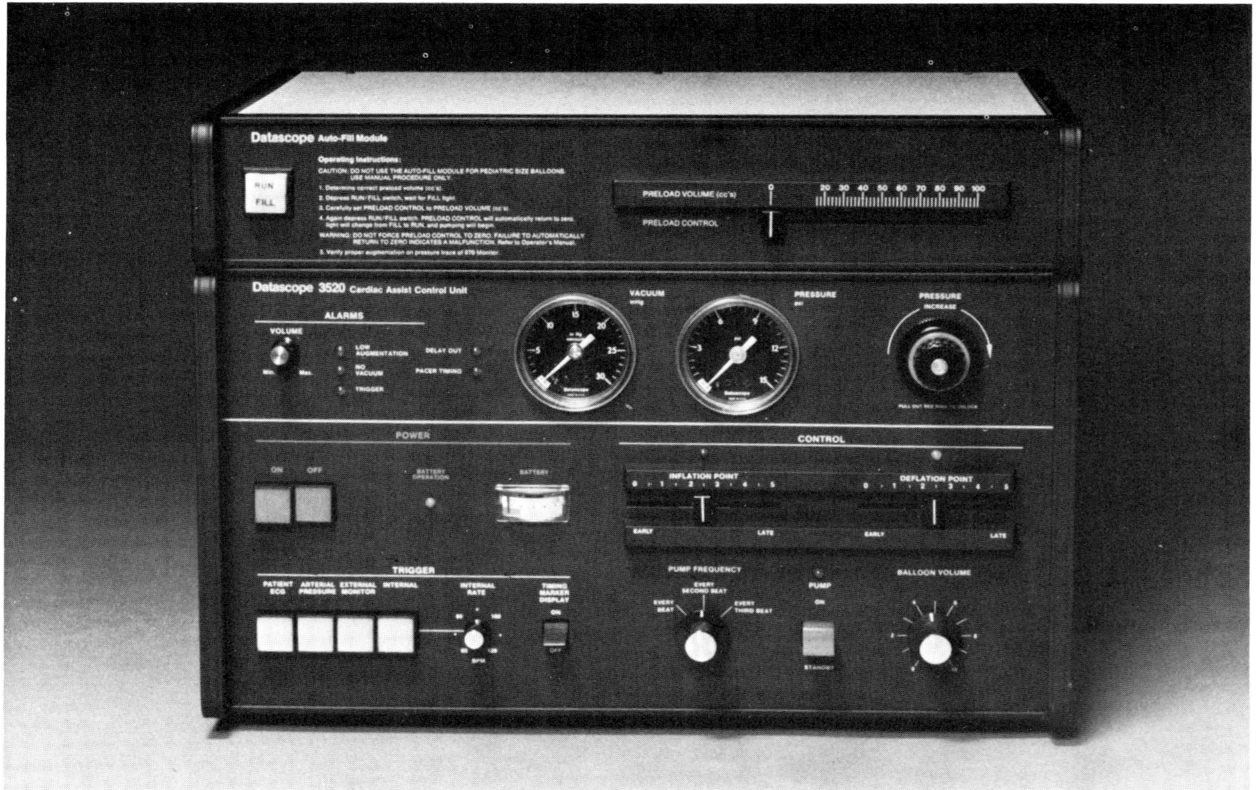

Figure 21.11 Close-up of cardiac assist control unit (3520) of the System 82. Note slide controls for balloon timing and the auto-fill module

System 82 utilizes a non-fade physiologic monitor, which gives excellent viewing of all pertinent data. In addition, it has the advantage of being able to freeze the tracing so that the pumping waves may be critically analysed. Furthermore, the System 82 incorporates an Electro-Surgical Interference Suppression Module (ESIS) which virtually eliminates interference from an electrocautery during surgery. The result is an ECG signal essentially free of noise and a reliable triggering of the balloon pump console even during the use of an electrosurgical unit. The balloon pump console is also considerably quieter than its predecessor. System 82 has built-in battery power which can easily enable transport of the patient.

Inflation and deflation of the balloon is accomplished by alternately applying pressure and vacuum to a closed circuit consisting of the intra-aortic balloon and a slave balloon within a safety chamber. This circuit is precharged with a fixed amount of carbon dioxide. Consequently the System is safe under virtually any conditions.

Safety chamber

Use of a fixed volume of CO_2 (closed system)

The slave balloon in the safety chamber is precharged with an effective volume of carbon dioxide equal to the volume of the intra-aortic balloon selected for clinical use (*Figure 21.12*). Because this is basically a closed system, the patient can never be exposed to more than 1 bolus of the

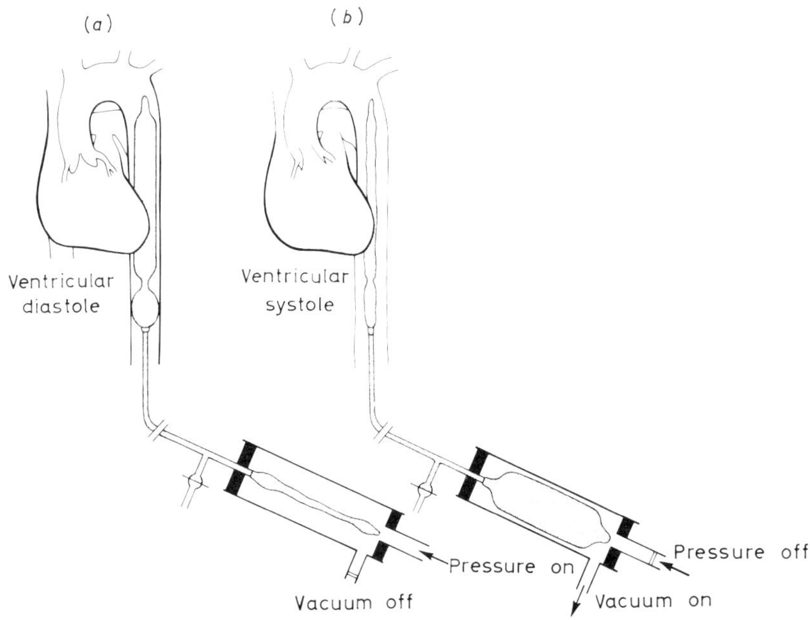

Figure 21.12 Dual-chambered balloon acting in tandem with slave balloon in safety chamber. (*a*) Transfer of CO_2 during diastole from slave balloon in safety chamber to intra-aortic balloon. (*b*) Complete deflation of intra-aortic balloon assisted by vacuum acting on slave balloon. (Reproduced from Bregman, Kripke and Goetz[43] by courtesy of *Transactions of the American Society of Artificial Internal Organs*)

driving gas. Lethal sequelae from intra-aortic balloon rupture with helium, both in animals[83] and in humans[144, 145, 147] have further convinced us that the use of carbon dioxide is a prudent choice as the driving gas for clinical intra-aortic balloon pumping. To our knowledge, there has been only one patient death as a result of a ruptured intra-aortic balloon when carbon dioxide was used.

Overdistension

Because the effective pumping volume of CO_2 introduced into the slave balloon in the safety chamber is never more than the displacement volume of the actual intra-aortic balloon, the intra-aortic balloon can never be overdistended. If the balloon is connected to a cylinder of the driving gas and inflation is then judged by the pressure build-up in the balloon, the intra-aortic balloon may become distended with each inflation cycle leading eventually to fatigue and balloon herniation and with subsequent weakness and eventual rupture.

Gas diffusion from balloon

Because of the ambient carbon dioxide tension in the arterial tree, there is minimal diffusion of carbon dioxide between the intra-aortic balloon and the patients's blood. However, a small amount of carbon dioxide is lost from the slave balloon in the safety chamber to the ambient external air under normal line-operated circumstances, since compressed air is the positive driving force within the safety chamber external to the slave balloon. This loss may amount to 1–2 ml/h. The loss would be accentuated if helium were used, since helium is a smaller molecular than CO_2 and because the arterial tension of helium is zero[38].

Vacuum

Not only is the intra-aortic balloon actively inflated, but it is actively deflated as well. By actively deflating the intra-aortic balloon, one has the advantage of precise timing of deflation and of a more completely deflated intra-aortic balloon which can never act as a partial intra-aortic obstruction during systole (*Figures 21.12, 21.13* and *21.14*)[39–43, 86].

Visual control and flexibility

Finally, the safety chamber provides accurate visual control of the intra-aortic balloon's performance by observing the slave balloon in the safety chamber. This feature has been found to be a useful adjunct in addition to monitoring the patient's ECG and blood pressure. It is particularly useful when initiating balloon pumping so that only the smallest augmentation can at first be applied to the patient to ensure that balloon pumping begins in the appropriate diastolic interval.

The safety chamber, which is supported by a flexible stainless steel arm, can be extended several inches beyond the pumping unit towards the patient's groin. Thus the pumping unit itself does not necessarily require close proximity to the operating table. This is particularly important in sterile surgical procedures where adequate draping of a large console next to the operating table would be cumbersome.

Battery operation

In light of the present clinical experience with intra-aortic balloon pumping[32, 38–43, 55–61, 75, 86, 127, 128, 151–156, 184, 196] it has become apparent

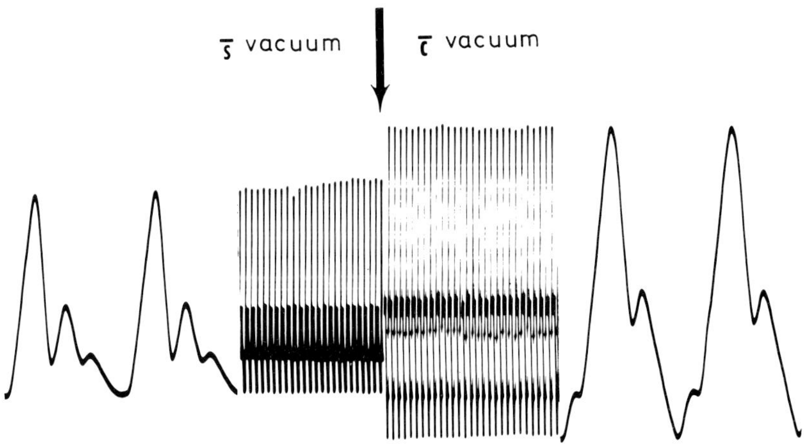

Figure 21.13 Advantage of using vacuum during IABP. Note completeness of deflation with vacuum (*on right*) and resultant greater pumping effectiveness of the balloon as demonstrated in a mock circulatory system. (Reproduced from Bregman, Kripke and Goetz[43], by courtesy of *Transactions of the American Society for Artificial Internal Organs*)

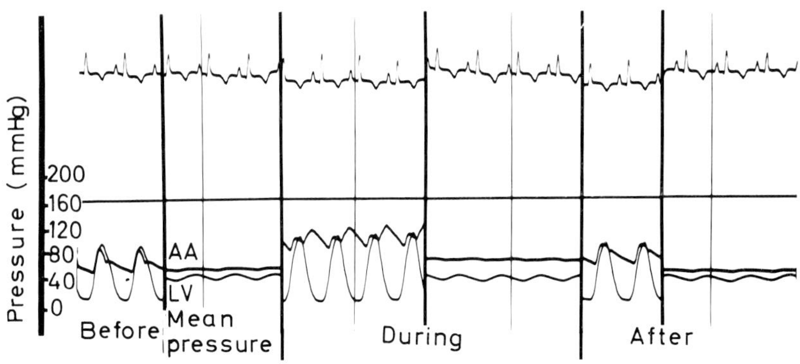

Figure 21.14 With systemic hypotension, complete collapse of the intra-aortic balloon just prior to ventricular systole cannot be assured if deflation is not uniformly assisted. In this animal experiment without vacuum assist, partial obstruction of the aorta, as evidenced by the rise in aortic and left ventricular systolic pressures during the assist, resulted from incomplete collapse of the balloon. A vacuum should be used at all times during IABP to assure total and complete balloon deflation

that quite frequently it is necessary to move the patient, and the cardiac assist console, from one part of the hospital to another. Therefore, it is necessary to have a system which is mobile and which can be readily battery operated. To initiate battery operation with the System 82, one need only turn on one of the two carbon dioxide cylinders on the rear of the cart. Once this is done, the unit can be immediately unplugged from the wall and the entire system will automatically be battery operated without any lapse in circulatory assistance. No further adjustments will be necessary to maintain the same diastolic augmentation. In the battery operated mode, the positive pressure for balloon pumping is derived from the carbon dioxide in the portable cylinders, and the vacuum is derived from routing the carbon dioxide through a small Venturi attachment. At a heart rate of 70 beats/min, each of the 2 cylinders provided on the cart will function for approximately 45 min.

Weaning feature

After the patient has become haemodynamically stable during balloon pumping, it may be desirable to wean him from the assist device. This can easily be accomplished with the System 82 because not only can the balloon volume be gradually decreased, but the assist can also operate in the 1:1, 1:2 and 1:3 modes so that the patient is assisted with every heartbeat, every second heartbeat, or every third heartbeat. Hence, by a combination of these features, the balloon volume and assist frequency can gradually and synchronously[15] be decreased until the assist has been discontinued.

Experience with intra-aortic balloon pumping

Clinical guidelines

The indications for IABP are changing almost daily. I will discuss initially the patient in *cardiogenic shock* whose management is summarized in *Table 21.1*.

All patients with an acute myocardial infarction diagnosed by the clinical picture, the ECG and enzyme studies should be admitted to the coronary care unit[33]. Those patients who demonstrate systolic hypotension (systolic blood pressure below 80 mmHg or systolic blood pressure less than 100 mmHg if formerly hypertensive) or, even without hypotension, a low output syndrome resulting in diminished tissue perfusion, peripheral cyanosis, cold clammy skin, oliguria (urine output less than 20 ml per hour, low sodium) and mental confusion or agitation are then evaluated for the possible effects of:

(1) Drug depression
(2) Arrhythmias
(3) Metabolic disturbances
(4) Volume depletion
(5) Gram-negative sepsis (*Table 21.1*)

If the hypotensive or low-output state is not related to any of these disturbances or if it persists after one or more of the disturbances have been corrected, then the patient is described as suffering from *cardiogenic shock as a result of myocardial infarction*.

Initially, patients should receive standard supportive therapy for 1 hour, including medications for pain, acidosis, hypoxia, and cardiac failure. Intravenous administration of digoxin should be undertaken or may be supplemented if the patient has already undergone digitalization. A central venous catheter should be inserted, a Swan–Ganz catheter positioned to monitor pulmonary artery wedge pressure, and a Foley catheter inserted. If the initial central venous pressure is less than 15 cm H_2O or the

TABLE 21.1

Management of cardiogenic shock

(A) Definition of cardiogenic shock
- (1) Low output syndrome
- (2) Systolic BP<80 mmHg *or* BP<100 mmHg if formerly hypertensive
- (3) Urine output<20 ml/h

↓

(B) Initial treatment
- (1) Standard supportive Rx–1 h
- (2) Digitalis
- (3) Volume (trial of D/W or albumin CVP >15 cmH_2O, PCWP >18 mmHg *or* deterioration)

↓

(C) Cardiac output studies
If: after (B),
- (1) Systolic BP<80 mmHg *or* BP<100 mmHg if formerly hypertensive or
- (2) Urine output<20 ml/h

↓

(D) Positive inotropic agent therapy.
Begun immediately after (B) while (C) is being arranged and performed.
- (1) Dopamine, Dobutamine
- (2) Levophed
- (3) Isuprel (least preferred)
- (4) Afterload reducing drugs

↓

THERAPEUTIC RESULTS

(E) If any two result, continue Rx
- (1) Low output syndrome improves
- (2) CI 2.2 ℓ/min per m^2 or greater
- (3) CVP falls 3 cmH_2O
- (4) PCWP falls 3 mmHg
- (5) Systolic BP>80 mmHg *or* 10 mmHg>basal level
- (6) Urine output 20 ml/h or >

(F) If any two result, assisted circulation
- (1) Low output syndrome persists
- (2) CI 2.0 ℓ/min per m^2 or less
- (3) Systolic BP<80 mmHg *or* BP<100 mmHg if formerly hypertensive
- (4) Urine output<20 ml/h

↓

DUAL-CHAMBERED INTRA-AORTIC BALLOON PUMPING

pulmonary capillary wedge pressure (PCWP) as measured with a Swan–Ganz catheter is less than 18 mmHg, a volume infusion should be started and given in increments of 100 ml of either dextrose in water or dextrose in water with salt-poor albumin added. If, after a trial of volume expansion, the systolic arterial pressure remains below 80 mmHg or is less than 100 mmHg in a formerly hypertensive patient or if the urine output remains below 20 ml per hour, then initial cardiac-output studies should be undertaken. While these are being arranged and performed, the patient should be given a therapeutic trial of inotropic agents, including dobutamine or dopamine. Isoproterenol (Isuprel), which was formerly used, is no longer advocated by most cardiologists[145]. The reason is that myocardial function basically depends upon the balance between oxygen supply and demand. Isoproterenol markedly increases the oxygen demand and decreases the oxygen supply by lowering the diastolic perfusion pressure. Therefore, although one may see transient improvement in haemodynamic parameters, the myocardium itself is essentially forced into a state of markedly negative oxygen balance.

Dobutamine (Dobutrex) is administered in increments of 5–20 μg/kg per min.

Dopamine (Intropin) should be administered in increments of 5–15 μg/kg per min. Tachycardia will usually signal the maximal rate of infusion. Afterload reduction by continuous administration of sodium nitroprusside can also be used either alone or in combination with the above inotropic drugs.

Therapy should be considered temporarily successful and continued if any two of the following measurements result from any agents:

(1) There is an improvement in the low output syndrome.
(2) The cardiac index is 2.2 ℓ/min per m^2 or greater.
(3) The central venous pressure is lowered by 3 cm H_2O or more.
(4) The pulmonary capillary wedge pressure falls by 3 mmHg or more.
(5) The systolic arterial blood pressure is greater than 80 mmHg or shows an increase of 10 mmHg from the prior basal level.
(6) The urinary output is 20 ml per hour or greater.

However, if any two of the following measurements apply, proceed to IABP:

(1) The low output syndrome clinically persists.
(2) The cardiac index remains persistently below 2 ℓ/min per m^2 after the therapeutic intervention.
(3) The systolic blood pressure persists at less than 80 mmHg or the blood pressure is less than 100 mmHg systolic in previously hypertensive patients.
(4) The urinary output persists at less than 20 ml per hour.

This entire diagnostic and therapeutic scheme can be performed in 2 to 3 hours.

Once the diagnosis of cardiogenic shock is established, these routine therapeutic procedures should be instituted as rapidly as possible, since the earlier the patient is referred for circulatory assistance, the better the result will be. Surrounding the actual area of the infarct, or the area of frank myocardial necrosis, there is a significant area of marginal myocardial ischaemia, the 'twilight zone'[69]. It is this zone of diminished myocardial perfusion that can be restored to viability by the early institution of IABP. Hence, more patients will survive from the circulatory assist alone, the earlier they are referred for treatment.

It should be stressed that this outline for patient selection is fairly rigid. At present most patients are being referred for pumping earlier, just as they require inotropic support.

Initially our cardiologists sometimes used diuretic agents during the period of observation and treatment. This only clouded the issue because, although an occasional patient did increase the urinary output with the use of furosemide or ethacrynic acid, this clinical improvement was transient and only served to delay the referral of the patient for circulatory assistance. We use the above protocol and attempt to refer the patient as early as possible for treatment with the intra-aortic balloon. If there is still confusion about the diagnosis (e.g., pulmonary embolus versus cardiogenic shock), a lung scan will not delay circulatory assistance greatly.

The only absolute contraindications to IABP are the presence of gross aortic insufficiency, cardiac standstill and the presence of an acute dissection of the aorta. Minor aortic insufficiency should not contraindicate the clinical use of balloon assistance[229]. A relative contraindication is the presence of an aortic aneurysm or the history of previous operation upon the aorta. This must be evaluated in light of the exigency of the clinical situation.

Patient preparation

After informed consent has been obtained (the possibilities of cardiac angiography and open-heart surgery should have been mentioned), the procedure should be performed in an area where other patients will not be disturbed (e.g., a side room in the coronary care unit or a special procedure room). Occasionally, because of the multiple electric circuits used, additional wiring may be necessary in the area designated for circulatory assistance.

The patient's respiratory function is critical during the procedure, and serial determinations of blood gases should be evaluated. Most of our patients have been treated with a Venturi mask, and occasionally the patients have required positive pressure ventilation via orotracheal or nasotracheal intubation. Gastric dilatation is not uncommon during the balloon pumping procedure, and when one evaluates a chest roentgenogram for balloon position, the stomach bubble should be noted. If it appears large, a nasogastric tube should be inserted without hesitation. If the patient is agitated, he should be sedated with small doses (2.5 mg) of intravenous diazepam (Valium). The patient himself should be arranged in the following manner. A radiolucent bed, if available, should be used. The balloon will be inserted through the common femoral artery in the groin with the strongest femoral pulse. The entire pubic area and both groins and upper thighs should be shaved. It is important to have an arterial blood pressure cannula above the balloon during IABP. This is best accomplished by inserting a small Teflon arterial catheter through a radial artery. A Swan–Ganz thermodilution catheter* is inserted in the antecubital fossa or through the internal jugular vein percutaneously and is threaded into the wedge position in the pulmonary artery. A peripheral intravenous line should be also inserted. It is important to have at least two intravenous lines running, one central and one peripheral. The fluids during balloon pumping will be given through the central venous catheter, and the inotropic agents through the peripheral intravenous drip.

* Edwards Laboratories, Santa Ana, California, USA

In addition, the following recommendations should be considered:

(1) Antibiotic coverage—routinely place the patient on broad-spectrum antibiotic coverage (i.e. cloxacillin).
(2) Digoxin should be supplemented as indicated.
(3) The urine output should be measured along with urinary electrolytes.
(4) The patient should be restrained gently on all four extremities.
(5) The patient should usually be maintained on either a dobutamine or a dopamine drip, possibly combined with sodium nitroprusside infusion.
(6) Type and cross-match the patient's blood for 2–4 units of packed red blood cells.

Parameters to be monitored

Urine output, urine specific gravity, central venous pressure, pulmonary artery wedge pressure, arterial blood pressure (which includes systolic pressure, peak diastolic pressure, mean pressure and end-diastolic pressure), thermodilution cardiac output, and heart rate, should be measured routinely. Fluid and haematological data should include a complete blood count and determinations of blood urea nitrogen, fasting blood sugar, electrolytes, clotting times, and platelet counts.

Comprehensive chemical profiles and serum enzyme determinations should be obtained at regular intervals.

Just prior to balloon insertion, the patient is heparinized with 50 mg (5000 units) of aqueous heparin intravenously. Routinely, our patients receive between 5000 and 7500 units of aqueous heparin intravenously every 4–6 hours, the dose depending upon their size.

Balloon insertion (dual-chambered intra-aortic balloon)

As suggested by Kantrowitz *et al.*[108], the balloon is usually inserted in either common femoral artery through a prosthetic graft, which is then snared to permit perfusion of the distal extremity during the period of cardiac assistance. The balloon is threaded centrally and its tip positioned just distal to the left subclavian artery (*Figures 21.15* and *21.16*).

Technique

The groin is palpated, and the side with the strongest femoral pulse is selected for insertion of the balloon.

After the skin is prepared and draped in the usual fashion, the skin and subcutaneous tissues are infiltrated with 1 per cent lidocaine (Xylocaine) without epinephrine. The skin incision should be vertical, beginning high in the groin over the inguinal ligament and carried inferiorly for approximately 6 cm. The incision is deepened, and the common femoral, profunda femoris, and superior portion of the superficial femoral arteries identified and secured with tapes (the proximal tape is encircled twice around the common femoral artery). If the patient is *in extremis*, the balloon must be inserted immediately and pumping instituted promptly. If however, the patient's condition is more stable, the arterial graft may be sutured on first and the balloon then inserted through the graft, which is the preferred method.

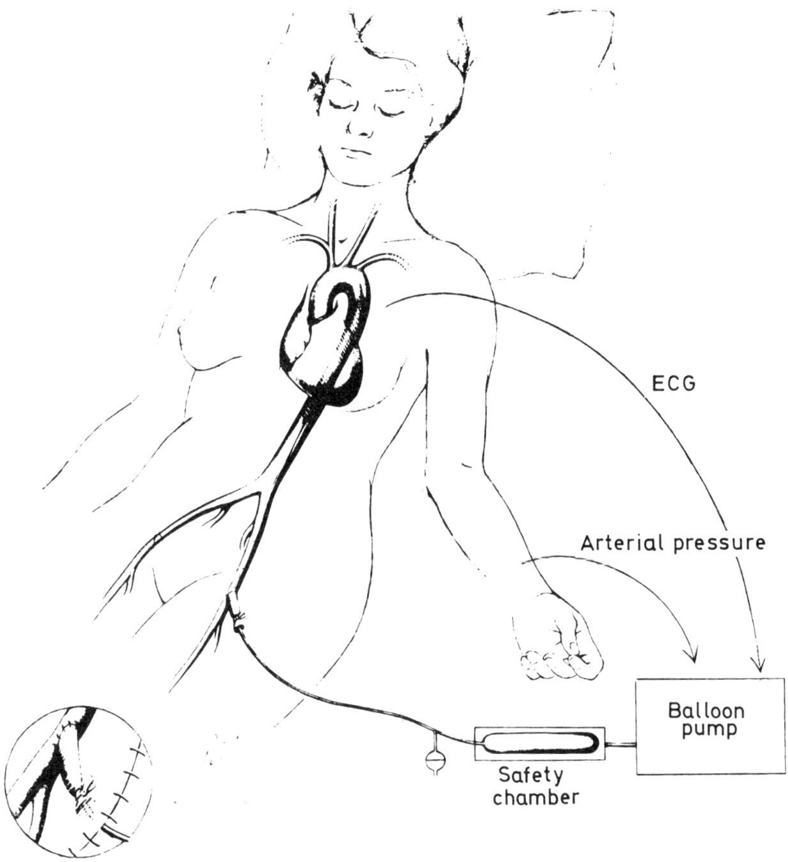

Figure 21.15 Artist's representation of clinical dual-chambered IABP

A 10 mm diameter woven Dacron tube graft is recommended. We personally use a segment approximately 8–10 cm long.

The dual-chambered balloons used in patients are available presterilized in two sizes—30 and 40 ml. If the subject is large and has a broad common femoral artery the 35 ml balloon is used.

If it is established that the patient must be assisted immediately, the graft is cut at one end at approximately 45 degrees so that its open longitudinal diameter will be about 2 cm. The graft is then placed over the balloon catheter so that the angled portion faces the balloon. Next, a three-way stopcock is attached to the end of the balloon catheter, and the balloon is completely deflated with a 50 ml syringe. The syringe is detached, and the stopcock is left attached to the balloon. Bulldog clamps are placed on the profunda and superficial femoral arteries, and a small curved vascular clamp is placed high on the common femoral artery. With a No. 11 knife blade, a vertical incision is begun in the common femoral artery. The arteriotomy is completed with an angled Potts scissors. The arteriotomy should be approximately 2 cm long and should be primarily in the *common femoral artery*. The most inferior aspect of this arteriotomy may overlie the profunda femoris orifice.

The desired position for the balloon is just distal to the left subclavian artery. The balloon and the catheter should be held over the patient to approximate this position, and a silk tie should be secured about the catheter at the proposed exit point from the groin. It is best to underestimate the amount of catheter to be inserted to avoid injury to the aortic arch. The balloon can easily be repositioned later. If a radiolucent bed and a portable image intensifier are available, they can be used for appropriate placement of the balloon.

The balloon is then immersed in saline, to which may be added a few ml of 1 or 2 mg/100 ml lidocaine to act as a lubricant. The polyurethane comprising the pumping (proximal) balloon is folded in half around the balloon catheter, and the tip of the balloon is inserted cephalad through the arteriotomy. The umbilical tape is loosened, and the vascular clamp removed from the common femoral artery. The balloon is then rapidly advanced. When the occluding (more distal) balloon is reached, the balloon is rotated clockwise as it is advanced. This will facilitate insertion of the more distal segment of the balloon. When the balloon has just been inserted and before the full selected amount of additional balloon catheter has been advanced, the double umbilical tape is snared. This will control blood loss, and the catheter can be advanced to the desired position. Following this, balloon pumping is begun.

At this point the graft is carefully sutured to the arteriotomy site with 4–0 or 5–0 cardiovascular suture material. Next, 2 heavy umbilical tapes are used to snare the graft and balloon catheter approximately 2 cm above the arteriotomy. These should be tied down snugly, but not tight enough to impinge upon the balloon catheter's diameter. The bulldog clamps and umbilical tapes are removed, and if blood is seen to escape between the catheter and the graft, an additional umbilical tape is tied on. The double tape around the common femoral artery is then removed. When the wound is dry the graft is trimmed so that only 3–4 cm will remain *in situ*. The wound can be irrigated with an antibiotic solution or saline, and the subcutaneous tissues and skin can be closed loosely with sutures. The balloon catheter usually exits in the middle of the wound. *No* suture should be placed around the catheter. If, after the portable chest roentgenogram is taken, the balloon is seen to be improperly positioned, the graft and catheter can be grasped and the balloon moved without removing the umbilical tapes. Neosporin is applied to the wound, which is then covered with a dry sterile dressing. The balloon catheter is taped to the wound dressing.

If there is time to suture the graft first, a similar arteriotomy is performed and the angled graft is attached to the common femoral artery. At this point the graft is cut approximately 5 cm above the arteriotomy site. Two mosquito clamps are placed on either side of the graft and are held by assistants. The balloon is prepared as previously described and is inserted through the graft into the artery. Again, when the occluding balloon is reached, the balloon catheter is rotated clockwise as the balloon is

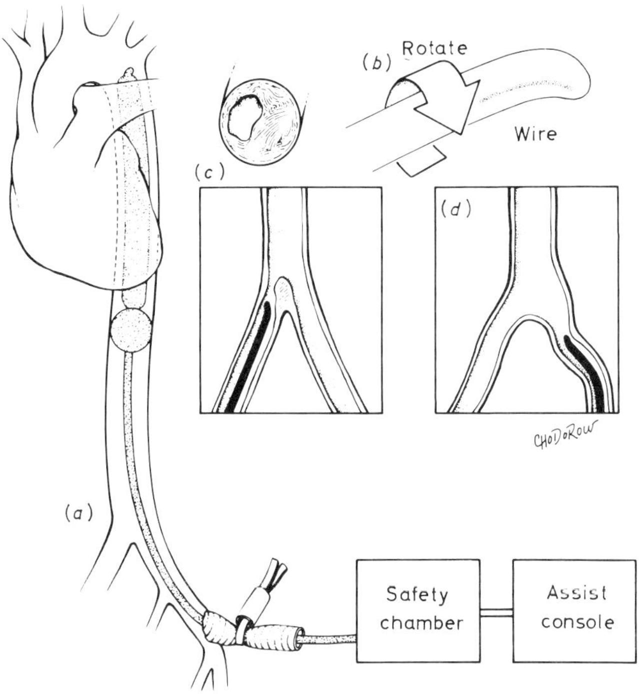

Figure 21.16 (*a*) A proper position of dual-chambered intra-aortic balloon just distal to left subclavian artery. Note that the balloon is inserted through a Dacron prosthesis that is snared, permitting perfusion of the distal extremity during the period of cardiac assist. (*b*) Technique of bending and rotating distal balloon catheter during insertion. (*c*) Balloon negotiating eccentric arteriosclerotic stenosis. (*d*) Balloon passing through an arterial tortuosity. (Reproduced from Bregman, Bolooki and Malm[37], by courtesy of *Annals of Thoracic Surgery*)

advanced. Balloon pumping is then initiated. Further wound management is similar.

If, after the arteriotomy has been negotiated, the balloon cannot be advanced, excessive force on the balloon catheter should not be exerted. Remove the balloon and manually bend the balloon catheter 0.5–1 cm distal to the lucite tip to a 45 degree angle or use a more gentle bend (*Figure 21.16*)[37]. The flexible stainless steel wire strut within the proximal pumping balloon will maintain the angulated position. Now reinsert the balloon and when the obstruction is reached, rotate the balloon and catheter. This manoeuvre will frequently permit the balloon to be passed through a tortuous or arteriosclerotic juncture. We have now had several patients in whom this technical improvement facilitated insertion of the balloon in the ipsilateral extremity, thereby sparing the patient a contralateral arteriotomy[41] while at the same time permitting earlier application of cardiac assistance[44].

If all the above measures fail, other routes of insertion such as the iliac artery[121] or the ascending aorta[175] have been successful alternatives.

The patient may exhibit limb ischaemia in the initial phase of balloon pumping when the cardiac output is low and the balloon catheter occupies a significant portion of the cross-sectional diameter of the common femoral artery. However, as cardiac output improves, blood flow increases in the extremity and this transient limb ischaemia usually abates.

A balloon should *never* be re-used clinically, for several reasons. After usage the balloon membrane may retain small deposits of foreign protein that may not be eliminated even with thorough washing. This foreign protein may serve as a nidus for the deposition of platelets and other formed elements of the blood and may cause eventual thrombosis. In addition there is the risk of serum hepatitis transferred from one patient to another. Finally, during balloon removal the balloon membrane may become damaged due to scratching as the balloon exits through the graft in the groin. With additional clinical usage this defect in the membrane could weaken its structural integrity and increase the risk of balloon rupture.

Balloon insertion (percutaneous intra-aortic balloon)

Technique

Employing the Seldinger method[192a] the percutaneous intra-aortic balloon is inserted utilizing the following technique. After the inguinal region is prepared and draped, the common femoral artery is punctured with a standard 18 gauge arterial needle, and a 0.038 inch (0.097 cm) J tip guidewire is introduced through the needle. After removal of the needle, an 8F dilator is passed over the guidewire to pre-dilate the subcutaneous tissues and the arterial puncture site. The dilator is then exchanged for a 12F dilator sheath combination, which is advanced over the guidewire into the artery. One inch of the sheath is left exposed to control bleeding.

Preparation of the percutaneous balloon. The balloon is moistened in saline solution and furled while an assistant holds the distal tip of the balloon catheter immobile. The deflated balloon is furled by wrapping it around the balloon catheter, starting at the distal end and proceeding proximally. Any air remaining in the balloon is completely evacuated with a syringe and stopcock. The guidewire and 12F dilator are then removed, leaving the 12F sheath in place. Bleeding is controlled by firmly compressing the exposed sheath. The furled balloon is then inserted through the sheath (*Figure 21.16A*) and positioned under fluoroscopy in the descending thoracic aorta. After removal of the stopcock, the balloon catheter is attached to the pumping console and intra-aortic balloon pumping is initiated. If resistance is encountered in passage through the aortoiliac bifurcation, the catheter can be rotated, but no force is imparted lest dissection occur. The appropriate length of catheter to be inserted may be estimated by placing the catheter on the patient's abdomen and chest with the tip 1 cm below the angle of Louis and marking the catheter at the end of the No. 12F intravascular sheath. Sometimes the tip of the catheter may be felt against the aortic arch and the catheter is withdrawn about 1 inch outward so that the tip will lie just below the left subclavian artery. Correct inflation and deflation of the balloon may be confirmed with

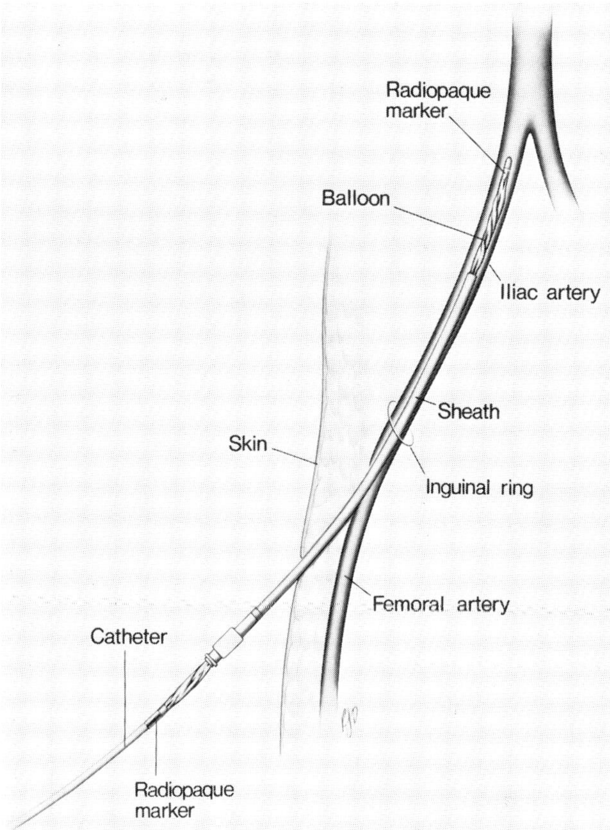

Figure 21.16A Insertion of percutaneous intra-aortic balloon

fluoroscopic visualization. The 12F sheath and balloon catheter are ligated with umbilical tape to prevent bleeding around the catheter, and a sterile dressing is applied to the sheath and balloon catheter assembly. Management of patients on the IABP has been described in detail elsewhere[33].

Percutaneous balloon removal. Before removal of the balloon catheter, the balloon is completely collapsed by aspiration with a syringe. The balloon is then withdrawn up into the 12F sheath, and the sheath and balloon are removed as a unit. Direct external pressure is applied to the puncture site for 30 minutes. After 20 minutes, external pressure is reduced to permit reperfusion of the limb. Reappearance of the distal pulses may be monitored by Doppler. A compression dressing is affixed to the puncture site for 24 hours. Weaning from percutaneous intra-aortic balloon pumping is accomplished in the same manner as previously described for the standard intra-aortic balloon pump[34].

For medical patients anticoagulation consists of 5000 to 7500 units of intravenous aqueous heparin every 4 to 6 hours. Postoperative patients requiring balloon assistance receive only 900 mg of rectal aspirin (ASA) every 4 to 6 hours. Cimetidine is administered prophylactically.

Long sheath insertion

A new technique for percutaneous insertion of intra-aortic balloon catheters in patients with tortuous or narrowed external iliac arteries was described by Nichols, Weiss, and Bregman[158a]. This method uses a long (45 cm) 12F sheath-dilator combination which extends up to the descending aorta and protects the iliac artery and aorta from injury during insertion of the balloon catheter. In patients with severe acute myocardial ischemia in whom insertion of intra-aortic balloon catheters is not possible by the conventional percutaneous technique, use of the long sheath approach permits rapid institution of circulatory support.

Placement of the intra-aortic balloon using the long sheath technique is performed in a manner similar to conventional percutaneous balloon insertion. However, following proper positioning of the balloon and catheter in the descending thoracic aorta, the long sheath is withdrawn into the iliac artery to allow complete unfurling of the balloon membrane.

Ideal balloon function

The primary goals of IABP are to implement the maximal increase in coronary blood flow during diastole and at the same time effect a decrease in left ventricular work[68]. Realization that these two beneficial effects are dependent upon one another permits maximal benefit to be obtained from each factor in the following fashion. The diastolic augmentation ordinarily begins at the dicrotic notch. One can encroach upon the dicrotic notch to begin balloon inflation slightly earlier in diastole. Provided the patient does not have premature ventricular contractions from this manipulation, it can be performed in patients who appear to be responding poorly to the balloon pumping to give them an additional benefit. The right-hand side or downslope of the augmentation is the part most intimately involved with the ventricular unloading aspect of balloon pumping. If the fall in end-diastolic pressure is too great, the following sequence of events occurs. Excessive fall in end-diastolic pressure essentially means that the balloon has collapsed too soon before the aortic valve has opened. Since blood must flow to occupy the space of the formerly expanded balloon, it flows retrograde from all branches of the aorta, including the coronary arteries if the fall in end-diastolic pressure caused by a prematurely collapsing balloon is excessive[68]. Therefore, one must effect a compromise and have some fall in end-diastolic pressure, but not an excessive one. Data from my experimental work, which has been substantiated by the clinical experience, established that this fall should not exceed 10 mmHg.

Usually, during balloon pumping with the unidirectional dual-chambered balloon the height of the diastolic augmentation is much greater than that of the patient's systolic pressure[43] (*Figure 21.17*). On occasion the two wave forms may be similar in height. This may occur under a variety of circumstances, but primarily when the aorta is much larger than the occluding balloon, in which case the dual-chambered balloon is basically acting as an improved unidirectional single-chambered balloon. A larger balloon can be inserted if desired. Also, the more normotensive the patient becomes, thc smaller will be the diastolic augmentation.

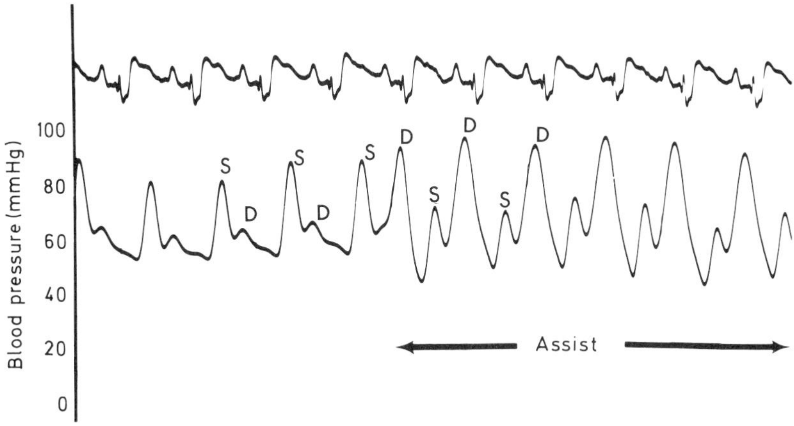

Figure 21.17 Unidirectional dual-chambered IABP in a patient with cardiogenic shock. S = systole; D = diastole augmentation. Note fall in systolic pressure, large diastolic augmentation, and fall in end-diastolic pressure. (Reproduced by permission from Bregman, D. 'Mechanical support of the failing heart.' In *Current Problems in Surgery*. Ed. M. M. Ravitch. Chicago: Yearbook Medical Publishers)

As far as the position of the balloon is concerned, we initially place the balloon as far proximally in the aorta as possible (that is, with the tip of the balloon just distal to the left subclavian artery). Be sure to feel the pulse in the left arm so that the tip of the balloon is not in the subclavian orifice and is not occluding the left subclavian inflow.

At rapid heart rates there is more dead space in the safety chamber balloon. Therefore one could increase the volume of carbon dioxide in the safety chamber balloon (e.g. to 45 ml with a 30 ml balloon in the patient) at heart rates over 120 beats per minute. This will improve intra-aortic balloon function[34].

In the clinical setting, heart rates of up to 140 beats per minute can usually be followed when a 30 ml balloon is used. If the rate is higher, simply assist on 1:2 (every other beat) until the rate slows, when 1:1 assist can be instituted.

If weaning a patient from IABP is undertaken by changing from a 1:1 to a 1:2 or a 1:3 assisting sequence, additional time will be present for the vacuum to build up, and the augmentation may demonstrate a deep 'sink'; the end-diastolic point may need elevation by a minor adjustment on the console.

Pharmacological management and expected haemodynamic sequelae

The suggested pharmacologic management of patients during IABP is outlined below.

Supportive measures—oxygen, analgesic, etc.

Fluids	Frusemide (Lasix)
Digitalis	Antiarrhythmics
Dobutamine	Anticoagulants
Nitroprusside	Antibiotics
Diazepam (Valium)	

The usual supportive measures for patients in cardiogenic shock are continued, and serial blood-gas determinations serve as a dual guide in patient management. If the blood-gas levels are poor, we do not hesitate to use nasotracheal or orotracheal intubation. In addition, the arterial pH is monitored carefully, since experience has shown that as balloon pumping commences there is a decrease in peripheral resistance and that as peripheral perfusion improves there is a washout of acid metabolic products, which must be corrected by the intravenous administration of sodium bicarbonate. Surprisingly, these cardiogenic shock patients who tolerate no fluid prior to balloon assist require many thousand millilitres of intravenous fluids within the first several hours of balloon pumping. Intravenous therapy is begun with 5 mg/100 ml dextrose in water to which may be added salt-poor albumin. As urinary output is resumed, a 5 mg/100 ml dextrose and 1/3 Normal saline solution is used, to which potassium is added. Digitalis therapy is continued, as is treatment with inotropic agents. Dobutamine is the usual agent used in the coronary care unit. Dopamine can also be tried and either drug can be used with nitroprusside. As indicated previously, isoproterenol is currently the least preferred inotropic agent in cardiogenic shock. Diazepam is given for agitation, 2.5–5 mg intravenously as necessary. Diuretic agents are usually not necessary during clinical dual-chambered IABP, since urinary excretions of more than 100 ml within the first hour of IABP are not unusual. Occasionally, it may be desirable to administer a single intravenous bolus of a diuretic such as frusemide.

Arrhythmias usually abate promptly during the initiation of balloon pumping. Otherwise they are treated with standard medical therapy. If a patient has a contraindication to heparin therapy, it is recommended that 10–25 ml per hour of low molecular weight dextran (Rheomacrodex) be administered intravenously as the sole anticoagulant therapy. For patients assisted in the immediate intraoperative or postoperative period, heparinization is reversed with protamine, and the aforementioned dextran regimen may be used, although more recently we have not employed it[34, 45]. Although the dextran therapy may help alleviate the thrombocytopenia reported by Leinbach *et al.*[130] during IABP, its use has also been associated with the finding of a diffuse background of subcellular particles on the balloon surfaces with a scanning electron microscope[191]. These particles may be related to the particular balloon material employed, but until the significance of this finding is clarified, the use of dextran during IABP should not be discouraged. Our present postoperative regimen is to use neither dextran nor heparin during the first 120 hours of IABP. The use of aspirin as the sole postoperative ‘anticoagulant’ is our current regimen. Cimetitidine is administered prophylactically. If a longer assist period is required, dextran or heparin or both can be used. In patients requiring IABP for prolonged preoperative or postoperative support, who can be expected to have a long hospitalization with a prolonged period of bed rest, longterm anticoagulation with warfarin sodium (Coumadin) is recommended after balloon removal. All patients undergoing dual-chambered IABP are treated with broad-spectrum antibiotics, which are continued for 2 days following balloon removal.

It is important to monitor the patient carefully during IABP, especially during the early phases. Central venous pressure and pulmonary artery wedge pressure will fall rather promptly and the administration of additional fluids will be required. The patient will usually become alert shortly after the beginning of balloon pumping.

During balloon pumping, if possible, we attempt to keep the peak diastolic pressure at 100–110 mmHg. At this level, urine excretion will start rather promptly in most patients. It is not wise to elevate the pressure much higher by means of inotropic agents, since balloon function may be impaired and usually the heart rate will be much higher. We keep the peak diastolic pressure at 100–110 mmHg and gradually taper off the inotropic agent. In some patients the inotropic drugs can be tapered very promptly.

As an additional pharmacological adjunct during IABP treatment of a patient in cardiogenic shock, one may administer small intravenous doses of propranolol, which has been shown to potentiate myocardial oxygen conservation[198]. This agent is primarily employed when the patient has tachycardia.

If the patient develops cardiac arrest during balloon pumping, the following procedure is recommended. If a pacemaker is present the balloon will continue to be activated. The chest should be massaged synchronously with the balloon so that every time the slave balloon in the safety chamber expands, the chest is manually compressed. Each time the chest is manually compressed, cardiac output increases, and every time the balloon expands, coronary blood flow is increased. After 30 to 60 seconds of this manoeuvre the heart frequently will begin beating spontaneously and balloon function will be automatically resumed. If a pacemarker is not present the machine can be turned to 'internal' and the trigger rate set at about 60 beats per minute to accomplish the same manoeuvre, or one can use the pressure trigger in the console. If the patient sustains ventricular fibrillation he can be defibrillated with the System 82 left on, since the components will not be damaged by direct current countershock. Most of these situations do not arise during adequate IABP but may occur at the beginning of the procedure before balloon timing or balloon function has been adjusted properly.

Duration of dual-chambered IABP

The duration of balloon pumping required in any particular patient may vary. However, in no instance is it wise to use balloon pumping continuously for more than 24 hours. The current experience has shown that a patient who cannot be weaned from the intra-aortic balloon before 24 hours certainly should have selective coronary arteriography and ventriculography and be considered as a candidate for operation[27]. Most patients are catheterized on IABP before 24 hours. The primary method of assessing whether a patient is ready to come off the intra-aortic balloon, aside from obvious clinical improvement, is by studying the cardiac output and its derivatives[196]. We obtained paired determinations off and on the intra-aortic balloon at intervals of 2 or 3 hours. When the outputs finally overlap, (that is, are approximately the same off and on the balloon), the balloon is turned off for approximately 30 minutes and the output is again determined. If the cardiac output is maintained, balloon pumping may be stopped.

In addition, it is now felt that the yield in treating medical patients with IABP alone has been so low that all patients on IABP should undergo cardiac catheterization and be considered for operation[189]. Another simple observation may be of help in deciding when to wean a patient from IABP. Significant systolic unloading occurs early in the IABP patients' course. The more significant the left ventricular failure, the greater the fall in the patients' systolic pressure with IABP. As clinical improvement is evident, this fall in systolic pressure (when the balloon is turned off to on at 1:1) is much less and may even be absent when the decision is made to terminate IABP[31].

Other clinical parameters of improvement are quite obvious. The patient will maintain his urine output; he will be awake and alert; the central venous pressure and left atrial pressure will be within the normal range; and the requirement for inotropic agents will be markedly diminished or absent at this point. The derivative of left ventricular pressure (dp/dt) will improve and will not change off or on the balloon. The presystolic ejection period is another parameter that can be evaluated[223]. This period shortens during balloon pumping and then remains shortened off the balloon, reflecting an improvement in haemodynamic performance.

If it is decided to perform arteriograms, the patient is moved to the radiology department. The study can be performed either through the upper extremity or through the contralateral femoral route. The only precaution with the femoral route is that the balloon must be turned off as the catheter is advanced up into the aortic arch. The balloon can then be turned on while the catheter is being manipulated and while the injections are done. One will note during arteriography that, when the balloon is turned on, the contrast material is flushed rapidly through the coronary tree. This may make it difficult to visualize the coronary vessels, and occasionally one may want to turn off the balloon during an injection or, as an alternative, to decrease the balloon volume. It is recommended that all patients requiring IABP be studied within the first 12–24 hours of the beginning of IABP.

Dual-chambered intra-aortic balloon pumping and cardiopulmonary bypass

For patients on cardiopulmonary bypass the following technique is recommended. The graft used should be woven Dacron and should be sutured to the femoral artery.

The ECG can be taken in the operating room either with the conventional limb leads or with a more rapid technique, an ECG pad*. The pad is simply placed under the patient's back by the anaesthesiologist and is connected to the patient cable. A crisp ECG is usually obtained. When the chest is closed, the standard ECG leads are applied and the ECG pad is disconnected prior to transporting the patient to the recovery room. The pressure trigger is valuable in the operating room primarily if there is ECG interference (that is, from an electrocautery) or if the ECG is not available or has very low voltage.

*V. Muller, Chicago, Illinois, USA

When the balloon is turned on during the weaning of a patient from cardiopulmonary bypass, the transition from partial bypass to the discontinuance of bypass should be gradual. If the patient has been pumped in the operating room and then cardiopulmonary bypass has been discontinued, we recommend the following policy concerning anticoagulation. The patient's heparin is reversed with protamine on the operating table, and bypass is discontinued in the usual manner. From this point on, no anticoagulants are used. Rectal aspirin is administered in the recovery room (600 mg every 4 hours). With this regimen we have experienced no clotting problems. Under no circumstance, however, should an intra-aortic balloon be left unpulsating *in vivo* for more than 1 hour. If a patient has been assisted preoperatively and it is desired to leave the balloon in place during operation with the expectation of further use when the patient comes off bypass or in the postoperative period, it is recommended that the balloon be synchronously inflated to create a bypass pulse pressure of 40–50 mmHg. When the heart fibrillates, the internal trigger is used at 80 beats per minute.

Presently, medical indications for intra-aortic balloon pumping have expanded, while the number of insertions in surgical patients has decreased[37a]. The decreased use of intra-aortic balloon pumping in intraoperative and postoperative patients is probably due to a greater awareness among surgeons that death from acute cardiac failure soon after cardiac operations is usually related to new and often extensive perioperative myocardial necrosis[110a]. Cardioplegia is now routinely employed during open-heart surgery. Furthermore, pulsatile flow during cardiopulmonary bypass results in better perfusion of the subendocardium[45]. However, until recently a pulsatile assist device capable of producing a traumatic phasic flow was not available. Thus, with the development of new techniques in myocardial protection the occurrence and extent of perioperative myocardial infarction has been reduced, and consequently there has been less need for the IABP.

Subendocardial ischaemia

Subendocardial ischaemia as a consequence of cardiopulmonary bypass has, prior to IABP, been recognized to contribute to more than one-half of the postoperative deaths[111, 158]. The low cardiac-output syndrome following cardiopulmonary bypass is not unlike the haemodynamic picture of cardiogenic shock. Both are self-perpetuating with progressive loss of myocardial contractility and ventricular performance. In both syndromes, when myocardial oxygen demand exceeds oxygen supply, myocardial efficiency deteriorates and low output (cardiogenic shock) ensues. Survival is influenced when the supply of oxygen equals or exceeds the myocardial demand.

Reliance upon systemic arterial pressure and central venous pressure in the postperfusion period as indicators of cardiac function may result in delayed diagnosis and treatment of severe myocardial ischaemia. On-line monitoring of the supply–demand ratio (EVR–endocardial viability ratio) in the immediate postperfusion period or in the coronary intensive care unit is an excellent method for the determination of subendocardial perfusion on a beat-to-beat basis. It is an accurate indicator of myocardial ischaemia and of potential patient survival.

Buckberg *et al.*[53] measured coronary blood flow and distribution during systole and diastole in dogs subjected to aortic constriction, atrial pacing, and arteriovenous fistulae. Results of these physiological stress studies verified that the adequacy of subendocardial perfusion as well as potential ischaemia could be predicted from indices derived from systolic and diastolic pressure measurements.

Sarnoff *et al.*[185] demonstrated that myocardial oxygen requirements are directly related to the area under the systolic pressure curve and termed this area tension–time index (TTI). This area has been shown to have a constant relationship to myocardial wall tension only if the geometry of the heart remains constant. McDonald, Taylor and Congolani[138] demonstrated that TTI and peak wall tension also both correlate well with myocardial oxygen consumption, and therefore the figures obtained from this index are accurate for determining myocardial oxygen demand.

Myocardial oxygen supply or the flow of blood to the subendocardial layers occurs predominantly during diastole. Diastolic duration, therefore, correlates well with myocardial blood distribution. The diastolic pressure–time index (DPTI), which describes the pressure–time events during diastole, accurately estimates diastolic and subendocardial blood flow. The ratio of DPTI to TTI, where TTI is the determinant of factors regulating demand, should therefore provide an accurate estimate of the oxygen supply–demand relationship[53] (*Figure 21.18*).

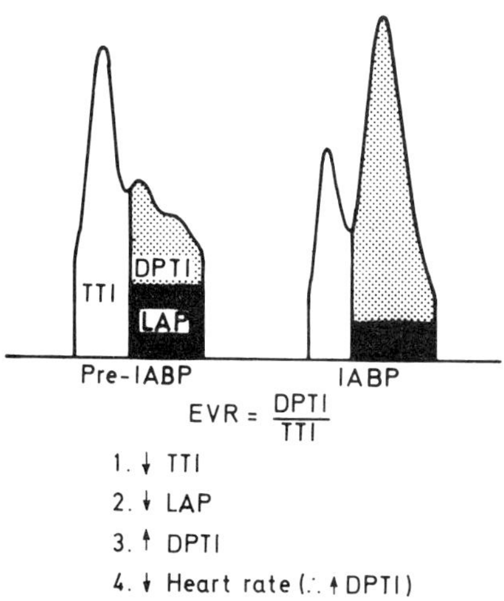

Figure 21.18 Effects of unidirectional IABP on the endocardial viability ratio (EVR). DPTI = diastolic pressure–time index; TTI = tension–time index; LAP = left atrial pressure

The work of Buckberg *et al.*[53] confirmed the efficiency of this ratio. With the use of microspheres 8–10 μm in diameter to determine flow distribution and with correlation of the hyperaemic response following periods of anoxia with subendocardial–subepicardial flow ratios, DPTI:TTI proved to be a highly accurate determinant of subendocardial ischaemia. Below a given ratio, for the experimental model, subendocardial blood flow decreased, the flow of coronary blood became predominantly systolic, and although in some instances there was an increase in coronary flow the distribution was subepicardial. Ischaemia of the subendocardium led to poor cardiac performance, characterized by inability to maintain cardiac output and aortic blood pressure, and to a rise in left atrial pressure.

Ischaemia more than any other single factor appears to be the most common cause of low cardiac-output syndrome[54]. Good subendocardial perfusion is necessary if the heart is to sustain the workload imposed upon it following operation. Early recognition of an ischaemic endocardium is imperative if proper therapy is to be initiated in time to prevent necrosis.

The concept of the EVR (Philips *et al.*[170, 172]) appears particularly well suited for use in monitoring patients undergoing unidirectional IABP, because there are at least four favourable alterations that the balloon imposes on this ratio (*Figure 21.18*).

(1) The area under the systolic pressure curve falls with balloon pumping. This is a reflection of the decrease in the impedance to left ventricular ejection caused by proper balloon deflation during IABP. The TTI is decreased, and therefore the EVR will increase.
(2) The left atrial pressure falls during IABP, and thus the resting left ventricular wall tension decreases.
(3) The area under the diastolic pressure curve will markedly rise during unidirectional IABP, which will increase myocardial oxygen supply or the DPTI.
(4) The heart rate will be slowed by reflex and other mechanisms, an effect that will primarily lengthen the diastolic period and also increase the EVR.

The applicability and reliability of the EVR as a monitoring index for subendocardial ischaemia and cardiac function are enhanced by observance of the ratio during periods of prolonged physiological stress. Low output problems secondary to cardiac dysfunction may be differentiated from other factors causing the shock state, and the cardiac response to stress can be measured in terms of subendocardial ischaemia. In shock secondary to volume depletion the effect on the myocardium can be followed, and signs of impending ischaemic dysfunction can be detected by a falling supply–demand ratio. Massive blood volume loss with associated falls in systemic and left atrial pressures may not be detrimental to subendocardial perfusion. With the combined fall in TTI and atrial pressures, and an increase in diastolic filling time, oxygen demand may not exceed supply and perfusion may be adequate for myocardial integrity. Although diastolic perfusion pressure may be low, intramyocardial compressive forces and left ventricular diastolic pressures are minimal, coronary dilation occurs, and subepicardial–subendocardial flow ratios remain constant[53]. The DPTI:TTI ratios indicate adequate perfusion, and ECGs do not show ischaemic patterns. Restoration of adequate blood volume restores normal haemodynamics, and good cardiac function is maintained.

On the other hand, low cardiac output secondary to pump failure is manifested by a stable or falling systemic pressure and a rising left atrial or left ventricular end-diastolic pressure. This change is reflected in a fall of the supply–demand ratio to levels where coronary flow is predominantly systolic and distribution is subepicardial. Subendocardial ischaemic deterioration occurs and may be detected by electrocardiographic ST-T segment depression. Increased lactate production has been reported[193].

With immediate application of IABP, ischaemic changes may be reversible, and the return to a balanced coronary flow pattern can be monitored by the EVR. By diastolic augmentation the amount of blood presented to the coronary arteries is increased. Equally important is the increase in the area under the diastolic pressure curve. With the associated fall in TTI (decrease in impedance to ventricular emptying), LVEDP and intramyocardial compression forces are lowered, and the subendocardial–subepicardial flow ratios return to normal. As the EVR rises, ST-T segments revert to normal, and lactate extraction is increased, indicating satisfactory reversal of the ischaemic state.

IABP therapy is more sound, physiologically, than is the administration of inotropic drugs[52, 222], which increase oxygen requirements. Balloon deflation reduces afterload and lowers oxygen demands while inflation simultaneously augments supply. In addition, intramural pressure is lowest at the end of diastole rather than at the beginning[6] as in the ventricular lumen. While unassisted systemic blood pressure decreases throughout diastole as blood drains off peripherally, IABP-supported diastolic blood pressure remains much higher, thus providing pressure during the period in which the myocardium is most amenable to accept blood flow.

The work of Buckberg *et al.*[54] and its application by Philips *et al.*[170, 171] is a significant advance in the care of the cardiac patient.

In summary, the supply–demand ratio (EVR = DPTI/TTI) has been shown to be an accurate determinant of subendocardial ischaemia. The use of this ratio for monitoring is facilitated by a simple electronic digital computer* that provides a beat-by-beat estimate of subendocardial viability. Continuous monitoring of patients under intensive care in whom Swan–Ganz catheters and radial or brachial arterial lines are placed will give early evidence of ischaemic deterioration and potential extension of infarction. The effects of therapeutic interventions designed to decrease myocardial ischaemia can be observed by the rise or fall of the EVR.

Balloon removal

When haemodynamic improvement is evident, the balloon can either be turned off rapidly or the patient can be weaned from the balloon pump.

Weaning can be performed in one of several ways. First, the volume of the safety chamber balloon can be decreased, which will result in less balloon action in the intra-aortic balloon and a consequent weaning of the patient. Another mode is to turn the selector switch from 1:1 to 1:2 and then to 1:3. This form of synchronous weaning decreases the frequency of intra-aortic balloon action. This can be used in conjunction with decreasing the balloon volume, and then the patient can be weaned from the balloon in any desired time. Perhaps the easiest method of weaning over several

* Datascope Corporation, Paramus, New Jersey, USA

hours is simply not to recharge the slave balloon in the safety chamber with carbon dioxide.

After catheterization, if it has been decided that the patient appears haemodynamically stable when the balloon is shut off, the balloon should not be left unpulsating *in situ* for more than 1 hour[15]. I usually leave the balloon in for 1 hour after balloon pumping is stopped and then remove it[181]. At this point I leave a 1.5 cm stump of arterial graft and oversew the graft. Should the patient's condition deteriorate, the graft stump would be readily available for balloon reinsertion. The graft can also be removed in its entirety, and the vessel repaired primarily. When the balloon is removed from the graft, I usually pass a Fogarty catheter through the graft proximally and distally to remove any foreign debris[181]. Generally none is present, but occasionally a small clot will be removed.

Sequelae of dual-chambered intra-aortic balloon pumping

In the days following the balloon pumping procedure the following should be kept in mind. There is no way of knowing whether microscopic intimal damage has been sustained in the aorta in a given patient, although none has been reported to date. We usually convert our cardiogenic shock patients to longterm anticoagulants. We repeat serial cardiac-output determinations to assess the state of the patient's haemodynamic functions. Should the patient deteriorate again, the balloon is reinserted without hesitation, but the need for this is unusual. If after several days of improvement the patient begins to deteriorate and he has not previously been catheterized, it may be wise to consider him for arteriography at this point, since other cardiac lesions, such as a ventricular aneurysm may have developed. Broad-spectrum antibiotic coverage is continued for at least 2 days following the procedure. All survivors are considered for elective coronary arteriography and ventriculography during the same hospital admission if this was not performed initially while on IABP, which is our current practice.

Clinical experience with dual-chambered intra-aortic balloon pumping at the Columbia Presbyterian Medical Center

In recent years the development of modern direct techniques for cardiac revascularization has resulted in a multitude of critically ill patients undergoing open-heart surgery. Before the initiation and use of counterpulsation techniques in open-heart surgery, left ventricular power failure and refractory ventricular arrhythmias had been associated with a postoperative mortality in excess of 90 per cent.

Patient selection

In the 74 month period from 1st February, 1972, until 1st April, 1978, 2100 adult patients had corrective open-heart operations at the Columbia Presbyterian Medical Centre. One hundred of these patients underwent unidirectional IABP in conjunction with open-heart operations during that period. The average age of the 100 patients was 55 years (range 15–75 years). There were 61 men and 39 women.

The patients undergoing IABP were categorized under three separate groups.

Group A

The 39 patients in group A had either crescendo angina refractory to medical therapy or were in the low cardiac-output state or cardiogenic shock prior to cardiac catheterization; all of the latter patients had New York Heart Association class IV disease. It was felt that the angiography would be extremely hazardous for these individuals, and therefore IABP was instituted prior to these studies and continued throughout the catheterization and into the postoperative period.

Group B

Group B consisted of 41 patients in whom cardiopulmonary bypass could not be discontinued after operation despite maximal pharmacological support. All patients in this category had evidence of inadequate systemic perfusion, a high ventricular filling pressure, the need for excessive inotropic drugs, or refractory ventricular tachyarrhythmias.

Group C

The 20 patients in group C were all assisted in the open-heart recovery room within the first 24 hours following operation. All exhibited the progressive clinical picture of a low cardiac-output syndrome, consisting of arterial hypotension, a high left atrial or central venous pressure, and a markedly decreased urinary output despite a requirement for high-dose inotropic support.

Materials and techniques

The Datascope System 80 (more recently the System 82) was used to drive the intra-aortic balloon (*Figure 21.10*); the unidirectional dual-chambered intra-aortic balloon (30 or 35 ml) was selected for these studies, and the techniques described in the preceding section were used.

In the group A patients, intravenous aqueous heparin was administered in a dose of 5000 to 7500 units every 4 to 6 hours. In the intraoperative and postoperative patients, aspirin, 600 mg given rectally every 4 hours, was the sole 'anticoagulant'.

Haemodynamic parameters were monitored, including arterial blood pressure, pulse, central venous pressure, and wedge or left atrial pressure. Cardiac ouput was measured by thermodilution[221] when practical*, as were intraoperative coronary graft blood flows†. An indication of subendocardial blood flow was calculated by the method of Buckberg *et al.*[53] and Philips *et al.*[171] by means of the DPTI:TTI ratio. An analog computer was used to measure the EVR. An EVR of less than 0.8 implies subendocardial ischaemia.

* Edwards Laboratories, Inc., Santa Ana, California, USA
† Carolina Medical Electronics, King, North Carolina, USA

Results

Group A

The 39 patients in group A were assisted an average of 14 hours prior to operation (*Figure 21.19*). These patients all underwent uneventful preoperative cardiac catheterization with balloon support and were assisted an average of 72 hours postoperatively. With the onset of balloon pumping the pulmonary artery wedge pressures fell an average of 15 mmHg.

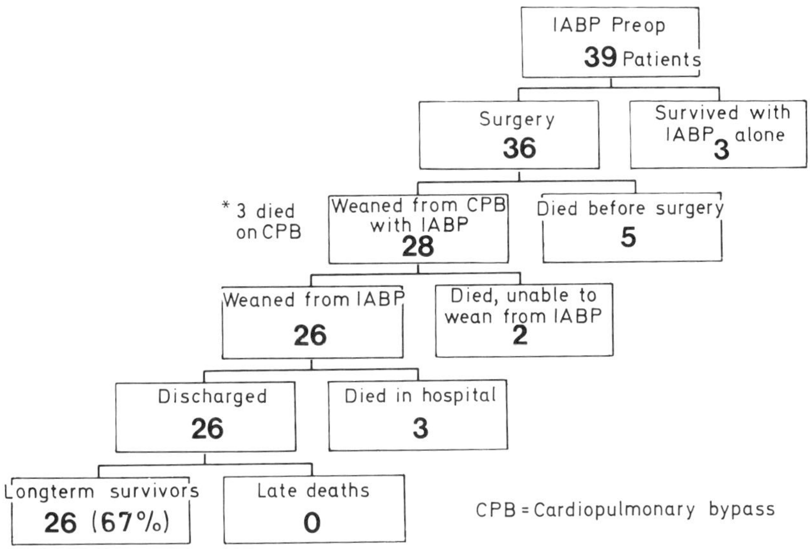

Figure 21.19 Columbia Presbyterian Medical Center. Preoperative unidirectional intra-aortic balloon pumping (IABP), 1972–78

Urinary output increased an average of 50 ml in the first hour of support, and the mean arterial pressure increased 25 mmHg. There was a marked decrease in the need for concurrent inotropic support. Twenty-six of the patients were longterm survivors (67%). The disease entities encountered in these patients included refractory heart failure with ventricular aneurysm, crescendo angina refractory to medical therapy, acute ventricular septal defects or acute mitral regurgitation after acute myocardial infarction, and early stages of cardiogenic shock.

Group B

The 41 patients in group B were assisted for an average of 48 hours after open-heart surgery (*Figure 21.20*). Fourteen patients incurred an acute intraoperative myocardial infarction, and 5 of these patients died. All 5 had diffuse subendocardial infarction of the left ventricle at autopsy.

The IABP effected an average rise in mean arterial pressure of 41 mmHg. Left atrial pressure fell an average of 16.5 mmHg in those patients who were weaned from cardiopulmonary bypass.

Eight of the patients had ventricular tachyarrhythmias after bypass that were resistant to high doses of antiarrhythmic drugs. The cessation of arrhythmias in this group was striking.

Thirty-six of the 41 patients in this group were successfully weaned from cardiopulmonary bypass, and 26 (63%) were discharged from the hospital.

The intraoperative responses of coronary graft blood flow to unidirectional IABP were measured in 12 of the group B patients. A uniform increase in coronary blood flow was observed in all patients when balloon

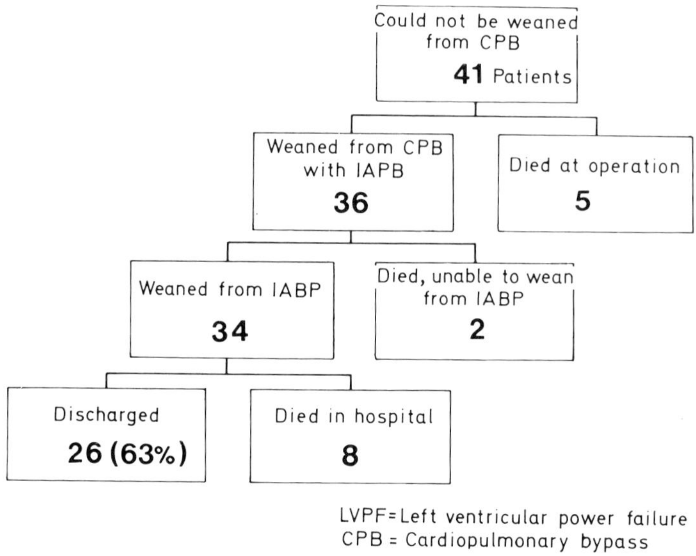

Figure 21.20 Columbia Presbyterian Medical Center. Intraoperative unidirectional intra-aortic balloon pumping (IABP), 1972–78

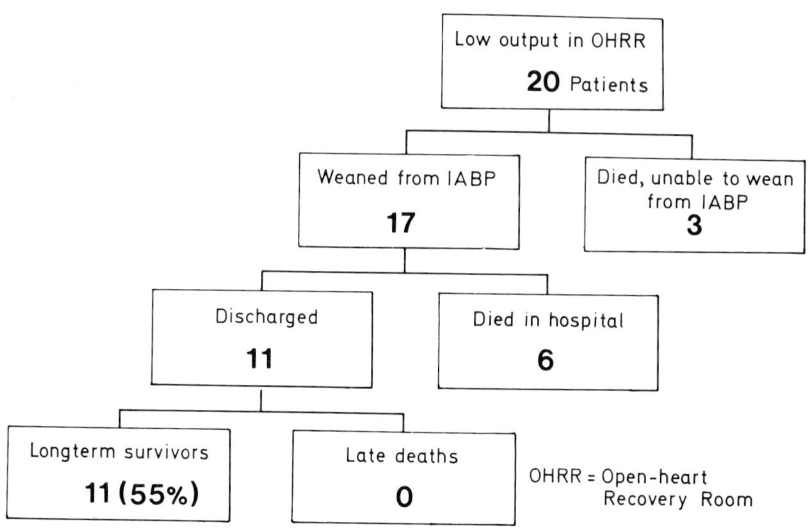

Figure 21.21 Columbia Presbyterian Medical Center. Postoperative unidirectional intra-aortic balloon pumping (IABP), 1972–78

assistance was instituted[44]. After the patient was weaned from cardiopulmonary bypass and the initial graft blood flow was measured during IABP, repeat measurements were also performed with the patient on and off assistance just prior to closure of the chest. The increase in coronary blood flow that can be attributed to the balloon alone was found to average 83 per cent (range 40–100 per cent, median 80 per cent). The increase in coronary blood flow was sustained during a 5 minute period of observation.

Group C

Group C consisted of 20 patients who were assisted an average of 14 hours after the completion of open-heart surgery (*Figure 21.21*). The duration of IABP averaged 64 hours, an increase of 33 per cent in time over the assist period for group B patients. With the onset of IABP the left atrial pressures fell an average of 13 mmHg and the central venous pressures fell an average of 7 cm H_2O in those patients who responded to the assist. Mean arterial blood pressure rose 38 mmHg. Urinary output increased an average of 36 ml per hour in the first hour of IABP. As in the other patient groups, there was a marked decrease in the concurrent requirement for inotropic support. Fifteen of the 20 patients in this category had a significant intraoperative acute myocardial infarction, and all of the patients undergoing coronary revascularization had at least one coronary graft in which the intraoperative blood flow measurement at the conclusion of cardiopulmonary bypass was less than 25 ml per minute. The changes in the course of these patients with acute myocardial ischaemia and its complications suggest that such patients can obtain the maximal beneficial response to IABP only if a careful early protocol is adopted so that the greatest mass of ischaemic myocardium will be preserved. Seventeen of the 20 patients assisted in this group could be weaned from the IABP, and 11 patients (55%) were discharged from the hospital.

An exciting report has been published from our institution by Reemtsma *et al.*[176], describing 3 balloon-dependent patients who underwent cardiac transplantation within 6 days of the requirement for the initiation of IABP. The intra-aortic balloon pump was removed in the operating room after the transplant was performed, and each of these 3 patients is alive and well at the time of writing, the longest follow-up being 14 months. Recently we have performed transplantation in a patient who had undergone emergency open-heart surgery for the closure of an acute ventricular septal defect secondary to a massive anteroseptal and lateral myocardial infarction. The patient was not improving on IABP support postoperatively, and transplantation was successfully performed on the fourth postoperative day.

Complications

Complications of IABP in the present series were relatively few and are reviewed in *Tables 21.2* and *21.3*. The balloon could not be inserted in 3 patients who would have been included in the group A category. In 25 patients the balloon tip required bending (*Figure 21.16*) so that it could be inserted in the ipsilateral extremity[37]. In one group B patient in whom the balloon could not be inserted in either extremity, the balloon was inserted

Table 21.2 Intra-aortic balloon insertions—100 patients at the Columbia Presbyterian Medical Center 1974–1978

Successful insertion at first attempt	94
Successful insertions contralateral extremity	2
Successful ascending aorta insertion	1
Unsuccessful insertion (1 extremity only)	3
Total	100

Table 21.3 Complications of balloon insertion—100 patients at the Columbia Presbyterian Medical Center 1974–1978

Lymph fistulas	2(2)*
Balloon rupture	0
Dissection (suspected)	1(1)
Femoral artery injury (surgical) with subsequent amputation	1
Femoral artery injury and infection with axillofemoral bypass graft	1(1)
Limb ischaemia with subsequent reinsertion	2
Total	7(4)

* Numbers in parentheses indicate survivors

directly in the ascending aorta[175]. This patient was successfully weaned from cardiopulmonary bypass and was returned to the operating room 3 days later for opening of the chest and removal of the balloon.

Relative limb ischaemia that abated after 1 hour was seen in 2 patients. There were 2 late peripheral vascular complications. In addition there was 1 local infection. Two lymph fistulae closed spontaneously within 2 months. In none of the patients undergoing valve replacement did sepsis develop. There were no patients with demonstrable emboli and arrhythmias were tracked without incident. Contraindications to IABP, which were not encountered in this series, are listed below.

Clinical experience with percutaneous intra-aortic balloon pumping

Results

From February 1979 to February 1981 percutaneous insertion of the single-chambered intra-aortic balloon pump by the Seldinger technique was attempted in 64 patients at the Columbia Presbyterian Medical Center. Successful percutaneous insertion was achieved in 57 of 64 patients (89%). In 7 of these 64 patients (11%) insertion by the percutaneous route could not be achieved.

If all patients with a cardiomyopathy are excluded from the present series, then percutaneous insertion of the intra-aortic balloon was attempted in 56 patients—in 50 (89%) it was successful, and in 6 (11%) it was unsuccessful.

There were 37 percutaneous insertion attempts in 37 male patients—32 (86%) which were successful and 5 (14%) which were unsuccessful. In comparison, percutaneous balloon insertion was attempted nineteen times in 19 female patients – in 18 (95%) it was successful and in 1 (5%) it was unsuccessful.

The location of percutaneous intra-aortic balloon insertion was varied. Nineteen balloons were placed in the cardiac care unit, 9 in the cardiac catheterization laboratory, 13 in the operating room and 9 in the open-heart recovery room.

Indications for percutaneous intra-aortic balloon pumping were broadly divided among surgical and medical groups. Of 56 patients undergoing percutaneous balloon insertion, 25 (45%) received the balloon for a surgical indication, whereas 31 (55%) required balloon support for a medical indication. Surgical indications were intraoperative low cardiac output in 16 patients, postoperative low cardiac output in 8, and cardiac arrest in 1. The medical indications for balloon counterpulsation were unstable angina, postinfarction angina, cardiogenic shock and ventricular septal defect following acute myocardial infarction in 8, 15, 5 and 3 patients, respectively.

Of the 31 patients in whom the intra-aortic balloon pump was inserted percutaneously for a medical indication, 24 (77%) ultimately underwent a cardiac surgical procedure.

Successful percutaneous balloon insertion was accomplished in 28 of 31 patients (90%) in the medical group and in 22 of 25 patients (88%) requiring balloon support for a surgical indication.

Fifty patients had successful insertion of the new single-chambered percutaneous balloon assist device and ultimately 44 (88%) underwent a cardiac surgical procedure, whereas 6 (12%) received medical treatment only. Of the 44 operative patients, 30 (68%) were discharged and 14 (32%) died. In the 6 patients undergoing medical therapy 5 (83%) were discharged and only 1 (17%) expired. In 6 patients the balloon could not be inserted by the percutaneous route. Five of these 6 patients (83%) underwent surgery and 3 (60%) were discharged, while 2 (40%) died. Only 1 of these 6 patients was treated medically and survived.

Of the 31 patients in whom the intra-aortic balloon pump was percutaneously inserted in the preoperative period for a medical indication, 28 (90%) were eventually discharged from the hospital. In contrast, only 11 of 25 patients (44%) undergoing percutaneous balloon counterpulsation for a surgical indication survived.

Of the 8 patients in whom the intra-aortic balloon was inserted for unstable angina, none died. Fourteen patients received the intra-aortic balloon for postinfarction angina and two died. In contrast, death occurred in 12 of 21 patients who required implantation of the intra-aortic balloon for low cardiac output either in the operating room or in the open-heart recovery room.

Complications associated with the percutaneous intra-aortic balloon were observed in 6 of the 56 patients. However, perforation of the aorta by the guidewire was the only insertion-related complication that occurred in our series. Complications related to balloon use and removal included iliac occlusion in 1 patient, femoral thrombi in 3 and weak dorsalis pedis pulses in 1. There was no balloon-related aortic dissection, sepsis, wound infection or false aneurysm. Extensive necropsy examination was not performed.

Contraindications to intra-aortic balloon pumping

(1) Severe aortic insufficiency.
(2) Cardiac standstill; ventricular fibrillation; profound hypotension (systolic blood pressure below 45 mmHg.
(3) Dissection of the aorta.
(4) Aortic aneurysm (thoracic, abdominal), aortic injury or both.
(5) Previous aortic surgery (relative contraindications).

Table 21.4 outlines the clinical summary for all 100 patients undergoing IABP. Seventy-four (74%) were weaned from IABP, and 63 (63 %) were discharged from the hospital.

Table 21.4 Unidirectional intra-aortic balloon pumping (IABP) and open-heart surgery at the Columbia Presbyterian Medical Center 1972–1978

Total patients	100
Number weaned from IABP	74 (74%)
Number discharged	63 (63%)

Clinical literature review

Myocardial infarction with shock

Initially it was believed that the IABP would be the physician's salvation in the management of patients with acute myocardial infarction and shock. In fact, when a given patient, who was in the shock syndrome secondary to acute myocardial infarction, was placed on IABP support, that patient invariably showed some clinical improvement. However, as the major experiences have evolved throughout the world with support of cardiogenic shock patients on intra-aortic balloons[7, 9, 65, 77, 99, 104, 119, 150, 224], certain basic and consistent observations have been made. Offering balloon support to patients who have been in shock for extended periods of time is not practical[189]. Although frequently there is an improvement in the patient's haemodynamics, organ function has usually reached irreversible deterioration, and the ultimate outcome of these patients is uniformly fatal. Therefore it appears more advisable to try to insert the intra-aortic balloon early during cardiogenic shock insult.

A more recent report by Hagemeijer *et al.*[93] involved 25 class III or IV myocardial infarction shock patients who were treated with IABP during a 4-year period. Twenty of these 25 patients were successfully weaned from the IABP, and 6 died within 3 months, 5 within the first 10 days of balloon weaning. Of the 14 patients who survived for more that 3 months, 13 were still alive at the time of the report, and 12 of the 13 were in functional class II. Six have resumed full activity. This report indicates that, even perhaps without surgery, with the early application of IABP a significant patient survival can be achieved.

An overall survival rate of approximately 50 per cent has been reported[22] for patients in cardiogenic shock secondary either to a mechanical defect complicating acute myocardial infarction or in shock patients treated with a combination of IABP and surgery. In a recent report[145] of IABP use in 728 patients, the rate of IABP-related mortality was only 0.8 per cent, and the survival of a large number of patients with acute myocardial ischaemia was attributed to the use of IABP. The success of this treatment modality, coupled with its low mortality rate has encouraged many authors[5, 8, 28, 66, 116, 129, 139, 178, 192, 220] to advocate the earlier institution of IABP support for cardiogenic shock. In all practical sense, it is recommended that all cardiogenic shock patients placed on IABP support undergo complete cardiac catheterization. This is usually performed within 12 hours of the insertion of the intra-aortic balloon pump. The unresolved question at this time is how next to proceed with the patient's care. If the patient is completely stable on the intra-aortic balloon pump, it has been suggested that the maximum benefit from the balloon will be achieved with 5 days of intra-aortic balloon pumping and accordingly the patient can then be weaned from the intra-aortic balloon. If the catheterization studies then dictate surgery, this can be performed usually within the same hospitalization. However, if the patient becomes balloon-dependent and cannot successfully be weaned from the intra-aortic balloon and from the associated pharmacological adjuncts, this situation has uniformly led to 100 per cent mortality even if surgical intervention is attempted. An exciting development in this regard has been the report by Reemtsma *et al.*[176]. If may evolve that cardiogenic shock patients who do well on IABP support and who have favourable anatomy during cardiac catheterization for revascularization, may do best with rather prompt surgical intervention which would include coronary revascularization and the avoidance of infarctectomy. The patients who may best profit from this therapeutic route seem to be those who respond most promptly to the balloon and who have major ischaemic changes on their electrocardiogram which return to normal with the onset of intra-aortic balloon pumping. At present, for the cardiogenic shock patient requiring intra-aortic balloon pump support and ultimately coronary revascularization surgery, the overall survival, as mentioned, is now being reported in excess of 50 per cent[13].

Myocardial infarction without shock

As evidence has accumulated supporting the use of IABP in postmyocardial infarction patients with shock, many authors[5, 8, 66, 116, 129, 139, 178, 192, 220] have supported the earlier institution of balloon pump therapy. Leinbach *et al.*[129] recently studied the reversibility of myocardial ischaemia through IABP use in patients with anterior myocardial infarction but without shock. Their criteria for selection were that the patients be under the age of 65 with pain and anterior ST segment elevation resistant to morphine, oxygen, and, in many cases, nitroglycerine. Continuous electrocardiographic monitoring was used, and, as soon as current therapy failure was observed, IABP therapy was instituted.

Five of the 11 patients studied responded with an 84 per cent fall in ST elevation in one hour, while maintaining precordial R waves and good ventricular function. The other 6 responded poorly, with a 40 per cent fall in ST elevation in one hour, Q wave development and poorer residual left ventricular function. Positive response correlated well with the presence or absence of complete left anterior descending coronary artery occlusion as demonstrated by coronary angiography. Thus, experimental documentation supports aggressive IABP therapy in the case of anterior infarction with residual anterior descending coronary artery patency.

High risk patients requiring cardiac catheterization

At present there is little doubt that a patient who has evidence of either a significant degree of left ventricular failure, ventricular tachyarrhythmia, or one of the acute mechanical complications of myocardial infarction, can be safely carried through cardiac catheterization without significant risk[90, 91,125,149,212]. Indeed, at the author's institution[34], 31 such intra-aortic balloon patients have been studied by the Judkins technique, and no patient with IABP support has incurred cardiac arrest or major complications in the Catheterization Laboratory. During the catheterization the balloon is momentarily switched off as the guidewire passes the balloon into the thoracic aorta. As soon as this procedure takes place, however, the balloon is returned to full function, and the catheterization proceeds uneventfully. Clearly, the intra-aortic balloon pump has significantly reduced the potential complications of cardiac catheterization in these critically ill patients. Cooper *et al.*[67] reported on 63 high risk myocardial revascularization patients who had preoperative IABP. Only 6 patients required rapid institution of cardiopulmonary bypass after anaesthetic induction despite marked drop in blood pressure in 50 per cent of the patients. There were 2 instances of post-pump power failure with 2 deaths in this series. The author concluded from this experience that preoperative IABP is a valid method of limiting morbidity associated with coronary surgery in high risk patients.

Preoperative IABP in high risk cardiac patients

The risks of early infarction and death in patients with acute coronary insufficiency are generally considered greater that in patients with stable angina. The most appropriate therapy, however, and the timing of that therapy, are points of significant controversy. Scully *et al.*[192] have recently studied the effects of preoperative IABP in 42 patients with acute coronary insufficiency complicated by abnormal left ventricular haemodynamics and refractory rest pain. Aggressive medical therapy had previously failed in all cases.

The perioperative mortality rate, when compared to that for similar patients treated before the use of IABP, was lowered from 25 to 8 per cent. Similar results have been achieved by Weintraub *et al.*[220], Langon *et al.*[123] and McEnany *et al.*[139]. In addition, inotropic support and duration of stay, both in intensive care and in the hospital, were decreased in the preoperative IABP group. Bolooki *et al.*[21] also report a shorter bypass time and Feola *et al.*[80] have noted an improvement in metabolic status as measured by decreased cardiac lactate production. Others have applied IABP[122, 126, 183] preoperatively in cases of decreased left ventricular function but the interpretation of the data is not as clear-cut as in the case of acute coronary insufficiency.

Perioperative intra-aortic balloon pumping

Myocardial failure following cardiopulmonary bypass constitutes a major complication of cardiac surgery, occurring in 4 per cent of all bypass operations performed at the Massachusetts General Hospital since 1971[139]. McEnany *et al.*[139] report that in their review of 728 cases in which IABP therapy has been instituted the most common indication (30.1%) for IABP therapy has been myocardial failure following cardiac surgery. Of these, 54.2 per cent survived.

Seventy-three per cent of the cases of perioperative IABP use were for coronary artery disease, while 24.4 per cent had undergone valve replacement. Survival was achieved in 55.5 per cent of the coronary artery disease group and 58.2 per cent in the valve replacement group. Of note is the fact that of the combined fatalities, 79 per cent occurred in the operating room while only 21 per cent took place after several days of IABP therapy and removal.

McEnany and his colleagues report that the most dramatic application of IABP is in helping wean those patients from cardiopulmonary bypass in whom intraoperative ischaemic damage or myocardial infarction precluded autonomous circulation. The group believes that the balloon acts as a temporizing device, supporting the patient at a lower level of myocardial work and oxygen demands, while the ischaemia can be reversed by normal coronary perfusion, perhaps augmented by the increased diastolic pressure. Still, surgical correction of lesions which inhibit adequate perfusion is essential. While perioperative IABP can reduce the occurrence of myocardial ischaemia during induction of anaesthesia and performance of an operation, it cannot compensate for inadequate surgical treatment. The use of IABP for weaning from cardiopulmonary bypass is clearly the most established use of balloon support. Most cardiac surgeons now believe that the availability of a balloon pump in a centre performing open-heart surgery should be mandatory.

Patients with crescendo angina refractory to medical therapy

The patient with recent onset of accelerated angina refractory to medical therapy or the patient in the immediate postinfarction period who continues to have chest pain is at major risk either to incur or to extend myocardial damage[8, 87, 201]. In a recent report by Levine *et al.*[131] 93 patients with severe unstable angina pectoris refractory to standard medical therapy which included beta-blockade, nitrates, heparin, oxygen, and bed-rest, were treated with IABP, early angiography, and myocardial revascularization surgery. Sixty patients were in the preinfarction group and 49 of these patients had complete relief of pain when the balloon was inserted. Forty-two of the 60 patients had typical ischaemic changes, and 18 had a variant pattern. Thirty-three patients were in the postinfarction angina group (less than 10 days), 25 had typical angina, and 8 had variant angina. Twenty-six of these patients had relief of pain with the IABP. Therefore, in 75 of the 93 patients, or 81 per cent, the balloon interrupted the ischaemic attacks, and in the remainder of the patients the frequency of ischaemic attacks was markedly reduced. In all 93 patients on balloon support angiography was uncomplicated. Of significance is that 52 per cent of the patients in this group had triple-vessel coronary artery disease. All patients underwent open-heart surgery and 2 of the 60 preinfarction patients expired; there was a total of 5 deaths or 4.5 per cent in this group. Two patients, one patient in each category, showed no postoperative Q waves (a 2.2 per cent incidence). In a late follow-up study of this group 74 per cent of the patients were angina-free. This experience and that of Weintraub *et al.*[220], Weintraub and Aroesty[219], Olinger *et al.*[162], Langon *et al.*[123] and McEnany *et al.*[139] demonstrate that IABP provides maximal perioperative myocardial protection in the patient with acute ischaemia before open-heart surgery and is certainly a major advance in the armamentarium of caring for these challenging patients. IABP does, however, carry with it a certain morbidity. McEnany *et al.*[139] have reported a decrease in their use of IABP for crescendo angina. The increased use of α- and β-blockade therapy, the increasing willingness to maintain propranolol therapy up to the time of operation, and the skilful use of vasodilators during induction of anaesthesia coupled with pulmonary artery wedge pressure monitoring, has allowed the satisfactory medical management of more patients with crescendo angina, and the safer administration of anaesthesia to patients with active myocardial ischaemia.

Postinfarction angina

Patients who have sustained a recent myocardial infarction and who subsequently develop anginal pain are at high risk to develop a second infarction in their already compromised myocardium. Bardet *et al.*[8] have reported a series of 21 patients with postinfarction angina (2 to 15 days after acute myocardial infarction) who did not respond to medical treatment. IABP therapy resulted in prevention of anginal pain and ST segment changes in all patients. Of note is that in 2 patients Q waves, which appeared during the anginal attack, disappeared without a shift of the QRS axis after a few hours of IABP therapy. Transient Q waves associated with angina pectoris and with Prinzmetal's angina have been attributed to reversible ischaemia. Bardet *et al.*[8] suggest that viable myocardium may be electrically silent and may recover normal activity when the balance between myocardial oxygen supply and demand is restored.

The great risk of death in patients with postinfarction angina and impending extension of a recent myocardial infarction unresponsive to medical treatment warrants more aggressive therapy. IABP stabilizes the clinical condition of such patients and thereby allows coronary arteriograms and operative intervention if the lesions are amenable to bypass surgery.

Tachyarrhythmias and ventricular irritability

The increase in coronary blood flow associated with IABP as well as the decrease in myocardial wall tension as a result of the acute reduction in left ventricular afterload is an ideal result in coping with ventricular tachyarrhythmias either in the setting of the coronary care unit or in the postoperative surgical patient[34]. The treatment of tachyarrhythmias after open-heart surgery with the IABP can frequently be definitive[225]. In the setting of the coronary care unit, however, many patients can be stabilized, and their arrhythmias will decrease significantly in frequency. It is the author's policy to catheterize every medical patient on an intra-aortic balloon whose indication for insertion has been ventricular tachyarrhythmias so that the patient's anatomy can be defined and surgical intervention can proceed if indicated.

Mundth[148] and Mundth *et al.*[150] have indicated that, in the medical setting, life-threatening, recurrent ventricular tachyarrhythmias in the acute postinfarct phase and in chronic coronary disease can be controlled initially with IABP as a prelude to cardiac catheterization and surgery. Ten patients with recurrent ventricular tachyarrhythmias were opeated upon, and seven survived.

Williams *et al.*[225] have reported success with IABP therapy even when no surgically correctable lesion is present, and recommend this therapy for all patients who develop ventricular or low nodal arrhythmias who are refractory to standard therapy.

High risk cardiac patients requiring major non-cardiac surgery

A few reports in the literature have suggested the use of IABP in high risk cardiac patients requiring major non-cardiac surgery. Investigators have reported the use of the IABP in high risk cardiac patients undergoing emergency gastrectomy[141], for other major abdominal surgery[9], and in peripartum cardiomyopathy[23]. An example of this technique is detailed in the following brief case report from this author's institution.

W.M., PH no. 2486872, a 64-year-old male, was admitted to the Columbia Presbyterian Medical Center with acute mitral insufficiency after a recent myocardial infarction. Despite a vigorous cardiotonic regimen, the patient was haemodynamically labile and at the borderline of pulmonary oedema. Routine chest x-ray revealed a coin lesion in the region of the right upper lobe. The patient was also anaemic, and further evaluation revealed an asymptomatic sigmoid carcinoma. Investigations for metastases were negative. The quandary in regard to this patient was that it would be ideal to know whether or not his carcinoma was resectable before performing a mitral valve replacement, but the instability of the patient seemed to preclude an exploratory laparotomy. On the day before surgery, the patient was taken to the surgical intensive care unit where a Swan–Ganz thermodilution catheter was inserted as well as the unidirectional intra-aortic balloon. The patient's haemodynamics improved on the IABP such that his wedge pressure fell and his cardiac output rose. The next day, the patient was taken electively to the operating room where an exploratory laparotomy revealed an isolated sigmoid carcinoma and no evidence of metastatic spread. A sigmoid resection was performed with a primary anastomosis. The abdomen was then closed, and the patient was returned to the surgical intensive care unit where he was gradually weaned off intra-aortic balloon support during the next 48 hours. He had an uneventful recovery and 3 weeks later he was returned to the operating room where, with the pulsatile assist device, his mitral valve was replaced. At this time the right pleural space was opened through the median sternotomy incision, and the coin lesion in the right upper lobe was easily palpable. There was no evidence of hilar adenopathy. The patient has successfully recovered from open-heart surgery and is now awaiting an elective pulmonary resection.

These new uses of IABP in patients with cardiac problems who require major non-cardiac surgery appear to have opened a new vista for the use of IABP as part of the routine surgical armamentarium in these high risk patients.

Septic shock

Sepsis is usually responded to by an increase in cardiac output, the limitation of which is posed by both Starling's law and the functional cardiac reserve of the individual patient. Ultimately the patient in septic shock will develop a low cardiac-output state; and, if the appropriate medical therapy fails, death will ensue. Berger *et al.*[13] reported on the fortuitous use of IABP in a septic shock patient who was initially thought to have a myocardial infarction with a low cardiac-output state. The distinct improvement in this patient prompted its use in a second individual. In both of these patients cardiac output could be maintained while the appropriate treatment including antibiotics and steroids, could be administered. The author's experience has also justified the concept of IABP in the low-output septic shock setting. Indeed, Berger's two initial patients ultimately were discharged from the hospital, and since then others[139, 163] have considered septic shock an indication for IABP therapy.

The author's experience would also suggest that the intra-aortic balloon can play a role in the management of patients in the low cardiac-output septic shock setting if used judiciously in regard to patient selection.

Paediatric intra-aortic balloon pumping

An obvious extension of counterpulsation would involve the paediatric age group. Two special balloon catheters have been designed*, one with a single-chambered 9 ml balloon and the second one with a 10 ml dual-chambered balloon[38, 40, 48]. Paediatric balloon pumping has been carried out three times at the Columbia Presbyterian Medical Center. In one instance the balloon was inserted directly into the ascending aorta of an infant. This patient was assisted for more than 48 hours postoperatively, and, although he initially responded to the balloon pump, he ultimately expired. A second, 5-year-old child with diphtheria myocarditis was assisted with IABP via the iliac artery through a 6 mm Dacron graft. Although the patient did respond haemodynamically to the balloon pump, she expired within 3 days, death ensuing from progressive pump failure. A third patient, aged 12, was assisted 48 hours postoperatively for a low cardiac output syndrome after a complex repair of a tetralogy of Fallot. An anomalous coronary artery crossing the pulmonary outflow tract was

*Datascope Corporation, Paramus, New Jersey, USA

identified, and therefore a Hancock conduit was employed to restore right ventricular-pulmonary artery continuity. However, the vessel most probably was injured because the patient sustained a massive postoperative myocardial infarction and was in a low cardiac-output state. The patient was assisted for 4 days postoperatively via the iliac route, and she survived.

There have been very few instances of paediatric intra-aortic balloon counterpulsation in the world literature[34, 35, 48]. Vascular access poses a significant problem in these children. With current technology, the only reasonable access in the infant is that directly through the ascending aorta with IABP. In dealing with children of a more advanced age, access can be accomplished through the peripheral route, as in two of the above cases. With paediatric IABP, the diastolic augmentation is usually at best equal to systole. However, systolic unloading is always achieved, as in the adult. With the passage of time and with improved techniques in balloon design, wider application of IABP in the paediatric age-group should take place.

Intra-aortic balloon pumping use for cardiac arrest of any aetiology

Another role for the intra-aortic balloon pumping made possible by the rapidity of the percutaneous approach is mechanical support during cardiac resuscitation. Conventional balloon insertion is not feasible during resuscitation because of the time required for surgical insertion. Because percutaneous insertion can be instituted in several minutes without interfering with resuscitative efforts or close chest massage, this approach can be used to provide mechanical circulatory support during resuscitation.

Time and scientific inquiry yield a more complete understanding of both the indications and contraindications for IABP support. Since it is simple in theory and practice[98], IABP insertion may be accomplished rapidly and efficiently, and thus appears ideal for the emergency situation. The haemodynamic effects of IABP actuation on left and right ventricular performance are immediate, and cannot be duplicated by pharmacological agents. These unique effects decrease right and left ventricular myocardial oxygen requirements (systolic unloading), increase biventricular indices of myocardial oxygen supply (diastolic augmentation), and increase right and left ventricular external performance (stroke volume) by the conversion of less efficient pressure work to more efficient volume work. Approximately one-third of the patients undergoing IABP support for postinfarction cardiogenic shock without additional surgery survive. As major institutions gain experience with the technique of IABP and confidence in their own capabilities with this therapeutic modality, there is a strong call in the literature[5, 8, 28, 66, 116, 129, 139, 178, 192, 220] for earlier initiation of IABP therapy. The realization that ischaemic heart disease is a reversible process inspires us to intercede before irreversible damage is done. Certainly IABP carries with it a certain morbidity and mortality [139] but its proven effectiveness and ease of initiation has led to the use of IABP as an adjunct in resuscitative measures following cardiac arrest of any aetiology[98]. Time and further study will delineate the safe and effective realm of IABP for this application.

Myocardial contusion

Myocardial contusion complicates approximately 20 per cent of cases of blunt anterior thoracic wall trauma[186]. Steering-wheel injuries are the most prevalent cause of myocardial contusion. Unfortunately, the diagnosis is frequently delayed or missed, complicating the treatment of the myocardial contusion which in turn may affect the treatment of associated injuries.

One of the most important physiological consequences which is always associated with severe myocardial contusions is decreased cardiac output. Proper treatment may be a major determinant of survival in some cases of severe myocardial contusion. While clinical IABP therapy for myocardial contusion has yet to be reported in the literature, Saunders and Doty[186] have applied this technique in dogs with experimentally induced myocardial contusion. The results of their study show that IABP does, in fact, improve left ventricular performance following myocardial contusion, especially when applied early after injury.

Community hospital use of intra-aortic balloon pumping

In most instances, in the medical setting, IABP use has ultimately been a prelude to cardiac catheterization and open-heart surgery. It is not practical to assume that every hospital with an intra-aortic balloon pump would have these facilities. With the advent of coronary care units, many patients with acute ischaemic and mechanical complications of myocardial infarction are being cared for in community hospitals. Accordingly, several community hospitals have purchased IABP equipment and have begun to insert intra-aortic balloons in selected patients in their coronary care units[11, 17, 139]. Patients included in early cardiogenic shock are primarily patients with preinfarction angina refractory to medical therapy and patients who have incurred one of the mechanical complications of acute myocardial infarction. These hospitals have formed a liaison with a major university hospital, and the patients are then transferred to that major hospital on balloon support for additional definitive therapy when it is required.

McEnany *et al.*[139] have reported that 32 of their 747 IABP's were started at peripheral community hospitals and the patients transported to the Massachusetts General Hospital while receiving diastolic augmentation support.

Recently, Bass, Katzman and Pois[11] have reported on their use of IABP in a private 280 bed hospital. After thoroughly training their nursing and supporting staff, they were able to report a survival rate of 44 per cent, comparable to that of major university centres.

Intra-aortic balloon pumping as a prelude to cardiac transplantation

Patients with low cardiac-output failure often require temporary mechanical circulatory support during evaluation and preparation for open-heart surgery. Occasionally, patients on the IABP have heart disease that is not amenable to usual surgical procedures. In addition, many patients on balloon support become balloon-dependent, and death usually ensues from progressive pump failure. At the Columbia Presbyterian Medical

Center the author and co-workers have begun to consider such patients for cardiac transplantation[4,21,37,64,80,105,126,159,176,202,228]. In five such patients, with a mean age of 47 years, we have maintained circulation with intra-aortic balloon support for an average of 7.8 days while a heart donor was found. Orthotopic cardiac transplantation was performed in all instances and circulatory assistance was discontinued immediately following transplantation. The Dacron graft was removed from the femoral artery with primary closure of the artery and meticulous closure of the wound. All patients were discharged from the hospital and the longest survivor has been 15 months to date. Disler, Scott Millar and Obel[71], have recently reported the maintenance of a cardiac transplant candidate on IABP for 30 days while a suitable donor was sought. In addition, the patient was transported, while on IABP support, 1400 kilometres by aeroplane.

Patients requiring IABP support are not ideal candidates for cardiac transplantation[176]. The incision in the groin, the femoral arteriotomy, and the use of a prosthetic graft on the artery—procedures well tolerated in other cardiac surgical patients—complicated the care of patients requiring immune suppression. Nevertheless, transplantation results in the immediate restoration of satisfactory circulation, which permits immediate removal of the balloon. Furthermore, the potential complications associated with the use of the balloon in patients on immunosuppression can be prevented.

It is the author's belief that this new approach to balloon dependency is a reasonable alternative to offer a patient whose death would otherwise be certain.

Effect of intra-aortic balloon pumping on right heart haemodynamics

The haemodynamic effect of IABP on left ventricular performance is well known. IABP support immediately decreases heart rate, left ventricular end-diastolic pressure and mean left atrial pressure[103]. It also causes a modest increase in cardiac output. Johnson *et al.*[103] have recently begun an in-depth haemodynamic assessment of IABP which includes right heart parameters as well. Actuation of IABP was consistently found to produce an instantaneous decrease in right atrial pressure averaging 11 per cent (reflecting a decrease in right ventricular preload). In addition, the major determinants of right ventricular afterload were found to decrease significantly. Pulmonary artery pressure decreased an average of 12 per cent and pulmonary vascular resistance decreased 19 per cent. These haemodynamic changes all occurred without a significant change in mean aortic pressure.

Reversed balloon to pump blood away from the heart

Pooley *et al.*[173] experimented with a unidirectional intra-aortic balloon in the downstream position so that blood would be pumped away from the heart. Downstream and standard unidirectional balloon pumping were compared in experiments with dogs. Downstream pumping effected a 32 per cent increase in cardiac index and a 24 per cent decrease in systemic vascular resistance. Upstream pumping in the normal animal did not significantly alter these parameters. This unique observation with reversed unidirectional IABP may perhaps have important implications for the treatment of low cardiac-output failure. Preliminary studies suggest that a baroreceptor reflex mechanism may be involved in this action.

Metabolic effects of intra-aortic balloon pumping

The metabolic effects of IABP are still under investigation and data are beginning to accumulate. Feola *et al.*[80] have examined myocardial lactate metabolism with pacing-induced tachycardia in seven patients. They found that lactate production changed from 0.24 ± 0.07 extraction at rest to 0.94 ± 0.01 production after pacing ($P < 0.001$) without IABP and from 0.10 ± 0.003 extraction at rest to 0.57 ± 0.001 production after pacing ($P < 0.001$) with counterpulsation. The difference between the lactate production levels occurring without and with counterpulsation was statistically significant ($P < 0.005$).

Spotnitz *et al.*[198] have examined levels of plasma catecholamines.

Previous studies have demonstrated that IABP or arterial counterpulsation reduces MVO_2 in the normal circulation by diminishing heart rate, peak LV systolic wall stress, and possibly, contractility[200, 205]. Wall stress in the left ventricle, an important determinant of oxygen consumption, can be decreased through reduction of either peak systolic pressure or of LVEDP and heart size[3]. Decreases in heart rate and reduction in frequency of ectopic beats suggest that IABP may reduce sympathetic tone and cardiac contractility through baroreceptor-mediated reflexes. This impression has been strengthened by observations of peripheral vasodilation[79] and increased frequency of discharge of the carotid sinus nerve[160] during IABP. The postulated reduction of sympathetic tone during IABP is further supported in the present study by observation of a decrease in circulating arterial epinephrine and norepinephrine during IABP.

Complications and other considerations

Major complications in the report by McEnany *et al.* of 728 cases occurred at a rate of 8.5 per cent[139]. IABP-related mortality was only 0.8 per cent. Other authors[126, 164, 210] have reported higher rates of both morbidity and mortality. Some acute complications[10, 97, 164] associated with IABP include arterial insufficiency of the catheterized limb, arterial emboli, retrograde aortic dissection, localized injury to the thoracic wall, balloon rupture with gas embolism, retroperitoneal aortoiliac haemorrhage, femoral artery false aneurysm, postischaemic neuritis, pericardial tamponade secondary to anticoagulants, thrombocytopenia, and certain immunological abnormalities. IABP can incur important hazards.

Our initial clinical experience suggests that the vascular complications associated with conventional surgical intra-aortic balloon insertion may be diminished by use of the percutaneous technique. Most previous reports of balloon-related complications of patients have indicated complications resulting from obstruction to the arteries supplying blood to the legs; less frequently, insertion of the device has been cited as the primary aetiologic factor. However, in a necropsy study of balloon-related complications, 60% resulted from conventional surgical insertion of the balloon[98a].

Whether the complications result primarily from obstruction of the arteries to the legs or insertion of the device, the ultimate determinant of balloon-related complications in most patients is the *status of the native arteries*[98a].

Several efforts have been directed at ameliorating complications of balloon use and insertion. Perhaps the most promising of these efforts has been the introduction of the percutaneous approach of balloon insertion, which obviates the need for surgical insertion and removal. Aortoiliofemoral angiography, Doppler monitoring, or both, have been recommended to access more optimally the distal arteries housing the device[1a,5a]. The addition of a central lumen to the intra-aortic balloon catheter to allow pressure monitoring or guidewire placement has also helped to avoid complications related to balloon insertion[228]. To maneuver around a tortous segment of the aortoiliac axis or negotiate passage through an eccentric arterial stenosis, the catheter tip may be bent and rotated into a modified J tip[37].

Complications occurred in 10.7% of our patients undergoing percutaneous balloon insertion[38]. In contrast to our experience Harvey *et al.*[95a] evaluated complications of percutaneous balloon pumping in 71 consecutive patients and found the number and magnitude of complications were comparable to their prior experience with conventional intra-aortic balloon insertion. They concluded that ease of insertion alone did not justify liberalizing indication for percutaneous intra-aortic balloon pumping among patients who can be managed effectively without counterpulsation.

Complications of percutaneous intra-aortic balloon pumping have been classified by Subramanian *et al.*[202a] into major and minor types and further subdivided into immediate and delayed[16]. Minor complications include malposition of the balloon in the ascending aorta, delay or difficulty in unfurling of the balloon within the aortic lumen, transient bacteraemia and transient loss of the dorsalis pedis pulse following percutaneous removal of the device. Major complications were those associated with haemorrhage at the attempted puncture site, renal embolism, dissection of the aortoiliac axis, ischaemic extremities or balloon-related death. In their series of 71 patients undergoing percutaneous balloon insertion, limb ischaemia without limb loss occurred in 9, haemorrhage at the puncture site in 2, aortic dissection in 2, renal embolism in 1 and pseudoaneurysm at the insertion site in 1. Asymptomatic loss of pedal pulses occurred in 6 patients. Malpositioning in the ascending aorta, which was encountered in 2 patients, and failure of the balloon to unwrap, which occurred in 10 patients, were successfully treated by repositioning of the device.

Immediate complications may be major or minor and included malpositioning of the balloon, persistent haemorrhage, and haematoma formation at the insertion site, transient bacteraemia, loss of dorsalis pedis pulse transiently, difficulty in unfurling the device, renal emboli and aortic dissection.

Necropsy evaluation of conventional intra-aortic balloon pumping has shown that patients with complications are not distinguishable from patients without complications either by the indications for insertion or the underlying cardiac disorder[98a]. Furthermore, the number of unsuccessful attempts at insertion does not necessarily predict a complication[98a].

Most complications appear to result from insertion of the device. One study suggests that insertion may be more difficult and attended by a higher complication rate in patients undergoing cardiac operations than in patients in whom a surgical procedure was not performed[98a].

There are several reasons why clinical studies may underestimate the true frequency of complications of intra-aortic balloon pumping. First, injury resulting from the use of the device may go unrecognized unless it results in a relatively catastrophic clinical consequence. Second, survival after attempted balloon insertion is often short; consequently, there may be inadequate time for the complications resulting from balloon insertion to evolve into clinically overt signs and symptoms. Third, most clinical studies of complications related to the balloon excluded patients in whom the balloon could not be successfully inserted. The frequency of complications in such patients is likely to be equal to, if not greater than, that in patients in whom balloon insertion was successful.

Aortoiliac dissection related to intra-aortic balloon insertion deserves special consideration. Aortoiliac arterial dissection has been reported as a complication of percutaneous balloon insertion. What is important to realize is that aortoiliac dissection is not always recognized clinically. In a group of 45 patients undergoing conventional intra-aortic balloon pump insertion dissection of the aortoiliac arterial axis occurred in 9[98a]. In none of these 9 patients was dissection suspected, much less recognized before death, and in 2 of the 9 patients the balloon functioned properly for 2 and 3 days, respectively, even though they were situated in the false channel. Thus, without necropsy, none of these 9 patients would have been classified as having had a complication. Only 3 of the 9 patients with a dissection survived more than 2 days after insertion. Wolfson *et al.*[10] have pointed out that there may be substantial delay in the appearance of clinical signs of dissection (pain, reduction in haematocrit, radiological abnormalities) despite injury to the arterial wall. Thus, in at least some patients, the limited survival after balloon insertion probably prevented the development of overt clinical signs of dissection that would have allowed clinical recognition of a balloon-related complication.

Isner *et al.*[98a] emphasized the difficulty of evaluating complications related to intra-aortic ballon pumping in patients whose baseline state is itself catastrophic. In the normotensive patient (one receiving the balloon prophylactically, for example) the precipitous onset of hypotension after balloon insertion would presumably be recognized as a catastrophic event. In contrast, in the patient who is hypotensive because of pump failure before balloon insertion, the persistence of hypotension after insertion would not be considered a new catastrophic event; more likely; it would be interpreted as pump failure refractory to counterpulsation.

In our experience with the percutaneous intra-aortic balloon, complications related to insertion of the device were observed in only 1 of 56 patients, and this resulted when the guidewire perforated the abdominal aorta. This represents a substantial reduction in insertion-related complications, however, none of our patients were subjected to an extensive necropsy analysis. Thus, percutaneous insertion of the intra-aortic balloon seems to diminish insertion-related complications. In contrast, complications associated with use and removal of the balloon are not decreased by percutaneous insertion.

Bemis *et al.*[11a] reported a complication rate of 5 per cent in a group of 44 patients in whom the IAB had been percutaneously implanted. Complications of percutaneous IAB were found in 18.5 per cent of 33 patients by Amsterdam *et al*[3a]. Insertion-related complications were not separated from complications occurring with balloon use and removal.

In conclusion, preliminary clinical experience suggests there may be a reduction of insertion-related complications by the percutaneous technique.

Initial reports of IABP use glowed with enthusiasm. Even though our own experiences have demonstrated the contraindications and limitations of this therapeutic modality, our own optimism transcends the literature. Scheidt[187] has offered some sobering observations:

(1) There exists no reported treatment series with a randomized (or any other) control group.
(2) The potential for bias in the medical literature may be quite significant. It seems likely that institutions with favourable results using IABP will be more likely to report their data, and it is further likely that manuscripts with positive rather than negative results will be accepted for publication. Many thousands of patients have received IABP during the past decade (one estimate is 5000 per year recently, calculated from the number of balloon catheters sold in 1976), yet the results of only a fraction of these have appeared in the medical literature.
(3) Nothing approaching a national registry, a large co-operative clinical trial, or even a single randomized study from one institution, exists to give us any confidence that we know the true efficacy of IABP for cardiogenic shock, postoperative ventricular failure, or any other indication. It seems premature to conclude, and authors do not, that we know the true role of IABP in limiting acute myocardial injury.
(4) There are significant complications associated with IABP therapy. The complication rates are acceptable in the shock patient whose mortality without IABP is exceedingly high, but might not be acceptable in the patient with acute myocardial infarction without shock, whose expected mortality is 6 per cent without cardiac failure or 17 per cent with mild-to-moderate congestive failure.
(5) Finally, there is the question of cost. Although the initial capital outlay for IABP is not great, surgeons, and operating room fees for insertion and removal of the balloon, the probable need for more intensive haemodynamic monitoring and nursing care, and a possible major increase in coronary angiography, all will inevitably greatly increase the cost of hospitalization for acute myocardial infarction. If IABP truly reduces mortality, complications, or disability resulting from myocardial infarction, the cost would be worthwhile.

Cost of intra-aortic balloon pumping

During the developmental years of IABP[76], haemodynamic effectiveness and reliability were emphasized. The cost was not prohibitive and has been only a peripheral consideration. However, increased utilization of IABP has stimulated the Texas Heart Institute[76] to establish a separate cost centre for its Circulatory Support Service and to undertake a study to determine the cost of IABP assistance.

Patient surveillance during IABP assistance, at the Texas Heart Institute, consists of continuous coverage by a registered nurse and a clinical engineer of the Circulatory Support Service. Patients were supported a total of 852 hours in 1975, 4176 in 1976 and 4446 through the first nine months of 1977. Because of this increased use of IABP and the concomitant increase in personnel time requirements, 2 biomedical engineering specialists have been added to the staff as well.

To generate an annual gross income sufficient to cover salary, expenses, supplies, equipment maintenance, and depreciation expenses, an IABP service charge of $100 for console set-up and the initial 2 hours of support was instituted, with an additional $20 per hour usage fee. A $100 charge for serial thermodilution cardiac output determinations includes the $75 cost of the necessary four-lumen catheter and use of the thermodilution cardiac-output computer. Professional fees and balloon cost are not included in these figures.

Direct IABP expenses include the cost of the balloon, console set-up and surveillance fees, thermodilution cardiac-output determinations, and additional operating room and anaesthesia expenses for balloon removal. When these direct fees are subtracted from the total, the expenses incurred by this group of patients is less than those with complicated recoveries. When compared to similar critically ill patients, the cost to a patient (including equipment and facility expenses, along with patient expenses) does not seem to prohibit its use.

New and future balloon designs

Because of the difficulty of balloon insertion by the peripheral route, Wolfson *et al.*[228] reported on a modified trisegment intra-aortic balloon with the addition of a 1 mm central lumen. This design would allow for arterial pressure measurement, contrast injection, and guidewire passage. This guidewire may be a useful adjunct in selected patients in whom the initial passage of the intra-aortic balloon meets with resistance. Our own experience with a hooked balloon[37] has led to successful insertion in more than 95 per cent of patients at the author's institution.

A modification of the unidirectional dual-chambered balloon has recently been developed and clinically tested (Datascope Corporation). This modification eliminates the catheter within the balloon proper and replaces the catheter leaving the stainless steel wire. This 'swivel balloon' can therefore be wrapped tightly about the stainless steel wire, and it allows for much easier peripheral balloon insertion. A recent advance has been the development of technology to insert this balloon percutaneously.

In our initial experience we found that the percutaneously inserted balloon catheter could not be easily inserted in patients with marked tortuosity of their iliac arteries. The stiff central wire, which forms the core of the percutaneous balloon catheter may prevent advancement of the catheter in such patients. Furthermore, negotiation of the aortic bifurcation is frequently not possible, particularly when the left iliac artery joins the aorta at a right-angle. To force the balloon catheter into the aorta may result in a dissection or perforation. Thus, to facilitate passage of the balloon catheter in patients with severe, aortoiliac disease a long sheath-dilator combination was designed[158a]. Since the long sheath-dilator is guided into the aorta by a safety wire, the likelihood that the dilator tip will dissect or perforate the arterial wall is reduced. As the long sheath-dilator combination is advanced over the guidewire, curves in the iliac artery are straightened. The long sheath extends beyond the diaphragm and thus provides for direct entry of the balloon catheter into the thoracic aorta.

Angiographic studies have demonstrated that mechanical dilation of severely stenotic peripheral arteries occurs with advancement of vascular dilators over guidewires[158a]. Although initial damage frequently results from this technique, arterial perforation is rare. Thus, this approach may permit insertion of the balloon catheter when other methods have failed and intra-aortic balloon pump support is desperately needed.

Several technical details should be carefully observed during insertion of the long sheath-dilator combination. Fluoroscopy is mandatory for observing the tip of the dilator as it transverses the aortoiliac arterial axis. Use of fluoroscopy also allows more precise positioning of the balloon in the aorta and permits evaluation of balloon inflation and deflation. Insertion of the long sheath-dilator apparatus requires a 0.038 inch guidewire; a smaller wire will not guide the tip of the 12F dilator and may cause arterial injury. After the balloon is positioned in the descending thoracic aorta, the sheath should be withdrawn before the balloon is inflated. Otherwise, the sheath may interfere with full inflation of the device or compromise distal perfusion of the contralateral extremity. Lastly, it should be remembered that the tapered tip of the dilator must be advanced ahead of the sheath during insertion into the femoral artery if crumpling of the sheath's tip is to be avoided.

Evaluating the safety of the long sheath-dilator will require experience with this technique in a larger series of patients. However, our initial application indicates this method is quite safe. One patient sustained thrombotic occlusion of the femoral artery and required surgical embolectomy. This complication was probably caused by prolonged occlusion of the femoral artery during compression of the puncture site after removal of the balloon catheter. It was not believed to be directly related to use of the long sheath-dilator and may occur with conventional balloon removal as well. Doppler monitoring of distal pulses during compression may avert such complications. If a doppler is not available, obliteration of the distal pulse with firm pressure should not be continued beyond 10 to 15 minutes.

We anticipate that use of the dilator-sheath combination in patients with severe tortuosity of the aortoiliac arterial axis will reduce the risk of arterial dissection or perforation during percutaneous balloon insertion. This 45 cm sheath provides a direct route into the descending thoracic aorta and protects the external iliac artery and aorta from injury during advancement of the intra-aortic balloon pump.

Ultimately, with advances in plastic technology, a blood-compatible elastic balloon material will be developed. This distensible balloon will lie flat on the catheter, and it should therefore be very easy to insert. An additional advantage of this balloon will enable the operator to vary the volume of the intra-aortic balloon once it is in place so that it will be more adaptable and haemodynamically effective over a wide range of aortic configurations.

Discussion

The importance of trying to achieve maximal coronary blood flow in a patient in cardiogenic shock secondary to an acute myocardial infarction is well understood. Acute major coronary occlusion with transmural infarction, rather than multicentric non-transmural infarction without coronary occlusion, is usually found in a patient with cardiogenic shock. The area of transmural infarction has the least blood flow, the greatest degree of muscle fibre destruction, and the poorest contractility. Adjacent to the area of frank infarction is a peripheral 'ischaemic zone' of myocardial tissue[69, 92] that presumably could maintain its viability if perfusion pressure were adequate to allow coronary collateral blood flow. There have been several reports in the literature regarding the effects of arterio-arterial counterpulsation and IABP in opening dormant coronary collateral channels[100, 101, 102]. This is particularly important in relation to the ischaemic zone of marginal myocardium. This zone could be preserved by the early institution of IABP, which would augment regional myocardial perfusion. The work of Jacobey *et al.* is further supported by other investigators who have clearly demonstrated that counterpulsation techniques can significantly reduce the extent of myocardial infarction[69, 157, 204]. If applied shortly after the coronary occlusion, before irreversible changes have taken place, IABP may be expected to minimize the area of myocardium that becomes necrotic and thereby improve the function of the ischaemic zone by improving the balance between myocardial oxygen supply and demand.

Kuhn *et al.*[118] demonstrated in dogs with acute myocardial infarction shock that increasing coronary blood flow by increasing coronary perfusion pressure through obstruction of the abdominal aorta for 1 hour was associated with an increase in cardiac output and an improvement in the mechanical efficiency of the ventricle. In some instances reversal of excess lactate production by the ventricle was demonstrated. Kuhn noted that left ventricular function was favourably affected by the pronounced increase in coronary blood flow despite the concurrent increase in the pressure load against which the left ventricle pumped. In general then, it would appear that deterioration of left ventricular performance in cardiogenic shock is largely related to diminished coronary blood flow. Under conditions of hypoxaemia, cardiac performance is coronary flow dependent, and unloading the heart does not necessarily improve myocardial muscular function by itself.

The primary beneficial effects of IABP are an increase in coronary blood flow and a decrease in left ventricular work[29, 31, 39–41, 43–48]. Clinical experience has failed to show that reducing left ventricular 'pressure work' alone reduces the mortality of patients having acute myocardial infarction with shock. However, coronary blood flow is apt to be pressure-dependent, since coronary arteriosclerosis is usually generalized and the vessels are narrowed proximally but dilated distally.

When the depressed coronary blood flow is restored to more normal levels, ventricular function is improved and susceptibility to arrhythmias is reduced.

The dual-chambered intra-aortic balloon was specifically designed for maximal increase of coronary blood flow. This balloon will increase coronary blood flow 66 per cent to 100 per cent over and above that obtained with a single-chambered balloon[206, 207]. It has been suggested that the intra-aortic balloon pump may not be effective during an extreme shock state when the arterial pressure is so low that the volume of blood in the aorta is on the flat portion of its pressure–volume curve[68]. However, this objection is obviated with the dual-chambered intra-aortic balloon because it phasically compartmentalizes the descending thoracic aorta in diastole and can thereby effectively increase coronary blood flow with even a minimal cardiac output[206, 207].

The single-chambered percutaneous balloon that is currently in use is more easily inflated and deflated than the conventional single-chambered balloon because the inlet and outlet gas ports at the end of the balloon are larger. Circulatory haemodynamics with the single-chambered percutaneous intra-aortic balloon were evaluated in 27 patients by Amsterdam *et al.*[3a] They found systolic blood pressure was unloaded from 121 to 108 mmHg ($P<0.025$), diastolic blood pressure was augmented from 65 to 123 mmHg ($P<0.001$) and cardiac index increased from 2.4 to 2.7 ℓ/min per m^2 ($P<0.001$) and stroke work index increased from 26 to 31 g-m/m^2 ($P<0.001$). Thus, percutaneous balloon pumping provides effective mechanical circulatory support. In addition, the percutaneous balloon is adaptable to any of the commercially available intra-aortic balloon pumping consoles.

Although IABP has been employed experimentally for the past 16 years[142, 143] and clinically for the past 10 years[109], only recently have data become available to evaluate its use in a variety of clinical settings. Initially it was felt that intervention with IABP in a patient with acute myocardial infarction and cardiogenic shock would lead to increased patient survival. However, although the shock syndrome is frequently reversed, the ultimate outcome has not been significantly altered[27]. There is no reason to expect an improved prognosis with conversion to the percutaneous approach, as circulatory haemodynamics are unchanged. However, some evidence is available which suggests that earlier institution of counterpulsation may enhance survival of patients with cardiac pump failure.

Ischaemic damage to the myocardium may be sublethal and reversible or more intense and prolonged, resulting in cell death. It is exceedingly difficult to define the boundaries which separate reversible from irreversible injury. Thus, the injured and failing heart exists along a continuum of progressive decompensation. Presumably, there is a point in time when the stressed myocardium still has the potential for recovery. By lowering the pressure at which the ventricle must expel its volume against and decreasing the pressure within the ventricle itself, the IAB reduces the work load of the ailing heart. In addition, the inadequate perfusion of the brain, heart and kidneys is augmented by counterpulsation with further reduction in myocardial work and oxygen consumption. Consequently, available chemical energy is diverted to synthetic and reparative cellular processes and the injured heart is allowed to recuperate.

Uses of unidirectional intra-aortic balloon pumping at the Columbia Presbyterian Medical Center

Surgical

(1) Intraoperative left ventricular power failure.
(2) Intraoperative and postoperative tachyarrhythmias refractory to medical therapy.
(3) Low cardiac-output state in the recovery room (within the first 12 hours).
(4) Evidence of severe postoperative subendocardial ischaemia.
(5) Intraoperative myocardial infarction with haemodynamic instability.
(6) Elective support of a preoperative high risk value or coronary patient.
(7) Elective support of high risk general surgical patients.

Combined medical and surgical

(1) Crescendo, preinfarction, or unstable angina refractory to medical therapy in preparation for coronary angiography and surgery.
(2) Preoperative support of patients with acute myocardial infarction complicated by a ventricular septal defect or acute mitral insufficiency.
(3) Support of unstable patients requiring cardiac catheterization and possible surgery.
(4) Support of patients incurring an acute myocardial infarction during cardiac catheterization.
(5) Cardiogenic shock patients within the first 12 hours after the onset of shock.
(6) Support of patients with uncomplicated myocardial infarctions with recurrent chest pain and evidence of infarct extension.
(7) Intractable tachyarrhythmias refractory to medical therapy.
(8) Support of medical or surgical patients in preparation for cardiac transplantation.

Other

(1) Support of patients with septic shock.
(2) Reduction of infarct size.
(3) Support of infants with myocarditis and intractable congestive heart failure refractory to medical therapy.

The most successful use of IABP to date has been as an adjunct to the preoperative, intraoperative, and postoperative support of patients undergoing open-heart surgery[27, 31, 38]. As can be seen in our group A patients, it is now possible to stabilize the condition of critically ill individuals, subject them to cardiac catheterization safely, and bring them to the operating room in a more stable condition. Also, high risk patients and those individuals with critical coronary artery lesions can undergo anaesthetic induction in relative safety with use of intra-aortic balloon support until cardiopulmonary bypass can be established. The results in our groups B and C patients demonstrate the success of IABP in weaning patients from cardiopulmonary bypass who have incurred either subendocardial ischaemia our infarction during the procedure and in supporting them in the postoperative period.

In our early experience with the conventional dual-chambered IABP 63 patients underwent balloon pumping for 1972 to 1976. Of these 63 patients, 17 patients (27%) received the balloon for a medical indication. None of these 17 patients died prior to operation and 11 (65%) were discharged from the hospital. In contrast, the IABP was inserted in 46 of 63 patients (73%) intraoperatively or shortly thereafter. Twenty-nine of these 46 patients (63%) subsequently left the hospital. Therefore, the percentage of patients undergoing preoperative percutaneous intra-aortic balloon pumping has expanded.

Reasons for the decreased survival rate in surgical patients assisted with the percutaneously inserted balloon are unclear, but probably are related to improvements in myocardial protection during cardiac surgical procedures. Consequently, a more seriously ill group of patients are receiving perioperative intra-aortic balloon support.

In our experience 45 per cent of patients received the intra-aortic balloon pump for surgical indication and 55 per cent were assisted preoperatively for a medical indication. Of the patients in whom the balloon pump had been placed for a surgical indication, 44 per cent survived. In contrast, 90 per cent of patients in our series undergoing preoperative intra-aortic balloon pumping for a medical indication ultimately were discharged from the hospital. Thus, it appears that preoperative implantation of the intra-aortic balloon pump for a medical indication is associated with a lower mortality rate than insertion of the device for a surgical indication.

In interpreting the above conclusions several points are worth mentioning. No data exists which suggests that the duration of counterpulsation affects outcome. Seventy-seven per cent of our patients initially assisted with the intra-aortic balloon for a medical indication eventually underwent a cardiac surgical procedure. Therefore, it is likely that surgery, itself, improved the survival of patients receiving preoperative balloon assistance. In summary, what is truly needed is a randomized, carefully controlled, prospective trial to determine whether preoperative balloon counterpulsation in patients with either unstable angina or postinfarction angina effects ultimate survival. What is clear to us, as well as to many cardiologists and cardiac surgeons throughout the world, is that such patients dramatically improve when intra-aortic balloon pumping is commenced.

Our clinical data confirm the theoretical and experimental observations of Buckberg *et al.*[53,54] who suggested that the adequacy of subendocardial perfusion and potential ischaemia could be predicted from indices of systolic and diastolic pressure measurements. Since ischaemia appears to be the most common cause of the low cardiac-output syndrome following open-heart surgery, it is imperative to recognize the condition early if proper therapy is to be initiated in time to prevent myocardial necrosis.

The increase in coronary blood flow during IABP, documented in our patients in conjunction with the improvement in EVR, suggests that a redistribution of transmural coronary blood flow has occurred and that the previously jeopardized subendocardial muscle is now being adequately perfused[44]. The hospital survival (74 per cent) and the longterm survival (63 per cent) in our series compares well with the encouraging data reported by other groups in similar patients.

An analysis of the data obtained in patients assisted with unidirectional IABP in conjunction with open-heart surgery at the Columbia Presbyterian Medical Center has led to 2 groups of criteria for employing intraoperative IABP[44].

The primary indications for intraoperative IABP as suggested by our data include any 2 of criteria 1 to 3 in conjunction with criterion 4 in patients in whom weaning from cardiopulmonary bypass has been attempted for one hour: (1) mean blood pressure 60 mmHg and falling; (2) cardiac index 1.8 ℓ/min per m^2 and falling; (3) left atrial pressure 25 mmHg and rising; and (4) requirement for high-dose inotropic support and/or afterload reduction.

Additional criteria include: (1) recurrent ventricular tachyarrhythmias; (2) evidence of a significant intraoperative myocardial infarction; and (3) subendocardial ischaemia (EVR less than 0.8 at the conclusion of bypass).

It is interesting in retrospect to see that most of our group C patients fell into these categories. They would now probably become group B patients. This will be particularly true when better methods for the detection and sizing of intraoperative myocardial infarcts become available.

Because of the potentially wide applicability of IABP, safety has been a major concern in our clinical set-up. The Datascope System incorporates a fail-safe system for tracking arrhythmias, an external safety chamber, an appropriately timed vacuum, adequate mobility to ensure that the patient can be transported safely during balloon pumping, and the facility for using a soluble gas (carbon dioxide) to drive the intra-aortic balloon[38]. Carbon dioxide is 20 times more soluble in plasma than is air or oxygen. Furman *et al.*[83] have clearly documented that when helium escapes from a ruptured intra-aortic balloon, death of the experimental animal is almost instantaneous and is certain. Also reported has been the clinical rupture of an intra-aortic balloon driven by helium gas, with the prompt death of the patient[144]. Turner *et al.*[208] have reported 100 cineangiocardiographic studies using 50 to 60 ml carbon dioxide with no morbidity. In our opinion this safe soluble gas, carbon dioxide, can and should be used during IABP. We believe its use is most effective if an appropriately timed vacuum is applied to the system to ensure complete and prompt balloon deflation.

It is apparent from the many indications for IABP that both the system and the balloon should be highly reliable, mobile, and fail-safe. It also appears that aortic insufficiency may not be an absolute contraindication to IABP[229].

There will continue to be patients who can be successfully supported by an intra-aortic balloon device but who will reach a plateau of stability and who will then be unable to be weaned from intra-aortic balloon assistance. It is our present feeling that all patients on IABP should then be studied with cinecoronary angiography and left ventriculography within 12 to 24

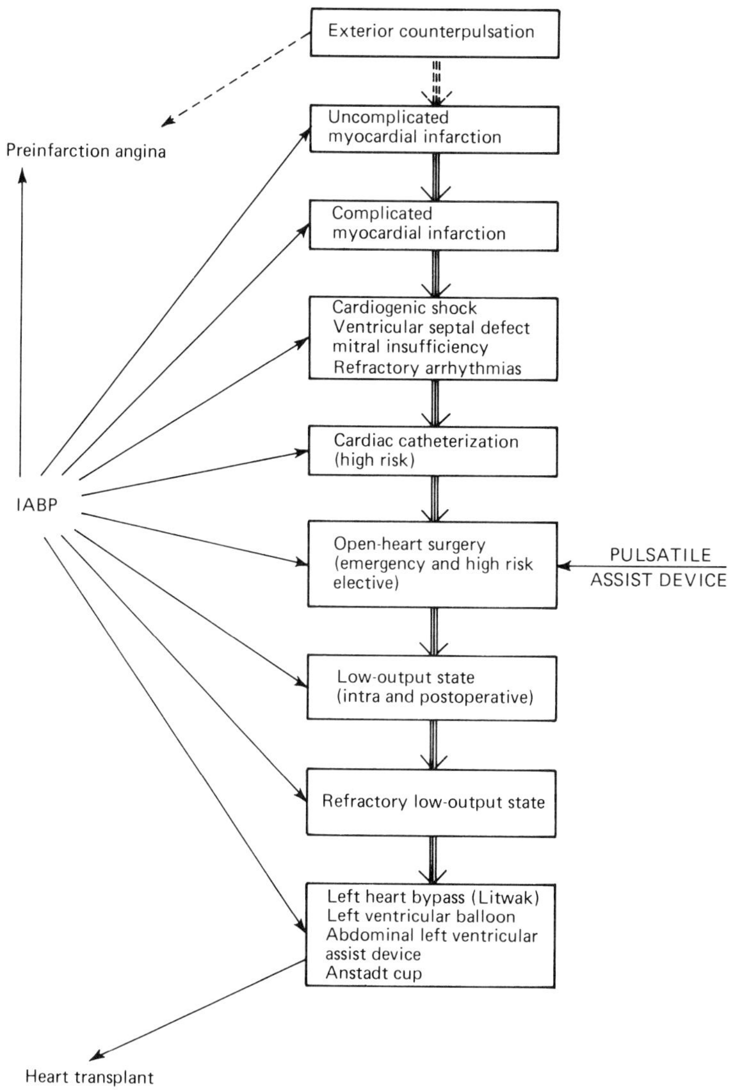

Figure 21.22 The role of left heart assist devices in clinical medicine

hours of balloon insertion and have definitive open-heart surgery performed on the basis of the radiographic findings. We also advocate angiographic study of patients surviving circulatory assistance during the same hospitalization who had not been studied in the acute phase. In conjunction with myocardial revascularization and the resection of ischaemic and non-contractile segments or ventricular aneurysms, it is anticipated that many patients who formerly could not be saved will now be brought to the operating room for definitive operation in a more viable state.

We have demonstrated that acutely ill patients can be supported with this mode of circulatory assistance and then be brought to the operating room for cardiac transplants. Eventually replacement of the heart with a total artificial heart will be feasible (*Figure 21.22*).

It is our impression that the use of IABP in selected patients undergoing open-heart surgery has led to greater patient survival and has enabled us to operate upon high risk patients with greater confidence and with improved clinical results. More significantly, use of the PAD has extended the role of counterpulsation in open-heart surgery and decreased the need for postoperative balloon pumping in these high risk patients.

The rapidity of insertion makes the percutaneously inserted balloon most useful in supporting patients with an acute coronary ischaemic syndrome. Using conventional surgical techniques, an experienced surgeon requires 30 to 45 minutes to insert the intra-aortic balloon, and must perform a second operative procedure for balloon removal. The percutaneous approach to intra-aortic balloon pumping facilitates insertion and removal and permits rapid institution of mechanical circulatory support. The availability of rapid percutaneous insertion of the intra-aortic balloon has broadened clinical indications for balloon pumping.

Comparing techniques of intra-aortic balloon insertion, Bemis *et al.*[11a] found that percutaneous insertion was unsuccessful in 91 per cent of 44 patients, whereas balloon insertion through a conventional arteriotomy was attended by a failure rate of 15 per cent. Amsterdam *et al.*[3a] were able to insert percutaneously the intra-aortic balloon in 27 of 33 patients for a failure rate of 18.2 per cent. The preliminary experience of Subramanian *et al.*[202a] with the percutaneous IAB, was unsuccessful insertion in only 4 of 37 patients (10.8%). In our own experience, insertion by the percutaneous route could not be accomplished in 7 of 64 patients (11%).

We did not find a higher failure rate for insertion in females as suggested by Isner *et al*[98a]. In fact, the number of unsuccessful insertion attempts in males was substantially greater in our series. A higher failure rate in older patients with more extensive aortoiliac atherosclerosis has been reported. Modifications in percutaneous IAB technology such as the long sheath-dilator combination and the dual-lumen balloon catheter promise further reductions in the number of unsuccessful insertions.

In patients with refractory angina after acute myocardial infarction, the risks of coronary arteriography are increased[15]. In this group of patients, the intra-aortic balloon may be inserted by the percutaneous technique in the catheterization laboratory just before coronary arteriography. This approach protects the patient during the angiographic study, and the balloon may be left in place to provide circulatory support for the patient during induction of anaesthesia and in the perioperative period.

Rapid percutaneous insertion of the intra-aortic balloon is particularly useful in patients experiencing severe myocardial ischaemia or acute myocardial infarction during coronary arteriography. In these patients the coronary catheter can be rapidly exchanged for the balloon pump through the same puncture site in the femoral artery. In patients experiencing acute myocardial infarction during coronary arteriography, percutaneous intra-aortic balloon placement and pumping rapidly reversed cardiogenic shock

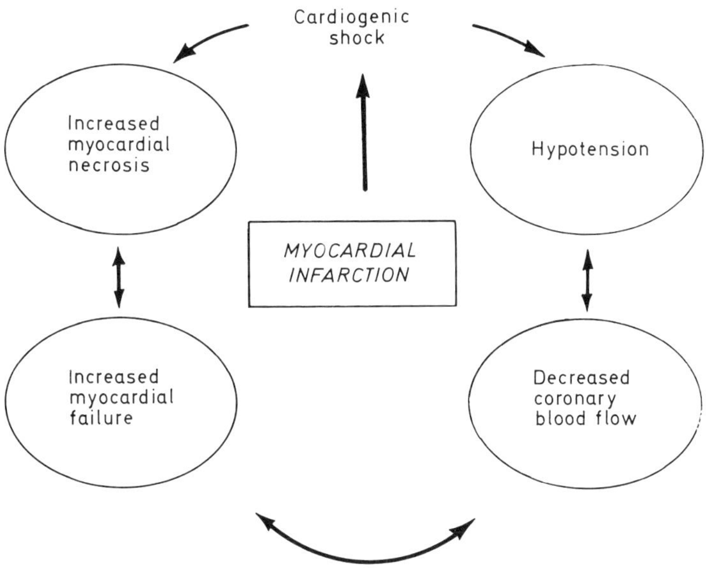

Figure 21.23 Vicious cycle of cardiogenic shock. IABP can interrupt the cycle at any point

and supported the patients during emergency revascularization and in the postoperative period.

Some patients continue to have severe angina after infarction despite aggressive medical therapy and are candidates for coronary artery bypass surgery. Good surgical results have been achieved in such patients with reduced operative mortality[8, 104a, 131a, 219a]. Some authors have attributed this reduction in mortality to the liberal use of postinfarction intra-aortic balloon pumping[8, 219a].

On the contrary, Brundage *et al.*[51a] infrequently use the intra-aortic balloon pump in the management of postinfarction angina. Only 3 of 30 patients (10%) required the IABP. They advocate use of the IABP only to control haemodynamic instability, not to control angina.

In our experience and that of others[3a, 11a], the majority of patients with unstable angina or postinfarction angina survive with intra-aortic balloon pumping. Amsterdam *et al.*[3a] found that patients with unstable angina or postinfarction angina who underwent preoperative counterpulsation had survival rates of 78 per cent and 100 per cent, respectively.

It is anticipated that the technique of IABP, as it becomes more widely accepted and indications for its use become more clearly defined, will be used earlier to break the vicious cycle (*Figure 21.23*) that entraps the patient in cardiogenic shock. Then clinical results of this encouraging mechanical assist technique will more accurately reflect survival rather than salvage figures.

Acknowledgements

The author wishes to thank Dr James R. Malm, Dr Keith Reemtsma, Dr Frederick O. Bowman, Jr., Dr Richard N. Edie, Dr Henry M. Spotnitz, Michael Bailin, and the entire professional staff of the Presbyterian Hospital in the City of New York at the Columbia Presbyterian Medical Center for their continued support of this work in both its clinical and experimental applications.

I would also like to express my thanks to Mr Donald Kurth for his assistance with the literature review.

References

1. Alonso, D. R., Scheidt, S., Post, M. and Killip, T. 'Pathophysiology of cardiogenic shock. Quantification of myocardial necrosis, clinical, pathologic and electrocardiograph correlations.' *Circulation*, **48,** 588 (1973)

1a. Alpert, J, Bhaktan, E. K., Gielchinsky, I., *et al.* 'Vascular complications of intra-aortic balloon pumping.' *Archives of Surgery*, **111,** 1190 (1976)

2. American Heart Association. *Heart Facts*. Dallas: American Heart Association (1981)

3. American Heart Association. *Heart Facts*. New York: American Heart Association (1976)

3a. Amsterdam, E. A., Low R. I., Bommer, *et al.* 'Mechanical circulatory assistence by the percutaneous intra-aortic balloon.' *Pump Clinical Research* (Abstract)

4. Avery, G. J., Spotnitz, H. M., Reemtsma, K., Malm, J. R. and Bregman, D. 'A new counterpulsation device for the treatment of acute pulmonary embolus and canine circulatory dynamics.' *Transactions of the American Society for Artificial Internal Organs*, **23,** 103 (1977)

5. Bahn, C. H. 'Cardiac catheterization and intra-aortic balloon counterpulsation.' (Letters to the Editor). *American Journal of Cardiology*, **42,** 873 (1978)

5a. Bahn, C. H., Vitikainin, K. J., Anderson, C. L. and Whitney, R. B. 'Vascular evaluation for balloon pumping.' *Annals of Thoracic Surgery*, **27,** 474 (1978)

6. Baird, R. J., Adiseshiah, M. and Okumori, M. 'The gradient in regional myocardial tissue pressure in the left ventricle during diastole: its relationship to regional flow distribution.' *Journal of Surgical Research*, **20,** 11 (1976)

7. Bardet, J., Masquet, C., Kahn, J. C., Gourgon, R., Bourdarias, J. P., Mathivat, A. and Bouvrain, Y. 'Clinical and haemodynamic results of intra-aortic balloon counterpulsation and surgery for cardiogenic shock.' *American Heart Journal*, **93,** 280 (1977)

8. Bardet, J., Rigaud, M., Kahn, J. C., Huret, J. F., Gandjbakhch, I. and Bourdarias, J. P. 'Treatment of post-myocardial infarction angina by intra-aortic balloon pumping and emergency revascularization.' *Journal of Thoracic and Cardiovascular Surgery*, **74,** 299 (1977)

9. Baron, D. W. and O'Rourke, M. F. 'Long-term results of arterial counterpulsation in acute severe cardiac failure complicating myocardial infarction.' *British Heart Journal*, **38,** 285 (1976)

10. Barsamian, E. M., Goldman, M. H., Crane, C., Felix, R., Jr., Braunwald, N. S., Buchholtz, T. and Smith, B. 'Femorofemoral bypass graft in intra-aortic balloon counterpulsation.' *Archives of Surgery*, **111,** 1070 (1976)

11. Bass, J., Jr., Katzman, L. and Pois, A. J. 'Experience with intra-aortic balloon counterpulsation in a community hospital.' *American Surgeon*, **44,** 324 (1978)
11a. Bemis, C. E., Mundth, E. D., Mintz, G. S., *et al.* 'Comparison of techniques for intra-aortic balloon insertion.' *American Journal of Cardiology*, (Abstract) **47,** 417 (1981)
12. Berger, R. L. and Saini, V. K. 'Conversion of nonpulsatile cardiopulmonary bypass to pulsatile flow by intra-aortic balloon pumping during myocardial revascularization for cardiogenic shock.' (Abstr.) *Circulation*, **45** and **46 (Suppl. II),** 130 (1972)
13. Berger, R. L., Saini, V. K., Long, W., Hechtman, H. and Hood, W., Jr. 'The use of diastolic augmentation with the intra-aortic balloon in human septic shock with associated coronary artery disease.' *Surgery*, **74,** 601 (1973)
14. Berger, R. L., Saini, V. K., Ryan, T. J., Sokol, D. M. and Keefe, J. F. 'Intra-aortic balloon assist for postcardiotomy cardiogenic shock.' *Journal of Thoracic and Cardiovascular Surgery*, **66,** 906 (1973)
15. Bernstein, E. F. and Murphy, A. E. 'The importance of pulsation in preventing thrombosis from intra-aortic balloons. A note of caution.' *Journal of Thoracic and Cardiovascular Surgery*, **62,** 950 (1971)
16. Bleifeld, W., Bussmann, W. D., Meyer, J. and Effert, S. 'Improved cardiac assistance with an aortic arch balloon.' *Cardiovascular Research*, **7,** 115 (1973)
17. Bolooki, H. *Clinical Application of Intra-aortic Balloon Pump*. New York: Futura Publishing Co. (1977)
18. Bolooki, H. 'Prolonged left ventricular pressure monitoring with a transducer catheter.' *Surgery*, **73,** 97 (1973)
19. Bolooki, H., Lemberg, L., Economides, C., Caldwell, T. and Jude, J. R. 'Clinical pathological and surgical correlation in patients with acute myocardial infarction and pump failure.' *Circulation*, **44**, 1034 (1971)
20. Bolooki, H., Mallon, S., Ghahramani, A., Sommer, L., Vargas, A., Slavin, D. and Kaiser, G. A. 'Objective assessment of the effects of aorto-coronary bypass operation on cardiac function.' *Journal of Thoracic and Cardiovascular Surgery*, **66,** 916 (1973)
21. Bolooki, H., Williams, W., Thurer, R. J., Vargas, A., Kaiser, G. A., Mack, F. and Ghahramani, A. R. 'Clinical and haemodynamic criteria for use of the intra-aortic balloon pump in patients requiring cardiac surgery.' *Journal of Thoracic and Cardiovascular Surgery*, **72,** 756 (1976)
22. Bourdarias, J. P., Gourgon, R. and Bardet, J. 'Mechanical circulatory assistance by intra-aortic balloon pumping for the treatment of cardiogenic shock.' *Intensive Care Medicine*, **4,** 29 (1978)
23. Brantigan, C. O., Grow, J. B., Sr. and Schoonmaker, F. W. 'Extended use of intra-aortic balloon pumping in peripartum cardiomyopathy.' *Annals of Surgery*, **183,** 1 (1976)
24. Braunwald, E. 'Control of myocardial oxygen consumption.' *American Journal of Cardiology*, **27,** 416 (1971)
25. Braunwald, E., Covell, J. W., Maroko, D. R. and Ross, J. R., Jr. 'Effects of drugs and of counterpulsation on myocardial oxygen consumption.' *Circulation*, **38** and **40 (Suppl. IV),** 220 (1969)
26. Bregman, D. Unpublished data
27. Bregman, D. 'Assessment of intra-aortic balloon counterpulsation in cardiogenic shock.' *Critical Care Medicine*, **3,** 90 (1975)
28. Bregman, D. 'Cardiac assist devices.' In *Blades' Surgical Diseases of the Chest*. 4th edition. Ed. D. B. Effler. St. Louis: C. V. Mosby Co. (1978)
29. Bregman, C. 'Clinical experience with a new pulsatile assist device (PAD) during open-heart surgery.' *Artificial Organs*, **2,** 3 (1978)

30. Bregman, D. 'Clinical experience with the dual-chambered intra-aortic balloon and system 80.' *Journal of Cardiovascular Surgery*, **15,** 193 (1974)
31. Bregman, D. 'Dual-chambered intra-aortic balloon counterpulsation.' In *Current Techniques in Extracorporeal Circulation*. Eds M. I. Ionescu and G. H. Wooler. pp. 407–516. London: Butterworths (1976)
32. Bregman, D. 'Intra-aortic balloon in open-heart surgery.' *New England Journal of Medicine*, **284,** 393 (1971)
33. Bregman, D. 'Management of patients undergoing intra-aortic balloon pumping.' *Heart and Lung*, **3,** 916 (1974)
34. Bregman, D. 'Mechanical support of the failing heart.' In *Current Problems in Surgery*. Ed. M. M. Ravitch. Chicago: Year Book Medical Publishers (1976)
35. Bregman, D. *Mechanical Support of the Failing Heart and Lungs*. New York: Appleton-Century-Crofts (1977)
36. Bregman, D. 'Technique of circulatory assistance.' *New England Journal of Medicine*, **285,** 1261 (1971)
37. Bregman, D., Bolooki, H. and Malm, J. R. 'A simple method to facilitate difficult intra-aortic balloon insertions.' *Annals of Thoracic Surgery*, **15,** 636 (1073)

37a. Bregman, D. and Cohen, S. R. 'Mechanical support of circulation: current status.' *Contemporary Surgery*. (In press)

38. Bregman, D. and Goetz, R. H. 'A failsafe cardiac assist system for intra-aortic balloon pumping.' *Transactions of the American Society for Artificial Internal Organs*, **17,** 505 (1972)
39. Bregman, D. and Goetz, R. H. 'A new concept in circulatory assistance – the dual-chambered intra-aortic balloon.' *Mount Sinai Journal of Medicine*, **39,** 123 (1972)
40. Bregman, D. and Goetz, R. H. 'Clinical experience with a new cardiac assist device – the dual-chambered intra-aortic balloon assist.' *Journal of Thoracic and Cardiovascular Surgery*, **62,** 577 (1971)
41. Bregman, D., Kripke, D. C., Cohen, M. N., Laniado, S. and Goetz, R. H. 'Clinical experience with the unidirectional dual-chambered intra-aortic balloon assist.' *Circulation*, **43** and **44 (Suppl. I),** 82 (1971)
42. Bregman, D., Kripke, D. C. and Goetz, R. H. 'Dual-chambered balloon assist in cardiogenic shock.' *Review of Surgery*, **288,** 221 (1971)
43. Bregman, D., Kripke, D. C. and Goetz, R. H. 'The effect of synchronous unidirectional intra-aortic balloon pumping on haemodyamics and coronary blood flow in cardiogenic shock.' *Transactions of the American Society for Artificial Internal Organs*, **16,** 439 (1970)
44. Bregman, D., Parodi, E. N., Edie, R. N., Bowman, F. O., Jr., Reemtsma, K. and Malm, J. R. 'Intraoperative unidirectional intra-aortic balloon pumping in the management of left ventricular power failure.' *Journal of Thoracic and Cardiovascular Surgery*, **70,** 1010 (1975)
45. Bregman, D., Parodi, E. N., Haubert, S. M., Szarnicki, R., Edie, R. N., Spotnitz, H. M., Bowman, F. O., Jr., Reemtsma, K. and Malm, J. R. 'Counterpulsation with a new pulsatile assist device (PAD) in open-heart surgery.' *Medical Instrumentation*, **10,** 232 (1976)
46. Bregman, D., Parodi, E. N., Haubert, S. M., Szarnicki, R., Edie, R. N., Spotnitz, H. M., Bowman, F. O., Jr., Reemtsma, K. and Malm, J. R. 'Unidirectional intra-aortic balloon pumping and counterpulsation during open-heart surgery.' In *Mechanical Support of the Failing Heart and Lungs*. Ed. D. Bregman. p. 17. New York: Appleton-Century-Crofts (1977)
47. Bregman, D., Parodi, E. N. and Malm, J. R. 'Left ventricular and unidirectional intra-aortic balloon pumping: effects on haemodynamics in canine cardiogenic shock.' *Journal of Thoracic and Cardiovascular Surgery*, **68,** 677 (1974)

48. Bregman, D., Parodi, E. N., Reemtsma, K. and Malm, J. R. 'Advances in Clinical Intra-aortic balloon pumping.' In *Coronary Artery Medicine and Surgery: Concepts and Controversies*. Ed. J. C. Norman. pp. 413–420. New York: Appleton-Century-Crofts (1975)
49. Bregman, D., Parodi, E. N., Reemtsma, K. and Malm, J. R. 'The effect of combined venous and arterial balloon pumping (counterpulsation) in canine cardiogenic shock.' *Journal of Thoracic and Cardiovascular Surgery*, (in press)
50. Brown, B. G., Goldfarb, D., Topaz, S. R. and Gott, V. L. 'Diastolic augmentation by intra-aortic balloon. Circulatory haemodynamics and treatment of severe left ventricular failure in dogs.' *Journal of Thoracic and Cardiovascular Surgery*, **53,** 789 (1967)
51. Brown, B. G., Gundel, W. D., Gott, V. L. and Covell, J. W. 'Haemodynamic determinants of retrograde arterial coronary flow following acute coronary occlusion'. (Abstr.). *Circulation*, **45** and **46 (Suppl II),** 100 (1972)
51a. Brundage, B. H., Ullyot, D. J., Winokur, S., Chatterjee, K., Ports, T. A. and Turley, K. 'The role of aortic balloon pumping in postinfarction angina; a different perspective.' *Circulation*, **62 (Suppl II),** I119 (1980)
52. Buckberg, G. D. 'Left ventricular subendocardial necrosis.' *Annals of Thoracic Surgery*, **24,** 379 (1977)
53. Buckberg, G. D., Fixler, D. E., Archie, J. P. and Hoffman, J. I. E. 'Experimental subendocardial ischaemia in dogs with normal coronary arteries.' *Circulation Research*, **30,** 67 (1972)
54. Buckberg, G. D., Towers, B., Paglia, D. E., Mulder, D. G. and Maloney, J. V. 'Subendocardial ischaemia after cardiopulmonary bypass.' *Journal of Thoracic and Cardiovascular Surgery*, **64,** 669 (1972)
55. Buckley, M. J., Craver, J. M., Gold, H. K., Mundth, E. D., Daggett, W. M. and Austen, W. G. 'Intra-aortic balloon pump assist for cardiogenic shock after cardiopulmonary bypass.' *Circulation*, **47** and **48 (Suppl III),** 90 (1973)
56. Buckley, M. J., Laird, J. D., Madras, P. N., Jones, R. T., Kantrowitz, A. R. and Austen, W. G. 'Left heart assist system: intra-aortic balloon pump.' *Surgical Clinics of North America*, **49,** 505 (1969)
57. Buckley, M. J., Leinbach, R. C., Kastor, J. A., Laird, J. D., Kantrowitz, A. R., Madras, P. N., Sanders, C. A. and Austen, W. G. 'Haemodynamic evaluation of intra-aortic balloon pumping in man.' *Circulation*, **41** and **42 (Suppl. II),** 130 (1970)
58. Buckley, M. J., Mundth, E. D., Daggett, W. M., De Sanctis, R. W., Sanders, C. A. and Austen, W. G. 'Surgical therapy for early complications of myocardial infarction.' *Surgery*, **70,** 814 (1971)
59. Buckley, M. J., Mundth, E. D., Daggett, W. M., Gold, H. K., Leinbach, R. C. and Austen, W. G. 'Surgical management of ventricular septal defects and mitral regurgitation complicating acute myocardial infarction.' *Annals of Thoracic Surgery*, **16,** 598 (1973)
60. Carlson, R. G., Baltaxe, H., Bregman, D., Bloch, J. H. and Lillehei, C. W. 'Veno-arterial perfusion with membrane lung and/or intra-aortic balloon during arteriography and surgery for coronary artery disease producing myocardial infarction with cardiogenic shock.' In *Coronary Artery Medicine and Surgery: Concepts and Controversies*. Ed. J. C. Norman. New York: Appleton-Century-Crofts (1974)
61. Carlson, R. G., Rees, J. R., Baltaxe, H., Levin, D., Lande, A. J., Bregman, D., Scheidt, S. and Lillehei, C. W. 'Mechanical cardiopulmonary support during arteriography and surgical correction of coronary insufficiency producing myocardial infarction with cardiogenic shock.' *Journal of the Association for the Advancement of Medical Instrumentation*, **6,** 244 (1972)

62. Caulfield, J. B., Dunkman, W. B. and Leinbach, R. C. 'Cardiogenic shock. Myocardial morphology with and without artificial left ventricular counterpulsation.' *Archives of Pathology*, **93**, 532 (1972)
63. Clayman, R. V., DeLaria, G. A., Johansen, K. H. and Bernstein, E. F. 'The hypertensive balloon: a beneficial synergism for salvage of ischaemic myocardium.' *Surgical Forum*, **24**, 152 (1973)
64. Cleveland, J. C., Lefemine, A. A., Madoff, I., Black, H., Amato, J., Sewell, D. H., Rheinlander, H. F. and Cleveland, R. J. 'The role of intra-aortic balloon counterpulsation in patients undergoing cardiac operations.' *Annals of Thoracic Surgery*, **20**, 652 (1975)
65. Cohn, L. H. 'Intra-aortic balloon counterpulsation in low cardiac output states.' *Surgical Clinics of North America*, **55**, 545 (1975)
66. Cohn, L. H., Alpert, J., Koster, J. K., Jr., Mee, R. B. B. and Collins, J. J., Jr. 'Changing indications for the surgical treatment of unstable angina.' *Archives of Surgery*, **113**, 1312 (1978)
67. Cooper, G. N., Jr., Singh, A. K., Vargas, L. L. and Karslon, K. E. 'Preoperative intra-aortic balloon assist in high risk revascularization patients.' *American Journal of Surgery*, **133**, 463 (1977)
68. Corday, E., Swan, J. J. C., Lang, T. W., Goldman, A., Matloff, J. M., Gold, H. and Meerbaum, S. 'Physiological principles in the application of circulatory assist for the failing heart.' *American Journal of Cardiology*, **26**, 595 (1970)
69. Cox, J. L., McLaughlin, V. W., Flowers, N. C. and Horan, L. G. 'The ischaemic zone surrounding acute myocardial infarction. Its morphology as detected by dehydrogenase staining.' *American Heart Journal*, **76**, 650 (1968)
70. Dilley, R. B., Ross, J., Jr and Bernstein, E. F. 'Serial haemodynamics during intra-aortic balloon counterpulsation for cardiogenic shock.' *Circulation*, **47** and **48 (Suppl. III)**, 99 (1973)
71. Disler, P. B., Scott Millar, R. N., and Obel, I. W. P. 'Prolonged circulatory support with the intra-aortic balloon pump after myocardial infarction.' *Thorax*, **33**, 504 (1978)
72. Doland, A. M., Metcalfe, J. B., Simani, A., Sterns, L. P. and Callaghan, J. C. 'Comparison of counterpulsation and balloon pumping for treating myocardial infarction.' *Transactions of the American Society for Artificial Internal Organs*, **16**, 455 (1970)
73. Donald, D. E. and McGoon, D. C. 'Circulatory support by a left ventricular balloon pump.' *Circulation*, **43** and **44 (Suppl. I)**, 96 (1971)
74. Dormandy, J. A., Goetz, R. H. and Kripke, D. C. 'Haemodynamics and coronary blood flow with counterpulsation.' *Surgery*, **65**, 311 (1969)
75. Dunkman, W. B., Leinbach, R. C., Buckley, M. J., Mundth, E. D., Kantrowitz, A. R., Austen, W. G. and Sanders, C. A. 'Clinical and haemodynamic results of intra-aortic balloon pumping for cardiogenic shock.' *Circulation*, **46**, 465 (1972)
76. Edmonds, C. H. and Hibbs, C. W. 'Costs of intra-aortic balloon pumping.' *Cardiovascular Diseases. Bulletin of the Texas Heart Institute*, **4**, 437 (1977)
77. Ehrich, D. A., Biddle, T. L., Kronenberg, M. S. and Yu, P. N. 'The haemodynamic response to intra-aortic balloon counterpulsation in patients with cardiogenic shock complicating acute myocardial infarction., *American Heart Journal*, **93**, 274 (1977)
78. Elkins, R. C. McCurdy, J. R., Brown, P. P. and Greenfield, L. J. 'Effects of coronary perfusion pressure on myocardial performance during endotoxic shock.' *Surgery, Gynecology and Obsetetrics*, **137**, 991 (1973)
79. Feola, M., Limet, R. R. and Glick, G. 'Direct and reflex vascular effects of intra-aortic balloon counterpulsation in dogs at four levels of aortic pressure.' *Clinical Research*, **19**, 313 (1971)

80. Feola, M., Wiener, L. Walinsky, P., Kasparian, H., Duca, P., Gottlieb, R., Brest, A. and Templeton, J. 'Improved survival after coronary bypass surgery in patients with poor left ventricular function: role of intra-aortic balloon counterpulsation.' *American Journal of Cardiology*, **39,** 1021 (1977)
81. Foster, E. D., Olsson, C. A., Rutenberg, A.M. and Berger, R. L. 'Mechanical circulatory assistance with intra-aortic balloon counterpulsation for major abdominal surgery.' *Annals of Surgery*, **183,** 73 (1976)
82. Fry, J., Jr. and Proctor, H. J., 'Effects of hypoxia, acidosis and peripheral vascular resistance on endocardial viability ratio.' *Surgery, Gynecology and Obstetrics*, **144,** 850 (1977)
83. Furman, S., Vijaynagar, R., Rosenbaum, R., McMullen, M. and Escher, D. J.W. 'Lethal sequelae of intra-aortic balloon rupture.' *Surgery*, **69,** 121 (1971)
84. Furman, S., Whitman, R., Stewart, J., Parker, B. and McMullen, M. 'Proximity to aortic valve and unidirectionality as prime factors in counterpulsation effectiveness.' *Transactions of the American Society for Artificial Internal Organs*, **17,** 153 (1971)
85. Gill, C. C., Wechsler, A. S., Newman, G. E. and Oldham, H. N., Jr. 'Augmentation and redistribution of myocardial blood flow during acute ischaemia by intra-aortic balloon pumping.' *Annals of Thoracic Surgery*, **16,** 445 (1973)
86. Goetz, R. H., Bregman, D., Esrig, B. and Laniado, S. 'Unidirectional intra-aortic balloom pumping in cardiogenic shock and intractable left ventricular failure.' *American Journal of Cardiology*, **29,** 213 (1972)
87. Gold, H. K., Leinbach, R. C, Buckley, M. J., Mundth, E. D. Daggett, W. M. and Austen, W. G. 'Refractory angina pectoris: follow-up after intra-aortic balloon pumping and surgery.' *Circulation*, **54 (Suppl. III),** 41 (1976)
88. Gold, H. K., Leinbach, R. C., Sanders, C. A., Buckley, M. J., Mundth, E. D. and Austen, W. G. 'Intra-aortic balloon pumping for control of recurrent myocardial ischaemia.' *Circulation*, **47,** 1197 (1973)
89. Gold, H. K., Leinbach, R. C., Sanders, C. A., Buckley, M. J., Mundth, E. D. and Austen, W. G. 'Intra-aortic balloon pumping for ventricular septal defect or mitral regurgitation complicating acute myocardial infarction.' *Circulation*, **47,** 1191 (1973)
90. Goldman, B. S., Gunstensen, J., Gilbert, B. W., Kelly, T. C., Scully, H., Williams, W. G. and Adelman, A. G. 'Increasing operability and survival intra-aortic balloon pumping assist.' *Canadian Journal of Surgery*, **19,** 69 (1976)
91. Gunstensen, J., Goldman, B. S., Scully, H. S., Huckell, V. F. and Adelman, A. G. 'Evolving indications for preoperative intra-aortic balloon pump assistance.' *Annals of Thoracic Surgery*, **22,** 535 (1976)
92. Haddy, F. J. 'Pathophysiology and therapy of the shock of myocardial infarction.' *Annals of Internal Medicine*, **73,** 809 (1970)
93. Hagemeijer, F., Laird, J. D., Haalebos, M. M. P. and Hugenholtz, P. G. 'Effectiveness of intra-aortic balloon pumping without cardiac surgery for patients with severe heart failure secondary to a recent myocardial infarction.' *American Journal of Cardiology*, **40,** 951 (1977)
94. Harken, D. E. *Presentation at the International College of Cardiology Meeting*, Brussels, Belgium (1958)
95. Harken, D. E., Soroff, H. S. and Birtwell, W. L. 'Assisted circulation: counterpulsation and coronary artery disease.' In *Surgery Annual.* Eds P. Cooper and L. M. Nyhus. pp. 165–189. New York: Appleton-Century-Crofts (1972)
95a. Harvey, J. C., Goldstein, J., McCabe, J. C., Hoover, E. L., Gay, W. A. and Subramanian, V. A. 'Complications of percutaneous intra-aortic balloon pumping.' (In press)

96. Housman, L. B., Bernstein, E. F., Braunwald, N. S. and Dilley, R. B. 'Counterpulsation for intra-operative cardiogenic shock. Successful use of intra-aortic balloon.' *Journal of the American Medical Association*, **224,** 1131 (1973)
97. Hyson, E. A., Ravin, C. E., Kelley, M. J. and Curtis, A. M. 'Intra-aortic counterpulsation balloon: radiographic considerations.' *American Journal of Roentgenology*, **128,** 195 (1977)
98. Igo, S. R., Hibbs, C. W., Trono, R., Fuqua, J. M., Edmonds, C. H., Leachman, C. J., Brewer, M. A., Holub, D. A. and Norman, J. C. 'Intra-aortic balloon pumping: theory and practice – experience with 325 patients.' *Artificial Organs*, **2,** 249 (1978)
98a. Isner, J. M., Cohen, S. R., Virmani, R., Lawrinson, W. and Roberts, W. C. 'Complications of the intra-aortic balloon counterpulsation device: clinical and morphologic observations in 45 necropsy patients.' *American Journal of Cardiology*, **45,** 260 (1980)
99. Jackson, G., Cullum, P., Pastellopoulos, A., Macarthur, A. and Jewitt, D. 'Intra-aortic balloon assistance in cardiogenic shock after myocardial infarction or cardiac surgery.' *British Heart Journal*, **39,** 598 (1977)
100. Jacobey, J. A. 'Results of counterpulsation in patients with coronary artery disease.' *American Journal of Cardiology*, **27,** 137 (1971)
101. Jacobey, J. A., Craddock, L. D., Wolf, P. S. and Beckwitt, H. J. 'Clinical experience with counterpulsation in coronary artery disease.' *Journal of Thoracic and Cardiovscular Surgery*, **56,** 846 (1968)
102. Jacobey, J. A., Taylor, W. J., Smith, G. T., Doorlin, R. and Harken, D. E. 'A new therapeutic approach to acute coronary occlusion. II. Opening dormant coronary collateral channels by counterpulsation'. *American Journal of Cardiology*, **11,** 218 (1963)
103. Johnson, M. D., Holub, D. A., Winston, D. S., Brewer, M. A., Hibbs, C. W., Leachman, C. J. and Norman, J. C. 'Retrospective analysis of 286 patients requiring circulatory support with the intra-aortic balloon pump.' *Cardiovascular Diseases. Bulletin of the Texas Heart Institute*, **4,** 428 (1977)
104. Johnson, S. A., Scanlon, P. J., Loeb, H. S., Moran, J. M., Pifarre, R. and Gunnar, R. M. 'Treatment of cardiogenic shock in myocardial infarction by intra-aortic counterpulsation and surgery.' *American Journal of Medicine*, **62,** 687 (1977)
104a. Jone, E. L., Douglas, J. S. Jr, Craver, J. M., King, S. B. III, Kaplan, J. A., Morgan, E. A. and Hatcher, C. R. 'Results of coronary revascularization in patients with recent myocardial infarction. *Journal of Thoracic and Cardiovascular Surgery*, **76,** 545 (1978)
105. Kaiser, G. C., Marco, J. D., Barner, H. B., Codd, J. E., Laks, J. and Willman, V. L. 'Intra-aortic balloon assistance.' *Annals of Thoracic Surgery*, **21,** 487 (1976)
106. Kantrowitz, A., Krakauer, J. S., Butner, A. N., Freed, P. S., Jaron, D., Rosenbaum, A. and Goodman, P. M. 'Phase-shift balloon pumping in cardiogenic shock.' *Progress in Cardiovascular Diseases*, **12,** 293 (1969)
107. Kantrowitz, A., Krakauer, J. S., Rosenbaum, A., Butner, A. N., Freed, P. S. and Jaron, D. 'Phase-shift balloon pumping in medically refractory cardiogenic shock: results in 27 patients.' *Archives of Surgery*, **99,** 739 (1969)
108. Kantrowitz, A., Phillips, S. J., Butner, A. N., Tjønneland, S. and Haller, J. D. 'Technique of femoral artery cannulation for phase-shift balloon pumping.' *Journal of Thoracic and Cardiovascular Surgery*, **56,** 219 (1968)
109. Kantrowitz, A., Tjønneland, S., Freed, P. S., Phillips, S. J., Butner, A. N. and and Sherman, J. L., Jr. 'Initial clinical experience with intra-aortic balloon pumping in cardiogenic shock.' *Journal of the American Medical Association*, **203,** 135 (1968)

110. Kantrowitz, A., Tjønneland, S., Krakauer, J. S., Phillips, S. J., Freed, P. S. and Butner, A. N. 'Mechanical intra-aortic cardiac assistance in cardiogenic shock. Haemodynamic effects.' *Archives of Surgery*, **97,** 1000 (1968)
110a. Kirklin, J. W., Conti, V. R. and Blackstone, E. H. 'Prevention of myocardial damage during cardiac operations.' *New England Journal of Medicine*, **301,** 135 (1979)
111. Kirklin, J. W. and Rastelli, G. C., 'Low cardiac output after open intracardiac operations.' *Progress in Cardiovascular Diseases*, **10,** 117 (1967)
112. Kolff, W. J., Moulopoulos, S. D., Kwan-Gett, C. S. and Kralios, A. 'Mechanical assistance to the circulation: the principle and the methods.' *progress in Cardiovascular Diseases*, **12,** 243 (1969)
113. Krakauer, J. S., Rosenbaum, A., Freed, P., Jaron, D. and Kantrowitz, A. 'Clinical management ancillary to phase-shift balloon pumping in cardiogenic shock.' *American Journal of Cardiology*, **27,** 123 (1971)
114. Kralios, A. C., Zwart, H. H. J., Moulopoulos, S. D., Collan, R., Kwan-Kett, C. S. and Kolff, W. J. 'Intra-pulmonary artery balloon pumping.' *Journal of Thoracic and Cardiovascular Surgery*, **60,** 215 (1970)
115. Kralios, A. C. Zwart, H. H. J., Yenching, W., Moulopoulos, S. D. and Kolff, W. J. 'Coronary flow supplementation in experimental myocardial infarction with shock.' *Chest*, **61,** 365 (1972)
116. Kuhn, L. A. 'Management of shock following acute myocardial infarction part II. Mechanical circulatory assistance.' *American Heart Journal*, **95,** 789 (1978)
117. Kuhn, L. A. 'Shock in myocardial infarction–medical treatment.' *American Journal of Cardiology*, **26,** 578 (1970)
118. Kuhn, L. A., Unger, A. H., Novick, S. A., Marano, A. J. and Rosenberg, A. S. 'Haemodynamics and cardiac metabolic effects of diastolic intra-aortic balloon obstruction combined with distal aortic "booster" occlusion in experimental acute myocardial infarction.' *American Journal of Cardiology*, **25,** 111 (1970)
119. Kveim, M., Cappelen, C., Jr., Frøysaker, T. and Hall, D. V. 'Intra-aortic balloon pumping in the treatment of cardiogenic shock follow-up in open-heart surgery.' *Scandinavian Journal of Thoracic and Cardiovascular Surgery*, **10**, 231 (1976)
120. Laird, J. D., Madras, P. N., Jones, R. T., Kantrowitz, A. R., Kothar, M. L., Buckley, M. J. and Austen, W. G. 'Theoretical and experimental analysis of the intra-aortic balloon pump.' *Transactions of the American Society for Artificial Internal Organs*, **14,** 338 (1968)
121. Lamberti, J. J., Cohn, L. H. and Collins, J. J., Jr. 'Iliac artery cannulation for intra-aortic balloon counterpulsation.' *Journal of Thoracic and Cardiovascular Surgery*, **67,** 976 (1974)
122. Lamberti, J. J. and Resnekov, L. 'Cardiac assist devices.' *Annual Review of Medicine*, **29,** 571 (1978)
123. Langon, R. A., Geha, A. S., Hammond, G. L. and Cohen, L. S. 'Surgical approach for patients with unstable angina pectoris: role of the response to initial medical therapy and intra-aortic balloon pumping in perioperative complications after aortocoronary bypass grafting.' *American Journal of Cardiology*, **42,** 629 (1978)
124. Laniado, S., Miller, H., Yellin, E., Barlow, B., Goetz, R. H. and Frater, R. M. 'Favourable effect of intra-aortic balloon pumping (IABP) on the distribution of total stroke volume in acute mitral regurgitation.' (Abstr.) *Circulation*, **46** and **46 (Suppl. II),** 118 (1972)
125. Lappas, D. G., Powell, W. M. J., Jr. and Daggett, W. M. 'Cardiac dysfunction in the perioperative period.' *Anesthesiology*, **47,** 117, (1977)
126. Lefemine, A. A., Kosowsky, B., Madoff, I., Black, H. and Lewis, M. 'Results and complications of intra-aortic balloon pumping in surgical and medical patients.' *American Journal of Cardiology*, **40,** 416 (1977)

127. Leinbach, R. C., Buckley, M. J., Austen, W. G., Petschek, H. E., Kantrowitz, A. R. and Sanders, C. A. 'Effects of intra-aortic balloon pumping on coronary flow and metabolism in man.' *Circulation*, **43** and **44 (Suppl. I),** 77 (1971)
128. Leinbach, R. C., Gold, H. K., Dinsmore, R. E., Mundth, E. D., Buckley, M. J., Austen, W. G. and Sanders, C. A. 'The role of angiography in cardiogenic shock.' *Circulation*, **47** and **48 (Suppl. III),** 95 (1973)
129. Leinbach, R. C., Gold, H. K., Harber, R. W., Buckley, M. J. and Austen, W. G. 'Early intra-aortic balloon pumping for anterior myocardial infarction without shock.' *Circulation*, **58,** 204 (1978)
130. Leinbach, R. C., Nyilas, E., Caulfield, J. B., Buckley, M. J. and Austen, W. G. 'Evaluation of haematologic effects of intra-aortic balloon pumping in man.' *Transactions of the American Society for Artificial Internal Organs*, **18,** 493 (1972)
131. Levine, F. H., Gold, H. K., Leinbach, R. C., Daggett, W. M., Austen, W. G. and Buckley, M. J. 'Management of acute myocardial ischaemia with intra-aortic balloon pumping and coronary bypass surgery.' (Abstr.) *Circulation*, **56 (Suppl. III),** 61 (1973)
131a. Madigan, N. P., Rutherford, B. D., Barnhorst, D. A. and Danielson, G. K. 'Early saphenous vein grafting after subendocardial infarction. Immediate surgical results and late prognosis.' *Circulation*, **56 (Suppl II),** II–I (1977)
132. Madras, P. N., Laird J. D., Iatridis, E., Kantrowitz, A. R., Buckley, M. J. and Austen, W. G. 'Effects of prolonged intra-aortic balloon pumping.' *Transactions of the American Society for Artificial Internal Organs*', **15,** 400 (1969)
133. Maroko, P. R., Bernstein, E. F., Libby, P., DeLaria, G. A., Covell, J. W., Ross, J., Jr. and Braunwald, E. 'Effects of intra-aortic balloon counterpulsation on the severity of myocardial ischaemic injury following acute coronary occlusion.' *Circulation*, **45,** 1150 (1972)
134. Maroko, P. R. and Braunwald, E. 'Modification of myocardial infarction size after coronary occlusion.' *Annals of Internal Medicine*, **79**, 720 (1973)
135. Mathivat, A., Bourdari, J. P., Bardet, J., Normand, J. P., Kahn, J. C., Rocha, P. and Brunet, A. 'Prolonged circulatory assistance by intra-aortic unidirectional counterpulsation in a state of shock following myocardial infarction.' *Nouvelle Presse Medicale*, **2,** 2663 (1973)
136. Matloff, J. M., Parmley, W. W., Manchester, J. H., Berkovits, B., Sonnenblick, E. H. and Harken, D. E. 'Haemodynamic effects of glucagon and intra-aortic balloon counterpulsation in canine myocardial infarction.' *American Journal of Cardiology*, **25,** 675 (1970)
137. Matsukura, H., Tamura, M., Matsuyama, M., Koh, S., Kato, H., Honma, J., Matsunami, O., Tamura, K., Sasa, T., Kawakami, T., Kuroshima, S. and Sugie, S. 'Haemodynamic effects of intra-aortic balloon counterpulsation on left heart failure. '*Japanese Circulation Journal*, **37,** 871 (1973)
138. McDonald, R. H., Taylor, R. R. and Congolani, H. E. 'Measurement of myocardial developed tension and its relation to oxygen consumption.' *American Journal of Physiology*, **211,** 667 (1966)
139. McEnany, M. T., Kay, H. R., Buckley, M. J., Daggett, W. M., Erdmann, A. J., Mundth, E. D., Rao, R. S., DeToeuf, J. and Austen, W. G. 'Clinical experience with intra-aortic balloon pump support in 728 patients.' *Circulation*, **58 (Suppl. I),** 124 (1978)
140. Miller, H., Laniado, S., Yellin, E., Frater, R. W. M. and Goetz, R. H. 'Effects of intra-aortic balloon pumping on the haemodynamics of acute mitral insufficiency.' *Surgical Forum*, **22,** 172 (1972)
141. Miller, M. G. and Hall, S. V. 'Intra-aortic balloon counterpulsation in a high-risk cardiac patient undergoing emergency gastrectomy.' *Anesthesiology*, **42,** 103 (1975)

142. Moulopoulos, S. D., Topaz, S. and Kolff, W. J.. 'Diastolic balloon pumping (with carbon dioxide) in the aorta – a mechanical assistance to the failing circulation.' *American Heart Journal*, **63,** 669 (1962)
143. Moulopoulos, S. D., Topaz, S. R. and Kolff, W. J. 'Extracorporeal assistance to the circulation and intra-aortic balloon pumping.' *Transactions of the American Society for Artificial Internal Organs*, **8,** 85 (1962)
144. Mueller, H., Ayres, S. M., Conklin, E. F., Giannelli, S., Jr., Massara, J. T., Grace, W. T. and Nealon, T. F., Jr. 'The effects of intra-aortic counterpulsation on cardiac performance and metabolism in shock associated with acute myocardial infarction.' *Journal of Clinical Investigation*, **50,** 1885 (1971)
145. Mueller, H., Ayres, S. M., Giannelli, S., Jr., Conklin, E. F., Mazzara, J. T. and Grace, W. J. 'Effect of isoproterenol, 1-norepinephrine and intra-aortic counterpulsation on haemodynamics and myocardial metabolism in shock following acute myocardial infarction.' *Circulation*, **45,** 335 (1972)
146. Mueller, H., Ayres, S. M., Gregory, J. J., Giannelli, S., Jr. and Grace, W. J. 'Haemodynamics, coronary blood flow, and myocardial metabolism in coronary shock; response to 1-norepinephrine and isoproterenol.' *Journal of Clinical Investigation*, **49,** 1885 (1970)
147. Mueller, H., Ayres, S. M., Mazzara, J., Giannelli, S. and Grace, W. 'Responses of haemodynamics and myocardial energetics to intra-aortic phase shift balloon pumping (IPSBP) in acute coronary shock.' (Abstr.) *Circulation*, **41** and **42 (Suppl. III),** 81 (1970)
148. Mundth, E. D. 'Mechanical and surgical interventions for the reduction of myocardial ischaemia.' *Circulation*, **53 (Suppl. I),** 176 (1976)
149. Mundth, E. D. 'Preoperative intra-aortic balloon pump assistance'. *Annals of Thoracic Surgery*, **22,** 603 (1976)
150. Mundth, E. D., Buckley, M. J., Daggett, W. M., McEnany, M. T., Leinbach, R. C., Gold, H. K. and Austen, W. G. 'Intra-aortic balloon pump assistance and early surgery in cardiogenic shock. Integrated medical-surgical care in acute coronary artery disease.' *Advances in Cardiology*, **15,** 159 (1975)
151. Mundth, E. D., Buckley, M. J., Daggett, W. M., Sanders, C. A. and Austen, W. G. 'Surgery for complications of acute myocardial infarction.' *Circulation*, **45,** 1279 (1972)
152. Mundth, E. D., Buckley, M. J., DeSanctis, R. W., Daggett, W. M. and Austen, W. G. 'Surgical treatment of ventricular irritability.' *Journal of Thoracic and Cardiovascular Surgery*, **66,** 943 (1973)
153. Mundth, E. D., Buckley, M. J., Gold, H. K., Daggett, W. M., Leinbach, R. C. and Austen, W. G. 'Intra-aortic balloon pumping and emergency coronary arterial revascularization for acute myocardial infarction with impending extension.' *Annals of Thoracic Surgery*, **16,** 435 (1973)
154. Mundth, E. D., Buckley, M. J. Leinbach, R. C., DeSanctis, R. W., Sanders, C. A., Kantrowitz, A. and Austen, W. G. 'Myocardial revascularization for the treatment of cardiogenic shock complicating acute myocardial infarction.' *Surgery*, **70,** 78 (1971)
155. Mundth, E. D., Buckley, M. J., Leinbach, R. C., Gol, H. K., Daggett, W. M. and Austen, W. G. 'Surgical intervention for the complications of acute myocardial ischaemia.' *Annals of Surgery*, **178,** 379 (1973)
156. Mundth, E. D., Yurchak, P. M., Buckley, M. J., Leinbach, R. C., Kantrowitz, A. and Austen, W. G. 'Circulatory assistance and emergency direct coronary artery surgery for shock complicating acute myocardial infarction.' *New England Journal of Medicine*, **283,** 1382 (1970)
157. Nachlas, M. M. and Sieband, M. P. 'The influence of diastolic augmentation on infarct size following coronary artery ligation.' *Journal of Thoracic and Cardiovascular Surgery*, **53,** 698 (1968)

158. Najafi, H., Henson, D., Dye, W. S., Javid, H., Hunter, J. A., Callaghan, R., Einstein, R. and Julian, O. C. 'Left ventricular haemorrhagic necrosis.' *Annals of Thoracic Surgery*, **7,** 550 (1969)
158a. Nichols, A. B., Weiss, M. B. and Bregman, D. 'Percutaneous intra-aortic balloon insertion in patients with aorto-iliac disease. (In preparation)
159. Norman, J. C., Cooley, D. A., Igo, S. R., Hibbs, C. W., Johnson, M. D., Bennett, J. G., Fuqua, B. S., Trono, R. and Edmonds, C. H. 'Prognostic indices for survival during post-cardiotomy intra-aortic balloon pumping; methods of scoring (0–16) and classification (A–C) with implications for left ventricular assist device utilization.' *Journal of Thoracic and Cardiovascular Surgery*, **74,** 709 (1977)
160. Norman, N. A. and Kennedy, J. H. 'Arterial baroreceptor responses to intra-aortic balloon assistance.' *Journal of Surgical Research*, **11,** 396 (1971)
161. Nyquist, O. 'Shock complicating acute myocardial infarction.' *Acta medica Scandinavica*, **(Suppl.)** 536 (1972)
162. Olinger, G. N., Bonchek, L. I., Keelan, M. H., Jr., Tresch, D. D., Siegel, R., Bamrah, V. and Tristani, F. E. 'Unstable angina; the case for operation.' *American Journal of Cardiology*, **42,** 634 (1978)
163. O'Rourke, M. F. 'Arterial counterpulsation in the management of ischaemic heart disease.' *Australian and New Zealand Journal of Surgery*, **47,** 1 (1977)
164. Pace, P. D., Tilney, N. L., Lesch, M. and Couch, N. P. 'Peripheral arterial complications of intra-aortic balloon counterpulsation.' *Surgery*, **82,** 685 (1977)
165. Page, D. L., Caulfield, J. B., Kastor, J. A., DeSanctis, R. W. and Sanders, C. A. 'Myocardial changes associated with cardiogenic shock.' *New England Journal of Medicine*, **285,** 133 (1971)
166. Parker, F. B., Jr., Neville, J. F., Hanson, E. L. and Webb, W. R. 'Intra-aortic balloon counterpulsation and cardiac surgery.' *Annals of Thoracic Surgery*, **17,** 144 (1974)
167. Parker, J. O., Chiong, M. A., West, R. O. and Case, R. B. 'Sequential alterations in myocardial lactate metabolism, S-T segments, and left ventricular function during angina induced by atrial pacing.' *Circulation*, **40,** 113 (1969)
168. Petrovsky, B. V. and Shumakov, V. I. 'Artificial heart implanted into the organism.' *Kardiologiia*, **7,** 14 (1967)
169. Petrovsky, B. V. and Shumakov, V. I. 'Employment of assisted circulation in myocardial ischaemia.' *Journal of Cardiovascular Surgery*, **12,** 202 (1971)
170. Philips, P. A. and Bregman, D. 'Intra-operative application of intra-aortic balloon counterpulsation determined by clinical monitoring of the endocardial viability ratio.' *Annals of Thorarcic Surgery*, **23,** 45 (1977)
171. Philips, P. A., Marty, A. T., Miyamoto, A. M., McCurdy, M. D., White, J. A., Morgan, B. J. and Brewer, L. A., III. 'A clinical method for detecting subendocardial ischaemia after cardiopulmonary bypass'. *Journal of Thoracic and Cardiovascular Surgery*, **69,** 30 (1975)
172. Piwnica, A., Gouigon, R., Masquet, C., Eisenma, B., Beaufils, P. and Bouvrain, Y. 'Aortic counterpulsation and arteriovenous bypass during prolonged circulation assistance.' (Letter) *Nouvelle Presse Medicale*, **2,** 2690 (1973)
173. Pooley, R. W., Truccone, N. J., Spotnitz, H. M., Parodi, E. N., Bregman, D., Malm, J. R. and Reemtsma, K. 'Increased cardiac output by downstream pumping with a reversed unidirectional intra-aortic balloon.' *Journal of Thoracic and Cardiovascular Surgery*, **73,** 647 (1977)
174. Powell, W. J., Jr., Daggett, W. M., Magro, A. E., Bianco, J. A., Buckley, M. J., Sanders, C. A., Kantrowitz, A. R. and Austen, W. G. 'Effects of intra-aortic balloon counterpulsation on caradiac performance, oxygen consumption and coronary blood flow in dogs.' *Circulation Research*, **216,** (1970)

175. Printup, C. A., Dietrick, W. R., Getzen, J. H., Penido, J. R. F., Golden, L. S., Johnson, P. E. J., Jr., Cotton, B. H. and Buggs, H. 'Ascending aorta insertion of the dual-chambered intra-aortic balloon for counterpulsation during cardiac operations.' *Annals of Thoracic Surgery*, **20**, 694 (1975)
176. Reemtsma, K., Drusin, R., Edie, R., Bregman, D., Dobelle, W. and Hardy, M. 'Cardiac transplantation for patients requiring mechanical circulatory support'. *New England Journal of Medicine*, **298,** 670 (1978)
177. Reemtsma, K., Parodi, E. N., Bregman, D., Edie, R. N., Bowman, F. O., Jr. and Mal, J. R. 'Clinical intraoperative coronary artery saphenous vein bypass graft pressure-flow relationship.' In *Coronary Artery Medicine and Surgery: Concepts and Controversies*. Ed. J. C. Norman. New York: Appleton-Century-Crofts (1974)
178. Roberts, A. J., Alonso, D. R., Combes, J. R., Jacobstein, J. G., Post. M. R., Cahill, P. T., Ho, S. T., Abel, R. M., Subramanian, V. A. and Gay, W. A., Jr. 'Role of delayed intra-aortic balloon pumping in treatment of experimental myocardial infarction'. *American Journal of Cardiology*, **41,** 1202 (1978)
179. Rosensweig, J., Chatterjee, S. and Merino, F. 'Treatment of acute myocardial infarction by counterpulsation. Experimental rationale and clinical experience.' *Journal of Thoracic and Cardiovascular Surgery*, **69,** 243 (1970)
180. Rubenfire, M., Krakauer, J., Ciborski, M., Wajszczuk, W., Malinowski, E., Jaron, D., Freed, P. and Kantrowitz, A. 'Prolonged circulatory support by intra-aortic balloon pumping.' (Abstr.) *Circulation*, **45** and **46 (Suppl. II)**, 214 (1972)
181. Saini, V. K. and Berger, R. L. 'Technique of aortic balloon catheter deployment with the use of a Fogarty catheter.' *Annals of Thoracic Surgery*, **14,** 440 (1972)
182. Saini, V. K., Wright, W., Hood, W. B., Hechtman, H. and Berger, R. L. 'Increase of nutrient myocardial blood flow by intra-aortic balloon pumping in experimental coronary ischaemia.' (Abstr.) *Circulation*, **45** and **46 (Suppl. II),** 99 (1972)
183. Sammel, N., O'Rourke, M. F. and Chang, V. 'Arterial counterpulsation: review of the first 100 patients.' *Medical Journal of Australia*, **2,** 802 (1976)
184. Sanders, C. A., Buckley, M. J., Leinbach, R. ., Mundth, E. D. and Austen, W. G. 'Mechanical circulatory assistance, emergency coronary angiography, and acute myocardial revascularization'. *Circulation*, **45,** 1292 (1972)
185. Sarnoff, S. J., Braunwald, E., Welch, G. H., Jr., Case, R. B., Stainsby, W. N. and Macruz, R. 'Haemodynamic determinants of oxygen consumption of the heart with special reference to the tension–time index'. *American Journal of Physiology*, **192**, 148 (1958)
186. Saunders, C. R. and Doty, D. B. 'Myocardial contusion: effect of intra-aortic balloon counterpulsation on cardiac output.' *Journal of Trauma*, **18,** 706 (1978)
187. Scheidt, S. 'Preservation of ischaemic myocardium with intra-aortic balloon pumping: modern therapeutic intervention or *Primum Non Nocere*?' *Circulation*, **58,** 211 (1978)
188. Scheidt, S., Ascheim, R. and Killip, T. 'Shock after acute myocardial infarction.' *American Journal of Cardiology*, **26,** 556 (1970)
189. Scheidt, S., Wilner, G., Mueller, H., Summers, D., Lesch, M., Wolff, G., Krakauer, J., Rubenfire, M., Fleming, P., Noon, G., Oldham, N., Killip, T. and Kantrowitz, A. 'Intra-aortic balloon counterpulsation in cardiogenic shock. Report of a co-operative clinical trial.' *New England Journal of Medicine*, **288,** 979 (1973)
190. Schoen, F. J., DeLaria, G. A. and Bernstein, E. F. 'Evaluation of intra-aortic balloon surfaces by scanning electron microscopy.' *Surgical Forum*, **22,** 167 (1972)

191. Schoen, F. J., DeLaria, G. A. and Bernstein, E. F. 'Morphology of blood surface interaction of intra-aortic balloons. An analysis of clinical and experimental specimens by scanning electron microscopy.' *Journal of Thoracic and Cardiovascular Surgery*, **65,** 304 (1973)
192. Scully, H. E., Gunstansen, J., Williams, W. G., Adelman, A. A., Baigre, R. S. and Goldman, B. S. 'Surgical management of complicated acute coronary insufficiency.' *Surgery*, **80,** 437 (1976)
192a. Seldinger, S. I. 'Catheter replacement of the needle in percutaneous arteriography: a new technique.' *Acta Radiologica* (*Stockh.*) **39,** 368 (1953)
193. Shea, T. M., Watson, R. M., Piotrowski, S. F., Dermksian, G. and Case, R. B. 'Anaerobic myocardial metabolism.' *American Journal of Physiology*, **203,** 463 (1962)
194. Shumakov, V. I. and Dragachev, S. P. 'An experimental study of the possibility of using a synchronous intra-aortic balloon pump for assisted circulation.' *Kardiologiia*, **9,** 13 (1969)
195. Shumakov, V. I., Tolpekin, V. E., Kasumov, A. H. and Dragachev, S. P. 'A comparative assessment of experimental counterpulsation and assisted circulation by means of an intra-aortic balloon pump.' *Kardiologiia*, **11,** 108 (1971)
196. Siegel, J. H., Farrell, E. J., Goldwyn, R. M. and Friedman, H. P. 'The surgical implications of physiologic patterns in myocardial infarction shock.' *Surgery*, **72,** 126 (1972)
197. Smith, G. H. and Morgan, W. E. 'Experience with counterpulsation in cardiac surgical patients.' *British Heart Journal*, **39,** 198 (1977)
198. Spotnitz, H. M., Beach, P. M., Bregman, D., Truccone, N., Parodi, E. N., Manger, W. M. and Malm, J. R. 'Oxygen conservation by propranolol and intra-aortic balloon pumping in the normal canine heart.' *Journal of Surgical Research*, **22,** 453 (1977)
199. Spotnitz, H. M., Beach, P. M., Manger, W. M., Bregman, D., Truccone, N. J., Parodi, E. N., Merker, C. and Malm, J. R. 'Propranolol potentiation of myocardial oxygen conservation during intra-aortic balloon pumping.' *Clinical Research*, **21,** 452 (1973)
200. Spotnitz, H. M., Covell, J., Ross, J., Jr. and Braunwald, E. 'Left ventricular mechanics and oxygen consumption during arterial counterpulsation.' *American Journal of Physiology*, **217,** 1352 (1969)
201. Steele, P., Pappas, G., Vogel, R., Jenkins, M. and Battock, D. 'Isosorbide dinitrate and intra-aortic balloon pumping in preinfarctional angina.' *Chest*, **69,** 712 (1976)
202. Stewart, S., Biddle, T. and DeWeese, J. 'Support of the myocardium with intra-aortic balloon counterpulsation following cardiopulmonary bypass.' *Journal of Thoracic and Cardiovascular Surgery*, **72,** 109 (1976)
202a. Subramanian, V. A., Goldstein, J. E., Sos, T. A., McCabe, J. C., Hoover, E. A. and Gay, W. A. Jr: 'Preliminary clinical experience with percutaneous intra-aortic balloon pumping.' *Circulation*, **62 (Suppl I),** I123 (1980)
203. Sugg, W. L., Rea, M. J., Webb, and Ecker, R. R. 'Cardiac assistance (counterpulsation) in ten patients.' *Annals of Thoracic Surgery*, **9,** 1 (1970)
204. Sugg, W. L., Webb, W. R. and Ecker, R. R. 'Reduction of extent of myocardial infarction by counterpulsation.' *Annals of Thoracic Surgery*, **7,** 311 (1969)
205. Summers, D. N., Kaplitt, M., Morris, J., Rubin, R., Nacht, R., Arieff, A., Lee, M., Wechsler, B. and Sawyer, P. N. 'Intra-aortic balloon pumping. Haemodynamic and metablic effects during cardiogenic shock in patients with triple coronary artery obstructive disease.' *Archives of Surgery*, **99,** 733 (1969)

206. Talpins, N. L., Kripke, D. C. and Goetz, R. H. 'Counterpulsation and intra-aortic balloon pumping in cardiogenic shock. Circulatory dynamics.' *Archives of Surgery*, **97,** 991 (1968)
207. Talpins, N. L., Kripke, D. C., Yellin, E. and Goetz, R. H. 'Haemodynamics and coronary blood flow during intra-aortic balloon pumping.' *Surgical Forum*, **19,** 122 (1968)
208. Turner, A. F., Meyers, H. I., Jacobson, G. and Lo, W. 'Carbon dioxide cineangiocardiography in the diagnosis of pericardial disease.' *American Journal of Roentgenology*, **97,** 342 (1966)
209. Tyberg, J. V., Keon, W. J., Sonnenblick, E. H. and Urschel, C. W. 'Effectiveness of intra-aortic balloon counterpulsation in the experimental low output state.' *American Heart Journal*, **80,** 89 (1970)
210. Tyras, D. H. and William, V. L. 'Paraplegia following intra-aortic balloon assistance.' *Annals of Thoracic Surgery*, **25,** 164 (1978)
211. Watson, J. T., Willerson, J. T., Fixler, D. E., Browning, R. M. and Sugg, W. L. 'Changes in collateral coronary blood flow (CCBF) distal to a coronary occlusion during intra-aortic balloon pumping (IABP).' *Transactions of the American Society for Artificial Internal Organs*, **19,** 402 (1973)
212. Webb, W. R., Parker, F. B., Jr., Neville, J. F., Jr. and Hanson, E. L. 'Acute mechanical complications of coronary arterial disease.' *Archives of Surgery*, **109,** 251 (1974)
213. Webb, W. R., Parker, F. B., Jr., Neville, J. F., Jr. and Hanson, E. L. 'Coronary artery disease: surgical management of acute emergencies.' *New York State Journal of Medicine*, **73,** 2572 (1973)
214. Weber, K. T. and Janicki, J. S. 'Coronary collateral flow and intra-aortic balloon counterpulsation.' *Transactions of the American Society for Artificial Internal Organs*, **19,** 395 (1973)
215. Weber, K. T. and Janicki, J. S. 'Intra-aortic balloon counterpulsation.' *Annals of Thoracic Surgery*, **17,** 603 (1974)
216. Weber, K. T., Janicki, J. S. and Walker, A. A. 'An assessment of intra-aortic balloon pumping in hypovolaemic and ischaemic heart preparations.' *Journal of Thoracic and Cardiovascular Surgery*, **64,** 869 (1972)
217. Weber, K. T., Janicki, J. S. and Walker, A. A. 'Intra-aortic balloon pumping: an analysis of several variables affecting balloon performance.' *Transactions of the American Society for Artificial Internal Organs*, **18,** 486 (1972)
218. Weikel, A. M., Jones, R. T., Dinsmore, R. and Petschek, H. E. 'Size limits and pumping effectiveness of intra-aortic balloons.' *Annals of Thoracic Surgery*, **12,** 45 (1971)
219. Weintraub, R. M. and Aroesty, J. M. 'The role of intra-aortic balloon pumping and surgery in the treatment of preinfarction angina.' (Editorial) *Chest*, **69,** 707 (1976)
219a. Weintraub, R. M., Aroesty, J. M., Paulin, S., Levine, F. H., Markis, J. E., LaRaia, P. J., Cohen, S. I. and Kurland, G. F.: 'Medically refractory unstable angina pectoris. I. Long-term follow-up of patients undergoing intra-aortic balloon counterpulsation and operation.' *American Journal of Cardiology*, **43,** 877 (1979)
220. Weintraub, R. M., Voukydis, P. C., Aroesty, J. M., Cohen, S. I., Ford, P., Kurland, G. S., LaRaia, P. J., Morkin, E. and Paulin, S. 'Treatment of preinfarction angina with intra-aortic balloon counterpulsation and surgery.' *American Journal of Cardiology*, **34,** 809 (1974)
221. Weisel, R. D., Berger, R. L. and Hechtman, H. B. 'Measurement of cardiac output by thermodilution.' *New England Journal of Medicine*, **292,** 682 (1975)

222. Weisel, R. D., Goldman, B. S., Teasdale, S. and Baigrie, R. S. 'Changing patterns of intra-aortic balloon pump assistance.' *Canadian Journal of Surgery*, **21,** 125 (1978)
223. Weissler, A. M., Harris, W. S. and Schoenfeld, C. D. 'Systolic time intervals in heart failure in man.' *Circulation*, **37,** 149 (1968)
224. Willerson, J. T., Curry, G. C., Watson, J. T., Leshin, S. J., Ecker, R. R., Mullins, C. B., Platt, M. R. and Sugg, W. L. 'Intra-aortic balloon counterpulsation in patients in cardiogenic shock, medically refractory left ventricle failure and/or recurrent ventricular tachycardias.' *American Journal of Medicine*, **58,** 183 (1975)
225. Williams, E. H., Tyers, G. F. O., Carter, S. L. and Williams, D. R. 'Ventricular arrhythmias following mitral valve replacement: control with intra-aortic balloon counterpulsation.' *Chest*, **68,** 641 (1975)
226. Windsor, H. M., O'Rourke, M., Shanahan, M. X. and Chang, V. P. 'Surgery and counterpulsation in cardiogenic shock.' *Medical Journal of Australia*, **2,** 841 (1973)
227. Wolff, G. A., Kamada, R. O., Collins, J. A., Kreisman, K. N. and Keith, J. I. 'Prolonged use of intra-aortic phase shift balloon pumping in cardiogenic shock.' *Chest*, **62,** 646 (1972)
228. Wolfson, S., Geha, A. S., Hammond, G. L., Langou, R. A. and Cohen, L. S. 'Preliminary report: modification of intra-aortic balloon for pressure measurement, contrast injection and guidewire passage.' (Abstr.) *American Journal of Cardiology*, **39,** 260 (1977)
229. Yellin, E., Levy, L., Bregman, D. and Frater, R. 'Haemodynamic effects of intra-aortic balloon pumping in dogs with aortic incompetence.' *Transactions of the American Society for Artificial Internal Organs*, **19,** 389 (1973)

22

Pulsatile Flow in Extracorporeal Circulation

David Bregman, Charles A. S. Marrin and Henry M. Spotnitz

And now I see with eye serene
The very pulse of the machine;
A being breathing thoughtful breath,
A traveller between life and death

William Wordsworth

The role of pulsatile perfusion during cardiopulmonary bypass has not yet been defined. However, recent technical advances and an improved understanding of the physiology of pulsatile flow have led to a greater appreciation of its importance.

The purpose of this chapter is to review the development of pulsatile perfusion, its physiology, technology and the role of new circulatory assist devices. The results of our own clinical experience with the pulsatile assist device at the Columbia Presbyterian Medical Center will be presented.

Evolution of pulsatile perfusion

The earliest systems for the artificial perfusion of organs were designed by physiologists for use in research laboratories. They attempted to reproduce normal circulatory physiology as closely as possible. The importance of fluctuations in perfusion pressure was first realized as long ago as 1868 by Ludwig and Schmidt, using a syringe injection technique[57]. In 1888 Hamel described a perfusion apparatus which delivered intermittent flow by means of a pendulum[38].

Carl Jacobj may properly be described as the 'father' of pulsatile perfusion in extracorporeal circulation. In 1890 he reported the use of a perfusion apparatus which delivered pulsatile flow by means of intermittent compression of a rubber balloon in the arterial end of the circuit[46].

In 1910 Hooker compared the effects of pulsatile and non-pulsatile perfusion on the function of the isolated kidney[45]. The pump that he used was capable of producing pulsatile flow by means of a cam, and the amplitude of the pulse pressure could be varied. He found that reducing the amplitude of the pulse pressure during perfusion of the isolated kidney lowered both the blood flow and the urinary output. Although Gesell was unable to confirm Hooker's observations concerning renal blood flow *in vivo*, he reported that lowering the pulse pressure caused a decrease in urinary output and in chloride excretion[33].

The pump oxygenators which were used in the early days of extracorporeal circulation were capable of producing pulsatile flow, but, because of problems with excessive haemolysis, this feature was not routinely employed. The use of non-pulsatile flow for perfusion of short duration did not appear to be deleterious and the problem of haemolysis was much less obvious.

In 1955 Wesolowski reported a series of experiments in which he compared the effects of pulsatile and non-pulsatile perfusion and he wrote that '. . . the entire systemic circulation appears to be maintained equally well by the use of pulsatile and non-pulsatile flows for periods up to six hours'[104]. Pulsatile perfusion reached its nadir, and non-pulsatile perfusion has become the standard technique of extracorporeal circulation used during cardiopulmonary bypass in most cardiac surgical centres today.

Since 1955 significant improvements have been made in the design of pumps for extracorporeal circulation. In 1961 Clauss *et al.*[21] introduced the concept of counterpulsation, but the early arterio-arterial counterpulsators were cumbersome and haemolysis was a major problem. In 1962 Moulopoulos, Topaz and Kolff[72] developed the concept of an intra-aortic balloon which could act as an arterial counterpulsator without the need for withdrawal and reinfusion of blood. This resulted in minimal haemolysis.

However, it was not until 1968 that Kantrowitz *et al.*[49] reported the first successful clinical use of intra-aortic balloon pumping. The development of tough, flexible plastics that are biologically inert, combined with the rapid advances made in cardiac surgery, ultimately led to the widespread and enthusiastic acceptance of intra-aortic balloon pumping.

In 1972 Berger and Saini reported the clinical use of an intra-aortic balloon to create pulsatile cardiopulmonary bypass[9], and others soon reported similar experiences[78]. The potential morbidity from the use of the intra-aortic balloon, however, obviated its routine use for the creation of pulsatile perfusion[2, 7, 10, 53, 58, 77, 103].

In 1975 a pulsatile assist device (PAD®) was introduced by Bregman[16]. It applied the balloon concept externally in the cardiopulmonary bypass circuit. The device made it possible to use pulsatile perfusion routinely during cardiopulmonary bypass without the problems of haemolysis or the complications associated with the insertion of an intra-aortic balloon.

Pump technology and pulsatile flow

The pumps used for perfusion during cardiopulmonary bypass may be divided into two broad groups:

(1) The positive displacement pumps

(a) Rotary pumps, in which a bolus of blood is trapped in a segment of tubing by rotating members and 'milked' towards the output. The *roller pump*, which is the most widely used of any of the pumps for routine extracorporeal circulation, is an example of this type.

(b) Reciprocating pumps, in which blood is allowed to collect in a valved cavity, from which it is ejected by the reciprocating action of a piston, diaphragm or similar device. This group includes the 'ventricle' pumps.

(2) The kinetic pumps
In these the velocity of the blood at the inlet is increased by the forced rotation of an impeller and then decreased at the outlet by a diffuser. The result is an increase in the kinetic energy (pressure head) of the blood at the outlet of the pump. The principal advantage of this concept is that the output is directly related to the input pressure and is inversely related to

the pressure head against which it works. Because the amount of kinetic energy imparted to the blood is directly proportional to the revolutions per minute (RPM) of the impeller, a given perfusion pressure can be maintained over a wide range of flow rates. Thus the greater the inflow, the greater the output, and, similarly, the greater the resistance to flow, the smaller the output. The centrifugal force-vortex pump is an example of this type. Improvements in the design of such 'load-sensitive' pumps have led to a reduction in haemolysis, which has been a problem in earlier models, and they are now considered the most suitable for use in artificial hearts[51].

Pulsatile flow may be defined as flow which is subject to periodic variations in velocity.

Thus, roller pumps actually deliver pulsatile flow but the pulses are of low amplitude and high frequency, depending upon the degree of occlusion, the number of rollers on the pump head, and the number of revolutions per minute. The pulsatile flow produced by standard roller pumps has aptly been described as 'ripple flow' as the pulses are rapidly eliminated by damping within the arterial tree.

The reciprocating pumps produce pulse waves analogous to those of the normal circulation.

Only the kinetic pumps produce truly non-pulsatile flow.

In the present discussion however, the flow produced by roller pumps will be considered as non-pulsatile, and the terms 'non-pulsatile' and 'continuous' will be used synonymously.

In addition to the combination of intra-aortic balloon pumping with otherwise non-pulsatile cardiopulmonary bypass circuits, three systems for pulsatile perfusion are available at present:

(1) The pulsatile assist device (PAD^{R*})

This is installed in the arterial line of the bypass circuit, and may be used with any of the pumps commonly used for extracorporeal circulation, including the centrifugal force-vortex type (*Figures 22.1*, *22.2* and *22.3*). It consists of a valveless, flexible inner blood conduit surrounded by a rigid plastic shell. Air is pumped in and out of the chamber between conduit and housing, resulting in compression and expansion of the balloon conduit. Synchronization with the R wave of the ECG is achieved by the electronic logic in the pumping console. During induced cardiac arrest or ventricular fibrillation the rate of pulsation may be controlled by using an internal trigger from the console.

Other devices based upon the same concept have also been developed[95].

(2) The 'bubble tube' system

This incorporates an especially dilated segment of tubing used in conjunction with a roller pump[30]. As the roller passes over the 'bubble' the stroke volume of the pump is increased. In this way pulsatile flow is created, but the frequency is dependent upon the number of rollers and the rpm of the pump head. The pulse pressure is fixed by the dimensions of the bubble used.

*Datascope Corporation, Paramus, New Jersey, USA

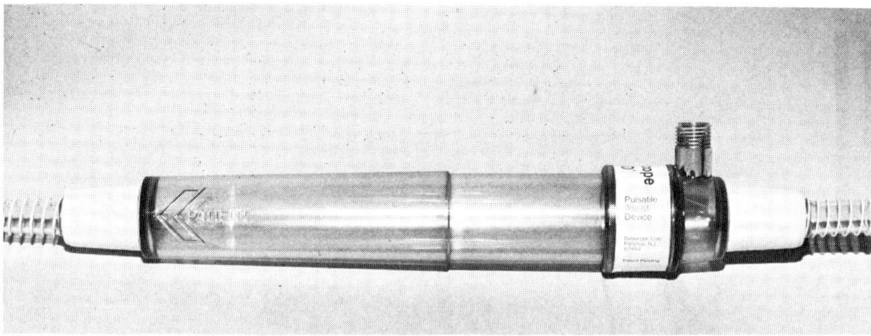

Figure 22.1 The pulsatile assist device (PAD^{R}). Maximum displacement of the balloon conduit is 80 ml

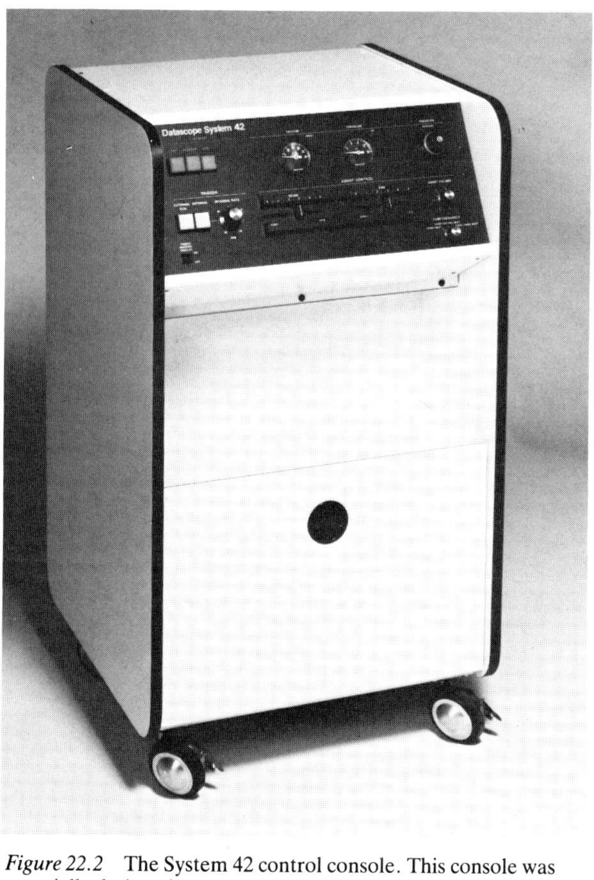

Figure 22.2 The System 42 control console. This console was especially designed to create pulsatile cardiopulmonary bypass by using any of the standard pumps in conjunction with the pulsatile assist device. However, the PAD can also be used with the standard intra-aortic balloon pumping console (System 80 or System 82)

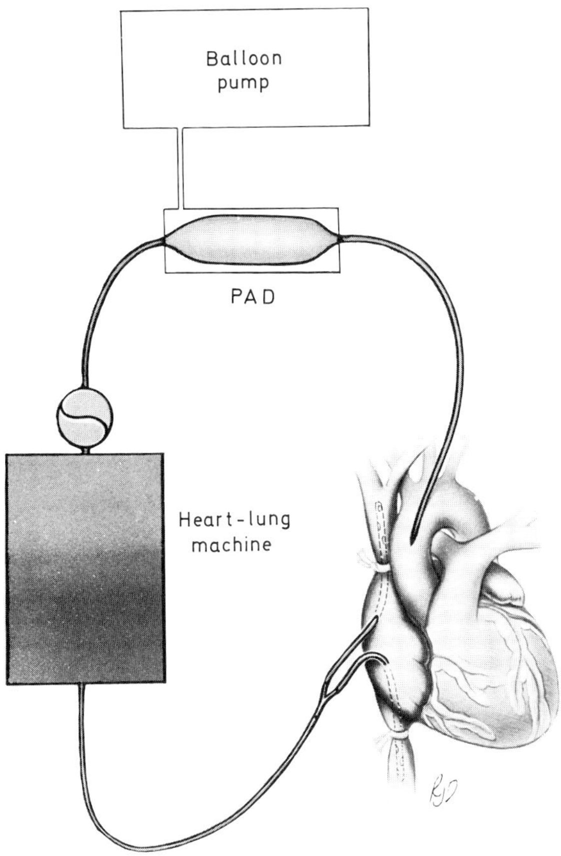

Figure 22.3 Schematic view of the pulsatile assist device in the cardiopulmonary bypass circuit. The PAD may be used to produce either synchronous counterpulsation through the arterial cannula or pulsatile cardiopulmonary bypass

Both the PAD and the 'bubble tube' are versions of the 'ventricle' pump, the difference being that no valves are used. Unidirectional flow is achieved by the forward impulsion and occlusion of the rollers on the pump head.

(3) The 'stepping' motor pump[44]

This is a modification of a standard roller pump with a motor capable of producing rapid acceleration and deceleration of the rollers. The system may be triggered either from the ECG or internally. The amplitude, frequency and duration of the pulse wave can be varied from the control console. A similar modification of the motor of the centrifugal force-vortex pump is also available.

Haemodynamic aspects of pulsatile flow

There have been several attempts to derive an equation to describe blood flow based on Poiseuille's Equation:

$$Q = \frac{dp \times \pi \times r^4}{8 \times \eta \times l}$$

where Q = volume flow rate; dp = pressure drop along the tube; r = radius of the tube; η = coefficient of viscosity of the liquid; and l = length of the tube.

However, the equation does not apply to the circulation of the blood for four reasons:

(1) Blood is not a Newtonian fluid*
(2) The radius of the blood vessels is not constant throughout their length, and the cross-sectional area of the vascular tree increases every time a vessel branches. Smooth muscle fibres in the vascular wall may also vary the calibre of the vessel.
(3) The walls of the blood vessels are elastic rather than rigid, and the elasticity is not uniformly distributed. Large arteries tend to be more elastic than small ones, and the vessels become progressively less distensible the further they are from the heart in the arterial tree.
(4) The flow of blood is not laminar.

It would therefore be difficult to describe blood flow in mathematical terms even if the velocity of blood flow were constant (i.e. continuous blood flow).

In the normal circulation, flow is pulsatile, however, and the flow is dependent upon the elasticity of the blood vessels as well as their calibre. The vascular elasticity determines the velocity at which the pressure and flow waves travel. The less elastic the vascular wall, the greater the velocity of the pressure and flow waves and therefore the less the pressure gradient and the less the flow.

The elastic recoil has the effect of amplifying the pulse wave as it travels towards the periphery and the pulse pressure is greater in the terminal aorta than in the ascending aorta. As the elastic properties of the vessel wall decrease with age the amplification diminishes and finally disappears so that the pulse pressure becomes the same throughout the aorta. The viscosity of the blood tends to reduce the amplitude of the pulse waves.

Because of the changes in the calibre and elasticity of the blood vessels, the pressure and flow waves are reflected within the arterial system at each branching so that the pressure and flow waves at any given point represent the summation of incident waves (travelling towards the periphery) and reflected waves (from the periphery).

*The coefficient of viscosity, η, is the ratio of the shear stress (which is proportional to the pressure drop along the tube) to the shear rate (the velocity gradient *across* the tube). For a Newtonian fluid, viscosity is independent of shear rate. However, the viscosity of blood varies greatly depending upon the shear rate.

The arterial tree may therefore be considered as being in a steady state of oscillation. The concept of mean flow is based upon continuous flow; in order to describe oscillatory flow it is necessary to introduce the concept of vascular impedance, which is the ratio of pulsatile pressure to pulsatile flow. The peripheral resistance depends upon the calibre of the blood vessels, but the vascular impedance depends upon both their calibre and their elasticity.

If it is assumed that the heart rate is regular, the wave forms of pulsatile pressure and flow may be mathematically reduced by harmonic analysis to a Fourier series. The pulse wave is represented by describing the true mean flow in terms of a sinusoidal wave at the frequency of the heart rate (fundamental or first harmonic) and in terms describing sinusoidal waves, whose frequencies are multiples of the heart rate (second, third, fourth, etc. harmonics). Harmonic analysis is a useful tool with which to study and compare the properties of the normal circulation with those of either the abnormal circulation, on the one hand, or of an extracorporeal perfusion system on the other.

The importance of comparing the wave forms in this way has been pointed out[69, 108]. The frequency and amplitude of the pulse wave are obviously most important in any consideration of pulsatile flow. If the characteristics of the pulse wave are not similar to those of the normal circulation it is doubtful whether such pulsatile flow is physiologically superior to non-pulsatile flow. Therefore pulsatile *flow* cannot be equated with pulsatile *perfusion*.

Hydraulic energy

Normally the arterial circulation is maintained by two pumps which are out of phase with one another. The first is the left ventricle and the second the elastic walls of the larger arteries. Similarly the venous circulation is maintained by two pumps, skeletal muscle and the thoracoabdominal pump, as well as by the '*vis a tergo*'. Pulsatile blood flow therefore requires more energy to move a given volume of blood in a given time than continuous flow. Hydraulic energy is of two kinds:

(1) Kinetic energy which can be calculated from the mass of the blood (stroke volume) and the square of its velocity*.
(2) Potential energy which is stored in the walls of the arteries and retransformed into kinetic energy by elastic recoil.

In this context calculations of stroke work based upon multiplying the mean pressure by the mean flow will clearly underestimate the true values, which can be more closely approximated in terms of the vascular impedance (the ratio of pulsatile pressure to pulsatile flow) calculated by using harmonic analysis. It has been estimated in this way that the energy required to deliver pulsatile flow is more than twice that required for non-pulsatile flow at the same mean arterial pressure[90]. It is postulated

* $e = \dfrac{m \times v^2}{2}$

that, as most of the dissipation of energy occurs at or beyond the arteriolar level in the circulation, the importance of the additional energy lies in maintaining perfusion by keeping capillary beds open and promoting lymphatic flow. This is merely un updated version of the concept of 'vascular shocks' introduced in 1913 by Gesell[33]. In other words, the concept of a 'critical closing pressure' should be applied to pulsatile as well as to mean flow.

For a more detailed discussion of pulsatile flow the reader is referred to McDonald's monograph[59].

Pathology and physiology

Although non-pulsatile perfusion had proved to be fairly satisfactory for short periods of cardiopulmonary bypass, it is well established that certain characteristic changes occur as a consequence of longer periods of non-pulsatile perfusion. They include:

(1) Disturbances of vasomotor control with alterations in the distribution of blood flow, arteriovenous shunting and venous pooling.
(2) Progressive increases in systemic and pulmonary vascular resistance leading to inadequate perfusion of the tissues.
(3) Accumulation of extracellular fluid causing interstitial oedema and further interference with blood flow.
(4) Anaerobic cellular metabolism manifested by metabolic acidosis, accumulation of lactate and reduced oxygen utilization.
(5) Disorders of endocrine function.
(6) Progressive dysfunction of various organs, notably the brain, kidneys, lungs and heart.

Experimental and clinical studies

The evidence in favour of and against pulsatile, as opposed to non-pulsatile, perfusion has recently been reviewed in detail by Mavroudis[68].

The published studies, especially the earlier ones, comparing the effects of pulsatile and non-pulsatile flow are confusing. The apparent inconsistencies in the results obtained by various investigators may be resolved by consideration of the flow rates used during perfusion.

Wesolowski[104], for example, used flow rates of 130 ml/kg per min and other workers have used flows as high as 200 ml/kg per min[11, 39, 83]. Ogata[76] pointed out that the differences between the effects of pulsatile and non-pulsatile flow only become obvious at flows less than 100 ml/kg per min, and it was only in the studies in which flow rates in this range were used that the differences between pulsatile and non-pulsatile perfusion were demonstrated in experimental animals[27, 82, 85, 89] and in humans[102]. Flows in the range of 50–100 ml/kg per min are routinely used for clinical cardiopulmonary bypass. Normal blood flow is about 110 ml/kg per min with a pulse pressure of 30–40 mmHg.

Vasomotor disturbances

It is well established in experimental animals that the increases in mean arterial pressure and peripheral vascular resistance seen with non-pulsatile perfusion do not occur during pulsatile perfusion[3–6, 9, 26, 27, 29, 34, 47, 52, 62, 74, 92, 101, 105]. Similar findings have been reported in humans[102].

Furthermore, Nakayama *et al.*[74] were impressed by the improvement in venous return during pulsatile, as opposed to non-pulsatile, cardiopulmonary bypass.

Similar responses to pulsatile and non-pulsatile perfusion have been reported in the pulmonary circulation[20].

The cause of the increase in pressure is not well understood. Elegantly designed experiments by Angell James and de Burgh Daly involving recordings from the aortic arch and carotid sinus baroreceptors with simultaneous recordings of pressure in the carotid artery and in the femoral artery have led to the suggestion that pulsatile flow, by stimulating the baroreceptors, plays an important role in normal reflex vasomotor control[3, 4, 5, 6, 26, 29, 34, 52, 92]. Mandelbaum and Burns, on the basis of equally impressive studies[62], have suggested that the pulse wave serves the more direct purpose of keeping the capillary beds open, and that non-pulsatile perfusion fails to perform this function, leading to precapillary shunting and an increase in peripheral resistance. This hypothesis is consistent with the finding that more energy is required to maintain pulsatile perfusion at a given mean arterial pressure[90].

Ssentjurin[93], in experiments on the isolated rabbit ear, observed that pulsatile perfusion produced a greater rate of flow than non-pulsatile perfusion, a finding confirmed more recently in humans by Trinkle *et al.*[102]. Similarly Long[56] and Ogata *et al.*[76] reported that non-pulsatile perfusion caused sluggish movement of erythrocytes and a tendency to intravascular aggregation, with marked impairment of capillary blood flow. Ogata *et al.*[76] studied the microcirculation of the omentum and demonstrated that capillary perfusion ceased after twenty minutes of non-pulsatile perfusion, as arteriolar flow was diverted by shunting. By contrast, pulsatile flow produced constant and more evenly distributed capillary perfusion.

Parsons and McMaster[60, 80, 81] demonstrated that dye injected into the tissue of rabbit ears cleared faster with pulsatile than with non-pulsatile flow and noted that oedema occurred more commonly during non-pulsatile flow. They also reported that the flow of lymph, which was quite rapid during pulsatile flow, was almost abolished by non-pulsatile perfusion.

Since then, other authors have remarked on the increased tendency towards the formation of oedema and the greater fluid requirements of experimental animals[24, 27, 47, 67, 74] and humans[102] during non-pulsatile cardiopulmonary bypass.

Capillary exchange depends not only on the mean capillary pressure and the pulsations, but also on the pressure gradient across the capillary wall. If the tissue pressure rises because of fluid accumulation in the extracellular space, whether due to protein leakage from damaged capillary endothelium or to the failure of lymphatic and venous drainage, the resulting interference with capillary exchange may initiate a vicious cycle of progressively increasing ischaemia and injury.

Metabolic disturbances

Shepard and Kirklin[89] measured whole-body oxygen consumption as an index of tissue perfusion during pulsatile and non-pulsatile perfusion in calves. They reported higher oxygen and lactate extraction and a decreased tendency to acidosis in the animals subjected to pulsatile perfusion. Other investigators have confirmed that the findings of reduced oxygen consumption and metabolic acidosis during non-pulsatile perfusion are absent during pulsatile perfusion, or, if present, are reversed by it[5, 27, 32, 47, 76, 102]

Endocrine disturbances

As part of the normal response to stress, plasma ACTH and cortisol levels rise following major surgery[96–98]. Although such increases have been demonstrated after closed cardiac surgery not involving the use of cardiopulmonary bypass, such as closed mitral valvotomy[19, 97], both adrenal and anterior pituitary function have been shown to be abnormal[17] following non-pulsatile cardiopulmonary bypass. The serum ACTH and cortisol levels are low and the pituitary fails to respond normally to thyrotropin-releasing hormone.

However, Taylor *et al.* have demonstrated a rise in plasma cortisol levels (i.e. normal stress response)[100] and a normal anterior pituitary response to thyrotropin-releasing hormone in humans during pulsatile cardiopulmonary bypass[99].

Pulsatile perfusion has also been shown to prevent or reduce the increases in circulating levels of renin[18, 22, 23, 35, 42, 50, 64–66, 91], vasopressin[55] and catecholamines[27, 40, 41, 82] which occur during non-pulsatile perfusion.

Specific effects

Central nervous system

Although disturbances of the cerebral function following cardiopulmonary bypass have been related to embolic phenomena, the use of filters has failed to entirely eliminate the problem[12, 43]. Several factors are certainly involved but inadequate perfusion must surely be one of the most important.

It was observed long ago that the cerebrospinal fluid pulsates with the heart beat[84] and de Langen[25] has shown that these pulsations can be increased or reduced in response to similar changes in the amplitude of the pulse in the carotid artery.

The brain is very vulnerable to inadequate perfusion and hypoxia. Halley, Reemtsma and Creech[37] reported decreased cerebral oxygen consumption following non-pulsatile perfusion, and Sanderson and Wright found evidence of diffuse nerve cell ischaemic injury after non-pulsatile perfusions which was not present following pulsatile cardiopulmonary bypass[85, 107]. Matsumoto reported improved cerebral and conjunctival perfusion in dogs during pulsatile flow, by comparison with non-pulsatile flow[67].

The kidney

The effect of pulsatile blood flow on the function of the kidney has been the subject of many investigations. It is well established that non-pulsatile flow is associated with abnormalities of renal function which do not occur during pulsatile perfusion[1, 63, 79, 88]. By comparison with non-pulsatile flow, pulsatile perfusion has been shown to improve the volume[70] and distribution[31, 35, 66] of renal blood flow, increase renal oxygen consumption[73], urine output[9, 11, 33, 45, 47, 48, 55, 79], creatine clearance[47], and reabsorption of water and electrolytes[44, 55, 79]. It is the pulse itself, rather than the mean pressure in the renal artery which is the critical factor.

Studies by Agishi, Peirce and Kent[1] and Belzer *et al.*[8] drew attention to the importance of pulsatile perfusion in the maintenance of renal structure and function with the result that most centres now preserve cadaveric donor kidneys with pulsatile pumps until transplantation.

The lungs

Clarke *et al.*[20] reported thickening of the alveolar walls and increased pulmonary vascular resistance following non-pulsatile blood flow. A significant amount of arteriovenous shunting is common after cardiopulmonary bypass, but, as similar changes occur following any major surgical procedure because of alveolar collapse, this phenomenon cannot be attributed to the effects of non-pulsatile perfusion alone.

The phenomenon of 'pump lung' was frequently a problem during the early days of cardiac surgery and several authors have reported reduced pulmonary compliance and alterations in the alveolar-capillary oxygen exchange. Although the 'pump lung' has been attributed to microemboli of damaged blood cells or platelets, denatured plasma proteins and fat emboli, the use of filters in the extracorporeal circuit has failed to prevent its occurrence[54]. Improved understanding of the pathophysiology of shock (and 'shock lung'), the use of haemodilution with colloids as well as crystalloids in the heart-lung machine prime, and shorter durations of extracorporeal circulation have played a major role in reducing such complications. However, no studies have so far been published on the effect of pulsatile perfusion in relation to these abnormalities.

There is some evidence that pulsatile flow causes less damage to the liver[78] and pancreas[70] than non-pulsatile perfusion, as assessed by changes in the plasma levels of SGOT and the serum and urinary amylase concentrations in the postoperative period.

Pulsatile flow and the myocardium

The effects of intra-aortic balloon pumping on the myocardium are discussed in Chapter 21.

There are conflicting reports concerning the effects of pulsatile perfusion on the heart itself. The number of reports is small, however, and different methods have been used to achieve pulsatile flow by different groups. Other variables, such as temperature, perfusion pressure and the duration of heart-lung bypass make it still more difficult to interpret the findings.

However, there is a small but growing body of evidence that pulsatile perfusion is beneficial, especially for the fibrillating heart. The literature will be briefly reviewed and will report our own clinical experience with the PAD at the Columbia Presbyterian Medical Centre.

Habal *et al.*[36] demonstrated that during prolonged ventricular fibrillation in dogs, pulsatile flow produced better subendocardial perfusion than non-pulsatile flow, a finding which was not confirmed in the studies of Steed *et al.*[94] or Moores *et al.*[71]. Furthermore, Habal reported higher coronary vascular resistances and relatively lower coronary blood flow to the left ventricle (indicating more effective perfusion) during pulsatile flow, as well as increased myocardial oxygen utilization and lactate extraction (implying less anaerobic metabolism), confirming the earlier clinical findings of Pappas *et al.*[78]

Similar studies have shown that the left ventricular ejection fraction in the early postoperative period is higher in patients undergoing aortocoronary bypass grafting with pulsatile perfusion, when compared with a similar group of patients treated with non-pulsatile cardiopulmonary bypass[61]. The same group of investigators, in an earlier publication, also reported a lower incidence of perioperative myocardial infarction in the patients subjected to pulsatile perfusion[78].

Laboratory studies by Dunn, Peterson and Kirsh[28] have shown that pulsatile flow is superior to non-pulsatile perfusion of the fibrillating heart in terms of maintenance of left ventricular contractility, compliance and reduced water content, While Schaff and his colleagues have demonstrated that pulsatile perfusion reduces the regional myocardial ischaemia which occurs with non-pulsatile perfusion in the presence of a critical stenosis of the anterior descending branch of the left coronary artery in the fibrillating ventricle[86, 87].

There is not yet any conclusive evidence of the superiority of pulsatile perfusion of the beating heart, but, on theoretical grounds, diastolic augmentation of the pulse might be expected to improve coronary perfusion and the benefits of counterpulsation in this respect are beyond doubt.

Applications

The technical details of the pulsatile assist device have already been described. The PAD may be used in various ways at different stages in the cardiac surgical procedure such as:

(1) To provide counterpulsation via the aortic cannula before the institution of extracorporeal circulation and during weaning from cardiopulmonary bypass.
(2) To augment the diastolic pressure and provide systolic unloading of the beating heart during cardiopulmonary bypass.
(3) To provide pulsatile perfusion of the fibrillating heart and/or the rest of the body during total cardiopulmonary bypass.

Experience with the pulsatile assist device at the Columbia Presbyterian medical center

The PAD was first evaluated in the laboratory by inducing cardiogenic shock in twelve dogs with intravenous injections of propranolol (3mg/kg of body weight). Representative tracings illustrating the efficacy of the PAD for counterpulsation and for providing pulsatile total cardiopulmonary bypass are presented in *Figures 22.4* and *22.5*, and the overall results obtained are summarized in *Table 22.1*.

Technical aspects

We routinely use roller pumps and bubble-type oxygenators for cardiopulmonary bypass. A No. 24 Bardic (U.S.C.I. Division of C.R. Bard

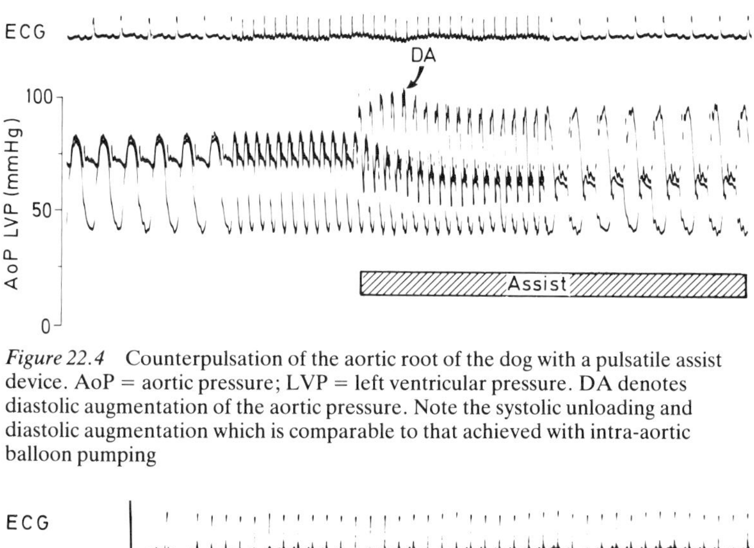

Figure 22.4 Counterpulsation of the aortic root of the dog with a pulsatile assist device. AoP = aortic pressure; LVP = left ventricular pressure. DA denotes diastolic augmentation of the aortic pressure. Note the systolic unloading and diastolic augmentation which is comparable to that achieved with intra-aortic balloon pumping

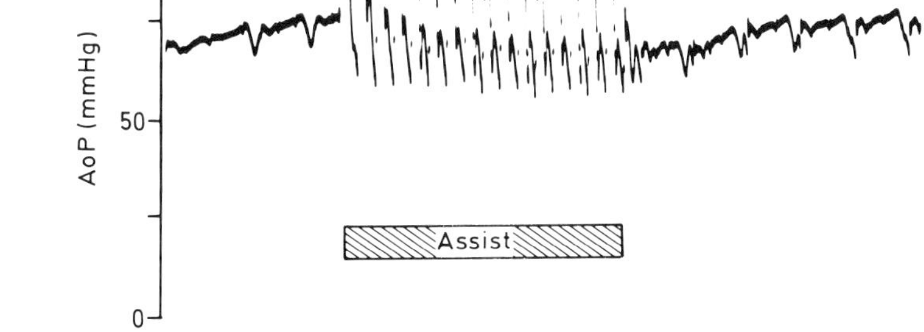

Figure 22.5 Pulsatile total cardiopulmonary bypass in the dog. AoP = aortic pressure. Pulse pressures of 40–50 mmHg are easily achieved

Table 22.1 Summary of the results of preliminary evaluation of the pulsatile assist device in the laboratory

Counterpulsation	
Cardiac output	↑ 62% (25–95%)
Diastolic augmentation	↑ 90% (35–140%)
Systolic pressure	↓ 10% (0–50%)
Haemolysis (2 hours) =	4–12 mg/100ml
Pulsation	
Pulse pressure	40–50 mmHg
Haemolysis (2 hours) =	10.5–17.5 mg/100ml

Incorporated, Billerica, Massachusetts, USA) arterial cannula is inserted in the ascending aorta. The tip of the cannula is directed towards the descending thoracic aorta at the beginning of the operation. However, turning the tip towards the aortic valve will maximize the effect of aortic root counterpulsation. During the insertion of the venous cannulae the triggering of the PAD is adjusted to alternate beats because of the frequency of atrial premature contractions.

The PAD is switched off during the initiation of cardiopulmonary bypass until the patient's bypass flow is stable.

It is *most important to switch off the PAD for a moment whenever the cross-clamp or partial occlusion clamp is applied to, or removed from, the ascending aorta.*

While heart-lung bypass is being discontinued at the end of the operation, PAD counterpulsation can be used with advantage to increase the coronary blood flow, to stabilize the patient with ventricular arrhythmias and to reduce the work of a functionally depressed left ventricle.

The PAD should be used with caution, if at all, in patients with significant disease of the aorta such as aneurysms, cystic medial necrosis etc. and in patients with significant aortic valvular insufficiency, in whom the PAD may tend to increase the ventricular work.

Since 1975, when it was introduced for clinical use, the PAD has been employed in more than 3000 patients at our institution and an analysis of the first 1000 has been detailed[13].

The haemodynamic effectiveness of the PAD for counterpulsation of the aortic root may be readily appreciated from the recording illustrated in *Figure 22.6*.

Figure 22.7 shows the effect of PAD counterpulsation on the flow in an aortocoronary bypass graft. The blood flow in the vein grafts was measured while the PAD was being used in a group of 17 consecutive patients undergoing coronary bypass grafting and it was found that the PAD produced an average increase in flow of 21.4 ± 6.1 per cent[15].

The urinary output during cardiopulmonary bypass was measured in another group of 100 patients. The PAD group had a mean urine output of 9.18 ± 0.68 ml/min, whereas the output of the group treated with non-pulsatile cardiopulmonary bypass was only 3.90 ± 0.35 ml/min ($P<0.001$).

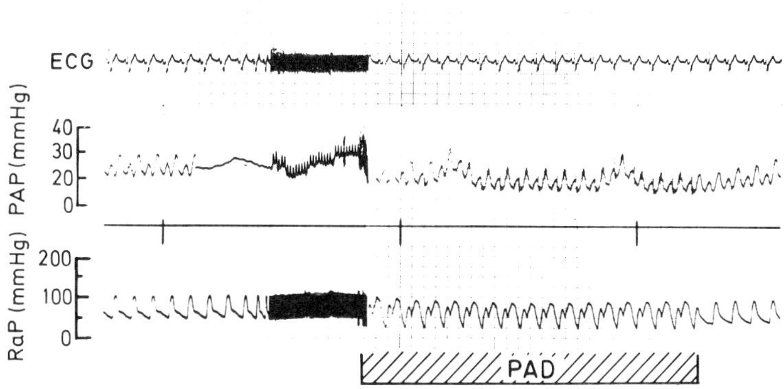

Figure 22.6 Aortic root counterpulsation with the PAD in the adult. The tracings were obtained before the institution of cardiopulmonary bypass in a patient undergoing coronary artery bypass grafting for ischaemic heart disease. PAP = pulmonary artery pressure; RaP = radial artery pressure. Note the systolic unloading and the diastolic augmentation of the arterial pressure and the reduction in pulmonary artery end-diastolic pressure produced by the pulsatile assist device

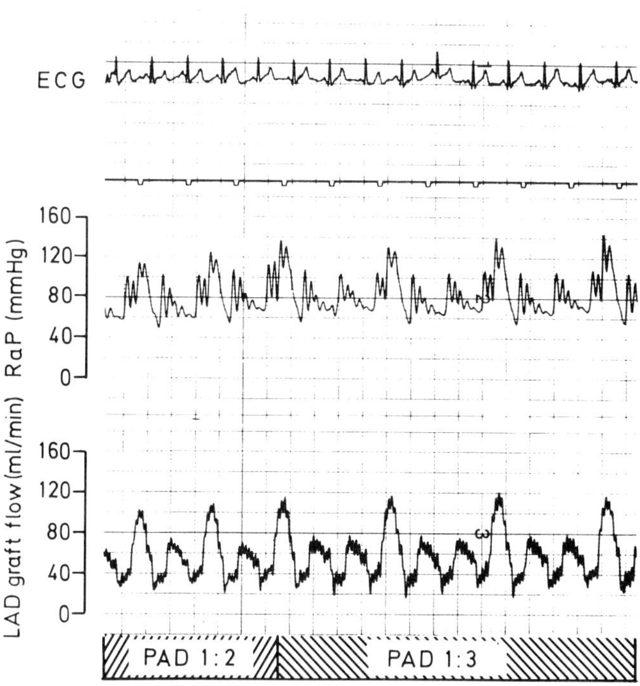

Figure 22.7 Flow augmentation by the PAD in a coronary bypass graft. This tracing was obtained in the same patient as the one in *Figure 22.6*, after termination of cardiopulmonary bypass. LAD graft = bypass graft to the left anterior descending coronary artery. The effect of the PAD on graft flow is shown with triggering on alternate (1:2) and on every third heartbeat (1:3)

Table 22.2 Summary of the experience using the pulsatile assist device in 1000 patients at the Columbia Presbyterian Medical Center (1975–1979)

Patients		
Age: 18–82 (Average = 59)		
Sex: 735 Males 265 Females		
(A) 776 Patients	NYHA Class III or IV	
	Ejection fraction less than 0.3	
	LVEDP more than 18 mmHg	
(B) 207 Patients	Left main (or equivalent) coronary lesion (158 in A)	
(C) 51 patients	Crescendo angina (47 in A)	
Operations		
Coronary bypass alone		519
Valve replacement alone		341
Ventricular aneurysm resection alone		12
Combined coronary bypass and valve replacement		105
Combined coronary bypass and resection of ventricular aneurysm		23
Results		
Number weaned from CPB		993 (99.3%)
(with PAD alone — 987)		
(with PAD + IABP — 6)		
Need for postoperative IABP		7 (0.7%)
Intraoperative myocardial infarction		15 (1.5%)
Postoperative hospital deaths (Within 4 weeks)		12 (1.2%)

Table 22.3 Summary of the experience using the pulsatile assist device with left main coronary artery disease at the Columbia Presbyterian Medical Center (1975–1977)

Number of patients: 50	
Age: 39–71 (Average = 58)	
Sex: 44 Males 6 Females	
Previous transmural myocardial infarction	25 (50%)
Crescendo angina	6 (12%)
NYHA Class II	12 (24%)
Class III	24 (48%)
Class IV	14 (28%)
Preoperative LVEDP ⩾ 18 mmHg	13 (26%)
Preoperative E, F, ⩽, 4	15 (30%)
Surgical results	
Number of patients	50
Preoperative left ventricular dysfunction	39 (78%)
Preoperative use of IABP	0
Number patients weaned from CPB with PAD	50 (100%)
Need for postoperative IABP	0
Perioperative myocardial infarctions	1 (2%)
Postoperative hospital deaths	1 (2%)

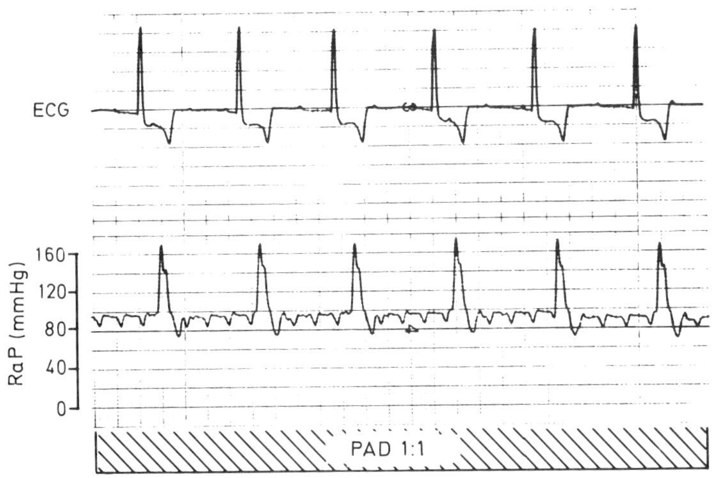

Figure 22.8 Pulsatile cardiopulmonary bypass with the PAD in children. The tracing was obtained during the repair of a ventricular septal defect in a five year old child on total cardiopulmonary bypass. RaP = radial artery pressure

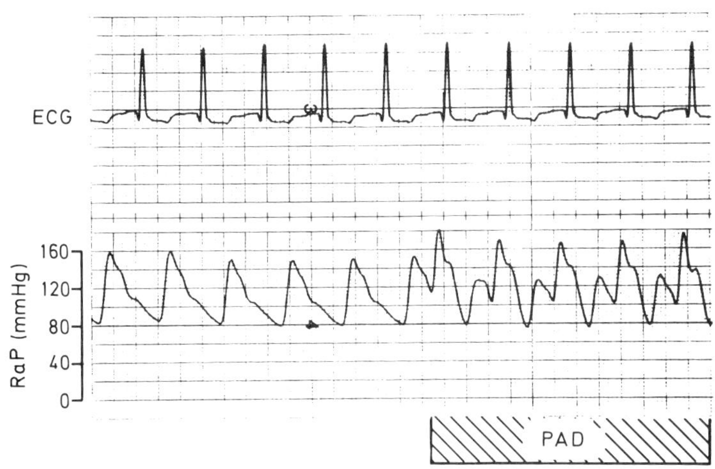

Figure 22.9 Aortic root counterpulsation with the PAD in children. This tracing was obtained from the same patient as in *Figure 22.8*, after termination of cardiopulmonary bypass. RaP = radial artery pressure

Table 22.2 summarizes our experience with the first 1000 patients. We have been particularly impressed by the reduction in the number of patients who require intra-aortic balloon pumping postoperatively[14]. At this institution the advent of the PAD had markedly reduced the incidence of postoperative low cardiac-output syndrome, and the great majority of patients can be weaned smoothly and uneventfully from cardiopulmonary bypass. The results are particularly impressive for those patients with severe or unstable ischaemic heart disease. The data from the subset of patients with critical left mainstem coronary artery disease are presented in *Table 22.3*.

Figures 22.8 and *22.9* show the effective use of the PAD in a 5-year-old child. Our experience with the PAD in children has been limited but encouraging. The use of profound hypothermia and circulatory arrest for cardiac surgery in infants has obviated the need for the PAD, although it has been suggested that more efficient cooling and rewarming of such patients could be achieved by pulsatile perfusion[106].

Conclusions

(1) Pulsatile flow is desirable for the preservation of normal function of various organs and systems of the body.
(2) The PAD safely creates pulsatile cardiopulmonary bypass.
(3) The PAD is effective when used for aortic root counterpulsation.
(4) The PAD is a simple alternative to intra-aortic balloon pumping for patients undergoing cardiac surgery.

References

1. Agishi, T., Peirce, E. C. II and Kent, B. B. 'A comparison of pulsatile and non-pulsatile pumping for *ex vivo* renal perfusion.' *Journal of Surgical Research*, **9,** 623 (1969)
2. Alpert, J., Bhaktan, E. K., Gielchinsky, I., Gilbert, L., Brener, B. J., Brief, D. K. and Parsonnet, V. 'Vascular complications of intra-aortic balloon pumping.' *Archives of Surgery*, **111,** 1190 (1976)
3. Angell James, J. E. 'The effects of altering mean pressure, pulse pressure and pulse frequency on the impulse activity in baroreceptor fibres from the aortic arch and right subclavian artery in the rabbit.' *Journal of Physiology (London)*, **214,** 65 (1971)
4. Angell James, J. E. 'The responses of aortic arch and right subclavian baroreceptors to changes of nonpulsatile pressure and their modification by hypothermia.' *Journal of Physiology (London)*, **214,** 201 (1971)
5. Angell James, J. E. and de Burgh Daly, M. 'Comparison of the reflex vasomotor responses to separate and combined stimulation of the carotid sinus and aortic arch baroreceptors by pulsatile and non-pulsatile and non-pulsatile pressures in the dog.' *Journal of Physiology (London)*, **209,** 257 (1970)
6. Angell James, J. E. and de Burgh Daly, M. 'Effects of graded pulsatile pressure on the reflex vasomotor reponses elicited by changes of mean pressure in the perfused carotid sinus–aortic arch regions of the dog.' *Journal of Physiology (London)*, **214,** 51 (1971)
7. Beckman, C. B., Geha, A. S., Hammond, G. L. and Baue, A. E. 'Results and complications of intra-aortic balloon counterpulsation.' *Annals of Thoracic Surgery*, **24,** 550 (1977)
8. Belzer, F. O., Ashby, B. S., Huang, J. S. and Dunphy, J. E. 'Etiology of rising perfusion pressure in isolated organ perfusion.' *Annals of Surgery*, **168,** 382 (1968)
9. Berger, R. L. and Saini, V. K. 'Conversion of nonpulsatile cardiopulmonary bypass to pulsatile flow by intra-aortic balloon pumping during myocardial revascularization for cardiogenic shock.' (Abstr.) *Circulation*, **45** and **46** **(Suppl. II)**, 130, (1972)

10. Biddle, T. L., Stewart, S. and Stuard, I. D. 'Dissection of the aorta complicating intra-aortic balloon counterpulsation.' *American Heart Journal*, **92,** 781 (1976)
11. Boucher, J. K., Rudy, L. W. Jr., and Edmunds, L. H., Jr. 'Organ blood flow during pulsatile cardiopulmonary bypass.' *Journal of Applied Physiology*, **36,** 86 (1974)
12. Branthwaite, M. A. 'Detection of neurological damage during open-heart surgery.' *Thorax*, **28,** 464 (1973)
13. Bregman, D. 'Clinical experience with a new pulsatile assist device (PAD) during open-heart surgery.' *Artificial Organs*, **2,** 244 (1978)
14. Bregman, D., Bailin, M., Bowman, F. O., Jr., Parodi, E. N., Haubert, S. M. Edie, R. N., Spotnitz, H. M., Reemtsma, K. and Malm, J. R. 'A pulsatile assist device (PAD) for use during cardiopulmonary bypass.' *Annals of Thoracic Surgery*, **24,** 574 (1977)
15. Bregman, D., Bowman, F. O. Jr., Parodi, E. N., Haubert, S. M., Edie, R. N., Spotnitz, H. M., Reemtsma, K. and Malm, J. R. 'An improved method of myocardial protection with pulsation during cardiopulmonary bypass.' *Circulation*, **56** (**Suppl. II**). 157 (1977)
16. Bregman, D., Parodi, E. N., Bowman, F. O. Jr., Edie, R. N., Reemtsma, K. R. and Malm, J. R. 'Clinical experience with a new cardiac assist device – the pulsatile assist device (PAD).' (Abstr.) *Clinical Research*, **24,** 211A (1976)
17. Bremner, W. F., Taylor, K. M., Baird, S., Thomson, J. A., Ratcliffe, J. G., Laurie, T. D. V. and Bain, W. H. 'Hypothalamo-pituitary-thyroid axis function during cardiopulmonary bypass.' *Journal of Thoracic and Cardiovascular Surgery*, **75,** 392 (1978)
18. Brull, L. 'Nouvelle Méthode pour l'Etude des Fonctions du Rein: L'Anastomose simultanée de la Circulation rénale avec la Circulation carotido-jugulaire de deux Donneurs.' *Comptes Rendus des Séances de la Société de Biologie et de ses Filiales* (*Paris*), **107,** 248 (1931)
19. Carveth, S. W., McGoon, D. C., Mattox, V. R. and Moffitt, E. A. 'Effect of surgery with and without whole body perfusion on plasma 17-hydroxy-corticosteroids in man.' *Annals of Surgery*, **161,** 105 (1965)
20. Clarke, C. P., Kahn, D. R., Dufek, J. H. and Sloan, H. 'The effects of non-pulsatile blood flow on canine lungs.' *Annals of Thoracic Surgery*, **6,** 450 (1968)
21. Clauss, R. H., Birtwell, W. C., Albertal, G., Lunzer, S., Taylor, W. J., Fosberg, A. M. and Harken, D. E. 'Assisted circulation. 1. The arterial counterpulsator.' *Journal of Thoracic and Cardiovascular Surgery*, **41,** 447 (1961)
22. Corcoran, A. C. and Page, I. H. 'Observations on relation of experimental hypertension to renal clearance and renal ischaemia.' *American Journal of Physiology*, **123,** 43 (1938)
23. Corcoran, A. C. and Page, I. H. 'Renal blood flow in experimental renal hypertension.' *American Journal of Physiology*, **135,** 361 (1942)
24. Dalton, M. L., Mosley, E. C., Woodward, K. E. and Barila, T. G. 'The effect of pulsatile flow on renal blood flow during extracorporeal circulation.' *Journal of Surgical Research*, **5,** 127 (1965)
25. de Langen, C. D. 'Die klinische Bedeuytung der Pulsdrückamplitude.' *Müchener Medizinische Wochenschrift*, **101,** 2132 (1959)
26. Douglas, W. W., Ritchie, J. M. and Schaumann, W. 'A study of the effect of the pattern of electrical stimulation of the aortic nerve on the reflex depressor responses.' *Journal of Physiology* (*London*), **133,** 232 (1956)
27. Dunn, J., Kirsh, M. M., Harness, J., Carroll, M., Straker, J. and Sloan, H. 'Haemodynamic, metabolic and haemotologic effects of pulsatile cardiopulmonary bypass.' *Journal of Thoracic and Cardiovascular Surgery*, **68,** 138 (1974)

28. Dunn, J., Peterson, A. and Kirsh, M. M. 'Effects of pulsatile perfusion upon left ventricular function.' *Journal of Surgical Research*, **25**, 211 (1978)
29. Ead, H. W., Green, J. H. and Neil, E. 'A comparison of the effects of pulsatile and non-pulsatile blood flow through the carotid sinus on the reflexogenic activity of the sinus baroreceptors in the cat.' *Journal of Physiology (London)*, **118**, 509 (1952)
30. Eguchi, S. and Asano, K. 'A new pulsatile pump controlled by a roller system.' *Surgery*, **63**, 490 (1968)
31. Finsterbusch, W., Long, D. M., Sellers, R. D., Amplatz, K. and Lillehei, C. W. 'Renal arteriography during extracorporeal circulation in dogs, with preliminary report upon effects of low molecular weight dextran.' *Journal of Thoracic and Cardiovascular Surgery*, **41**, 252 (1961)
32. German, J. C., Chalmers, G. S., Hirai, J., Mukherjee, N. D., Wakabayashi, K. A. and Connolly, J. E. 'Comparison of nonpulsatile and pulsatile extracorporeal circulation on renal tissue perfusion.' *Chest*, **61**, 65 (1972)
33. Gesell, R. A. 'On the relation of pulse pressure to renal secretion.' *American Journal of Physiology*, **32**, 70 (1913)
34. Giron, F., Birtwell, W. C., Soroff, H. S. and Deterling, R. A. 'Hemodynamic effects of pulsatile and nonpulsatile flow.' *Archives of Surgery*, **93**, 802 (1966)
35. Goodman, T. A., Gerard, D. F., Bernstein, E. F. and Dilley, R. B. 'The effects of pulseless perfusion on the distribution of renal cortical blood flow and on renin release.' *Surgery*, **80**, 31 (1976)
36. Habal, S. M., Weiss, M. B., Spotnitz, H. M., Parodi, E. N., Wolff, M., Cannon, P. J., Hoffman, B. F. and Malm, J. R. 'Effects of pulsatile and nonpulsatile coronary perfusion on performance of the canine left ventricle.' *Journal of Thoracic and Cardiovascular Surgery*, **72**, 742 (1976)
37. Halley, M. M., Reemtsma, K. and Creech, O. Jr. 'Cerebral blood flow, metabolism and brain volume in extracorporeal circulation.' *Journal of Thoracic Surgery*, **36**, 506 (1958)
38. Hamel, G. 'Die Bedeutung des Pulses für den Blutstrom.' *Zeitschrift für Biologie (Munich)*, **25**, 474 (1898)
39. Harken, A. H. 'The influence of pulsatile perfusion on oxygen uptake by the isolated canine hind limb.' *Journal of Thoracic and Cardiovascular Surgery*, **70**, 237 (1975)
40. Harrison, T. S., Chawla, R. C., Seaton, J. F. and Robinson, B. H. 'Carotid sinus origin of adrenergic responses compromising the effectiveness of artificial circulatory support.' *Surgery*, **68**, 20 (1970)
41. Harrison, T. S. and Seaton, J. F. 'An analysis of pulse frequency as an adrenergic excitant in pulsatile circulatory support.' *Surgery*, **73**, 868 (1973)
42. Hawthorne, E. W., Perry, S. L. C. and Pogue, W. G. 'Development of experimental renal hypertension in the dog following reduction of renal artery pulse pressure without reducing mean pressure.' *American Journal of Physiology*, **174**, 393 (1953)
43. Heimbecker, R., Robert, A. and McKenzie, F. N. 'The extracorporeal pump filter – Saint or sinner?' *Annals of Thoracic Surgery*, **21**, 55 (1976)
44. Hoffman, B. F., Klopp, E. H., Jacobs, L. A., Seamone, W. and Gott, V. L. 'A pulsatile roller pump for cardiac bypass.' *IEEE Transactions on Bio-medical Engineering*, **17**, 78 (1970)
45. Hooker, D. R. 'A study of the isolated kidney: The influence of pulse pressure upon renal function.' *American Journal of Physiology*, **27**, 24 (1910)
46. Jacobj, C. 'Apparat zur Durchblutung isolirter überlebender Organe.' *Archiv für experimentelle Pathologie und Pharmakologie (Leipzig)*, **26**, 388 (1890)
47. Jacobs, L. A., Klopp, E. H., Seamone, W., Topaz, S. R. and Gott, V. L. 'Improved organ function during cardiac bypass with a roller pump modified to deliver pulsatile flow.' *Journal of Thoracic and Cardiovascular Surgery*, **58**, 703 (1969)

48. Judson, W. E. and Rausch, N. H. 'Effects of acute reduction of renal artery blood pressure on renal haemodynamics and excretion of electrolytes and water.' *Journal of Laboratory and Clinical Medicine*, **50,** 923 (1957)
49. Kantrowitz, A., TjØnneland, S., Freed, P. S., Phillips, S. J., Butner, A. N. and Sherman, J. L. Jr. 'Initial clinical experience with intra-aortic balloon pumping in cardiogenic shock.' *Journal of the American Medical Association*, **203,** 135 (1968)
50. Kohlstaedt, K. G. and Page, I. H. 'The liberation of renin by perfusion of kidneys following reduction of pulse pressure.' *Journal of Experimental Medicine*, **72,** 201 (1940)
51. Kolff, W. J. and Lawson, J. 'Status of the artificial heart and cardiac assist devices in the United States.' *Transactions of the American Society for Artificial Internal Organs*, **21,** 160 (1975)
52. Koushanpour, E. and McGee, J. P. 'Effect of mean pressure on carotid sinus baroreceptor response to pulsatile pressure.' *American Journal of Physiology*, **216,** 599 (1969)
53. Lefemine, A. A., Kosowsky, B., Madoff, I., Black, H. and Lewis, M. 'Results and complications of intra-aortic balloon pumping in surgical and medical patients.' *American Journal of Cardiology*, **40,** 416 (1977)
54. Lesage, A. M., Tsuchioka, H., Young, W. G., Jr. and Sealy, W. C. 'Pathogenesis of pulmonary damage during extracorporeal perfusion.' *Archives of Surgery*, **93,** 1002 (1966)
55. Levine, F. H., Philbin, D. M., Coggins, C. H., Emerson, C. W., Austen, W. G. and Buckley, M. J. 'Plasma vasopressin and urinary sodium ion excretion during cardiopulmonary bypass: A comparison of pulsatile and nonpulsatile flow.' *Surgical Forum*, **29,** 320 (1978)
56. Long, D. Discussion of: Sanger, P. W., Robicsek, F., Taylor, F. H., Reese, T. T. and Stan, R. E. 'Vasomotor regulation during extracorporeal circulation and open-heart surgery.' *Journal of Thoracic and Cardiovascular Surgery*, **40,** 355 (1960)
57. Ludwig, C. and Schmidt, A. 'Das Verhalten der Gase, welche mit dem Blut durch den reizbaren Säugethiermuskel strömen.' *Arbeiten aus der Physiologischen Anstalt zu Leipzig*, **3,** 1 (1868)
58. McCabe, J. C., Abel, R. M., Subramanian, V. A. and Guy, W. A., Jr. 'Complications of intra-aortic balloon insertion and counterpulsation.' *Circulation*, **57,** 769 (1978)
59. McDonald, D. A. *Blood Flow in Arteries*. Baltimore: Williams and Wilkins Company (1960)
60. McMaster, P. D. and Parsons, R. J. 'Effect of pulse on spread of substances through tissues.' *Journal of Experimental Medicine*, **68,** 377 (1938)
61. Maddoux, G., Pappas, G., Jenkins, M., Battock, D., Trow, R., Smith, S. C., Jr. and Steel, P. 'Effect of pulsatile and nonpulsatile flow during cardiopulmonary bypass on left ventricular ejection fraction early after aortocoronary bypass surgery.' *American Journal of Cardiology*, **37,** 1000 (1976)
62. Mandelbaum, I., and Burns, W. H. 'Pulsatile and nonpulsatile blood flow.' *Journal of the American Medical Association*, **191,** 657 (1965)
63. Many, M., Birtwell, W. C., Giron, F., Wise, H., Soroff, H. S. and Deterling, R. A., Jr. 'The effects of pulse wave pattern on renal function.' *Transactions of the American Society for Artificial Internal Organs*, **13,** 157 (1967)
64. Many, M., Giron, F., Birtwell, W. C., Deterling, R. A., Jr. and Soroff, H. S. 'Effects of depulsation of renal blood flow on renal function and renin secretion.' *Surgery*, **66,** 242 (1969)
65. Many, M., Soroff, H. S., Birtwell, W. C. and Deterling, R. A., Jr. 'Effects of bilateral renal artery depulsation on renin levels.' *Surgical Forum*, **19,** 387 (1968)

66. Many, M., Soroff, H. S., Birtwell, W. C., Wise, H. M. and Deterling, R. A., Jr. 'The physiologic role of pulsatile and nonpulsatile blood flow. III. Effects of unilateral renal artery depulsation.' *Archives of Surgery*, **97,** 917 (1968)
67. Matsumoto, T. Wolferth, C. C., Jr. and Perlman, M. H. 'Effects of pulsatile and non-pulsatile perfusion upon cerebral and conjunctival microcirculation in dogs.' *American Surgeon*, **37,** 61 (1971)
68. Mavroudis, C. 'To pulse or not to pulse.' *Annals of Surgery*, **25,** 259 (1978)
69. Min, B. G., Abbassi, M. Z., Welkowitz, W., Kostis, J. B., Fich, S. and Mackenzie, J. W. 'Significance of left ventricular power waveform on changes in stroke work during pulsatile left ventricular bypass.' *Journal of Surgical Research*, **24,** 544 (1978)
70. Moores, W. Y., Gago, O., Morris, J. D. and Peck, C. C. 'Serum and urinary amylase levels following pulsatile and continuous cardiopulmonary bypass.' *Journal of Thoracic and Cardiovascular Surgery*, **74,** 73 (1977)
71. Moores, W. Y., Kahn, D. R., Kirsh, M. M., Gago, O., Carr, E. A., Jr. Abrams, G. D., Dufek, J. and Sloan, H. 'Mechanical support of the circulation by a modified pulsatile roller pump.' *Annals of Thoracic Surgery*, **12,** 262 (1971)
72. Moulopoulos, S. D., Topaz, S. and Kolff, W. J. 'Diastolic balloon pumping (with carbon dioxide) in the aorta – a mechanical assistance to the failing circulation.' *American Heart Journal*, **63,** 669 (1962)
73. Mukhgerjee, N. D., Beran, A. V., Hirai, J., Wakabayashi, A., Sperling, D. R., Taylor, W. F. and Connolly, J. E. '*In vivo* determination of renal tissue oxygenation during pulsatile and nonpulsatile left heart bypass.' *Annals of Thoracic Surgery*, **15,** 354 (1973)
74. Nakayama, K., Tamiya, T., Yamamoto, K., Izumi, T., Akimoto, S., Hashizume, S., Iimori, T., Odaka, M. and Yazawa, C. 'High-amplitude pulsatile pump in extracorporeal circulation with particular reference to haemodynamics.' *Surgery*, **54,** 798 (1963)
75. Ninomiya, I. and Irisawa, H. 'Aortic nervous activities in response to pulsatile and non-pulsatile pressure.' *American Journal of Physiology*, **213,** 1504 (1967)
76. Ogata, T., Ida, Y., Nonoyama, A., Takeda, J. and Sasaki, H. 'A comparative study of the effectiveness of pulsatile and nonpulsatile blood flow in extracorporeal circulation.' *Nippon Geka Hokan* (*Kyoto*), **29,** 59 (1960)
77. Pace, P. D., Tilney, N. L., Lesch, M. and Couch, N. P. 'Peripheral arterial complications of intra-aortic balloon counterpulsation.' *Surgery*, **82,** 685 (1977)
78. Pappas, G. Winter, S. D., Kopriva, C. J. and Steel, P. P. 'Improvement of myocardial and other vital organ functions and metabolism with a simple method of pulsatile flow (IABP) during clinical cardiopulmonary bypass.' *Surgery*, **77,** 34 (1975)
79. Paquet, K. J. 'Haemodynamic studies on normothermic perfusion of the isolated pig kidney with pulsatile and non-pulsatile flows.' *Journal of Cardiovascular Surgery*, **1,** 45 (1969)
80. Parsons, R. J. and McMaster, P. D. 'Effect of pulse upon formation and flow of lymph.' *Journal of Experimental Medicine*, **68,** 353 (1938)
81. Parsons, R. J. and McMaster, P. D. 'Normal and pathological factors influencing spread of vital dye in connective tissue.' *Journal of Experimental Medicine*, **68,** 869 (1938)
82. Replogle, R., Levy, M., Dewall, R. A. and Lillehei, R. C. 'Catecholamine and serotonn response to cardiopulmonary bypass.' *Journal of Thoracic and Cardiovascular Surgery*, **44,** 638 (1962)
83. Rudy, L. W., Heyman, M. A. and Edmunds, L. H. 'Distribution of systemic blood flow during cardiopulmonary bypass.' *Journal of Applied Physiology*, **34,** 194 (1973)

84. Ryder, H. W., Espey, F. F., Kimbell, F. D., Penka, E. J., Rosenauer, A., Podolsky, B. and Evans, J. P. 'Modification of effect of cerebral blood flow on cerebrospinal fluid pressure by variations in craniospinal blood volume.' *Archives of Neurology and Psychiatry*, **68,** 170 (1952)
85. Sanderson, J. M., Wright, G. and Sims, F. W. 'Brain damage in dogs immediately following pulsatile and non-pulsatile blood flows in extracorporeal circulation.' *Thorax*, **27,** 275 (1972)
86. Schaff, H. V., Ciardullo, R. C., Flaherty, J. T., Brawley, R. K. and Gott, V. L. 'Regional ischaemia distal to a cirtical coronary stenosis during prolonged fibrillation – Improvement with pulsatile perfusion.' *Circulation*, **56** (**Suppl. II**), 25 (1977)
87. Schaff, H. V., Flaherty, J. T., Ciardullo, R. and Gott, V. L. 'Effects of a critical coronary stenosis on regional myocardial blood flows in a fibrillating heart.' *Journal of Thoracic and Cardiovascular Surgery*, **73,** 746 (1977)
88. Senning, A., Andres, J., Bornstein, P., Norberg, B. and Anderson, M. N. 'Renal function during extracorporeal circulation at high and low flow rates in dogs.' *Annals of Surgery*, **151,** 63 (1960)
89. Shepard, R. B. and Kirklin, J. W. 'Relation of pulsatile flow to oxygen consumption and other variables during cardiopulmonary bypass.' *Journal of Thoracic and Cardiovascular Surgery*, **58,** 694 (1969)
90. Shepard, R. C., Simpson, D. C. and Sharp, J. F. 'Energy equivalent pressure.' *Archives of Surgery*, **93,** 730 (1966)
91. Skinner, S. L., McCubbin, J. W. and Page, I. H. 'Renal baroceptor control of renin secretion.' *Science*, **141,** 814 (1963)
92. Spickler, J. W. and Kezdi, P. 'Dynamic response characteristics of carotid sinus baroreceptors.' *American Journal of Physiology*, **212,** 472 (1967)
93. Ssentjurin, B. S. 'Ueber die Wirkung von Giften auf die Gefässe des isolierten Ohrs bei konstantem und pulsierendem Flüssigkeitsstrom.' *Pfluger's Archiv für die gesamte Physiologie des Menschen und der Tiere* (*Bonn*), **215,** 683 (1927)
94. Steed, D. L., Follette, D. M., Foglia, R., Maloney, J. V. and Buckberg, G. D. 'Effects of pulsatile assistance and non-pulsatile flow on subendocardial perfusion during cardiopulmonary bypass.' *Annals of Thoracic Surgery*, **26,** 133 (1978)
95. Tamari, Y., Frantz, S. L., Vagnini, F. J., Beil, A. R., Jr., Degnan, T. J., Seidman, S., Garfinkle, T. J., Newman, J. C. and Kaplitt, M. J. 'Experimental evaluation and clinical application of intraoperative counterpulsation without balloon pumping.' *Journal of Cardiovascular Surgery*, **17,** 398 (1976)
96. Taylor, K. M., Bain, W. H., Jones, J. V. and Walker, M. S. 'The effect of haemodilution on plasma levels of cortisol and free cortisol.' *Journal of Thoracic and Cardiovascular Surgery*, **72,** 57 (1976)
97. Taylor, K. M., Jones, J. V., Walker, M. S., Rao, L. G. S. and Bain, W. H. 'The cortisol response during heart-lung bypass.' *Circulation*, **54,** 20 (1976)
98. Taylor, K. M., Walker, M. S., Rao, L. G. S., Jones, J. V. and Gray, C. E. 'Plasma levels of cortisol, free cortisol and corticotrophin during cardiopulmonary bypass.' *Journal of Endocrinology*, **67,** 29 (1975)
99. Taylor, K. M., Wright, G. S., Bain, W. H., Caves, P. K. and Beastall, G. S. 'Comparative studies of pulsatile and non-pulsatile flow during cardiopulmonary bypass: III. Response of anterior pituitry gland to thyrotropin-releasing hormone.' *Journal of Thoracic and Cardiovascular Surgery*, **75,** 579 (1978)
100. Taylor, K. M., Wright, G. S., Reid, J. M., Bain, W. H., Caves, P. K., Walker, M. S. and Grant, J. K. 'Comparative studies of pulsatile and nonpulsatile flow during cardiopulmonary bypass: II. The effects on adrenal secretion of cortisol.' *Journal of Thoracic and Cardiovascular Surgery*, **75,** 574 (1978)

101. Trank, J. W. and Visscher, M. B. 'Carotid sinus baroreceptor modification associated with endotoxin shock.' *Journal of Physiology (London)*, **202,** 971 (1962)
102. Trinkle, J. K., Helton, N. E., Wood, R. E. and Bryant, L. R. 'Metabolic comparison of a new pulsatile pump and a roller pump for cardiopulmonary bypass.' *Journal of Thoracic and Cardiovascular Surgery*, **58,** 562 (1969)
103. Tyras, D. H. and Willman, V. L. 'Paraplegia following intra-aortic balloon assistance.' *Annals of Thoracic Surgery*, **25,** 164 (1978)
104. Wesolowski, S. A., Sauvage, L. R. and Pinc, R. D. 'Extracorporeal circulation: The role of the pulse in maintenance of the systemic circulation during heart-lung bypass.' *Surgery*, **37,** 663 (1955)
105. Wilkens, H., Regelson, W. and Hoffmeister, F. S. 'The physiologic importance of pulsatile blood flow.' *New England Journal of Medicine*, **267,** 443 (1962)
106. Williams, G. D., Callaway, J. K., Seifen, A. B., Norton, J. B., Dungan, W. T. and Readinger, R. 'Repair of Swiss cheese ventricular septal defect utilizing core cooling with pulsatile bypass and hypothermic arrest.' *Motion Picture Session on Surgical Techniques, Fifteenth Annual Meeting of the Society of Thoracic Surgeons*, Phoenix, Arizona (1979)
107. Wright, G. and Sanderson, J. M. 'Brain damage and mortality in dogs following pulsatile and non-pulsatile blood flow in extracorporeal circulation.' *Thorax*, **27,** 738 (1972)
108. Wright, G., Sanderson, J. M. and Furness, A. 'Pulsatile pumps for open-heart surgery.' *Lancet*, **1,** 217 (1978)

23

Prolonged Extracorporeal Oxygenation for Pulmonary Insufficiency

J. Donald Hill

pondere, non numero

Introduction

Twenty years have now passed since the first clinical open-heart procedures were performed using extracorporeal oxygenation. This marked the beginning of a new technology that eventually affected many areas of medicine and industry. The whole field of intensive-care medicine, respiratory care, pacemakers and angiography were to be influenced when routine open-heart surgery became a reality. Medical engineering arose as a strange alliance between two disciplines, and eventually became a vital component in any serious research and development in cardiac surgery.

The early heart-lung machines were crude and unsophisticated but were used successfully for perfusions of 2 to 3 hours. The late 1950s and early 1960s were spent in learning the limitations of perfusion and the basic principles of management. Total body perfusion lasting longer than 6 hours was almost always followed by serious postoperative problems and, more commonly, death.

The time limitation of perfusion was linked to the denaturization of plasma proteins resulting from the large areas of blood-gas interfaces which were inherent in all the early oxygenator designs. Surgeons, who foresaw the usc of longterm extracorporeal circulation as a means of supporting a patient in respiratory and/or cardiac failure, awaited the development of a membrane oxygenator.

This was first accomplished in 1958 by Clowes, Hopkins and Neville[2]. His device was used clinically but never became available to the medical community as a whole. In 1964, Bramson designed and developed a membrane oxygenator which has been clinically used continuously since that time[1, 9]. In recent years a number of other satisfactory membrane oxygenators have been developed[6, 14, 17, 19].

Their availability has opened up a new era in critical care medicine. We have this new tool, primitive though it may be, and now we must learn how to use it. In the following pages, the clinical application of this new technology in the treatment of acute respiratory insufficiency is presented.

Potential applications of prolonged extracorporeal oxygenation

Most investigators have defined their immediate goal for this procedure as the extracorporeal support of patients in acute respiratory insufficiency. This is a problem we are being faced with every day in intensive care units, very often involving a young adult who is dying from acute respiratory failure and its complications. The eventual potential for the application of these new procedures is broader. At least three avenues of application are possible.

Treatment of reversible pulmonary pathology

This can involve either acute or chronic pathology. Patients suffering from acute pulmonary insufficiency constitute the single largest group that would benefit from this procedure now. It includes patients suffering from viral or bacterial pneumonia, aspiration pneumonia, pulmonary fat emboli, respiratory burns, lung contusion and shock lung, or respiratory failure after open-heart surgery. The projected mortality for acute respiratory insufficiency in the United States in 1977 is between 75 000 and 85 000[15]. The mean age of these patients will be 46 years. Many of these patients would be candidates for artificial support.

The use of extracorporeal oxygenation in chronic pulmonary insufficiency is less obvious, but there is a definite place for its use. For example, the patient with emphysema, who decompensates due to a pulmonary infection, can be supported for several days until the infection resolves itself.

Irreversible pulmonary pathology

This includes patients suffering from acute and chronic pulmonary disease as well. Lung transplantation is the only foreseeable solution to irreversible pulmonary pathology. It would find its principal use in chronic lung failure. Acute respiratory insufficiency often eventually leads to irreversible pulmonary destruction. In this situation no amount of time on extracorporeal oxygenation will allow the lung to recover[10]. The availability of an implanted artificial lung is probably years away. Lung transplantation, itself, has not been clinically successful over a long period of time, but is a potential therapy.

Where would extracorporeal oxygenation technology fit into a transplantation programme? There are three potential areas of application: (1) Support of the patient who has irreversible pulmonary pathology and lethal hypoxaemia until such time as a donor lung can be found. (2) Support of a patient immediately after a lung transplant until the transplanted lung has resumed satisfactory gas transfer function. (3) Support of the patient during a rejection crisis.

Organ salvage

Transplantation programmes are limited by the availability of organs in satisfactory condition. Extracorporeal circulation with oxygenation is a feasible means of preserving all body organs in good condition until the disposition of these organs can be arranged.

Rationale of prolonged extracorporeal oxygenation

The original premise that prompted clinicians to endeavour to use extracorporeal oxygenation in respiratory failure was the assumption that, if the gas exchange function of the biological lung can be substituted by extracorporeal oxygenation, a patient whose lung function is acutely impaired can be kept alive until his lungs heal and eventually take over their function again.

This was a rather simplistic approach to a very complicated problem. It was based on the same pattern of thinking that preceded development of the artificial kidney for acute renal failure. The kidney, however, is exceptional in that the pathology is nearly always some variant of acute tubular necrosis which invariably heals itself. Second, renal dialysis support is only required intermittently.

Therefore, in acute respiratory insufficiency certain other aspects have to be taken into account. These complicating factors became more apparent as experience was gained in clinical extracorporeal oxygenation. Two areas are foremost amongst these problems and they require better definition.

The premise. It is not enough just to support the patient and wait for the lungs to recover. One must make the pulmonary environment conducive to healing. This involves primarily the management of the respirator and the lungs during perfusion.

The selection of patients. The selection of patients for perfusion is difficult since there is a variety of aetiologies accompanied by little knowledge of the natural course of the individual diseases in the absence of extracorporeal oxygenation. If extracorporeal oxygenation is not introduced before irreversibility occurs, there will be little chance of the therapy bringing ultimate benefit to the patient. One is therefore faced with the dilemma of deciding whether to place a patient on perfusion early in the disease process in the hope of bringing about a reversal, knowing that the process itself can be dangerous, or to wait too long and risk the lung regressing. The selection of the patients and timing for the initiation of the procedure are, therefore, very important.

These problems are examined separately in the following sections.

Physiological criteria for the selection of patients for perfusion

There are no precise indications for the initiation of perfusion. Indeed, there are considerable divergencies in the criteria adopted by different clinical investigators.

Our early clinical perfusions were performed on desperately hypoxaemic patients in whom the prognosis was hopeless if conventional therapy was continued. After this beginning, we adopted specific guidelines for the initiation of bypass. These were:

(1) An a$P\text{O}_2$ of less than 35 mmHg consistently while using maximum respiratory support.
(2) Hypoxaemic myocardial depression.
(3) Hypoxaemic central nervous system depression.
(4) The knowledge that the natural course of the disease is one of potential reversal.
(5) No contraindications to systemic anticoagulation.

These were quite stringent criteria and required that the patient be extremely ill before extracorporeal oxygenation was used.

We observed a distinct pattern of response among patients who were treated with extracorporeal oxygenation. If the patient was so treated early in the disease process out of necessity due to hypoxaemia, the pulmonary pathology could be reversed. Conversely, if the patient developed lethal

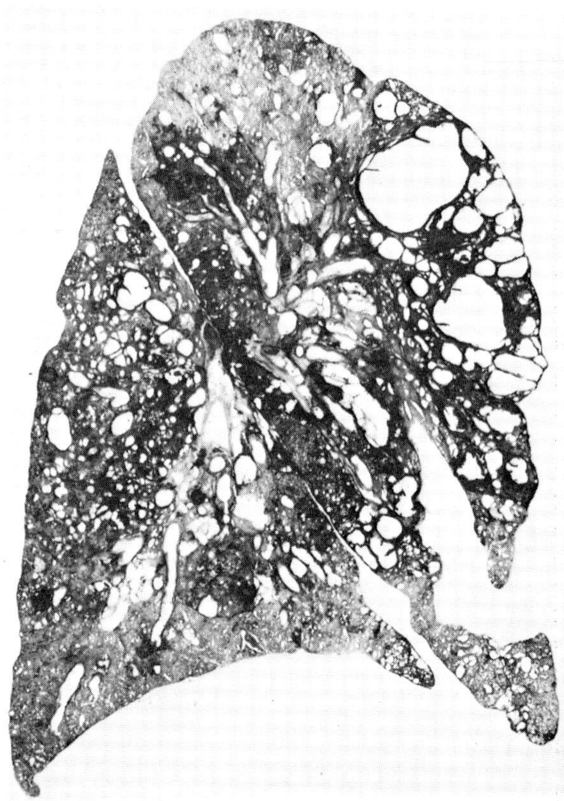

Figure 23.1 This is a Gough section of a lung following 10 days of venoarterial extracorporeal oxygenation. The patient was placed on bypass at the 12th day of her illness. This type of pathology represents irreversible pulmonary changes

hypoxaemia in the 10th or 12th day of illness and was then treated with extracorporeal oxygenation, the lungs were usually irreversibly damaged and the patient could not be taken off perfusion (*Figure 23.1*). It seemed therefore advisable to use extracorporeal oxygenation early in the disease, if in fact this therapy could alter the natural course of the disease. Clinical confirmation that it could, plus a growing confidence in the methods we were using, resulted in our altering the criteria for the initiation of bypass. The new, more comprehensive indications now are:

(1) An aP_{O_2} of less than 50 mmHg, or an aP_{O_2} less than 60 mmHg with a mixed venous oxygen saturation of less than 40 per cent, at a normal blood pH using maximum respiratory support with an F_{IO_2} of 1.0 for over 24 hours. If rapid clinical deterioration supervenes such as hypoxaemic cerebral or myocardial depression, this period would be shortened.
(2) No evidence of terminal disease from which the patient cannot survive. Example: cancer or irreversible neurological damage.

(3) No haematological contraindications to anticoagulation. Example: active bleeding from the gastrointestinal tract, trachea or pharynx. Some types of central nervous system damage would be contraindications to anticoagulation.
(4) No major secondary organ involvement of a chronic nature. Example: cirrhosis of the liver or degenerative neurological disease.
(5) The patient must be less than 60 years of age.
(6) The patient must have been in acute respiratory disease less than 21 days.

As experience is gained, these indications will, no doubt, be further modified. The final solution for the selection of patients will depend upon our ability to predict accurately the natural course of an individual case of acute respiratory insufficiency so that extracorporeal oxygenation can be initiated at the most opportune time. This decision will be made even easier when extracorporeal oxygenation becomes completely safe and physiological. At present, we must balance the risk of extracorporeal oxygenation against the as yet unknown positive curative aspects of a new therapy.

Techniques of extracorporeal oxygenation

There are three methods of accomplishing extracorporeal oxygenation: venovenous, venoarterial and arteriovenous perfusion. Each is aimed at improving the oxygen–gas tension in the systemic blood.

Venous perfusion

We and other investigators have used this technique[11, 21]. The object is to preoxygenate the venous blood before it goes to the lung. The chief advantage is that the method is simple and does not affect the arterial phase of the circulation. The cannulation technique is shown in *Figure 23.2*. The principal disadvantages of this method are: (1) there is a limit to the percentage of the total cardiac output one can obtain by bypass; (2) there is no reduction in the pulmonary hypertension; and (3) it requires cannulation of both the neck and the groin vessels. This method will provide the patient with adequate oxygen but does not allow one to provide a more suitable environment to enhance pulmonary healing. To attain this, one must obtain 80 to 90 per cent of the cardiac output so that the patient is in no way dependent upon an artificial ventilator and one may work on the lungs directly without fear of producing hypoxaemia. We have therefore switched to venoarterial perfusion.

Venoarterial perfusion

Cannulation technique for partial venoarterial bypass is illustrated in *Figure 23.3*. In most instances of respiratory insufficiency, the heart will function satisfactorily unless hypoxaemic myocardial depression occurs. This type of myocardial depression can be reversed by perfusion with

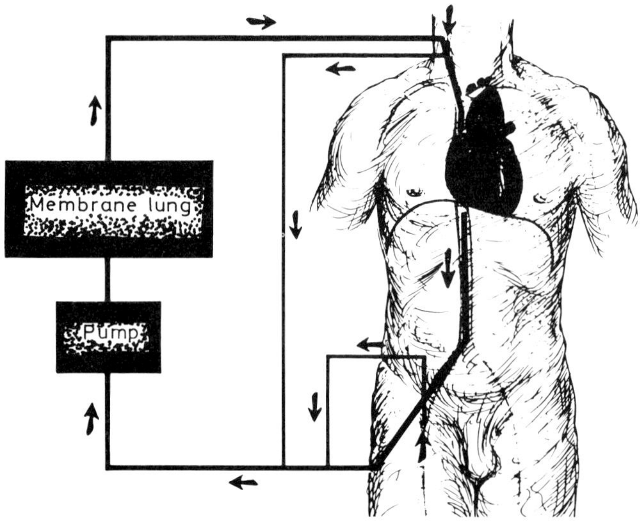

Figure 23.2 Venous blood is removed from the inferior vena cava via a vinyl wire-reinforced cannula (8 to 12 mm outside diameter) that is introduced into the femoral vein, advanced proximally and positioned just below the diaphragm. Blood is removed oxygenated and returned fully saturated to the superior vena cava via a cannula introduced into the internal jugular vein. The distal femoral vein and the distal internal jugular vein are also cannulated to prevent formation of oedema

oxygenated blood. It is usually only necessary to assist the lungs and not the heart. By diverting a large proportion (60 to 75 per cent) of the total venous return through the heart-lung machine, and thence direct to a femoral artery, we reduce substantially the pulmonary hypertension which is, in most cases, contributory to the patient's pulmonary pathology. The 25 to 40 per cent which is not diverted extracorporeally will traverse the patient's lungs and be pumped into the aorta by the left ventricle. It has been suspected that bidirectional flow into the aorta might interfere with pulsatility, the maintenance of which in prolonged perfusion is probably important. However, in our cases, there has been normal pulsatile flow in each patient in spite of the greatly reduced left ventricular stroke volume. A normal pulse can be felt in the dorsalis pedis pulse in the foot of the leg that is not cannulated for perfusion. In patients whose kidneys were normal before perfusion, urine output remained normal. We have not seen any clinical detrimental effects from prolonged retrograde femoral artery perfusion.

A second possible technical difficulty in venoarterial pumping for respiratory insufficiency is of more immediate importance. The blood leaving the left ventricle supplies the patient's head and heart. It could be substantially desaturated since it may have been insufficiently oxygenated in the patient's own lungs. We have been aware of this possible complication in our cases, but we have had no instance in which there was any

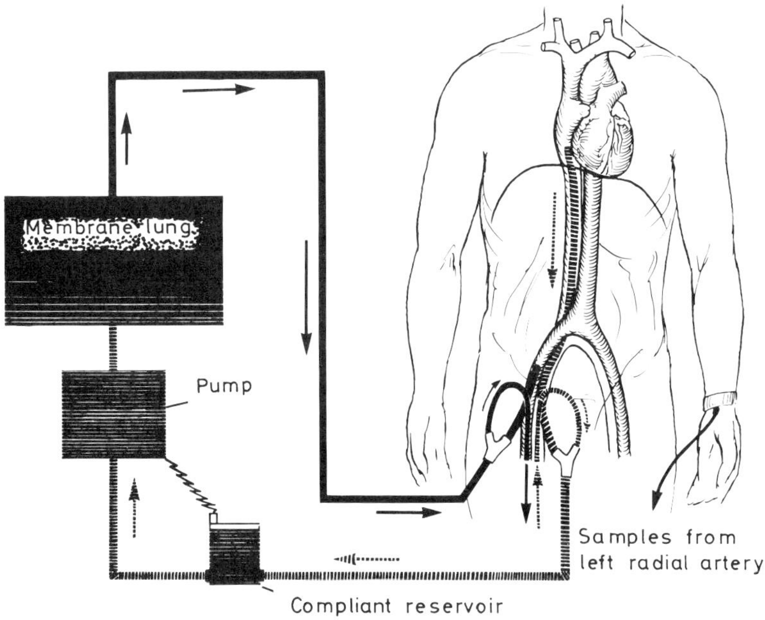

Figure 23.3 Venoarterial perfusion technique. Venous blood is removed from the right atrium by way of a cannula introduced into the right common femoral vein. The distal common femoral vein is cannulated as well. The venous blood is pumped through the membrane oxygenator and returned to the body by way of retrograde perfusion through the right common femoral artery. The distal femoral artery is perfused as well. The groin incision is closed while the patient is on perfusion. Arterial samples are drawn from the left or right radial artery. This ensures sampling at a point where the potentially lowest levels of aP_{O_2} will be found. Deceptively high values from the lower part of the body are thus avoided

serious desaturation of blood in the aortic arch. During perfusion, the left or right radial artery is always cannulated and all systemic blood-gas samples are drawn from it so that we may know the level of saturation in the aortic arch. This will be the point in the arterial circulation at which blood is most desaturated. We have always been able to maintain the saturation of the blood in the aortic arch between 88 and 92 per cent or higher. The blood flow to the lower part of the body is usually fully saturated.

Using this technique of a single cannula in the right atrium, and obtaining between 60 and 75 per cent of the cardiac output, we have been able to reduce the F_{IO_2} of the respirator to between 0.4 and 0.6 and reduce the peak airway pressures by 15 to 20 cm of water. Mean pulmonary artery pressure has also been reduced, but to varying degrees of from 5 to 23 mmHg. Our future intent is to increase the percentage of total systemic flow diverted through the heart-lung machine, thereby acquiring better control of the patient's lungs so that we may manage the respirator at any level we desire.

Table 23.1 Cardiopulmonary haemodynamics during perfusion (range and average)

	Venovenous perfusion	*Venoarterial perfusion*
Increase aP_{O_2} (mmHg)	22 (13–31)	57 (32–95)
Cardiac output through oxygenator (%)	48 (31–65)	55* (50–68)
O_2 exchange (%)	55 (41,70)	65 (34–80)
CO_2 exchange (%)	38 (37,39)	61 (44–80)
Decrease PAP (mmHg)	0,1	16 (10–23)

*This represents the average of all patient data. We now can routinely direct over 65 per cent of the cardiac output through the extracorporeal circuit

Table 23.1 shows the comparison of cardiopulmonary data obtained during venovenous and venoarterial bypass. *Figure 23.4* shows changes in the aP_{O_2} before, during and after venovenous and venoarterial bypass. The arterial gas tensions have been much better using venoarterial technique and the reduction in the pulmonary artery hypertension has been felt to be instrumental in providing a better pulmonary environment. On the basis of these data, we have judged venoarterial bypass to offer better hope of keeping patients alive and of improving the pulmonary environment for healing.

We hope to increase the amount of venous return diverted through the membrane oxygenator to 80 or 90 per cent by using balloon cannulae. This would relieve the patient of the necessity for artificial respiration. If this can be accomplished, the following untested therapies would become feasible in the attempts to alter the natural course of the disaease and should enhance the likelihood of reversal of the pulmonary pathology:

(1) The F_{IO_2} could be reduced to 0.2.
(2) The mean tracheal pressure could be set at physiological levels.
(3) Total pulmonary lobe irrigation and suctioning would be possible.
(4) Direct instillation of mucolytic agents or detergents would be possible and may be helpful in certain disease states.
(5) Direct application of steroids or antibiotics, if they are applicable, could be easily accomplished.
(6) The inspection of small bronchioles using a fibre-optics bronchoscope would be feasible, and specimens of secretions from selected segments of the lung could be obtained.

Arteriovenous perfusion

This is a method devised to produce preoxygenation of the blood on the venous side of the circulation. Its chief advantage is that there is no pump required in the circuit since the patient's systemic circulation supplies the pressure needed to propel blood through the artificial oxygenator. There is

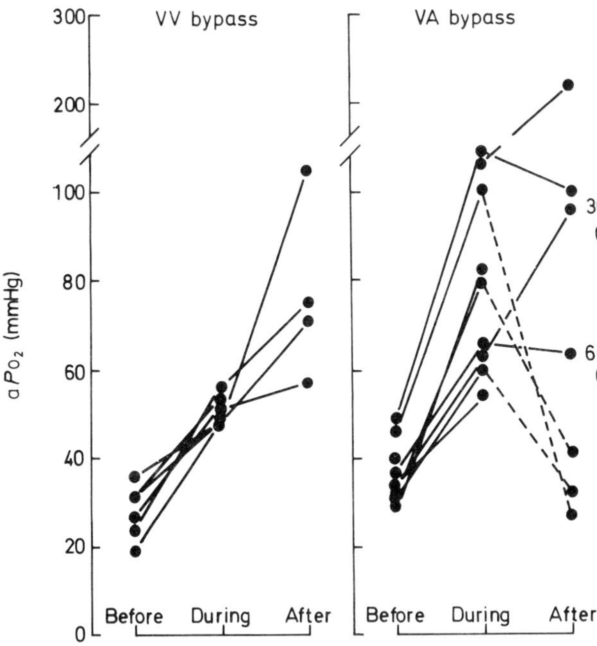

Figure 23.4 This graph indicates the aP_{O_2} levels before, during and after perfusion. The dotted lines delineate the aP_{O_2} obtained after perfusion but prior to death in 3 different patients. Lung function had clearly not been improved in these 3 patients, but their perfusions were discontinued for other reasons. In the other patients (solid lines) substantial improvements in the A–a (alveolar-arterial) gradient were found. VV = venovenous; VA = venoarterial. The postperfusion aP_{O_2} was taken with an F_{IO_2} of 1 except where otherwise indicated

however a major disadvantage that outweighs this: there is a limit to the bypass flow one can obtain because the circuit constitutes a large arterio-venous fistula. This method has had limited clinical application.

Haematological considerations

The possibility of serious bleeding is the single biggest risk of extracorporeal oxygenation. There are three sources of this bleeding potential. Patients who are candidates for extracorporeal oxygenation may already have a predisposition to develop stress ulcers and/or disseminated intravascular coagulation. The foreign surface of the extracorporeal circuit necessitates the use of systemic heparin anticoagulation to prevent clotting in the system. Patients undergoing extracorporeal oxygenation quickly lose a substantial proportion of their circulating blood platelets. The questions of heparin administration and platelet losses merit separate discussion.

Originally, we used levels of systemic heparin anticoagulation that produced clotting times of 'infinity'. This was excessive and subjected the patient to unnecessary risk. We now know that a Lee–White clotting time of between 25 and 40 minutes is sufficient to prevent the blood from producing thrombogenesis in the Bramson membrane oxygenator during prolonged perfusion. Following an initial intravenous injection of 100 units/kg, a 10 mg/100ml solution of lung bovine heparin in saline is continuously infused, using an infusion pump into the venous line leading to the membrane oxygenator. The rate of infusion is adjusted frequently according to the level of anticoagulation as measured by the 'activated clotting time'[8, 3]. The activated clotting time system provides a quick and efficient method of measuring the level of anticoagulation in the circulating blood. We maintain an activated clotting time of about 200 seconds which is approximately equivalent to 25 to 40 minutes Lee–White clotting time.

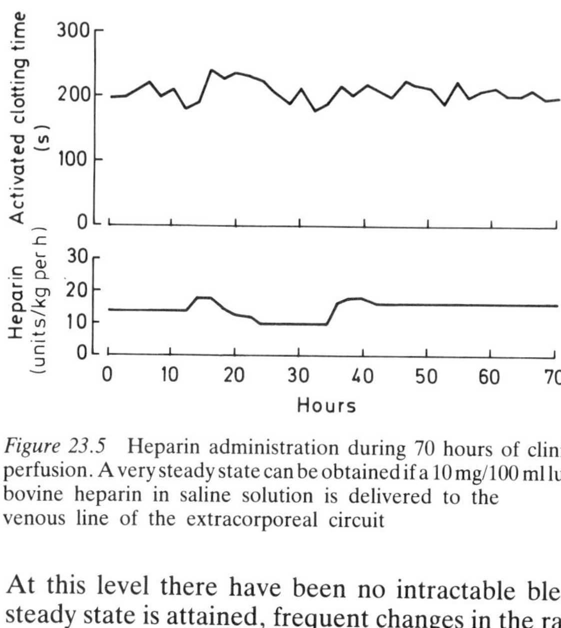

Figure 23.5 Heparin administration during 70 hours of clinical perfusion. A very steady state can be obtained if a 10 mg/100 ml lung bovine heparin in saline solution is delivered to the venous line of the extracorporeal circuit

At this level there have been no intractable bleeding problems. Once a steady state is attained, frequent changes in the rate of infusion are seldom necessary (*Figure 23.5*). The heparin requirements vary from 15 to 45 units/kg per hour. Oliguria will reduce heparin requirements and, conversely, diuresis will increase them. It is probable that lower levels of circulating heparin would be acceptable. In over 600 hours of clinical prolonged extracorporeal oxygenation, we have never seen any incidence of thrombogenesis within the Bramson oxygenator. The ultimate solution to this problem, of course, is the development of a good antithrombogenic surface.

Platelets

The platelet counts fall consistently during clinical perfusion[12]. Most patients have a platelet count of less than 100 000/mm^3 before perfusion begins. Following the initiation of perfusion, a drop of 30 to 50 per cent in the circulating platelets will occur. Platelets will then continue to drop at a slower rate which varies from patient to patient. The final platelet count at

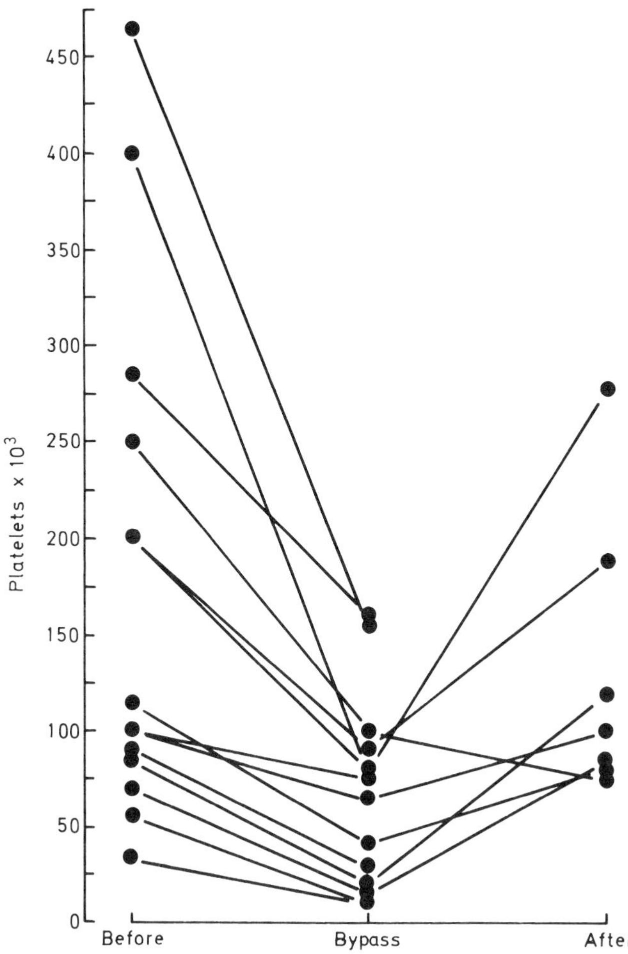

Figure 23.6 The specific platelet count before, during and after perfusion in 14 patients

which a patient tends to stabilize also varies considerably. Sometimes this level is dangerously low (less than 20 000/mm^3). *Figure 23.6* shows the platelet counts in perfusion patients before, during, and after perfusion. Platelet transfusions have been given to patients with very low platelet counts; however, the platelet count is only temporarily increased by this and within several hours returns to a low level once again. We now prefer not to give platelet transfusions because of several detrimental side-effects. Platelet transfusions produce platelet antibodies and there is other particulate matter in platelet transfusions that is not necessarily good for the patient. Furthermore, the transfusions are, of course, very demanding on the blood bank. The initial platelet loss is a reversible phenomenon, and is explained in detail in Chapter 14. A practical solution to this clinical problem is urgently needed; to find it one will probably have to search for pharmacological agents that will inhibit the sensitizing of the platelet which eventually occurs during its passage through the extracorporeal circuit. This, in turn, eventually causes it to be sequestrated in the liver[4]. The development of antithrombogenic surfaces will probably not solve the problem of low platelet counts during perfusion since these platelets are influenced by the internal geometry of the oxygenators as well as by their contact with large foreign surfaces.

Other haematological phenomena

Fibrinogen levels during bypass are not seriously affected. Disseminated intravascular coagulation has not been a contraindication to perfusion and, in fact, several patients have been placed on bypass while a consumption coagulopathy was in progress. They subsequently improved during perfusion.

Metabolic aspects of extracorporeal circulation

Patients subjected to extracorporeal oxygenation very often have varying degrees of pre-existing renal failure and are also developing the early effects of starvation. We have attempted to maintain certain standards of metabolic care in these patients. Special situations may prevent us from attaining them. In those cases preference is given to whatever we consider the highest clinical priority.

Patients suffering from acute respiratory insufficiency are kept in mild dehydration. This is accomplished with furosemide and ethacrynic acid. We do not allow the serum molality to rise above 330 mmol/kg or the serum sodium above 150 mmol/litre. The condition of the skin and the mental status are also used in determining the degree of dehydration. Intravenous fluids are given in sufficient quantities to ensure a urinary output of 1000 to 1500 ml per day. One must not forget that a great deal of water vapour from the patient's blood will diffuse through the membranes separating the blood from the oxygen in the oxygenator, if dry oxygen is used. This can greatly increase the 'insensible fluid loss'. Salt-poor human serum albumin is administered daily to maintain the serum protein above 4 g/100ml. The effects of starvation are minimized by using 15 to 20 g/100ml dextrose intravenous solutions. If the patient's kidney function is good, hyperalimentation can be used. We have never used this therapy during perfusion but we have employed it immediately afterwards. Potassium and magnesium are administered as required. Vitamins are also given daily.

The patient is sedated with morphine at regular intervals so that a satisfactory level of consciousness is maintained. The patients have not encountered any difficulty in metabolizing these drugs except if there has been renal or liver dysfunction. The body temperature is kept at 37°C, which is easily maintained by means of the heat exchanger which is integral with the oxygenator.

Clinical results of extracorporeal oxygenation

Considerable data has been accumulated in the treatment of acute respiratory insufficiency with prolonged partial extracorporeal oxygenation[5, 7, 10, 16, 18, 20]. There are approximately 256 cases collected in the world with a survival rate of 10–15 per cent. Clinical investigators who have considerable experience with prolonged extracorporeal oxygenation and who have accumulated more than 20 cases have similar survival rates. The most comprehensive study performed was a clinical controlled study in the United States sponsored by the National Institutes of Health between 1974 and 1977 (in press). In this controlled study the survival rate was 10 per cent in the group treated with prolonged extracorporeal oxygenation as well as in the control group. One of the conclusions of the study was that often acute respiratory insufficiency is a non-reversible disease due to the progressive nature of the pulmonary pathological lesion. This reaffirms the need for careful selection of patients and for directing the therapy towards patients with reversible pulmonary disease. The future success of this therapy will depend upon this approach.

Another important consideration for the future is improvement in the technology. Specifically, non-thrombogenic surfaces are needed to minimize the need for heparinization. This would reduce the morbidity of the therapy and allow it to be used earlier and more safely with improved results.

References

1. Bramson, M. L., Osborn, J. J., Main, B. F., O'Brien, M. F., Wright, J. S. and Gerbode, F. 'A new disposable membrane oxygenator with integral heat exchange.' *Journal of Thoracic and Cardiovascular Surgery*, **50,** 391 (1965)
2. Clowes, G. H. A. Jr., Hopkins, A. L. and Neville, W. E. 'An artificial lung dependent upon diffusion of oxygen and carbon dioxide through plastic membranes.' *Journal of Thoracic and Cardiovascular Surgery*, **32,** 630 (1956)
3. de Laval, M., Dontigny, L., Hill, J. D. and Mielke, C. H. Jr. 'A simple method of heparin management during prolonged extracorporeal circulation.' *Presented at the American Association for Medical Instrumentation Conference, Las Vegas, April 24–26, 1972* (1972)
4. de Leval, M., Hill, J. D., Mielke, H., Bramson, M. L., Smith, C. and Gerbode, F. 'Platelet kinetics during extracorporeal circulation.' *Transactions of the American Society for Artificial Internal Organs*, **18,** 355 (1972)
5. Drinker, P. Personal communication
6. Dutton, R. C., Mather, F. W., III, Walker, S. N., Lipps, B. J., Jr., Rudy, L. W., Severinghaus, J. W. and Edmunds, L. H., Jr. 'Development and evaluation of a new hollow fibre membrane oxygenator.' *Transactions of the American Society for Artificial Internal Organs*, **17,** 331 (1971)
7. Gannon, P. Personal communication
8. Hattersely, P. G. 'Activated coagulation time of whole blood.' *Journal of the American Medical Association*, **196,** 436 (1966)
9. Hill, J. D., Bramson, M. L., Hackel, A., Deal, C. W., Sanchez, P. A., Osborn, J. J. and Gerbode, F. 'Laboratory and clinical studies during prolonged partial extracorporeal circulation using the Bramson membrane lung.' *Circulation*, **37** and **38 (Suppl. II)**, 139 (1968)

10. Hill, J. D., de Leval, M., Fallat, R. J., Bramson, M. L., Eberhart, R. C., Schulte, H. D., Osborn, J. J., Barber, R. and Gerbode, F. 'Acute respiratory insufficiency. Treatment with prolonged extracorporeal oxygenation.' *Journal of Thoracic and Cardiovascular Surgery*, **64,** 551 (1972)
11. Hill, J. D., de Leval, M., Mielke, C. H., Jr., Bramson, M. L. and Gerbode, F. 'Clinical prolonged extracorporeal circulation for respiratory insufficiency: haematological effects.' *Transactions of the American Society for Artificial Internal Organs*, **18,** 546 (1966)
12. Hill, J. D., Fallat, R. J., Cohn, K., Eberhart, R., Dontigny, L., Bramson, M. D., Osborn, J. J. and Gerbode, F. 'Clinical cardiopulmonary dynamics during prolonged extracorporeal circulation for acute respiratory insufficiency.' *Transactions of the American Society for Artificial Internal Organs*, **17,** 355 (1971)
13. Hill, J. D., Fallat, R. J., de Leval, M. R. and Bramson, M. L. 'Prolonged extracorporeal oxygenation: some special problems.' *Mount Sinai Journal of Medicine*, **40,** 199 (1973)
14. Kirsh, M. M., Peirce, E. C., II, Gago, O., Dufek, J., Lee, R., Jordan, F., Reinish, J., Straker, J., Roloff, D., Rhodes, L. and Sloan, H. 'Clinical use of Peirce–General Electric membrane oxygenator.' *Annals of Thoracic Surgery*, **14,** 140 (1972)
15. Kitrilakis, S., Lutch, J. and McIlroy, A. *Systems Analysis Study for Respiratory Devices*, Prepared for Medical Devices Applications Program by Tecna Corporation for the US Department of Health Education and Welfare, Public Health Service, National Institutes of Health, March 24 1972 (1972)
16. Kolobow, T. Personal communication
17. Kolobow, T., Spragg, R. G., Pierce, J. E. and Zapol, W. M. 'Partial extracorporeal blood gas exchange with the spiral membrane lung in unanaesthetized lambs.' *Transactions of the American Society for Artificial Internal Organs*, **17,** 350 (1971)
18. La Frak, E. and Qvist, J. Personal communication
19. Landé, A. J., Edwards, L., Block, J. H., Carlson, R. G., Subramanian, V., Ascheim, R. S., Scheidt, S., Fillmore, S., Killip, T. and Lillehei, C. W. 'Clinical experience with emergency use of prolonged cardiopulmonary bypass with a membrane pump-oxygenator.' *Annals of Thoracic Surgery*, **10,** 490 (1970)
20. Schulte, H. D., Birks, W. and Dudziak, R. 'Erste Erfahrungen mit der Bramson-Membran-Lunge.' *Thoraxchirurgie*, **20,** 54 (1972)
21. Zapol, W., Pontoppidan, J., McCullough, N., Schmidt, V., Bland, J. and Kitz, R. 'Clinical membrane lung support for acute respiratory insufficiency.' *Transactions of the American Society for Artificial Internal Organs*, **18,** 553 (1972)

24

Arteriovenous Extracorporeal Membrane Oxygenation for Partial Respiratory Support

Harvey S. Borovetz, Robert L. Hardesty, Bartley P. Griffith, G. Michael Deeb and Tin-Kan Hung

aude sapere

Introduction

The successful application of prolonged extracorporeal membrane oxygenation (ECMO) in 1971 by J. D. Hill is a benchmark in the two decades of developing this advanced technique of respiratory support[34]. Less than 15 per cent of over 300 patients have survived prolonged ECMO[24], but survival has recently improved due to better selection of patients and increased technical experience[6, 8, 21, 35, 36]. Positive pressure respiratory techniques fail annually in 40 000 adults and 12 000 infants in the United States[52]. Associated with conventional ventilation using positive pressure are the barotrauma and the toxicity of oxygen which compound the injury related to the primary disease. A mortality of 41 per cent is reported for patients with acute respiratory insufficiency who require ventilation with positive pressure and inspired oxygen content ($F\text{IO}_2$) $\geqslant 0.5$ for 24 hours[51]. The concomitant use of ECMO with conventional ventilation avoids the deleterious effects of the latter. The membrane lung permits life-sustaining oxygenation at lower ventilatory pressures and diminished concentrations of oxygen[2, 8, 48, 53, 64].

The emergence of ECMO as a system of pulmonary support has resulted from development of both membrane oxygenators and techniques of extracorporeal perfusion (arteriovenous, venovenous, venoarterial, or mixed combinations). While the venoarterial mode of perfusion which allows total cardiopulmonary support is the current preferred method for the clinical application of ECMO, there are potential advantages associated with the use of arteriovenous (A-V) perfusion. First, arteriovenous perfusion may be conducted without the assistance of a mechanical pump if the total resistance in the extracorporeal circuit (cannulae, tubing, and oxygenator) is sufficiently low. 'Pumpless' perfusion is technically simple and increases the potential for conducting bypass without systemic anticoagulation with heparin. Tubing and oxygenator components can be surfaced with thromboresistant coatings while systems using extracorporeal blood pumps are more difficult to anticoagulate. Secondly, oxygenated blood delivered to the pulmonary arteries may provide a beneficial milieu for healing of injured pulmonary parenchyma and reduction of hypoxic vasoconstriction. Lastly, A-V perfusion may result in a distribution of oxygenated blood to the critical cerebral, coronary, and renal vascular beds without the need for either retrograde aortic cannulation with a long femoral artery catheter or direct cannulation of carotid or axillary arteries.

Low flow arteriovenous extracorporeal support has been employed successfully for the elimination of CO_2 but its use to date as a method of oxygenation has been unrewarding[7]. A primary objection to the use of the arteriovenous mode is that less oxygen transfer occurs than would be obtained in the venoarterial mode for the same rate of extracorporeal perfusion. This implies that high rates of arteriovenous flow are necessary to deliver adequate oxygen support with commercially available membrane oxygenators. High flow arteriovenous perfusion has been condemned due to the theoretical consideration that it imposes an obligate increase in venous return which in turn produces an increase in cardiac output. A rise in cardiac output could place an additional burden on the heart and especially on the right ventricle, should pulmonary hypertension exist[7, 58, 63].

The ongoing development of an efficient pulmonary assist membrane oxygenator has prompted an investigation of the haemodynamic consequences and potential for transfer of gases in the arteriovenous mode. Biomechanical features of design of the pulmonary assist membrane oxygenator make it an attractive unit for use as an additional assist in the A-V mode along with conventional ventilation techniques.

Pulmonary assist membrane oxygenation

A pulmonary assist membrane oxygenator has been developed for potential clinical support to infants and small children when CPAP, PEEP, and oxygen-enriched mechanical ventilation fail to provide adequate support to lung function. The oxygenator is designed to be used as an additional assist in parallel with conventional ventilation techniques when the latter alone become inadequate.

The oxygenation assist unit, designed originally by Michael H. Weissman, M.D., Ph.D. in 1969 at Carnegie-Mellon University, employs the efficient mass exchange processes of blood flowing through impermeable microchannels with membrane placed across the diametric plane of the channel for gas

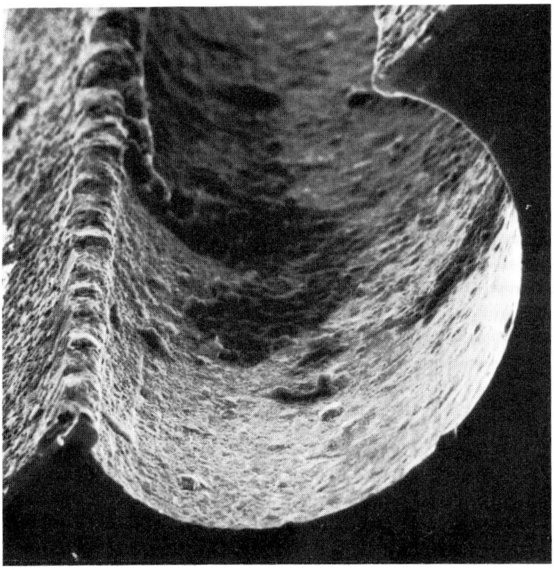

Figure 24.1 Scanning electron photomicrograph of a typical etched microchannel plated with a thin nickel layer (magnification × 400)

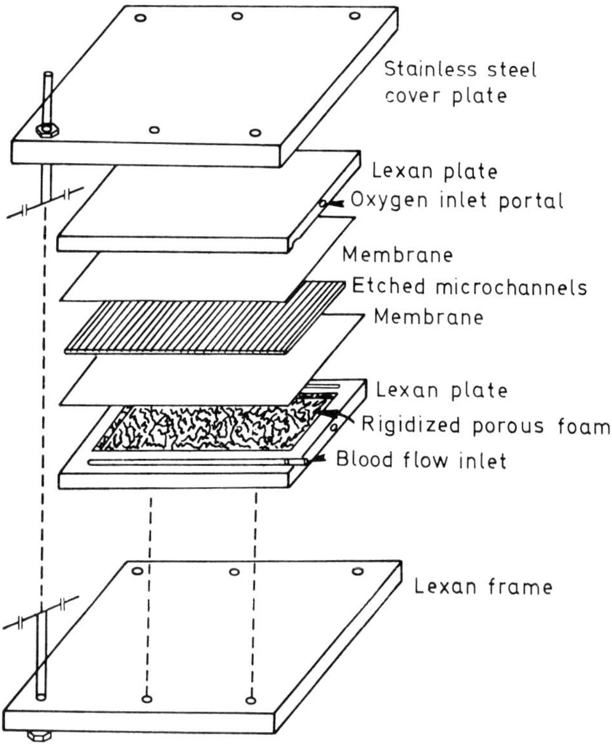

Figure 24.2 Schematic drawing of the components of the pulmonary assist membrane oxygenator. (From Borovetz *et al.*[12] by courtesy of *The International Journal of Artificial Organs*)

exchange. The microchannels are photochemically etched* onto both sides of a stainless steel or copper plate. Each side of the plate (11 × 5 × 0.015 inches in dimensions) contains 665 channels. The channels are approximately semicircular in shape (*Figure 24.1*) with a radius of 115 ± 20 μm or 150 ± 20 μm. Direct contact between the flowing blood and copper substrate is prevented by electroplating the copper sheets with a thin nickel layer approximately 1 μm thick. Microporous membranes† with nominal pore sizes of 0.2 μm and sheet thickness of 50–100 μm are placed flush with both surfaces of the plate and are sandwiched in two rigidized porous foams which are encased in 1 inch thick lexan plates (*Figure 24.2*). Two or three sets of these components or sandwiches are mounted in a stack to form a pulmonary assist membrane oxygenator for potential neonatal support (*Figure 24.3a*). The design perfusion rate *in vivo* for a three-plate unit is 180–240 ml/min [42].

*Magnetics Inc., Butler, Pennsylvania, USA
†Gelman Instrument, Ann Arbor, Michigan, USA

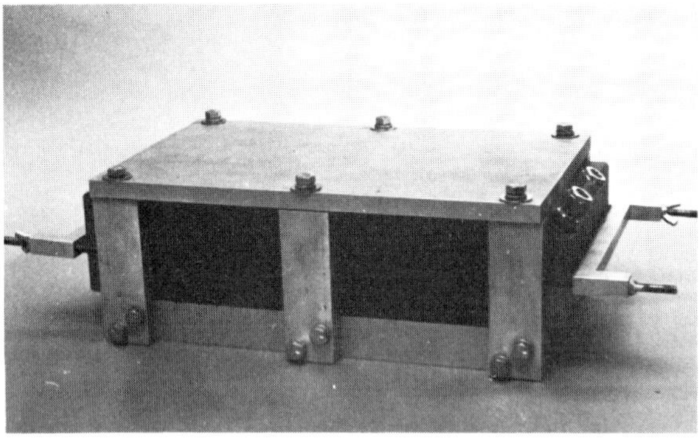

(a)

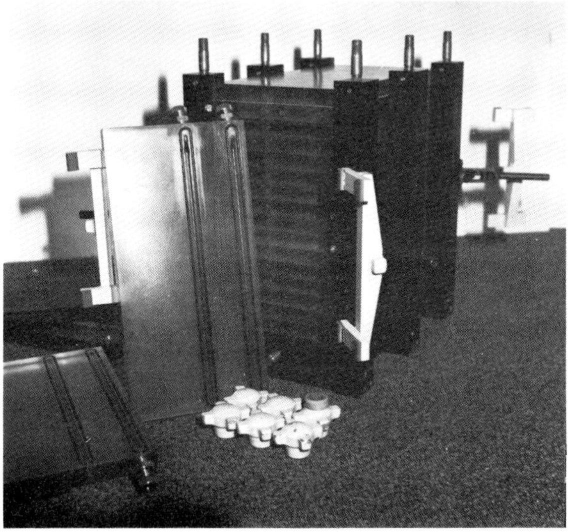

(b)

Figure 24.3 (*a*) Pulmonary assist membrane oxygenator for neonatal support. (*b*) Sixteen-plate pulmonary assist membrane oxygenator. (From Borovetz *et al.*[12] by courtesy of *The International Journal of Artificial Organs*)

The distribution of blood flow in a typical microchannel plate unit is illustrated in *Figure 24.4*. Blood flow is introduced into a manifold and then to an entrance membrane conduit which is formed by the deformation of two membrane sheets into semicircular grooves, 12 inches long and 0.125 inches wide, in the lexan plate. Because of its relatively large dimensions (as compared to that of an etched channel), the entrance conduit provides a uniform blood distibution among the individual etched channels. Arterialized blood is collected in an exit membrane conduit with the outflow through a stainless steel tube into the outlet fluid manifold. It should be noted that

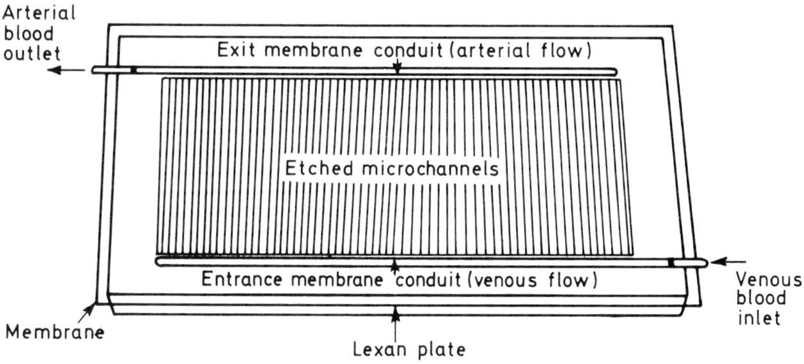

Figure 24.4 Distribution of blood flow in a typical microchannel plate unit. (From Borovetz *et al.*[12] by courtesy of *The International Journal of Artificial Organs*)

arterial blood is introduced into the plate unit shown in *Figure 24.4,* if the pulmonary assist membrane oxygenator were being used in the arterio-venous mode of support.

For partial support of respiratory distress syndrome in small children, a much larger assist unit will be required. The optimal perfusion rate will depend on the degree of respiratory distress and the total cardiac output of the patient. By the vertical arrangement of sixteen sets of the components shown in *Figure 24.2*[62] a pulmonary assist membrane oxygenator is formed with a designed flow capacity of 1 to 1.4 ℓ/min and priming volume of 80 ml which includes 20 ml for both the inflow and outflow manifolds (*Figure 24.3b*).

Biomechanical design criteria of the pulmonary assist oxygenator and associated bypass system are based upon the following principles: (1) keeping shear stress in the blood flow below the critical value that may lead to blood trauma; (2) low blood flow resistance for potential pumpless bypass in the arteriovenous mode; (3) low priming volume; and (4) optimal oxygen and carbon dioxide exchange[43]. The pressure drop across a channel with a radius of 150 ± 20 μm will be as low as 20 to 30 mmHg at a perfusion rate per etched plate of 50 ± 10 ml/min. The same pressure drop can be maintained for a smaller size of microchannel (115 ± 20 μm) when the perfusion rate per plate is reduced to 30–35 ml/min. It has been reported previously[11, 43] that the pressure drop for blood flowing in the microchannels is about 40–60 per cent smaller than the theoretical value for the Newtonian flow case. This reduction is caused by the Fåhraeus–Lindqvist effect related to erythrocyte migration toward the core region thus leaving a peripheral layer of low resistance near the wall of the channel. The formation of a peripheral layer also reduces shear stress which is estimated in the microchannels to be in the range of 300–500μN (30–50 dynes)/cm^2. This magnitude is about 30 per cent of the critical shear that would damage platelets for rich platelet suspensions in plasma free of red blood cells[17, 41].

For the reduction of blood trauma due to the interface between flowing blood and the pulmonary assist membrane oxygenator, the blood-contacting surfaces were treated with various antithrombotic agents.

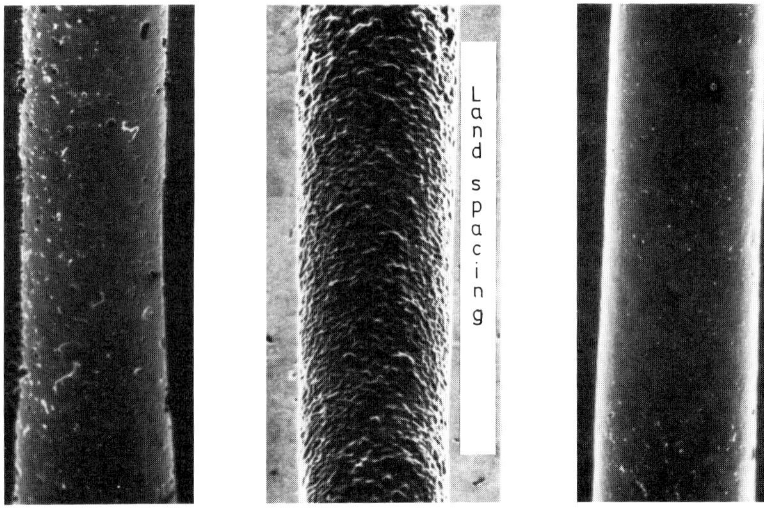

(*a*) (*b*) (*c*)

Figure 24.5 Scanning electron photomicrographs showing: (*a*) a microchannel covered with a thin layer of nickel (magnification × 100); (*b*) the attachment of the TDMAC-heparin coating to a microchannel plated with nickel (magnification × 100); (*c*) The ULTI carbon adherent to the nickel plating (magnification × 100). The land spacings between adjacent channels, identified in (*b*), are not in contact with the blood flow

Specific attention was focused upon the effects of tridodecylmethylammonium chloride (TDMAC) and Ultra Low Temperature Isotropic (ULTI) carbon*. The former was attached to the membranes and microchannels following a modified one-step procedure developed at Battell Memorial Institute[28]. Scanning electron microscopy (SEM) and sequential surface analytic techniques were employed to study the composition and uniformity of these surface coatings prior to blood perfusion[13].

Figure 24.5 compares the surface topography of a microchannel covered with a thin nickel coating, a microchannel first plated with nickel and then treated with TDMAC-heparin, and a microchannel with ULTI carbon attached to the nickel metallic surface. Whereas the channel coated with TDMAC appears to contain diffuse and random micro-areas void of heparin coating, the ULTI carbon can be uniformly applied to the channel surface. At magnification × 1000 (*Figure 24.6*) topographic details of the coating layers are distinguished. The TDMAC-heparin coating is seen to have irregular thickness and density as compared to the smoother carbon surface. It is postulated that a wetting agent or compound may be needed in order to secure a uniform coating of TDMAC-heparin to a metallic surface[15].

*Biolite Carbon, Trademark of Carbo Medics Inc., Austin, Texas, USA

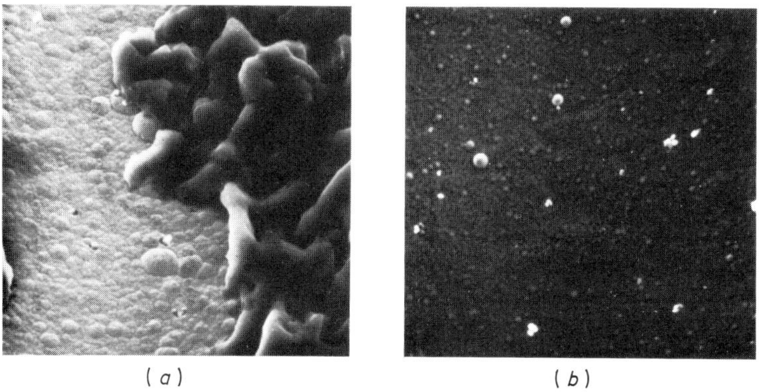

Figure 24.6 (*a*) Surface non-uniformities and void areas in the TDMAC-heparin coating of an etched channel plated with nickel (magnification × 1000). (*b*) Topographic details of the ULTI carbon (magnification × 1000)

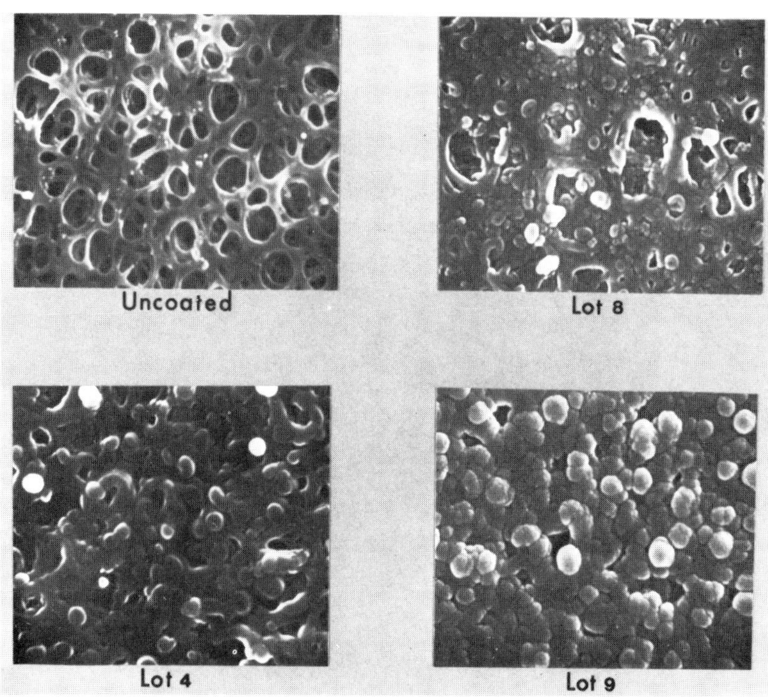

Figure 24.7 Attachment of the ULTI carbon coating to microporous membrane material. For comparison the surface view of the base (uncoated) microporous membrane is presented. The three lot numbers correspond to a particular date of fabrication of the carbon-surfaced membranes. The thickness of the carbon coating varied between 0.5 and 2.0 μm

Attachment of the ULTI carbon coating to the microporous membrane material is illustrated in *Figure 24.7*. The beaded appearance of these sample coatings is typical of other thin carbon films[33, 59]. Uniform coverage of the membrane surface with ULTI carbon films of a thickness between 0.5 and 2.0 μm was verified by SEM techniques.

Investigations of the blood-pulmonary assist oxygenator material interface in *ex vivo* perfusion experiments using dog models revealed noticeable differences in the interactions of blood with various biosurfaces. *Figure 24.8a* exemplifies the attachment of platelets, both singularly and in small

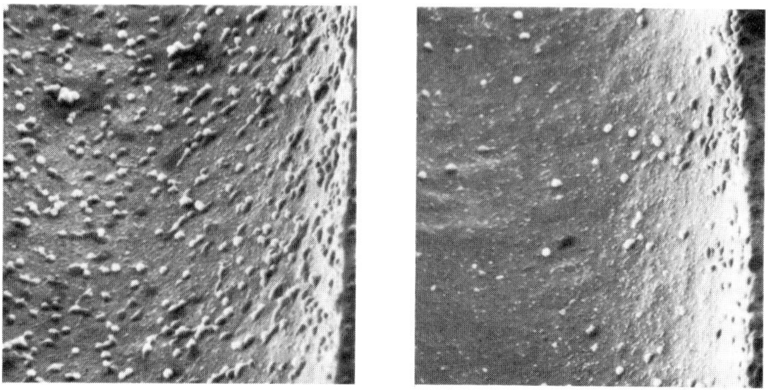

(*a*) (*b*)

Figure 24.8 (*a*) Deposition of cellular elements upon an etched channel plated with nickel following 4 hours of blood perfusion (magnification × 500). (*b*) Paucity of cellular adhesion to a carbon-surfaced channel for the same perfusion period *ex vivo* of 4 hours

aggregates, to etched microchannel surfaces plated with nickel after four hours of perfusion. By comparison a paucity of cellular adhesion can be identified for a carbon-surfaced channel for the same perfusion period *ex vivo* of four hours (*Figure 24.8b*). Similar findings are available for the blood–membrane material interface (*Figures 24.9* and *24.10*). The minimal platelet adherence to a micorporous membrane covered with ULTI carbon is impressive, although cytoplasmic extensions are apparent suggesting some degree of platelet activation (*Figure 24.9*). For comparison, a higher density of white blood cells, distorted platelets, and fibrin masses can be seen attached to the base microporous substrates (*Figure 24.10*). We conclude that for the particular haemodynamic conditions of low Reynolds number blood flow in these *ex vivo* experiments, the ULTI carbon attracted fewer and less distorted cellular elements than uncoated microporous membranes and microconduits, and in contrast to the uncoated materials, the coated surfaces mitigated fibrinogen conversion and blood clotting.

A second important feature of the ULTI carbon, as relates to its use in the fabrication of the blood contacting components of the pulmonary assist membrane oxygenator, regards the permeability to oxygen (PmO_2) of the carbon-surfaced microporous membrane. The presence of the ULTI carbon film on the microporous membrane was found not to reduce significantly the

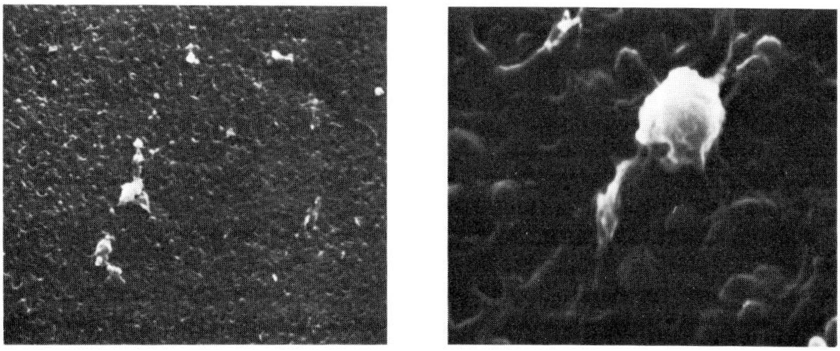

(*a*) (*b*)

Figure 24.9 (*a*) Low magnification image showing minimal cellular debris attached to a carbon-surfaced microporous membrane following 4 hours of perfusion *ex vivo* (magnification × 1000). (*b*) Cytoplasmic extensions and morphological details of a platelet adherent to the ULTI surface. Note that the general beaded appearance and porous structure of the membrane remain as shown in *Figure 24.7* following 4 hours of contact with blood (magnification × 10 000). (From Borovetz *et al.*[13] by courtesy of *Scanning Electron Microscopy*)

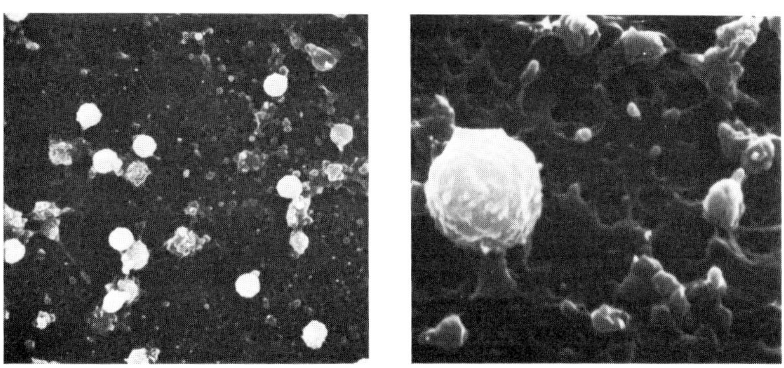

(*a*) (*b*)

Figure 24.10 Attachment of cellular debris to the uncoated microporous substrate for the same perfusion period of *Figure 24.9*. (*a*) Magnification × 1000. (*b*) Magnification × 10 000. (From Borovetz *et al.*[13] by courtesy of *Scanning Electron Microscopy*)

permeability to oxygen (PmO_2) of the base material[14]. *Table 24.1* summarizes the results of 27 measurements of PmO_2 for the carbon-surfaced membranes and uncoated micorporous material. The range of permeabilities presented correspond to the upper and lower bounds of data taken for each material in a multi-compartment diffusion cell using a modern chromatograph for measurement and analysis of oxygen exchange. Only a slight reduction in PmO_2 below that obtained for the uncoated membrane is seen for the carbon-surfaced membranes. When compared with data presented by Ketteringham *et al.*[45], the PmO_2 of the carbon-surfaced membrane was found to be two orders of magnitude above that measured

Table 24.1 Experimental membrane PmO_2

Material	*No.*	*Range of values*[2]
Uncoated	5	7.0–8.4
ULTI carbon	27	5.9–8.0

Number of measurements

2×10^6 ml (STP)–cm/cmHg–cm^2–sec

for silicone rubber membrane (polydimethylsiloxane and polydimethylsiloxane/polycarbonate copolymer). Thus ULTI carbon-surfaced microporous membranes may effectively be used for gas exchange in the pulmonary assist membrane oxygenator.

Gas exchange characteristics in the microchannel flow have demonstrated the efficiency of the pulmonary assist device for blood oxygenation. Data for O_2 uptake and CO_2 removal obtained both *in vitro*[11, 43] and *in vivo*[12] are found to exceed theoretical predictions of mass exchange. The disagreement between the calculated rates of O_2 and CO_2 exchange and the experimental data probably reflects the augmentation of gas transfer due to the shear induced rotation of red blood cells or micromixing[11, 43]. The rates of gas transfer may also be increased if velocities adjacent to the membrane are augmented because of the presence of the peripheral plasma layer (which has been identified as the cause for the low resistance to blood flow in the microchannels).

Of the two gases (oxygen and carbon dioxide) the transfer of oxygen controls the design of the pulmonary assist membrane oxygenator as an exchange device. The permeability of the microporous membranes to carbon dioxide is adequate to reduce the $P\text{CO}_2$ of blood flowing in the pulmonary assist oxygenator from 67 mmHg to 45 mmHg at the designed perfusion rate *in vitro*[43]. The implication is that should the pulmonary assist oxygenator be used for partial respiratory support in the arteriovenous mode, a near normal $P\text{aCO}_2$ can be anticipated even at low rates of extracorporeal flow.

Figure 24.11 shows the relationship between the oxygen transfer per unit membrane area exposed to blood and the rate of blood flow to the same area for various types of oxygenators[60]. The former was calculated for the 16-plate unit pulmonary assist membrane oxygenator (*Figure 24.3(b)*) from *in vitro* data taken at room temperature (20°–22°C). The membrane material used was uncoated microporous membrane. Based on the above findings of PmO_2 for carbon-surfaced microporous membranes (*Table 24.1*), similar oxygen transfer to that shown in *Figure 24.11* can be anticipated with the replacement of the base microporous material with carbon-surfaced membranes. The other data of this figure were obtained from *in vivo* studies at 37°C. When the 'effective' membrane area (i.e. the portion contacting blood and excluding the area in contact with the land spacings (*Figure 24.5*) between adjacent channels) is used to assess the

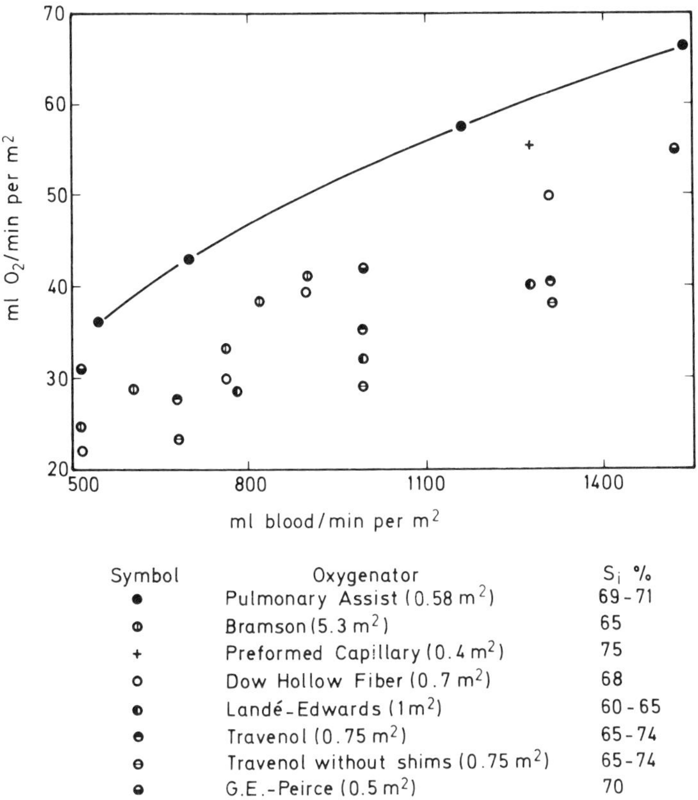

Figure 24.11 Relationship between the rate of oxygen transfer per unit membrane area exposed to blood and the rate of blood flow to the same area for various types of oxygenators. The single data point for the preformed capillary oxygenator represents the oxygen transfer at the rated flow of the device. Si = Venous blood O_2 saturation

oxygen transfer rate, the oxygen transfer per unit membrane area of the 16-plate pulmonary assist device (with 0.58 m^2 of 'effective' membrane area) is about twice that of the Travenol oxygenator without shims[61], and 25 per cent higher than the General Electric–Peirce lung. Oxygen transfer for the Dow SRO hollow fibre oxygenator[22] lies between the Peirce lung and the Travenol oxygenator without shims. Oxygen delivery to blood flowing in the preformed capillary oxygenator[18] falls slightly below that indicated for the pulmonary assist membrane oxygenator.

Biomechanical design features of the pulmonary assist membrane oxygenator make it an attractive unit for use as an additional assist in parallel with conventional ventilation techniques. The low resistance to blood flow and efficient oxygen and carbon dioxide exchange make it ideally suited for arteriovenous and potentially pumpless bypass. Treatment of the blood contacting surfaces with ULTI carbon has produced an antithrombogenic interface for the microchannel flow of blood.

Arteriovenous mode of extracorporeal membrane oxygenation

Arteriovenous oxygenation with the pulmonary assist membrane oxygenator

The feasibility of using the pulmonary assist membrane oxygenator for partial respiratory support in arteriovenous bypass was demonstrated in an experimental study in which small mongrel dogs (2.8–5 kg) which were rendered hypoxic (Pa_{O_2} = 27–50 mmHg) by oxygen depression served as the animal model. Arteriovenous flow was instituted between carotid artery, femoral artery, or infrarenal aorta with return via the external jugular vein or the inferior vena cava. The rates of arteriovenous perfusion $\dot{Q}av$ through the pulmonary assist oxygenator (as regulated by a roller pump) were between 18 and 33 per cent of the total cardiac output $\dot{Q}t$ as measured on bypass (i.e. $\dot{Q}av/\dot{Q}t$ = 0.18–0.33). The 16-plate oxygenator assist shown in *Figure 24.3b* was employed in this series of experiments.

The effect of the ratio of the arteriovenous rate of flow to the total cardiac output ($\dot{Q}av/\dot{Q}t$) upon blood arterialization is demonstrated in *Figure 24.12*. Here the solid parallel lines represent upper and lower bounds for the *in vivo* data. From a mean depressed Pa_{O_2} of 43 mmHg arterial oxygen tensions *in vivo* were upgraded by an average of 20 mmHg at $\dot{Q}av/\dot{Q}t$ ratios of 0.18–0.33. The partial pressure for oxygen of the blood exiting the pulmonary assist oxygenator exceeded 250 mmHg for data shown in this figure. As expected, the increase in Pa_{O_2} was greater as the rate of arteriovenous flow increased. For example at $\dot{Q}av/\dot{Q}t$ equal to 0.83, Pa_{O_2} rose from 50 mmHg initially to a normal arterial value of 95 mmHg.

The data from *Figure 24.12* may be replotted to indicate directly the oxygen tension in the arterial blood following initiation of arteriovenous flow through the pulmonary assist oxygenator (*Figure 24.13*). The data points which lie at the bottom of each vertical line represent the initially depressed Pa_{O_2} (prior to the bypass) while those at the top show the upgraded values for various $\dot{Q}av/\dot{Q}t$ ratios. In all cases the Pa_{O_2} values fell to within ± 5 per cent of their preperfusion values.

Based upon the data for the upgrade in Pa_{O_2} presented in *Figures 24.12* and *24.13*, calculation of the extracorporeal rate of oxygen delivery can be made. For $\dot{Q}av/\dot{Q}t$ equal to 0.18–0.33 in this experimental study, the rate of oxygen delivery by the pulmonary assist membrane oxygenator ranged between 4 and 11 ml/min. This compares with the estimated basal metabolic requirements of these animals of 2–5 kg body weight of 10–20 ml O_2/min. For this series of experiments the pulmonary assist membrane oxygenator permitted the satisfactory upgrade of poorly oxygenated arterial blood for rates of arteriovenous perfusion equal to 33 per cent of the total cardiac

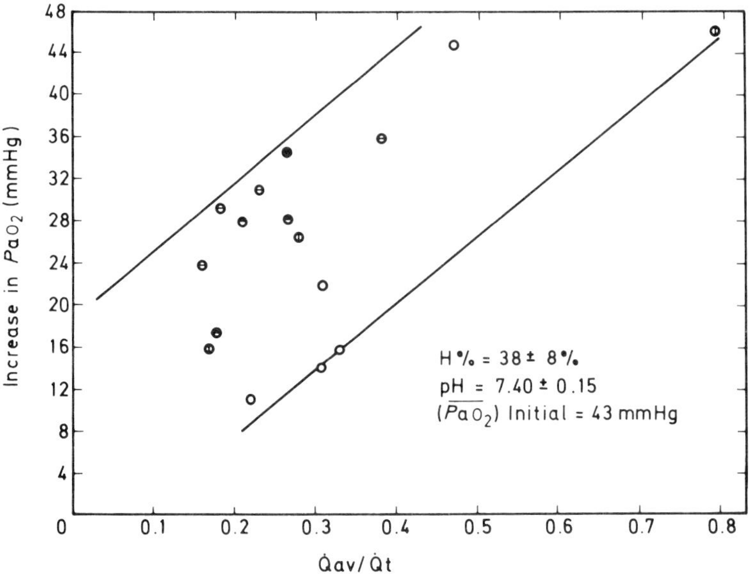

Figure 24.12 The effect of arteriovenous perfusion on the increase in arterial oxygen tension Pa_{O_2}. The ratio $\dot{Q}av/\dot{Q}t$ defines the percentage of the total cardiac output as measured on bypass which is circulated through the pulmonary assist oxygenator (H per cent = the blood haematocrit). (From Borovetz *et al.*[12] by courtesy of *The International Journal of Artificial Organs*)

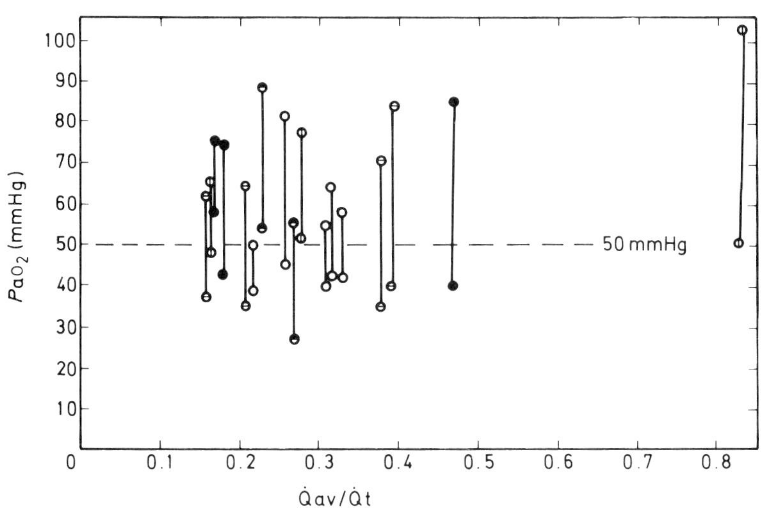

Figure 24.13 Arterial oxygenation for various percentages of cardiac output circulated through the pulmonary assist membrane oxygenator. Experimental conditions are the same as for *Figure 24.12*. (From Borovetz *et al.*[12] by courtesy of *The International Journal of Artificial Organs*)

output. Similar findings have previously been reported by Rashkind *et al.*[54, 55] for a disposable plastic bubble oxygenator. Their results show that at $\dot{Q}av$ equal to 34 per cent of the total cardiac output, a 30 per cent increase in Pa_{O_2} (from 43 mmHg to 56 mmHg) occurred.

Haemodynamic response to A-V perfusion

The effects of arteriovenous perfusion on myocardial performance, pulmonary circulatory dynamics, and organ preservation were studied in dogs in order to evaluate the applicability of arteriovenous ECMO for partial respiratory support. Studies were made on normally oxygenated dogs and on dogs with pulmonary injury and moderate pulmonary hypertension induced by injection of oleic acid into the right ventricle. The latter group was included to assess the changes which occur in cardiopulmonary dynamics in the presence of moderate pulmonary hypertension. The pulmonary assist membrane oxygenator (16-plate unit) was employed to provide partial respiratory support to those animals with pulmonary injury. The results indicate that no deleterious haemodynamic changes occurrred in either of the groups of animals during arteriovenous (A-V) flow for periods of up to five hours at perfusion rates corresponding primarily to 15–35 per cent of the total cardiac output. Adequate systemic oxygenation was provided by the pulmonary assist oxygenator at these rates of arteriovenous perfusion.

Animal model

Myocardial performance and pulmonary circulatory dynamics were studied in five animals with normal oxygenation and in seven dogs in whom haemorrhagic 'shock lung' and moderate pulmonary hypertension were induced by injection of oleic acid (0.3 ml/kg) into the right ventricle[23]. Organ preservation studies were conducted in an additional group of normoxaemic animals. In six dogs the effect of A-V perfusion upon the brain was assessed by measurement of carotid and vertebral blood flow, EEG monitoring, and recordings of intracranial pressure. Renal blood flow and urine volume, molarity, and electrolytes were recorded in eight animals. All animals of this study were 18–25 kg in body weight.

The arteriovenous circuit was constructed from polyvinyl chloride tubing connecting a catheter in the common iliac artery with one in the external jugular or femoral vein. Catheters (size 8 Fr. O.D./6 Fr. I.D.) constructed of polyurethane reinforced with spring wire were employed for cannulation[49]. The arterial catheter in the common iliac artery permitted rates of flow in excess of 100 ml/kg per min. Regulation of arteriovenous flow between 15 and 35 per cent of the total cardiac output was possible by interposition of a roller pump. The pulmonary assist membrane oxygenator was positioned between the roller pump and the venous return catheter for the dogs with haemorrhagic 'shock lung' in order to provide arteriovenous ECMO for partial respiratory support (*Figure 24.14*).

Anaesthesia was provided by halothane (1 per cent) and muscle relaxation was induced by pancuronium (0.1 mg/kg). Mechanical ventilation was maintained with a volume-regulated respirator. High tidal volumes (30 ml/

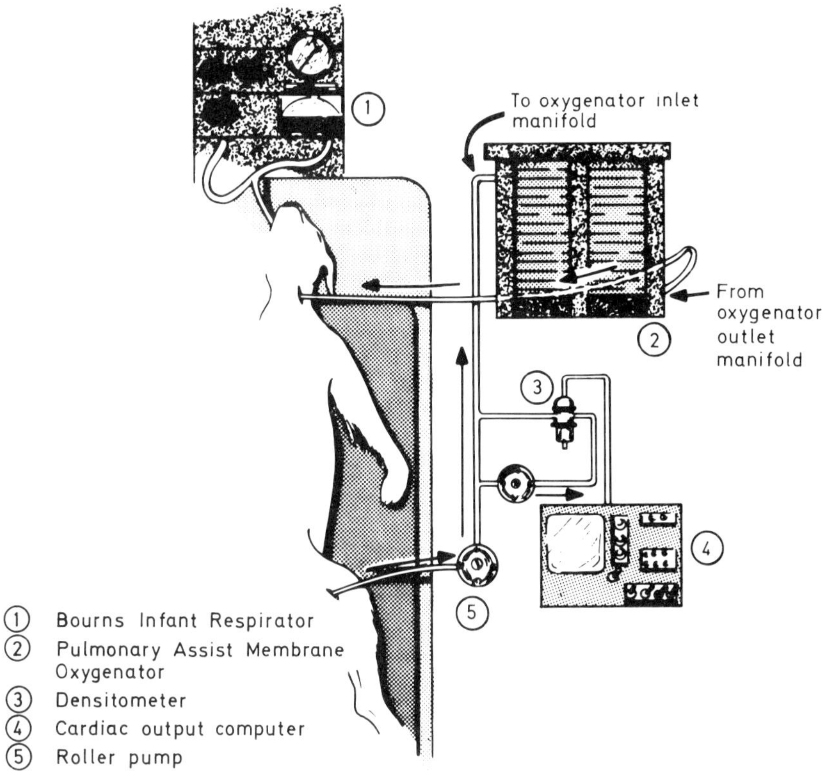

Figure 24.14 Bypass circuitry for arteriovenous ECMO

kg) with 99 per cent oxygen, elevated respiratory rate (15–20/min), and positive end-expiratory pressure (5–10 cm H_2O) were necessary prior to arteriovenous ECMO in order to support those animals whose lungs were injured with oleic acid.

The arterial oxygen saturation of animals injured with oleic acid ranged between 55 and 70 per cent and the arterial $P\text{CO}_2$ between 20 and 45 mmHg prior to perfusion. During arteriovenous ECMO systemic arterial saturations were elevated to between 60 and 90 per cent, and those in the pulmonary artery between 55 and 82 per cent. The increase in oxygen saturation depended upon the ratio of the arteriovenous flow to total cardiac output and the degree of hypoxia present prior to ECMO[12].

Transfusions of a balanced electrolyte solution and whole blood were administered to those animals with the oleic acid injury to replete loss of intravascular volume from pulmonary oedema. Calcium chloride was given to replace calcium bound by the fatty acids, and infusions of sodium bicarbonate were occasionally necessary to buffer acidosis. Anticoagulation with heparin (3mg/kg) was monitored in all animals to maintain an activated clotting time between 2 to 5 times the control value. Heating blankets maintained the rectal temperature at 34° to 39°C.

Measurement of experimental data

Cardiac output was determined by the indocyanine green dye dilution method using a continuous sampling technique developed to minimize volume loss[25]. A circuit including a densitometer and a small roller pump was positioned in parallel with the arteriovenous tubing (*Figure 24.14*). Blood was siphoned continuously through the densitometer at a constant rate of 20 ml/min.

Number 7 French catheters with 2 lumens (Swan–Ganz) were placed under fluoroscopic control to measure the pulmonary capillary wedge (PCW), pulmonary arterial (PA), and right atrial pressures* (RA). A size 5 French catheter positioned in the right ventricle provided pressure measurements and served as a site for injection of oleic acid. Aortic pressure was measured proximal to the perfusion cannula.

Carotid, vertebral, and renal blood flows were measured on a Carolina 501 – Square Wave Flow Meter from electromagnetic probes. A metal pressure screw was inserted into the subarachnoid space for measurement of intracranial pressure. EEGs were monitored from scalp electrodes.

The haemodynamic consequences of arteriovenous perfusion, including myocardial performance, pulmonary vascular resistance, as well as carotid and renal perfusion, were assessed for periods of up to four to five hours. Parameters of myocardial performance included cardiac output, PCW, RA and right ventricular pressures (RVP) and stroke work (RVSW). RVSW is defined here as the product of the stroke volume and the difference between peak right ventricular pressure and mean RA pressure. Pulmonary vascular (PV) resistance was calculated as the mean PA pressure minus the PCW divided by the cardiac output[29]. The parameters measured prior to initiation of arteriovenous flow were used as preperfusion conditions for all animals. Subsequent observations made at various rates of arteriovenous perfusion were compared with the preperfusion data by Student's t-test for paired observation with equal variance. A two-tailed significance level was assigned to the *P* values. The magnitude of the arteriovenous perfusion ($\dot{Q}av$) was varied in each group of animals between rates corresponding primarily to 15–35 per cent of the total cardiac output ($\dot{Q}t$) as measured during A-V flow.

Results

A rise in cardiac output ($\dot{Q}t$) was noted upon initiation of arteriovenous flow ($\dot{Q}av$) in each group of animals for the ranges of perfusion tested ($\dot{Q}av/\dot{Q}t$ = 0.15–0.35 corresponding to 20–65 ml/kg per min). A linear relationship existed between the rise in cardiac output and the incremental elevations of arteriovenous flow from the preperfusion levels with $\dot{Q}av$ = O. Cardiac outputs were not maintained above preperfusion levels when arteriovenous flow was kept at a constant rate for periods beyond one hour. These trends persisted in spite of marked minute-to-minute variability in cardiac output associated with small animal experimentation. $\dot{Q}t$ is related to arteriovenous perfusion for one normoxaemic animal in *Figure 24.15*. The cardiac output

*Statham transducers (P-23 Series)

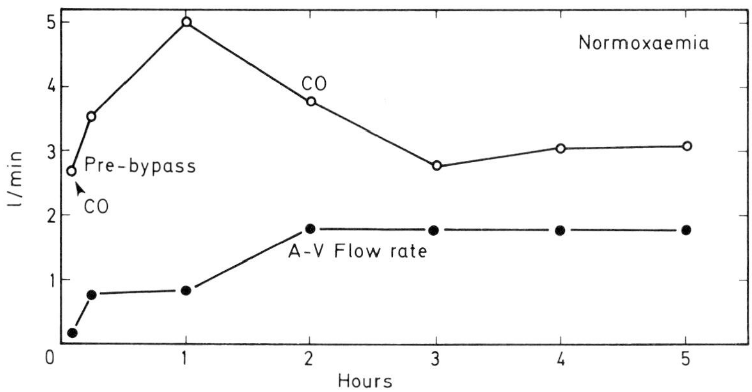

Figure 24.15 Variation in cardiac output in one normoxaemic animal during arteriovenous perfusion. The absence of a persistent elevation in cardiac output above preperfusion values was seen in all of the animals of this study. CO = cardiac output

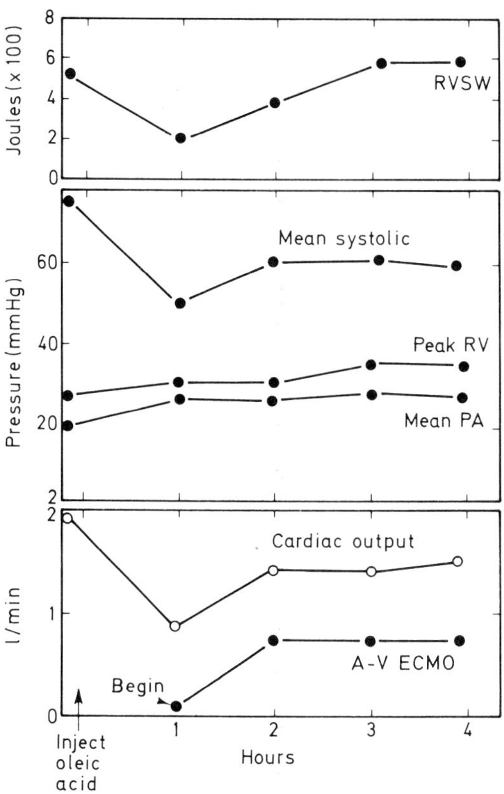

Figure 24.16 Haemodynamic consequences of oleic acid injury in one typical experiment. Upon the initiation of arteriovenous ECMO, RVSW and cardiac output rose toward pre-injury levels. Mean PA and peak RV pressures did not increase significantly ($P > 0.05$) in any of the animals with lung injury for the range of perfusions tested

rises with initiation of arteriovenous flow and beyond one hour nears the preperfusion level. This same trend in cardiac output was noted in all animals of this study.

Immediately after the injection of oleic acid, cardiac output, RVSW, and systemic pressures fell, while a slight elevation was noted in mean PA pressures (10 mmHg), and pulmonary vascular resistance (0.5 PRU) relative to those of normoxaemic animals. PCW and RA pressures fell within twenty minutes because of marked intravascular loss of volume in the form of pulmonary oedema. Transfusions of whole blood and salt solutions were directed to maintain the preperfusion values of RA and PCW pressures. Following the initiation of arteriovenous ECMO a moderate elevation in cardiac output and RVSW occurred (*Figure 24.16*). Pulmonary vascular resistance, mean systemic and mean PA pressures did not increase ($P > 0.05$) in any of the animals from this group during perfusion periods lasting up to five hours.

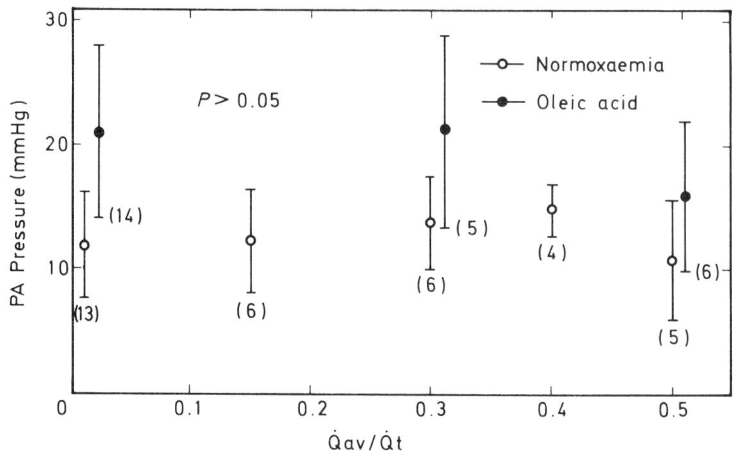

Figure 24.17 Mean pulmonary artery pressure (PA) in normoxaemic animals and those with lung injury during arteriovenous flows. Results are plotted as the mean value ± SD for *n* data points (indicated in parentheses below each bar) at a particular ratio of the arteriovenous flow rate (Q̇av) to the total cardiac output (Q̇t)

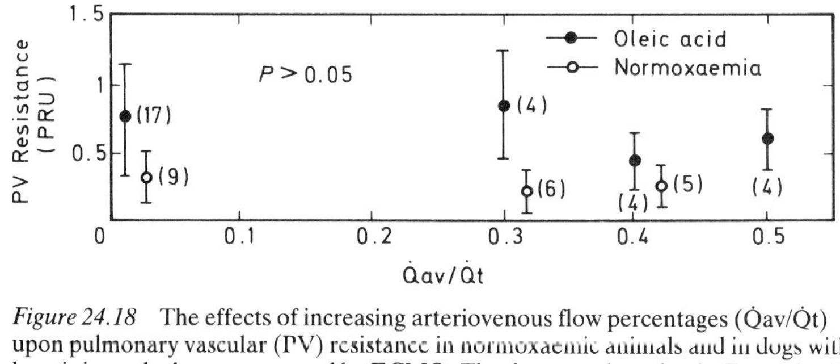

Figure 24.18 The effects of increasing arteriovenous flow percentages (Q̇av/Q̇t) upon pulmonary vascular (PV) resistance in normoxaemic animals and in dogs with lung injury, the latter supported by ECMO. The data are plotted as in *Figure 24.17*

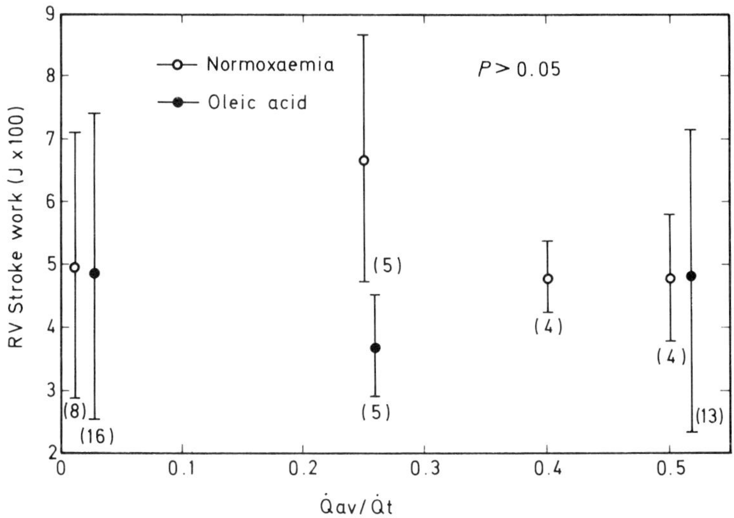

Figure 24.19 Right ventricular stroke work during arteriovenous perfusion in normoxaemic animals and those with lung injury. (From Griffith *et al.*[27] by courtesy of *Surgical Forum*)

Mean PA pressure, pulmonary vascular resistance, and RVSW of both normoxaemic animals and those whose lungs were injured with oleic acid did not change significantly ($P > 0.05$) from preperfusion levels with increasing ratios of arteriovenous perfusion to total cardiac output level (*Figures 24.17* and *24.18*). Little difference was seen in the preperfusion value for right ventricular stroke work in these two groups of animals even though RV pressure was elevated by 11 mmHg in animals with induced pulmonary injury (*Figure 24.19*).

During the experiments of organ preservation, A-V flows were regulated between 30–35 per cent of the total cardiac output. Mean baseline cerebral flow was 740 ml/min (25 per cent of $\dot{Q}t$). The flow fell to a mean value of 645 ml/min (20 per cent of $\dot{Q}t$) at one hour before rising to a mean of 890 ml/min (28 per cent of $\dot{Q}t$) at three hours and 860 ml/min at four hours. None of the changes was significant ($P > 0.05$) (*Figure 24.20*). The mean intracranial pressure (ICP) prior to arteriovenous flow was 24 mmHg and it remained essentially unchanged for the four hour period of perfusion (*Figure 24.21*). No EEG changes were noted in any of the animals during the four hour test period. Mean renal blood flow prior to initiation of A-V flow was 495 ml/min (19 per cent of $\dot{Q}t$). After one and two hours of A-V perfusion, renal flows remained unchanged with mean values of 440 ml/min and 435 ml/min respectively (*Figure 24.22*). The measurements were concluded after two hours in these animals because of excessive extravascular volume loss into the retroperitoneum. Urine volume (15 ml/h), molarity (780 mmol), and electrolytes remained unchanged and within normal physiological ranges during the two hour test period.

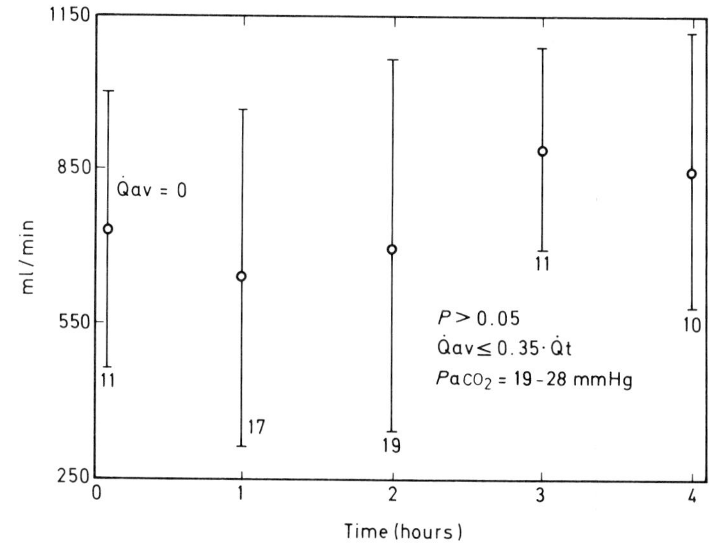

Figure 24.20 Variation in cerebral blood flow during arteriovenous perfusion $\dot{Q}av$ was maintained at 20–35 per cent of $\dot{Q}t$ as measured at baseline. Results are plotted as the mean value ± SD for *n* data points indicated below each bar

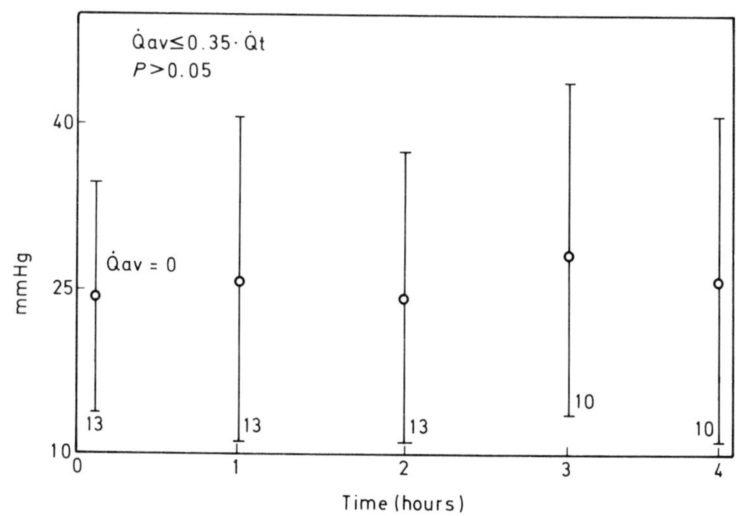

Figure 24.21 Intracranial pressure measurement in six animals during A-V flow. The arteriovenous flow rate was set as in *Figure 24.20*

Discussion

Arteriovenous perfusion at flow rates corresponding to less than 35 per cent of the cardiac output did not produce significant haemodynamic changes even in the presence of moderate pulmonary hypertension. An explanation of this finding was the surprising but consistent lack of a persistent elevation in cardiac output during A-V flow in any of the groups of animals (*Figure*

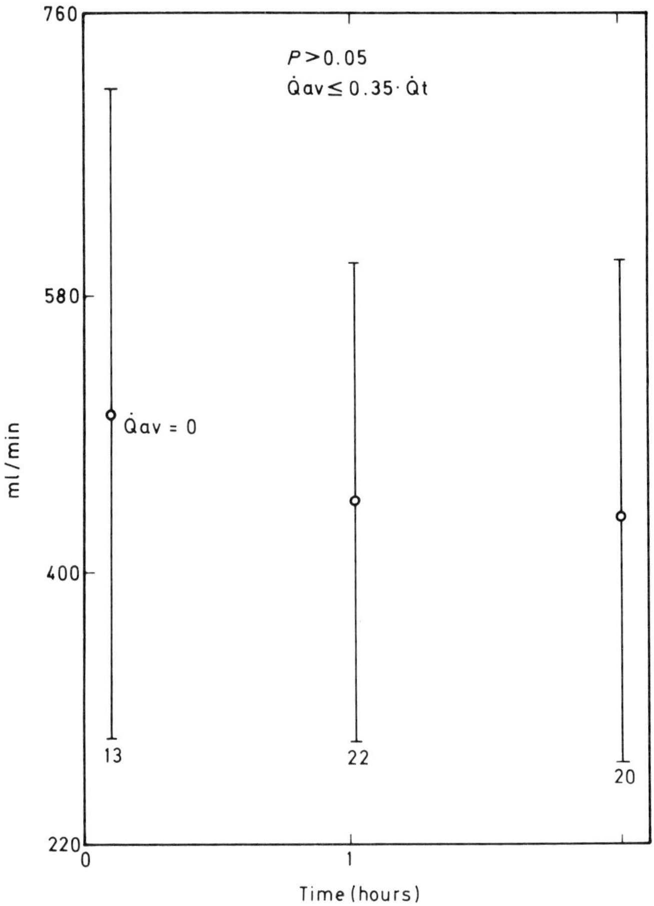

Figure 24.22 Renal blood flow during the two hour period of arteriovenous perfusion ($\dot{Q}av/\dot{Q}t = 0.30–0.35$)

24.15). Upon initiation of arteriovenous flow a linear increase in cardiac output was observed with increasing rates of arteriovenous flow analogous to that which occurs for an arteriovenous fistula. As perfusion times progressed beyond the initial periods a lack of any persistent increase in the cardiac output above preperfusion values was noted in all animals. The lack of continuing elevation in cardiac output could have resulted from either deterioration of myocardial function or from an accommodation by the peripheral circulation to the arteriovenous flows. The absence of any significant change in either PCW, RA or ECG in any of the animals throughout the five hours of perfusion suggests that myocardial function was preserved. Rather the stabilization of cardiac outputs near preperfusion levels during constant arteriovenous flow suggests that an adjustment has occurred in peripheral vascular resistance as mediated by tissue blood flow requirements. Because of the presence of the arteriovenous circuit, peripheral vascular resistance could not be measured directly during arteriovenous perfusion. Its change is implied by the variation in cardiac output.

Awad and Morin have recently employed the arteriovenous mode of perfusion with dogs in a study using the Awad capillary tubular membrane lung[3]. They report that initially a rise in cardiac output occurs which is equal to the arteriovenous rate of flow. Their results further confirm that cardiac output returns to values obtained prior to perfusion within two hours of the initiation of arteriovenous flow and remains essentially constant during a subsequent period of 23 hours of bypass.

Pulmonary injury induced by the injection of oleic acid provided a suitable animal model of respiratory distress for employment of the pulmonary assist membrane oxygenator. The obstruction of the pulmonary capillaries by oleic acid resulted in a decrease in cardiac output along with a moderate rise in peak right ventricular and PA pressures[46]. Right ventricular stroke work fell as a consequence of the decrease in cardiac output. With the initiation of arteriovenous ECMO ($\dot{Q}av/\dot{Q}t < 0.35$) cardiac output and RVSW rose toward the levels measured prior to infusion of oleic acid, while RV and PA pressures remained essentially unchanged. The rise in RVSW during arteriovenous ECMO reflected the elevation in cardiac output. The lack of significant change in RA and RV pressures during ECMO suggests that the upgrade in pulmonary arterial oxygenation mitigated the effects of a diminished pulmonary capillary reserve. The vasodilatory effects of oxygen upon the pulmonary arteriolar sphincters have been well documented.

Of particular concern during prolonged extracorporeal membrane oxygenation is the problem of organ preservation. In contrast to the conventional venoarterial mode of ECMO, pulse pressure is preserved (or increases) during arteriovenous perfusion (*Figure 24.23*). Previous studies have indicated that a pulse pressure of 15 mmHg is required for preservation of renal function during venoarterial ECMO at flows equal to 100 ml/kg per min[16, 20, 30, 32, 40, 54]. In the present investigation cerebral blood flow and ICP remained at preperfusion values for up to four hours and EEG tracings did not reflect change. Renal blood flow remained at preperfusion levels for two hours and no significant changes in urine volume, osmolarity, or electrolytes were noted. The maintenance of brain and kidney function at A-V rates of flow equalling 30–35 per cent of cardiac output suggests that organ preservation is accomplished by limiting flow to the less critical capillary beds (skin and muscle).

Gross and microscopic examination of the kidneys showed no pathologic changes. Although flow to the brain was maintained, pathohistologic findings were present in the tissue of all specimens. Because the brains were fixed by immersion rather than perfusion with fixative, the interpretation of the neuronal findings becomes difficult, but early ischaemic–hypoxic change must be considered possible. The anatomical distribution of the neuronal alterations is consistent with the pattern attributed to global cerebral ischaemia in a number of mammalian species. Whether these histologic findings would alter function of the brain if A-V flow were continued for longer periods, or whether they are reversible, requires further investigation.

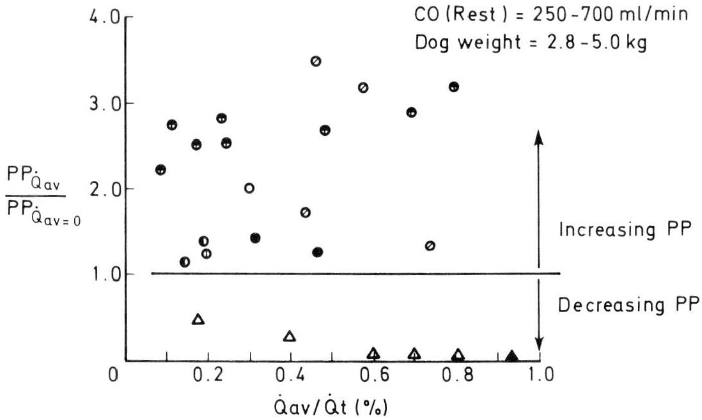

Figure 24.23 Variation in pulse pressure (PP) amplitude during arteriovenous and venoarterial perfusion modes. The circular symbols are taken from the study of *Figure 24.12* and *24.13*. The triangular points represent those reported in venoarterial perfusions with the Landé–Edwards oxygenator (△) and the pulmonary assist membrane oxygenator (▲). All data is normalized to the resting conditions of pulse pressure prior to bypass ($PP_{\dot{Q}av=0}$). (From Borovetz *et al.*[12] by courtesy of *The International Journal of Artificial Organs*)

Arteriovenous ECMO partial support of neonatal lambs

To investigate the applicability of the arteriovenous mode of perfusion with the pulmonary assist membrane oxygenator for partial support of neonatal respiration, perigestational lambs were delivered by Caesarean section and served as an animal model of respiratory distress. Arteriovenous flow was accomplished between a single umbilical artery and vein. Total systemic flow, pulmonary blood flow, and pulmonary vascular resistance were assessed at various rates of arteriovenous perfusion and correlated with systemic oxygenation. A reduction in right-to-left shunting of blood and pulmonary vascular resistance occurred as arterial oxygenation rose from conditions of hypoxaemia to Pa_{O_2} above 50 mmHg. Myocardial performance was not impaired at rates of arteriovenous perfusion below 30 per cent of the total systemic flow as evidenced by normal ECG tracings and pulmonary capillary wedge and central venous pressures.

Animal model

A Caesarean section was performed on 10 pregnant ewes in order to deliver premature lambs (0.8–0.9 of term) weighing 2.5–3.5 kg. Regional anaesthesia (½ per cent Xylocaine) was administered. The fetal pelvis was palpated through the uterus and served as the landmark for the hysterotomy. Once delivered, the lamb was placed on the abdomen of the ewe without obstructing or stretching the umbilical vessels, and immediate tracheal intubation was performed with a No. 18 French endotracheal tube. Irregular spontaneous respirations occurred upon delivery. Catheters were placed in the aortic arch and right atrium through a femoral artery and vein, and pressures were measured on P-23 Statham transducers. An umbilical artery

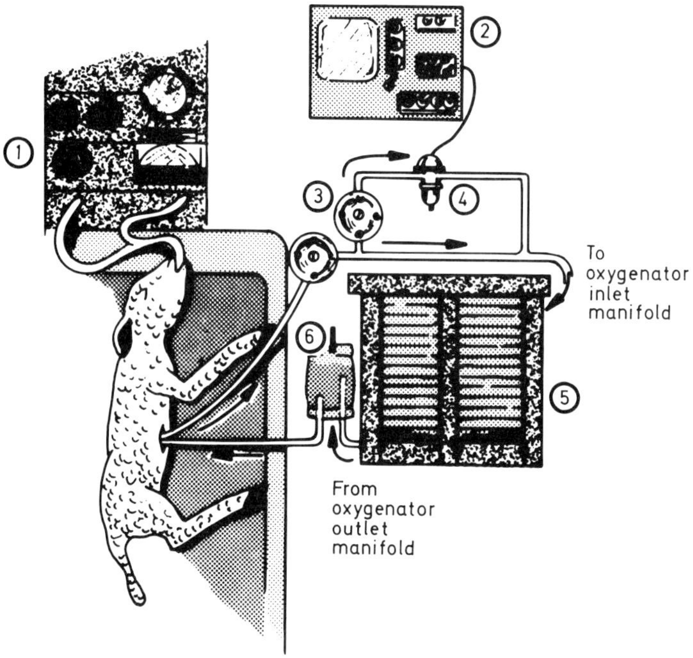

Figure 24.24 Perfusion circuit for arteriovenous ECMO. Nomenclature: (1) Bourn's respirator; (2) cardiac output computer; (3) roller pump; (4) densitometer and minicircuit; (5) pulmonary assist oxygenator; (6) bubble-trap

and vein were isolated. A polyurethane catheter reinforced with thin wire[49] and employed in the study of the haemodynamics of A-V perfusion was introduced through an arteriotomy after the artery was physically dilated. The catheter was coated with a surgical lubricant to compensate for vascular spasm and friability. The stylet was removed as the arterial catheter was advanced beyond the acute angle formed where the umbilical artery passed retroperitoneally. A similar technique was performed on the umbilical vein, and the catheter was positioned 3 cm into this vessel. Between 10 and 20 minutes were required for cannulation during which time partial placental circulation through the remaining umbilical artery and vein supported inadequate spontaneous respirations.

The extracorporeal circuit was constructed similarly to that shown in *Figure 24.14* and consisted of the pulmonary assist membrane oxygenator (16-plate unit), a small roller pump, a bubble-trap and interconnecting Tygon tubing. The roller pump was employed in the present study solely to guarantee a constant rate of arteriovenous flow for acquisition of data. All interconnecting tubing was shortened to minimize the priming volume (150–220 ml). The priming solution consisted of whole blood which was anticoagulated with heparin and balanced appropriately for pH, Na^+, K^+, and Ca^{++} ions.

Prior to the initiation of arteriovenous ECMO, the remaining umbilical vessels were ligated, the cord was severed, and the animal was positioned adjacent to the ECMO circuit (*Figure 24.24*). The lamb was paralyzed with pancuronium (0.1 mg/kg) and ventilated on room air with a tidal volume of 30 ml/kg and at a respiratory rate between 18–30/min in order to maintain normal $Pa\text{CO}_2$. Transfusions of whole blood were given to maintain the peak arterial pressure above 50 mmHg and a central venous pressure between 5 and 10 mmHg. Sodium bicarbonate was administered to correct acidosis. A No. 5 French balloon tip catheter (Swan–Ganz) was inserted via the right external jugular vein into the pulmonary artery (PA). The position of the catheter was verified by pulse contours and later by examination at autopsy. Systemic heparin was administered in an initial dose of 5 mg/kg to maintain the whole-blood activated clotting time at 3 to 5 times the control value. Rectal temperature was maintained at 36° ± 3°C by heating blankets and infrared lamps. The ECG was monitored using the standard limb leads. Arteriovenous flow was then initiated for periods of 4–6 hours (*Figure 24.24*). At the conclusion of each experiment autopsies were performed to verify the position of the cannulae and to assess organ morphology.

Indocyanine green dye dilution curves were used qualitatively to demonstrate patterns of blood flow and to estimate total systemic flow. The latter is the sum of blood flow through the patent foramen ovale, patent ductus arteriosus, and blood which is passed normally through the circulation. The continuous sampling method developed to minimize volume loss in small animals[25] and described in the previous section was again employed for determination of total systemic flow. A quantity of 1.25 mg of dye was injected into the right atrium and concentration changes at the distal aorta were measured by the densitometer in the minicircuit (*Figure 24.24*). A dye curve with two peaks was inscribed. The initial peak represented that portion of the circulation that was shunted right-to-left (R→L) while the second peak was produced by the normal circulation of blood. The forward triangle method was used to calculate total systemic flow (or venous return) from the area inscribed by both peaks[56]. The right-to-left shunting of blood through both the patent foramen ovale and the ductus arteriosus was expressed as a percentage of the total systemic flow[56]. Pulmonary blood flow (PBF) was determined from the difference between total systemic flow and the R→L shunt. The pulmonary vascular (PV) resistance[29] was calculated as the mean PA pressure minus the PCW divided by the pulmonary blood flow. As in the previous study of haemodynamics of A-V perfusion, $\dot{Q}$av was determined by precalibrating the flow generated by the ECMO roller pump.

Data obtained for R→L shunting and PV were correlated to the oxygen tension in the aorta ($Pa\text{O}_2$). The t-test for paired observations with equal variance was used to calculate the significance of changes in the percentage of flow shunted R→L and PV resistance at various levels of aortic oxygenation.

Results

Experimental data was obtained from 8 of the 10 newborn lambs. Technical problems early in the development of the animal model associated with the cannulation of the umbilical vessels resulted in prolonged acidosis and death of 2 of the lambs, before arteriovenous support could be initiated.

The delivery of arteriovenous flow to the ECMO circuit requires satisfactory myocardial performance. The limiting factors for establishing satisfactory arteriovenous ECMO flows were mean arterial pressure in excess of 30 mmHg and central venous pressure between 4 and 10 mmHg. Pulmonary and systemic arterial P_{O_2} varied directly with the rate of arteriovenous perfusion. At the higher arterial Pa_{O_2}s (>50 mmHg) pulmonary blood flow rose while PV resistance and the percentage of flow shunted R→L decreased.

Arteriovenous ECMO was begun at rates of flow of 20 to 30 ml/kg per min. At these low rates an initial 7 to 15 mmHg reduction in peak arterial pressure from 50 to 65 mmHg was noted in all experiments. Simultaneously

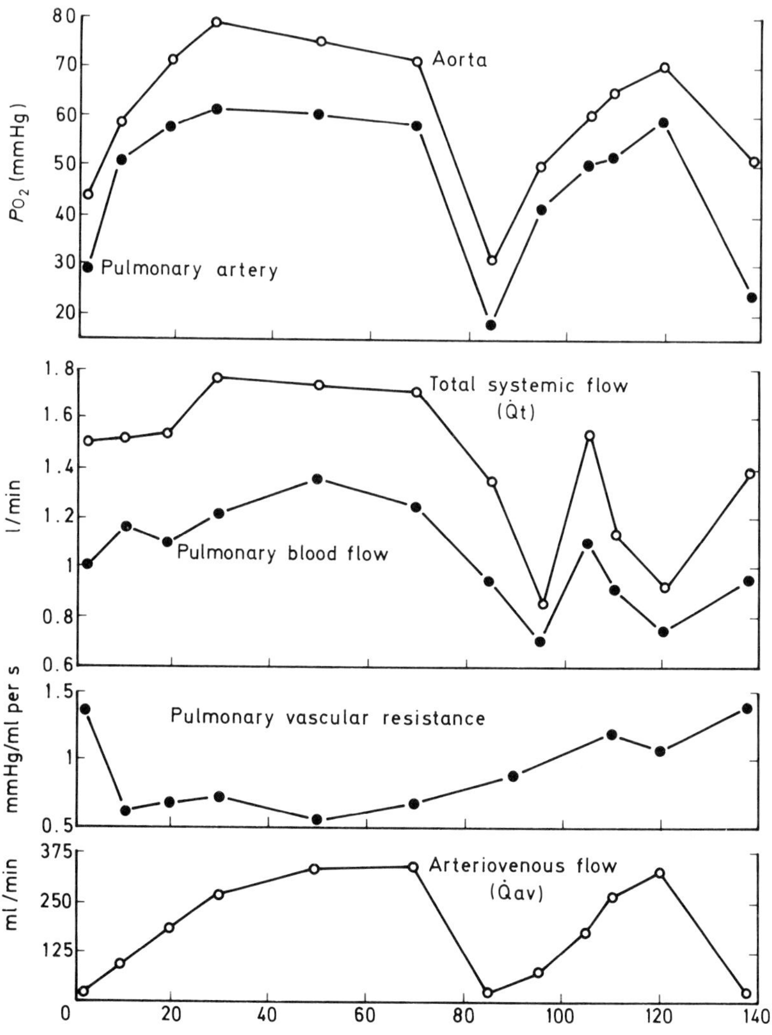

Figure 24.25 Oxygenation and haemodynamic parameters monitored during a 140 minute period of a five hour ECMO study. Arteriovenous ECMO flow was increased from zero to rates equalling 20–30 per cent of the total systemic flow, i.e. $\dot{Q}av/\dot{Q}t = 0.2–0.3$. The cessation of arteriovenous flow was carried out periodically to check baseline measurements

the central venous pressure fell below 5 mmHg. Transfusions of 50–150 ml of whole blood raised the central venous pressure to 5–10 mmHg and produced stable peak arterial pressures above 50 mmHg. Arteriovenous ECMO was continued at these rates of flow for 15–30 minutes in order to permit cardiovascular stabilization. Perfusion was subsequently raised incrementally to values of 100–150 ml/kg per min.

The variations in aortic and pulmonary arterial Po_2, total systemic flow, PBF and pulmonary vascular resistance at different rates of arteriovenous flow are shown for a typical experiment in *Figure 24.25*. In the absence of arteriovenous perfusion ($\dot{Q}av$ = O) arterial oxygenation was severely depressed and PV resistance was three times the normal value for lambs at term. As arteriovenous perfusion was increased from zero conditions to rates equalling 20–30 per cent of the total systemic flow $\dot{Q}t$ ($\dot{Q}av/\dot{Q}t$ = 0.2–0.3), pulmonary artery Po_2 rose from baseline values of 17–35 mmHg to

Table 24.2 Variations in aortic and pulmonary arterial Po_2, total systemic flow, PBF and pulmonary vascular resistance at different rates of arteriovenous flow for a typical experiment

$\dot{Q}av/\dot{Q}t$ (%)	PA* pH	PA* Po_2 (mmHg)	PA* Pco_2 (mmHg)	Aorta* pH	Aorta* Po_2 (mmHg)	Aorta* Pco_2 (mmHg)	O_2 transfer (ml O_2/min)
0	7.40	29	35	7.50	44	29	—
7	7.48	52	30	7.51	59	34	1.4
11	7.52	57	28	7.49	72	30	1.4
15	7.55	62	26	7.54	78	25	1.7
17	7.55	60	25	7.58	75	24	2.2
20	7.58	57	22	7.57	72	21	2.2
0	7.34	17	42	7.36	31	40	—
9	7.40	43	34	7.38	50	36	2.1
11	7.47	50	29	7.46	60	30	2.5
24	7.50	52	25	7.50	64	25	3.0
34	7.54	57	19	7.53	70	18	2.5
0	7.36	18	45	7.42	27	40	—
44	7.57	60	21	7.49	64	23	4.5

*Measured at 37°C

52–60 mmHg. A corresponding rise in Po_2 was measured in the aorta (*Table 24.2*). The elimination of carbon dioxide was proportional to the arteriovenous ECMO flow: at $\dot{Q}av/\dot{Q}t > 0.2$, $Paco_2$ was reduced by 15–20 mmHg from the baseline conditions in which $\dot{Q}av$ = O (*Table 24.2*).

Right-to-left shunting of blood through the patent foramen ovale and ductus arteriosus varied with arterial oxygenation (*Figure 24.26*). The data compiled from the 8 animals in this study was taken for ratios of $\dot{Q}av/\dot{Q}t$ ranging from 0 to 45 per cent. A reduction in the percentage of flow shunted R→L from 38 per cent under conditions of hypoxaemia (Pao_2 = 30–38 mmHg) to 20–25 per cent occurred at higher levels of Pao_2 (>50 mmHg). This reduction is significant ($P<0.001$).

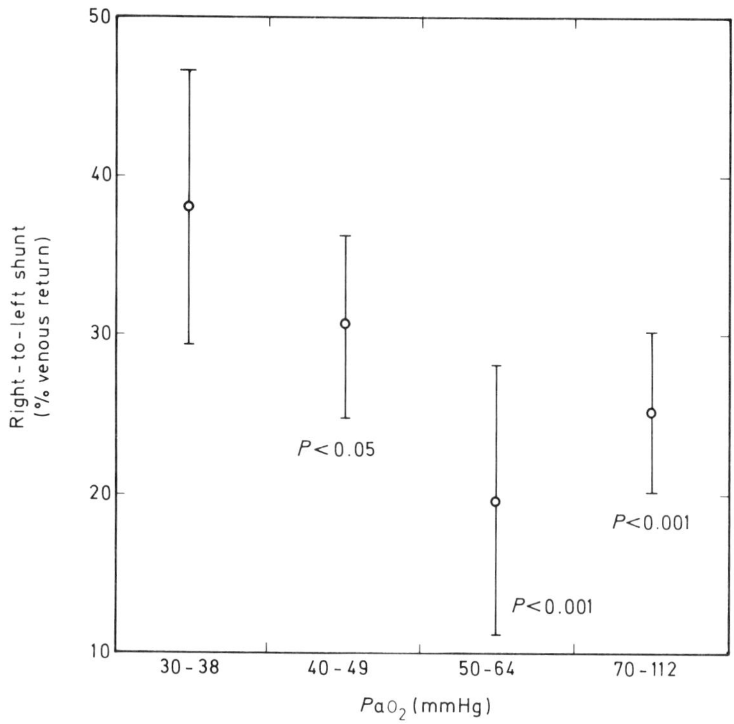

Figure 24.26 Variation in the right-to-left shunting of blood through the patent foramen ovale and ductus arteriosus with arterial oxygenation. Results are plotted as the mean ± SD for data compiled from all animals of this study

An inverse relationship existed between the PV resistance and the level of systemic arterial oxygenation (*Figure 24.27*). PV resistance was 40 per cent lower at Pa_{O_2} above 66 mmHg than at Pa_{O_2} below 38 mmHg. The mean PA pressure was not elevated from pre-bypass conditions (48/27 mmHg) at arteriovenous ECMO flows corresponding to less than 30 per cent of the total systemic flow ($P > 0.05$).

Discussion

This series of experiments was conducted to identify the acute response to arteriovenous ECMO in an animal model of neonatal respiratory distress. The results of these acute experiments can be used as a guide for an improved chronic model. A single distal aortic cannula inserted from an umbilical artery sustained blood flows in excess of 100 ml/kg per min for periods of up to 6 hours. The bypass rates of flow were periodically between 175 and 200 ml/kg per min. The pressure drop across the polyurethane catheter at flow rates equal to 100 ml/kg per min was estimated from Poiseuille's law to be 30 mmHg. This implies that the minimum arterial pressure required to establish arteriovenous perfusion at these flows is 30 mmHg. In the absence of a mechanical pump this value would be increased to 40–50 mmHg in order to include the low resistance to flow in the pulmonary assist membrane oxygenator (10–20 mmHg).

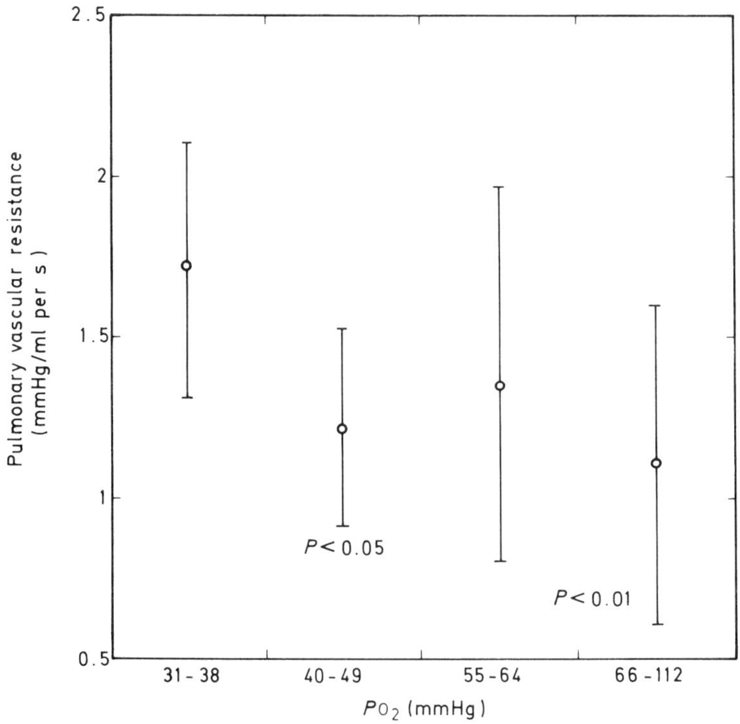

Figure 24.27 Reduction in pulmonary vascular resistance with increasing levels of arterial oxygenation. The data are plotted as described in *Figure 24.26*

The rate of oxygen transferred by the pulmonary assist oxygenator at arteriovenous ECMO flows between 20 and 45 per cent of the total systemic flow ranges between 1.4 and 4.5 ml O_2/min (*Table 24.2*). This compares with the requirements of oxygen for lambs at 130 days of gestation of 18 ml O_2/min for normoxaemic conditions[65]. For lambs in the present study which were hypothermic and treated with muscle relaxants the rate of oxygen delivery in the extracorporeal circuit was sufficient to increase the arterial oxygenation to life-sustaining levels. The therapeutic effects of delivering highly oxygenated blood to the pulmonary vasculature include a reduction in the percentage of flow shunted R→L, an elevation in PBF, and a decrease in resistance (*Figures 24.26* and *24.27*). The fall in PV resistance with an elevation of PBF suggests that there occurs a vasodilatory effect at the precapillary sphincter level mediated by elevation in pulmonary arterial oxygenation[10]. When pulmonary and systemic arterial pressures are the same, the ratio of flow through the ductus to that in the pulmonary circulation varies directly with the systemic and pulmonary vascular resistances. In neonates with elevated PV resistance and equal pulmonary and systemic arterial pressures a fetal pattern of circulation exists characterized by marked R→L shunting of blood through the ductus, diminished pulmonary blood flows, and consequential systemic hypoxia. The partial respiratory support provided by the arteriovenous ECMO with the pulmonary assist oxygenator causes a therapeutic reversal in this circulatory pattern through delivery of sufficient increments of oxygen to the pulmonary vasculature. Zapol and Kolobow presented cineangiographic evidence that the diameter of the ductus arteriosus markedly narrowed at arterial oxygen tensions above 35 mmHg[65]. This implies that the reduction in R→L shunting observed in the present study Pa_{O_2} above 50 mmHg may be in part a consequence of the narrowing of the ductus. The reversal in the fetal circulation pattern rapidly occurred following the initiation of extracorporeal support and was dependent upon the continuation of ECMO (*Figure 24.25*). A lack of variation in ECG tracings, PCW and central venous pressures suggests that myocardial performance was not impaired with the initiation of arteriovenous ECMO for partial respiratory support.

Conclusions

The attraction of the arteriovenous mode of perfusion for prolonged extracorporeal membrane oxygenation is its simplicity. Laboratory[1, 4] and clinical experiences[2, 19, 44, 58] have identified advantages and disadvantages of this mode, but the considerations are either theoretical or controversial based on current data. The possible advantages include simplicity, duplication of the placental circulation for neonates, a uniform oxygen tension in the systemic arterial tree, and the therapeutic effect of increasing pulmonary arterial oxygen saturation. The possible disadvantages are the less efficient transfer of oxygen by an oxygenator receiving arterial rather than venous blood, an increase in cardiac output, and an increase in pulmonary arterial pressure as pulmonary flow increases. As these considerations are theoretical and current evidence is not conclusive, each possibility warrants examination individually.

Simplicity is the hallmark of a device which can be operated easily and safely for an extended period of time. The ideal is a thromboresistant system which requires no anticoagulation and no extracorporeal pump. Thromboresistance is a problem of 'haemocompatibility'. Arteriovenous perfusion without an extracorporeal pump using an oxygenator having low resistance to flow is a unique feature of this mode of perfusion. Pumpless perfusion has been used primarily in the laboratory as a method of evaluating membrane oxygenators. It has also been applied clinically with Awad's tubular membrane oxygenator[3] and is possible, with the low resistance to flow through the pulmonary assist membrane oxygenator described in previous sections of this chapter. The General Electric–Peirce, Kolobow, Bramson, and Travenol lungs have a higher resistance to flow and require a pump to propel blood.

Pumpless arteriovenous perfusion for partial respiratory support is attractive for both oxygenation and elimination of carbon dioxide. In acute respiratory insufficiency, partial respiratory support for oxygenation and removal of carbon dioxide could be used to reduce barotrauma[5, 50]. Its 'prophylactic' use in these circumstances is contingent upon developing a system which could be applied and continuously operated both safely and easily for an extended period of time. Criteria for its application could then be redefined to permit its use early in the course of acute respiratory insufficiency. For chronic pulmonary insufficiency pumpless arteriovenous perfusion could be used as a partial support to eliminate carbon dioxide under conditions of chronic respiratory insufficiency associated with hypercarbia. An implantable artificial lung for use as a replacement or for use in parallel with existing lungs could be powered by the right or left ventricles in the arteriovenous mode.

Arteriovenous perfusion is attractive as the mode for respiratory support of neonates because it mimics the placental circulation. Cannulation of the umbilical vessels for perfusion at rates of flow adequate to maintain oxygenation and normocarbia has been successful even though there has not been a survivor of this technique[19]. The use of a thin-walled polyurethane cannula reinforced with spring wire[49] aids in obtaining and maintaining adequate rates of flow. The theoretical objection to the increase in cardiac output that might occur as a consequence of the increased venous return could be countered by demonstration that adequate partial support can be sustained at rates of flow effecting cardiac outputs not in excess of those which existed *in utero*[57]. Experimental evidence suggests that such conditions can be met[26].

Uniformity of the oxygen tension in the systemic arterial tree during prolonged extracorporeal membrane oxygenation is a relevant consideration in order to assure that oxygenated blood perfuses the coronary and cerebral circulations. Arteriovenous perfusion assures complete mixing of the patient's blood with that from the artificial lung prior to ejection into the aorta.

The last advantage of arteriovenous perfusion for consideration is the possible therapeutic effect of increasing oxygenation of the blood in the pulmonary artery. Two possibilities exist: it could be therapeutic haemodynamically or it could aid in the healing process of diseased pulmonary parenchyma. No evidence exists relative to the second possibility. Experimental evidence suggests that the former may occur. Arteriovenous perfusion with a membrane lung in premature lambs having immature lungs rapidly reverses the fetal circulatory pattern and the reversal is dependent upon continuation of the arteriovenous extracorporeal membrane oxygenation. Pulmonary vascular resistance decreases, pulmonary blood flow increases, and right-to-left shunting through the patent foramen ovale and ductus arteriosus decreases. The assumption is that the decrease in pulmonary vascular resistance is a consequence of the associated increase in pulmonary arterial oxygenation which results in vasodilation effected by the precapillary sphincters[26, 65].

The therapeutic advantage of increasing the pulmonary arterial saturation is especially attractive as a consideration in treating neonates with respiratory disease resulting in a fetal pattern of circulation. This includes persistent fetal circulation with or without a congenital diaphragmatic hernia and infant respiratory distress syndrome. Its advantage in other respiratory diseases is a possibility only if the pulmonary hypertension is potentially reversible.

A distinct disadvantage to arteriovenous perfusion is that the rate of transfer of oxygen by a membrane lung is inherently less efficient since the oxygenator receives arterial blood for oxygenation. The volume of gas transferred per unit of time is thus less in the arteriovenous mode than it would be in the venoarterial one. Consequently higher rates of flow through the artificial lung are necessary if total respiratory support is to be achieved. The arteriovenous mode is not ideal for total respiratory support because of this limitation and the improbability of conveniently obtaining and sustaining these high flows without impairment of myocardial performance and systemic perfusion. This disadvantage could be circumvented if low rates of flow were adequate to achieve the anticipated therapeutic goal.

Arteriovenous perfusion at low flow rates is applicable as a partial support of respiration. Experimental evidence suggests that arteriovenous perfusion with the pulmonary assist membrane oxygenator at rates of flow corresponding to 35 per cent of the cardiac output can provide up to 50 per cent of the basal metabolic need for oxygen. Total extracorporeal removal of carbon dioxide in the absence of ventilation is another form of partial respiratory support which has been feasible in the laboratory. A normal composition of alveolar gases and normal systemic arterial gases have been maintained during apnoeic oxygenation and removal of carbon dioxide by arteriovenous perfusion at low flow rates through an extracorporeal carbon dioxide membrane lung[47]. A current application would be the use of apnoeic oxygenation and removal of carbon dioxide by an artificial lung to stop the air leak associated with mechanical ventilation and a bronchopleural fistula. The 'prophylactic' use of partial respiratory support using an artificial lung to reduce barotrauma is contingent upon developing a system which can be applied easily and continuously operated for an extended period of time.

A second potential disadvantage of arteriovenous perfusion is the theoretical consideration that an increase in venous return results which then produces an increase in cardiac output that may be deleterious. Previous investigations of unregulated arteriovenous fistulae (with flows not set by a mechanical pump) have documented the occurrence of and increase in cardiac output which is proportional to the magnitude and velocity of the flow through an arteriovenous communication[9, 31, 37,39]. Laboratory studies employing the arteriovenous mode of ECMO confirm that cardiac output initially rises in an amount which is equal to the rate of arteriovenous perfusion but that this increase is transient[3].

The last objection to the arteriovenous mode of perfusion is that an increase in pulmonary blood flow may augment pulmonary arterial pressure and be deleterious in the presence of pulmonary hypertension. Experimental data indicate that the use of A-V ECMO for partial respiratory support at flow rates corresponding to less than 35 per cent of the cardiac output does not produce significant haemodynamic changes even in the presence of moderate pulmonary hypertension[27]. In premature lambs having immature lungs pulmonary blood flow increases but pulmonary vascular resistance decreases for reasons discussed in the previous section.

Prolonged extracorporeal membrane oxygenation using the arteriovenous mode of perfusion is attractive for providing partial respiratory support because of its unique potential simplicity in including pumpless perfusion, easy vascular access, and low rates of flow. In neonates with respiratory disease producing a fetal pattern of circulation, the therapeutic effects of reducing pulmonary vascular resistance and right-to-left shunting add to its attractiveness. Its limitation is that total respiratory support using this mode is impractical and circulatory support is not possible. Defining the appropriate application of A-V ECMO for partial support of the failing lung is the challenge of the future. Arteriovenous perfusion has a great probability of achieving the idea of a simple system which can be safely interfaced with a patient.

Abstract

The feasibility of employing the arteriovenous (A-V) mode of extracorporeal oxygenation (ECMO) for partial respiratory support has been evaluated in animal models using an oxygenator characterized by the flow of blood through etched microconduits for gas exchange. Particular emphasis is focused upon the haemodynamic consequences and gas exchange characteristics of partial A-V support. Among the haemodynamic parameters monitored during incremental rates of A-V perfusion are cardiac output, ECG, pulmonary artery, pulmonary capillary wedge, right atrial, and mean arterial pressures, renal and cerebral blood flows, intracranial pressure, EEG, electrolytes, urine volume and molarity, pulmonary vascular resistance, and right ventricular stroke work. The results indicate that for rates of arteriovenous flow below 35 per cent of the cardiac output no deleterious effects of A-V perfusion on myocardial performance and organ blood flow occur. Application of arteriovenous ECMO to partial support of neonatal respiration was studied using perigestational lambs as an animal model of infant respiratory distress. At rates of extracorporeal flow which did not produce haemodynamic derangements in these frail animals (35 per cent of the cardiac output) a reduction in the fetal pattern of circulation was found to occur with the delivery of oxygenated blood to the pulmonary artery.

Acknowledgements

The authors wish to acknowledge the financial support of the Western Pennsylvania Heart Association, Health Research and Services Foundation, and American Philosophical Society (Grant Number 8055 from the Penrose Fund) during the course of this research. Special thanks are extended to Axel Haubold of Carbo Medics Inc. Austin, Texas for his able participation in the fabrication and evaluation of carbon-surface components for the pulmonary assist oxygenator. The continued encouragement and support of Henry T. Bahnson, M.D. for membrane oxygenator research at the University of Pittsburgh are deeply appreciated. The authors also wish to thank Mrs Mary Ann Charlton for typing the manuscript and Mr Frank McSteen, BS, for assistance in conducting the animal experiments.

References

1. Awad, J. A., Brassard, A., Roy, J., Nadeau, P. and Caron, W. M. 'Arteriovenous perfusion with the disc oxygenator. Treatment of acute respiratory failure.' *Archives of Surgery*, **99,** 69 (1969)
2. Awad, J. A., Cloutier, R., Paradis, B., Dorval, J., Martin, L. and Horin, P. S. 'Prolonged pulmonary assistance with the membrane gas-exchanger: a case report.' *Journal of Pediatric Surgery*, **8,** 871 (1973)
3. Awad, J. A. and Morin, P. J. 'Arteriovenous partial perfusion.' In *Artificial Lungs for Acute Respiratory Failure*. Eds W. M. Zapol and J. Quist. p. 329. New York: Academic Press (1976)
4. Awad, J. A., Roy, J., Brassard, A. and Caron, W. M. 'Arteriovenous perfusion with a disposable bubble oxygenator for the temporary support of respiration.' *Annals of Thoracic Surgery*, **6,** 535 (1968)
5. Baeza, O. R., Wagner, R. B. and Lowery, B. D. 'Pulmonary hyperinflation. A form of barotrauma during mechanical ventilation.' *Journal of Thoracic and Cardiovascular Surgery*, **70,** 790 (1975)
6. Bartlett, R. H., Drinker, P. A., Hill, J. D., Hill, R. N. and Wetmore, N. 'Indications for ECMO support: quantitating pulmonary insufficiency.' In *Artificial Lungs for Acute Respiratory Failure*. Eds W. M. Zapol and J. Quist. p. 373. New York: Academic Press (1976)
7. Bartlett, R. H. and Gazzaniga, A. B. 'Extracorporeal circulation for cardiopulmonary failure.' *Current Problems in Surgery*, **15,** 3 (1978)
8. Bartlett, R. H., Gazzaniga, A. B., Fong, S. W., Jefferies, M. R., Roohk, H. V. and Haiduc, N. 'Extracorporeal membrane oxygenator support for cardiopulmonary failure.' *Journal of Thoracic and Cardiovascular Surgery*, **73,** 375 (1976)
9. Binak, K., Regan, T. J., Christensen, R. C. and Hellems, H. K. 'Arteriovenous fistula: haemodynamic effects of occlusion and exercise.' *American Heart Journal*, **60,** 495 (1960)
10. Bohr, D. R. 'The pulmonary hypoxic response.' *Chest*, **71,** 244 (1977)
11. Borovetz, H. S. 'An *in vitro* and *in vivo* study of an etched channel membrane oxygenator.' *Ph.D. Thesis, Carnegie-Mellon University* (1976)
12. Borovetz, H. S., Griffith, B. P., Hung, T-K., Hardesty, R. L. and Weissman, M. H. 'Arteriovenous perfusion with the pulmonary assist membrane oxygenator.' *The International Journal of Artificial Organs*, **1,** 232 (1978)
13. Borovetz, H. S., Griffith, B. P., Phillips, L. V., Haubold, A. D., Hercules, D. M., Hung, T-K. and Hardesty, R. L. 'Scanning electron microscopic and surface analytical study of an isotropic vacuum vapour deposited carbon on microporous membranes.' *Scanning Electron Microscopy II*, **85,** (1978)
14. Borovetz, H. S., Mateer, D. D., Hardesty, R. L. and Haubold, A. 'Oxygen permeability of carbon-surfaced microporous membranes.' *Journal of Biomedical Materials Research*, **14,** 145 (1980)
15. Borovetz, H. S., Matta, R. K., Griffith, B. P., Hung, T-K., Weissman, M. H. and Hardesty, R. L. 'A scanning electron microscopic study of blood-material interfaces in extracorporeal capillary flow. In Eighth International Congress on X-Ray Optics and Microanalysis. Eds D. R. Beaman, R. E. Ogilvie, and D. B. Wiffry. p. 501. Midland, Michigan: Pendell Publishing Co. (1980)
16. Boucher, J. K., Rudy, L. W. and Edmunds, L. H. 'Organ blood flow during pulsatile cardiopulmonary bypass.' *Journal of Applied Physiology*, **36,** 86 (1974)
17. Brown, C. H., Lemuth, R. F., Hellums, J. D., Leverett, L. B. and Alfrey, C. P. 'Response of human platelets to shear stress.' *Transactions of the American Society for Artificial Internal Organs*, **21,** 35 (1975)

18. Dantowitz, P., Borsanyi, A. S., Deibert, M. C., Snider, M. T., Scherler, M., Lipsky, M. H. and Galletti, P. M. 'Blood oxygenation with pre-formed membrane-lined capillary channels.' *Transactions of the American Society for Artificial Internal Organs*, **15,** 139 (1969)
19. Dorson, W., Heyer, B., Baker, E., Cohen, M., Elgis, R., Molthan, M. and Trump, D. 'Response of distressed infants to partial bypass lung assist.' *Transactions of the American Society for Artificial Internal Organs*, **16,** 345 (1970)
20. Dunn, J., Kirsch, M., Harness, J., Carroll, M., Steaker, J. and Sloan, H. 'Haemodynamic metabolic and haematologic effects of pulsatile cardiopulmonary bypass.' *Journal of Thoracic and Cardiovascular Surgery*, **68,** 138 (1974)
21. Fallat, R. J., Lany, H., Koeniger, E. and Hill, J. D. 'Use of physiologic and pathologic correlations in evaluating adult respiratory distress syndromes.' In *Artificial Lungs for Acute Respiratory Failure*. Eds W. M. Zapol and J. Quist. p. 391. New York: Academic Press (1976)
22. Galletti, P. M., Richardson, P. D., Snider, M. T. and Friedman, L. I. 'A standardized method of defining the overall gas transfer performance of artifical lungs.' *Transactions of the American Society for Artificial Internal Organs*, **18,** 359 (1972)
23. Gemer, H., Dunegan, L. J., Bruner, J. D., Stetz, C. W., Don, H. F., Hayes, J. A. and Drinker, P. A. 'Pulmonary insufficiency induced by oleic acid in the sheep.' *Journal of Thoracic and Cardiovascular Surgery*, **69,** 793 (1975)
24. Gille, J. P. 'World census of long-term perfusions for respiratory support.' In *Artificial Lungs for Acute Respiratory Failure*. Eds W. M. Zapol and J. Quist. p. 525. New York: Academic Press (1976)
25. Griffith, B. P., Borovetz, H. S. and Hardesty, R. L. 'Continuous indocyanine green dye determination of cardiac output through an arteriovenous shunt.' *Proceedings of the Association for the Advancement of Medical Instrumentation, 13th Annual Meeting*, p. 109 (1978)
26. Griffith, B. P., Borovetz, H. S., Hardesty, R. L., Hung, T-K and Bahnson, H. T. 'Arteriovenous ECMO for neonatal respiratory support: A study in perigestational lambs.' *Journal of Thoracic and Cardiovascular Surgery*, **77,** 595 (1979)
27. Griffith, B. P., Hardesty, R. L., Borovetz, H. S., Hung, T-K. and Bahnson, H. T. 'Arteriovenous extracorporeal membrane oxygenation for respiratory support.' *Surgical Forum*, **29,** 192 (1978)
28. Grode, G. S., Falb, R. D. and Crowley, J. P. 'Biocompatible materials for uses in the vascular system.' *Journal of Biomedical Materials Research Symposium*, **3,** 77 (1972)
29. Guyton, A. C. *Textbook of Medical Physiology*. p. 206. Philadelphia: W. B. Saunders (1971)
30. Guyton, A. C. *Textbook of Medical Physiology*. p. 314. Philadelphia: W. B. Saunders (1971)
31. Harrison, T. R., Dock, W. and Holman, E. 'Experimental studies in arteriovenous fistulae: Cardiac output.' *Heart*, **11,** 337 (1924)
32. Harrison, T. S. and Seton, J. F. 'An analysis of pulse frequency as an adrenergic excitant in pulsative circulatory support.' *Surgery*, **73,** 868 (1973)
33. Haubold, A. 'Carbon in prosthetics.' *Annals of New York Academy of Sciences*, **283,** 383 (1977)
34. Hill, J. D., O'Brien, T. G. and Murray, J. J. 'Prolonged extracorporeal oxygenation for acute post-traumatic respiratory failure (Shock Lung Syndrome).' *New England Journal of Medicine*, **286,** 139 (1972)

35. Hill, J. D., Ratliff, J. L., Parrot, J. C. and Lang, M. 'Pulmonary pathology in acute respiratory insufficiency; lung biopsy as a diagnostic tool.' *Journal of Thoracic and Cardiovascular Surgery*, **71,** 64 (1976)
36. Hill, R. N., Shible, E. M., Spragg, R. G. and Moser, K. M. 'Adult respiratory distress syndrome: early predictors of mortality.' *Transactions of the American Society for Artificial Internal Organs*, **21,** 199 (1975)
37. Holman, E. 'Abnormal arteriovenous communications: Great variability of effects with particular reference to delayed development of cardiac failure.' *Circulation*, **32,** 1001 (1975)
38. Holman, E. 'The anatomic and physiologic effects of an arteriovenous fistula.' *Surgery*, **8,** 362 (1940)
39. Holman, E. 'The vicissitudes of an idea: The significance of total blood volume in the story of arteriovenous fistula.' *Reviews of Surgery*, **20,** 152 (1963)
40. Hukberjee, N. D., Berran, A. V., Hirai, J., Wakabryashi, A., Sperling, D. R., Taylor, W. F. and Connolly, J. E. '*In vivo* determination of renal tissue oxygenation during pulsatile and left heart bypass.' *Annals of Thoracic Surgery*, **15,** 354 (1973)
41. Hung, T. C., Hochmuth, R. M., Joist, J. H. and Sutera, S. P. 'Shear-induced aggregation and lysis of platelets.' *Transactions of the American Society for Artificial Internal Organs*, **22,** 285 (1976)
42. Hung, T-K., Borovetz, H. S., Hardesty, R. L. and Weissman, M. H. 'Toward the development of a neonatal pulmonary assist membrane oxygenator.' *The South African Mechanical Engineer*, **28,** 112 (1978)
43. Hung, T-K., Borovetz, H. S. and Weissman, M. H. 'Transport and flow phenomena in a microchannel membrane oxygenator.' *Annals of Biomedical Engineering*, **5,** 343 (1977)
44. Jung, R. C., Lubiate, P., Kay, J. G. and Balchum, O. J. 'Partial pumpless pulmonary bypass in respiratory insufficiency.' *Chest*, **62,** 365 (1972)
45. Ketteringham, J., Zapol, W., Birkett, J., Nelsen, L., Massucco, A. and Raith, C. 'A high permeability, nonporous, blood compatible membrane for lungs: *In vivo* and *in vitro* performance.' *Transactions of the American Society for Artificial Internal Organs*, **21,** 224 (1975)
46. King, E. G., Wagner, W. W., Ashbaugh, D. G., Latham, L. D. and Halsey, D. R. 'Alterations in pulmonary microanatomy after fat embolism.' *Chest*, **59,** 524 (1971)
47. Kolobow, T., Gattinoni, L., Tomlinson, T. and Pierce, J. E. 'An alternative to breathing.' *Journal of Thoracic and Cardiovascular Surgery*, **75,** 261 (1978)
48. Kolobow, T., Stool, E. W., Sachs, K. L. and Vyrek, G. G. 'Acute respiratory failure.' *Journal of Thoracic and Cardiovascular Surgery*, **69,** 947 (1975)
49. Kolobow, T. and Zapol, W. 'A new thin walled non-kinking catheter for peripheral vascular cannulation.' *Surgery*, **68,** 625 (1970)
50. Kumar, A., Pontoppidan, H., Falke, K. H., Wilson, R. and Laver, M. 'Pulmonary barotrauma during mechanical ventilation.' *Critical Care Medicine* I, 181 (1973)
51. NHLI-ECMO Study: 'Extracorporeal support for respiratory insufficiency: selection on natural history of acute respiratory insufficiency.' *DHEW Publication* (1980)
52. NHLI Respiratory Diseases: 'Task Force Report on Prevention, Control, Education.' *DHEW Publication NIH 771248*, (1977)
53. Pyle, R. B., Helton, W. C., Johnson, F. W., Hornung, J. R., Hunt, C. E., Turnball, H. R., Lindsay, W. G. and Nichloff, D. M. 'Clinical use of the membrane oxygenator.' *Archives of Surgery*, **110,** 996 (1975)
54. Rashkind, W. J., Freeman, A., Klein, D. and Toft, R. W. 'Evaluation of a disposable plastic, low volume, pumpless oxygenator as a lung substitute.' *Journal of Pediatrics*, **66,** 94 (1965)

55. Rashkind, W. J., Miller, W. W., Falcone, D. and Toft, R. 'Haemodynamic effects of arteriovenous oxygenation with a small volume artificial extracorporeal lung.' *Journal of Pediatrics*, **20,** 425 (1967)
56. Rudolph, A. M. 'Cardiac catheterization and angiocardiography.' In *Congenital Diseases of the Heart*. New York: Yearbook Medical Publishers (1974)
57. Rudolph, A. M. 'Changes in the circulation after birth.' In *Congenital Diseases of the Heart*. New York: Yearbook Medical Publishers (1974)
58. Schenkar, D. L., Lanae, A. J., Subramanian, M. and Lillehei, C. W. 'Arteriovenous partial support for respiratory distress support.' *Circulation*, **39** and **40 (Suppl. III)**, 179 (1969)
59. Shim, H. S. and Meyer, C. H., Jr. 'The microstructure of isotropic vapour-deposited carbon films.' *Journal of Bioengineering*, **1,** 99 (1977)
60. Smeby, L. and Grimsrud, L. 'Theoretical investigations of mass transfer in membrane oxygenators.' *Medical and Biological Engineering*, **12,** 698 (1974)
61. Trudell, L. A., Friedman, L. I., Kakvan, M., Galletti, P. M. and Richardson, P. D. 'Evaluation of a disposable membrane oxygenator.' *Transactions of the American Society for Artificial Internal Organs*. **18,** 538 (1972)
62. Weissman, M. H., Hung, T-K. and Borovetz, H. S. 'The development of the etched channel membrane oxygenator.' *Proceedings of the Annual Conference of Engineering in Medicine and Biology*, **17,** 740 (1975)
63. White, J. J. 'Membrane lung extracorporeal bypass for prolonged respiratory support in infants.' In *Artificial Lungs for Acute Respiratory Failure*. Eds W. M. Zapol and J. Quist. p. 465. New York: Academic Press (1976)
64. White, J. J., Andrews, G. N., Risemberg, H., Mazur, D. and Haller, J. A. 'Prolonged respiratory support in newborn infants with a membrane oxygenator.' *Surgery*, **70,** 288 (1971)
65. Zapol, W. and Kolobow, T. 'Isolated extracorporeal placentation of the fetal lamb.' In *The Mammalian Fetus In Vitro*. Ed. C. R. Austin, p. 147. London: Chapman and Hall (1973)

25

Future Developments and Potential Applications of Extracorporeal Circulation in Medicine and Surgery

Hans H. J. Zwart and Willem J. Kolff

dum vita est, spes est

Introduction

Isolated organ perfusion has been studied for more than a century[22]. Blood was rendered incoagulable by whipping. Around the middle of the eighteenth century, it was discovered that blood turned red by thoroughly mixing it with air[3] and that organ function could be sustained better with bright red blood. In 1885, a detailed description appeared[31] of an apparatus for continuous perfusion with oxygenated blood. This machine functioned much like a modern heart-lung machine although on a smaller scale and in a cruder fashion. Great improvements were made possible in perfusion experiments by the discovery of heparin in 1916[23] and by the development of blood transfusion, anaesthesia and antimicrobial techniques.

The adaptation of laboratory perfusion techniques to clinical use must be credited to Gibbon[11] for the heart-lung machine and to Kolff[16] for the artificial kidney. With the heart-lung machine, venous blood is drained from the great veins or the right atrium, oxygenated and returned via a cannula inserted into a peripheral artery or directly into the aorta (*Figure 25.1*). Gibbon envisioned that his machine could be used for the treatment of severe cardiac failure and that it would make open-heart surgery possible. It has been the latter application that greatly stimulated further development of the heart-lung machine. In 1953, Gibbon[12] performed the first successful clinical open-heart operations with the heart-lung machine.

At present, cardiopulmonary bypass for open-heart surgery is a commonly accepted and safe procedure although much remains to be improved. However, for the treatment of cardiac failure the bypass was initially only sporadically used. Extracorporeal blood handling and oxygenation caused too much damage to be tolerated for more than a few hours. In order to be beneficial for the treatment of cardiac failure it was thought that the bypass would have to be applied for much longer periods, possibly days or even weeks. It was hoped that during the period of assistance, while the circulation was maintained by the heart-lung machine, the heart would be rested and given a chance to recover.

The frightful death toll from coronary arteriosclerotic heart disease has continued to stimulate researchers to refine bypass techniques to enable safe prolonged perfusion. A major achievement in decreasing blood damage during bypass was the introduction of membrane oxygenators. In these artificial lungs, the blood is separated from the gas by a membrane which results in less blood damage, and decreases the risk of emboli formation and contamination with micro-organisms. Early membrane oxygenators were bulky, cumbersome and unreliable devices. Gradually, performance was improved and over the last five years practical, disposable oxygenators became available. Simultaneously, interest in using the heart-lung machine for the treatment of cardiac failure revived. And still another field of possible application emerged—that of clinically refractory pulmonary failure such as occurs during the course of hyaline membrane disease, fulminating pulmonary infections and after pulmonary trauma. In fact, it has been with the latter clinical conditions that most experience has been gained recently with prolonged cardiopulmonary bypass. A detailed review was recently published covering the worldwide experience with extracorporeal oxygenation for respiratory insufficiency[13].

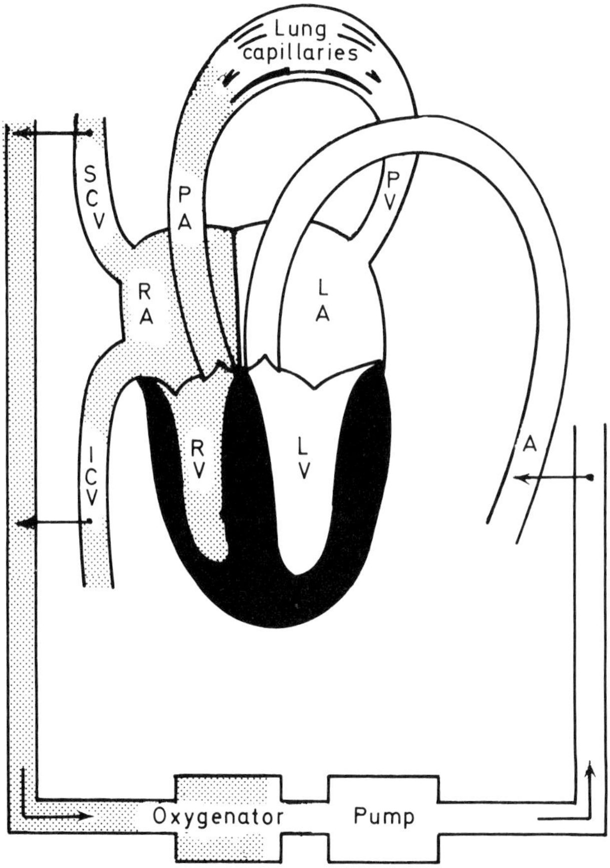

Figure 25.1 Schematic drawing of the function of the heart-lung machine. Blood is drained from the large veins (SCV and ICV, superior and inferior caval veins) and led to the oxygenator of the heart-lung machine. After being oxygenated and decarbonized, the blood is pumped back to the arterial vascular bed. A = aorta; LA and RA = left and right atria; LV and RV = left and right ventricles; PA and PV = pulmonary arteries and veins

Prior to these fantastic achievements, several bypass techniques were developed in an effort to circumvent the necessity of artificial oxygenation. Simple shunting of the blood from the veins to the arterial system, it was thought, would relieve the heart and if the venous blood were pumped to the lower half of the body, this so-called venoarterial bypass might improve cardiac function without depriving vital organs of adequate oxygenation (*Figure 25.2*). This idea now seems naive in view of the commonly known fact that blood mixes thoroughly so that serious tissue oxygen debt with development of intractable metabolic acidosis and circulatory deterioration would be expected. That this indeed happens was demonstrated in animal models where the bypass was applied to treat left ventricular failure with shock: if left alone, dogs would survive; when treated, they surely died[25].

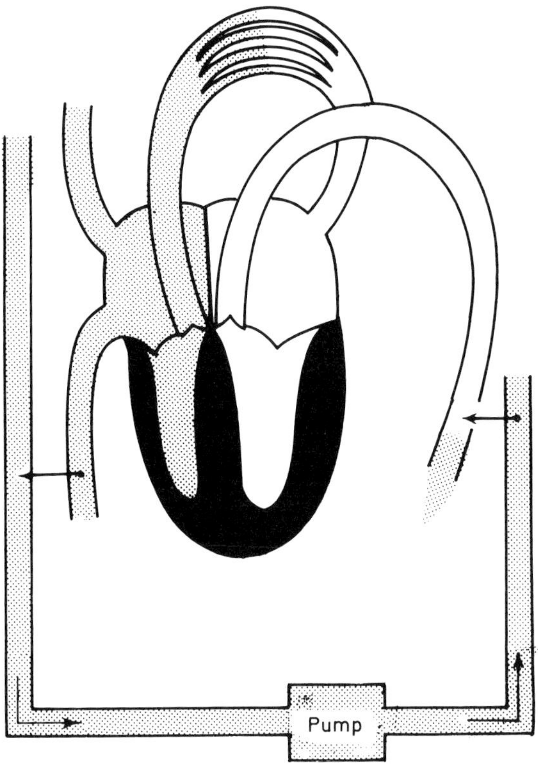

Figure 25.2 Venoarterial bypass. Blood is drained from veins and pumped back to the arterial system without being oxygenated

Another bypass was much more rational. It involved diverting the blood from the circulation only after it had passed through the lungs by cannulating the left atrium or ventricle and returning it to the arterial vascular system (*Figure 25.3*). This so-called left heart bypass seemed promising in animal experiments. Shock, produced by compromising left ventricular function, could be treated effectively and the heart showed signs of recovery. However, for many years, the bypass was thought impractical for clinical use because the chest had to be opened in order to cannulate the left side of the heart. Several techniques have since been developed for closed-chest left heart bypass and sporadic reports have appeared of its application in patients with intractable cardiac failure. Circulation could often be improved but the heart did not recover. The same holds for recent attempts to treat these patients with the heart-lung machine using a membrane oxygenator. Indeed, all presently available methods for mechanical assistance to the failing heart have this in common. Even balloon counterpulsation, considered by many to be the best assist device available, produces disappointing end-results[28]. To recover, the heart apparently needs more than just the assist. This subject will be dealt with in more detail later.

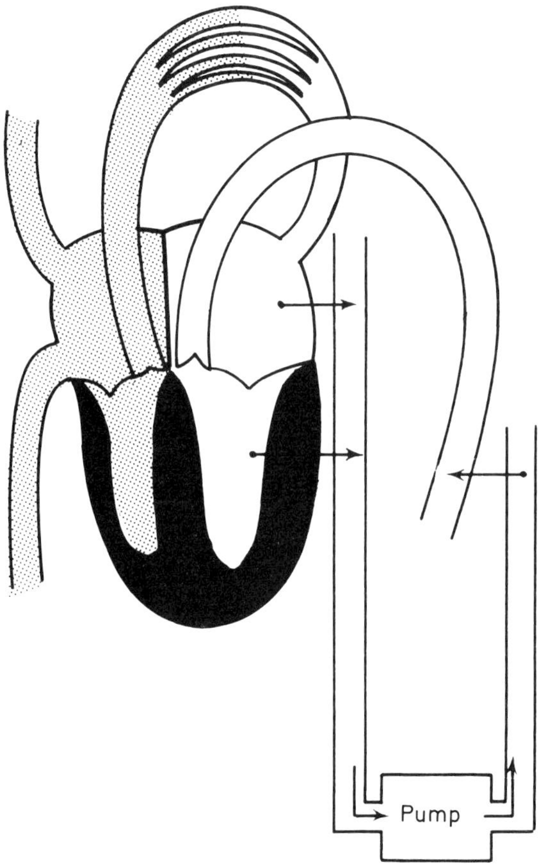

Figure 25.3 Left heart bypass. Blood is drained from the left atrium or the left ventricle and pumped back to the arteries. Oxygenation is not necessary

As more experience was gained with extracorporeal blood handling, other applications were investigated. The artificial kidney, as mentioned earlier, paralleled in its development the heart-lung machine and technological improvements in the one were applied in the other and vice versa. A striking example is the observation by Kolff and Berk[16] that venous blood turned red as it passed through the artificial kidney which led him to develop one of the first membrane oxygenators. Technology of membrane oxygenator fabrication in turn stimulated the development of a simple disposable artificial kidney. Selective perfusion of parts of the body or of organs has been developed for organ preservation, cancer treatment and for the protection of organs that had to be deprived temporarily of blood supply (coronary perfusion). Total body perfusion is used for rapid cooling in heart and brain surgery. The heart-lung machine has been used to enable complicated reconstruction of the tracheobronchial tree. Left heart bypass is commonly applied to protect the spinal cord and the heart during surgery of the thoracic aorta. Bypass circuits to assist or possibly substitute the function of the uterus, the liver and the bowels are under investigation. It is not difficult to imagine future efforts to aid in the function of still other internal organs with extracorporeal blood circuits[27].

The ultimate goal in the development of many of these devices is to make them portable and even totally implantable. In this field, those who are involved in research on heart-assist devices are most active. Partly implantable assist devices and totally implantable artificial hearts are being developed. Calves survived for more than 6 months with the circulation being maintained by an artificial heart[14]. Investigations have also been undertaken to design implantable artificial kidney and lungs. A description of all applications of extracorporeal circulation is beyond the scope of this chapter. Further discussion will be limited to those devices that were designed for assistance of the heart and the circulation.

The main indication for mechanical circulatory support is cardiogenic shock. Shock from cardiac origin is defined as a state of inadequate circulation, incompatible with life, caused by insufficient cardiac output. Under such circumstances the function of even vital organs deteriorates. The condition is further aggravated by massive metabolic acidosis, intravascular sludging and coagulation and pulmonary oedema with desaturation. If appropriate medical management fails to result in some improvement, the mortality rate is 100 per cent.

Cardiogenic shock is encountered most often in the course of myocardial infarction. In the United States of America, more than 600 000 people die each year from arteriosclerotic heart disease. It is estimated that shock develops in 10–20 per cent of patients with myocardial infarction. The mortality rate approximates 90 per cent under these circumstances.

The use, in these patients, of some mechanical device which is capable of substituting the function of the heart seems an obvious measure of great promise. And, indeed, many of the assist devices that were developed over the years have been proved, experimentally and clinically, to be beneficial to the circulation. Some can be applied without any or with only minor surgical procedures. They are relatively safe and often very effective in the treatment of the shock. The circulation can be restored, blood pressure increases, right and left atrial pressures decrease, pulmonary oedema subsides, urine production increases and patients wake up from coma.

However, if the assist device is switched off, left ventricular failure occurs again in the majority of the cases. The hope that, during the period of assistance, the heart will recover spontaneously, apparently is not justified. At autopsy, it appears that the heart is infarcted so extensively in many a case that recovery in retrospect is considered impossible.

Where assist devices were applied only if the condition of the patient was considered hopeless (intractable cardiogenic shock) these results are, on second thought, not surprising. If, for many hours, parts of the myocardium are kept deprived of blood supply, it is unlikely that the heart will recover. The first method of improving late results is, therefore, earlier application of the apparatus, preferably before cardiogenic shock develops. However, it would be highly impracticable and medically unjust to treat all patients with myocardial infarction with mechanical assistance. If patients who develop serious left ventricular failure could be recognized before shock actually appears and in particular if those who will die from it could be selected, then early mechanical assistance would be justified in this group. Fortunately, studies have recently been undertaken to enable this kind of patient selection. It now seems possible to detect patients susceptible to shock with a better than 90 per cent reliability before cardiac failure occurs[29]. Earlier application of assist devices will, it is hoped, improve the late results, but data on more than a few patients thus treated are as yet not available.

Even if mechanical assist is applied at an early stage it still seems unrealistic to expect good results. Complete or near total obstruction of major coronary arteries cannot be expected to disappear spontaneously, nor is it reasonable to hope for collateral circulation of adequate capacity to develop in a few hours, or even days or weeks. With the present state of the art in cardiac surgery it would seem indicated to remove or bypass such obstructions in the coronary circulation surgically. Therefore, patients selected to be treated with mechanical assist devices must be subjected to coronary angiography and subsequently be operated upon to reconstitute myocardial blood supply. This approach has now been followed in a few patients with decidedly better results[9]. The next question that arises is how long the myocardium can survive or regenerate after its blood supply is cut off or greatly diminished. Clinical experience would seem to indicate that it is unsafe to interrupt coronary blood supply beyond a period of 30 minutes at normothermia. At moderate hypothermia (30°C) this time-limit can be extended to about 1 hour[10]. Relevant conclusions drawn from animal experiments are surprisingly divergent. Myocardial recovery was observed after ischaemic periods of up to 12 hours. If, after 24 hours of myocardial ischaemia, blood supply was reinstituted, the effect was harmful rather than beneficial[5]. Results are undoubtedly influenced by development of collateral circulation and the general condition of the body. In patients, too, regeneration capability can be expected to be divergent, depending on the blood-carrying capacity left in the myocardium. For practical purposes, it would seem proper to proceed with the management as outlined earlier as quickly as possible.

As previously indicated, many of the assist devices are certainly capable of restoring the circulation. Little attention is paid to the influence of the methods on the heart. It is generally assumed that if application of the assist results in a decrease of myocardial work and if it increases coronary flow, then it is of benefit to the heart. This axion has, however, not been proven to be true. It may well be that rest is of no benefit to the heart, and as is the case with skeletal muscle, it might even be harmful. Abundance of coronary flow might similarly be less beneficial than assumed. To reach an answer to these basic questions it is necessary first to document the haemodynamic changes produced by assist devices in and around the heart.

Application of the heart-lung machine results in relief of the heart from pumping blood proportional to bypass flow. However, the pressure against which the left ventricle has to pump the non-bypassed blood is increased as a result of the bypass. Realizing that pressure work costs more energy than volume work, it is not surprising that, in actuality, workload on the heart may increase as cardiopulmonary bypass is applied. This explains the observation that failure, as evidenced by an increase in left ventricular end-diastolic pressure is aggravated as the heart-lung machine is switched on[9, 21]. On the other hand, it is the common experience of cardiac surgeons that a heart which fails to take over the circulation after surgery, improves its function when bypass is reinstituted. Apparently the end-result depends upon the amount of blood bypassed, the severity of myocardial failure and the increase in aortic pressure. Much is unpredictable in patients and therefore it is advisable to measure left ventricular pressure during treatment of cardiogenic shock with a heart-lung machine. If left ventricular end-diastolic pressure is found to increase, the left ventricle needs to be decompressed or bypass has to be discontinued. Clinical experience in the treatment of cardiogenic shock with a heart-lung machine is limited to a few incidental cases[20, 21, 30]. Circulation could be restored in nearly all cases but most patients did not survive beyond a few hours.

With left heart bypass, all of the blood entering the left ventricle can be diverted so that the aortic valve remains closed. The work performed by the heart then largely depends on the peak systolic pressure that is still generated by the left ventricle. If this pressure remains below 25 mmHg, myocardial oxygen consumption decreases substantially. The bypass has the additional advantages that pulmonary venous congestion is effectively relieved and that artificial oxygenation is not necessary. When, in 1962, Dennis *et al.*[8] described a method by which left heart bypass could be applied without thoracotomy (*see Figure 25.4*), interest in the bypass revived. The left atrium is cannulated with a wide-bore thin-walled stainless steel cannula which is inserted via the right internal jugular vein, passed down to the right atrium and forced through a small opening which is punched in the interatrial septum. Blood is drained from the left atrium and returned via a femoral artery. It has been demonstrated in animal experiments that the left ventricle can be bypassed completely, oxygen consumption decreases substantially as the peak systolic left ventricular pressure drops below arterial diastolic pressure, the bypass offers protection against arrhythmias and shock can be effectively treated. It should be realized that with this bypass the left ventricle cannot be decompressed maximally as long as the mitral valve is competent. Small amounts of blood remain trapped for a while in the left ventricle so that now and then the ventricle has to empty against the aortic pressure. Another problem is that shunting can occur along the cannula tip from right to left atrium resulting in serious desaturation[32]. Clinical experience has been obtained in more than 30 patients where the bypass was applied by different investigators for various reasons[6]. Closed-chest cannulation appeared rather difficult and in one case, the right atrial wall was inadvertently perforated[7]. The circulation could commonly be restored but most patients nevertheless died after bypass was discontinued.

Another technique to bypass the left ventricle without thoracotomy was developed by Zwart in 1966[32] (*Figure 25.4*). Blood is removed from the left ventricle with a flexible, thin-walled cannula which is inserted via the right subclavian artery and advanced past the aortic valve. With this technique it appeared possible to substitute left ventricular function completely (*Figure 25.5*). The left ventricular pressure could be decreased to atmospheric pressure, cardiogenic shock could be reversed and infarcted hearts showed signs of recovery[33]. The aortic valve remained competent during and after

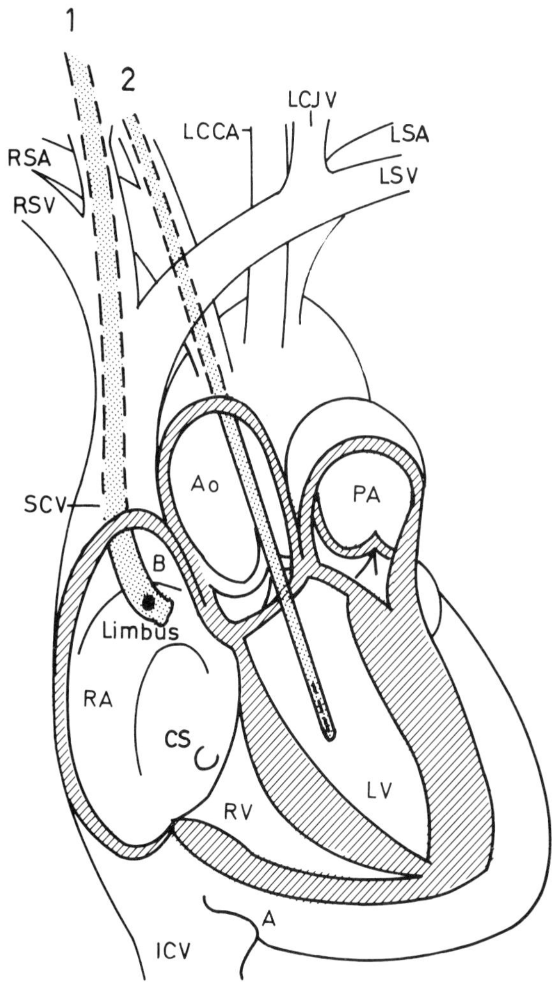

Figure 25.4 Two techniques for closed-chest left heart bypass. (1) A thin-walled stainless-steel cannula is inserted via the right internal jugular vein to the right atrium. After perforation of the interatrial septum the cannula tip is advanced into the left atrium. Blood is drained from the left atrium and returned to the arteries. (2) A thin-walled flexible cannula is inserted via the right subclavian artery, past the aortic valve into the left ventricle (LV). Blood is removed from the LV and returned to the arteries. RSA, RSV, LSA, LSV = right and left subclavian arteries and veins; CS = coronary sinus; LCCA = left common carotid artery; LCJV = left common jugular vein

bypass. This technique has the advantage that intracardiac manipulation is minimal and perforation of the interatrial septum is not necessary. In addition, the left ventricle can be decompressed more effectively. A disadvantage is that only small-sized cannulae can be fitted in the subclavian artery which limits maximum flow to around 4 litres/min. Clinical

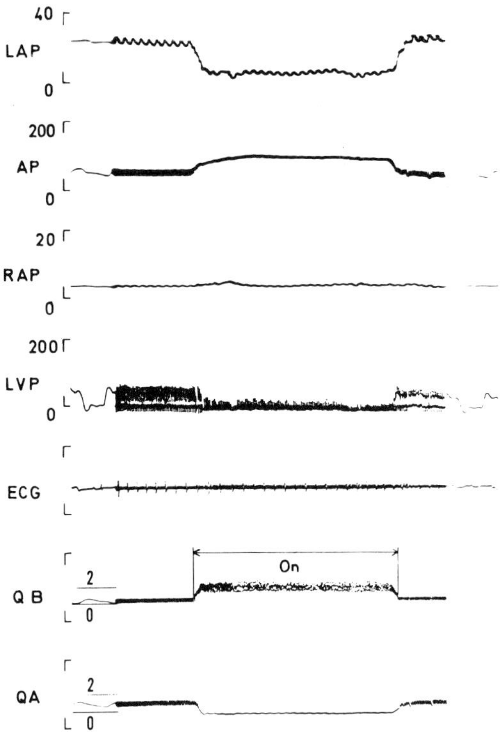

Figure 25.5 Tracings obtained during an experiment with transarterial left heart bypass on a sheep. LAP = left atrial pressure; AP = arterial pressure; RAP = right atrial pressure: LVP = left ventricular pressure (all in mmHg); ECG lead aVF × 1; QB and QA = flow (ℓ/min) of bypass circuit and in aorta. Left ventricular failure has been produced by ligation of coronary arteries. As the left heart bypass is switched on (QB from 0 to 2), LAP and LVP decrease, AP increases and QA falls below 0 (negative flow indicates retrograde aortic flow to coronary arteries). The left ventricle is completely bypassed and total flow to the arterial system is increased by 100 per cent (QA1 to QB2). Arterial pressure increases

experience is limited to only 3 patients. In 2, cardiogenic shock could be reversed but the patients died nevertheless[34]. In 1 patient, the cannula tip could not be inserted past the aortic valve.

Still another technique to divert left atrial blood was suggested by Kralios and Zwart in 1970[17]. A flexible, thin-walled cannula is inserted into the right internal jugular vein and passed down via the right side of the heart to the pulmonary arteries. After the cannula tip is wedged there, suction is applied to the cannula. It appeared possible to drain left atrial blood by retrograde flow through parts of the lung. Experimental evidence suggests that substantial flow can be obtained only if left atrial pressure rises above 20 mmHg. Assuming that up to this pressure the left heart and the lungs are not in danger and that diastolic filling pressure is optimal, the bypass could be beneficial in that a pressure rise above 20 mmHg would be prevented. The assumption, however, remains to be proven true.

Recently a left ventricular bypass technique was described which could be of benefit to patients who cannot safely be disconnected from the heart-lung machine following cardiac surgery[26]. Before closing the chest, a wide-bore cannula is inserted into the left ventricle through a stab-wound in the apex. After closing the chest, blood can still be removed from the left ventricle and is pumped back via a femoral artery. If the bypass can safely be discontinued, the left ventricular cannula is disconnected and a solid obturator is inserted so as to fill up its lumen completely. Thus the build-up of clots in the cannula is prevented. If bypass needs to be reinstituted, the obturator is removed and the cannula can be connected to the blood circuit again.

Over the past five years several groups of investigators have developed implantable devices to bypass the left ventricle over prolonged periods of time. These are meant to be applied in patients who develop intractable cardiac failure after heart surgery. Compressed air is commonly used to drive the assist device. A ventricle-type pump, fitted with an inlet and outlet valve, is inserted between the left ventricular apex and the descending aorta. The pump is synchronized to fill during systole and empty during diastole. This provides for maximal unloading of the left ventricle which ejects part of the stroke volume into the pump against only atmospheric pressure. A host of other devices have been studied, some completely implantable, others paracorporeal. Major problems encountered are the construction of an implantable energy source and the development of blood-compatible inner linings for the pumps. These will be dealt with in more detail with the description of the artificial heart. In a recent review the world-wide clinical experience with semipermanent assist pumps has been described[2].

If, even with the most advanced management of heart failure, including modern diagnostic, surgical and mechanical assist techniques, the heart does not recover, only one measure remains if the patient is to be saved. The heart has to be replaced with either a transplant or a mechanical heart. The problems encountered in heart transplantation are beyond the scope of this chapter. Suffice it to state that rejection is still a serious threat and that the supply of donor hearts will remain short of the demand. Insertion of a mechanical heart, if a reliable device were available, would certainly be more convenient than transplantation. However, the development of mechanical hearts is still in an early stage. Modern artificial hearts are made up of four chambers analogous to the natural heart (*Figure 25.6*). The ventricles consist of an inner collapsible chamber within a rigid housing. Inlet and outlet valves ensure unidirectional flow. During diastole the space between blood chamber and housing is vented to room air or connected to a vacuum. Systole is initiated by building up pressure in that space which results in collapse of the blood chamber so that the blood in the chamber is pumped out. Main problems encountered include: construction of durable and reliable pumps, fabrication of a blood-contact surface compatible with blood, and improvement of pump efficiency. Survival has been so short so far that durability testing has hardly been

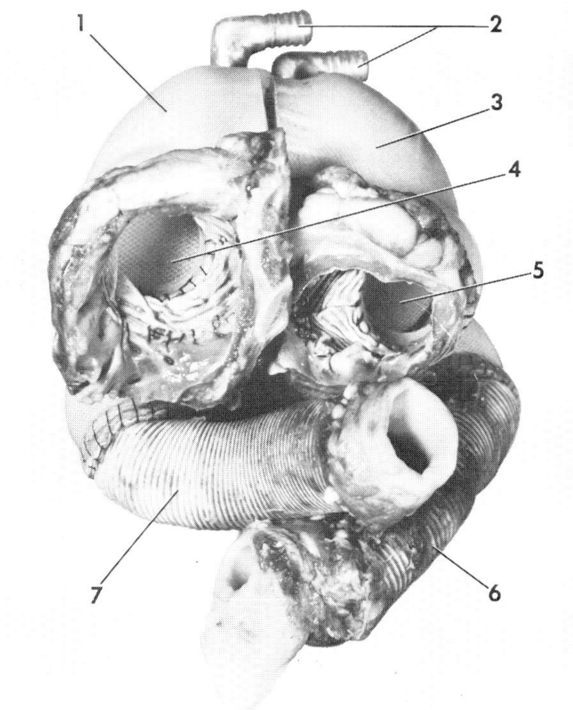

Figure 25.6 Implantable artificial heart. 1 = right ventricle; 2 = connections for high pressure lines to initiate systole; 3 = left ventricle; 4 = right atrium with inflow valve (flap type); 5 = left atrium with valve; 6 = aorta; 7 = pulmonary artery. This heart was implanted in a calf. It survived for 7 days and then died from congestive liver failure with massive oedema

studied yet. For many years, artificial heart experiments were plagued with massive embolization from thrombi formed within the devices. Blood damage caused by the pumps was considerable. Recent developments have led to surfaces and pumping techniques where these problems have been eliminated to a great extent[15]. Surprisingly, how to design safe pumps with adequate efficiency has now appeared as a difficult problem. The atrial pressure necessary to fill the artificial heart adequately during systole needs to be from 15 to 20cmH_2O. Although in humans with heart disease such pressures probably would not be harmful, in previously healthy experimental animals this atrial pressure leads to congestion of lungs and liver and the formation of oedema. Much attention is now being paid to the development of an artificial heart which can pump adequate flows (5–15 litres/min) at normal atrial pressures. Lengths of survival with an artificial heart after removal of the natural heart is now more than 6 months[14]. Death is commonly caused by embolization, pulmonary and liver failure, infection and technical breakdown. Only once has an artificial heart been implanted in a human[4]. It functioned properly for 62 hours after which it was replaced by a heart transplant. For the time being, in view of the present state of development, this is probably the only indication for use of an artificial heart. Even if the pumps proper reach a state of reliability, a total implantable power source needs to be available prior to routine clinical use. In this field recent developments have shown promising results[24].

References

1. Bardet, J., Rigaud, M., Kahn, J. C., Huret, J. F., Gandjbakhch, J. and Bourdarias, J. P. 'Treatment of post-myocardial infarction angina by intra-aortic balloon pumping and emergency revascularization.' *Journal of Thoracic and Cardiovascular Surgery*, **74,** 299 (1977)
2. Bregman, J. and Norman, J. C. 'Mechanical circulatory support: evolving perspectives.' *Transactions of the American Society for Artificial Internal Organs*, **24,** 782 (1978)
3. Brown-Sequard, E. 'Recherches experimentales sur les proprietes physiologiques at les usages du sang rouge et du sang noir et leurs principaux elements gazeux, l'oxygene et l'oxide carbonique.' (Experimental study on the physiological properties and the application of red and black blood and the main gaseous elements, oxygen and carbonic acid.) *Journal de Physiologie de l'Homme,* **1,** 95, 353, 729 (1858)
4. Cooley, D. 'Discussion on artificial hearts.' *Transactions of the American Society for Artificial Internal Organs*, **15,** 252 (1969)
5. Deloche, A., Fontaliran, F., Fabiani, J. N. and Carpentier, A. 'Surgical revascularization of myocardial infarction.' *Seventh Congress of the European Society for Experimental Surgery*, (Abstracts), 125 (1972)
6. Dennis, C. 'Assisted circulation.' In *Surgery of the Chest*. Eds J. H. Gibbon, Jr., D. C. Sabiston, Jr. and F. C. Spencer. Ch. 28, p. 674. London: W. B. Saunders (1969)
7. Dennis, C., Grosz, C., Wesolowski, S. A. and Chin, C. J. 'External circulatory support in acute heart failure.' *Journal of Cardiovascular Surgery*, **5,** 626 (1964)
8. Dennis, C., Hall, D. P., Moreno, J. R. and Senning, A. 'Left atrial cannulation without thoracotomy for total left heart bypass.' *Acta chirurgica Scandinavica*, **123,** 267 (1962)
9. Drinkman, W. B., Buckley, M. J., Leinbach, R. C., Mundth, E. D., Kantrowitz, A. R., Austen, W. G. and Sanders, C. A. 'Effects of intra-aortic balloon pumping for cardiogenic shock.' (Abstract) *Circulation*, **43** and **44 (Suppl. II)**, 103 (1971)
10. Enright, L. P., Staroscik, R. M. and Reis, R. L. 'Left ventricular function after occlusion of the ascending aorta.' *Journal of Thoracic and Cardiovascular Surgery*, **60,** 737 (1970)
11. Gibbon, J. H. 'Artificial maintenance of circulation during experimental occlusion of the pulmonary artery.' *Archives of Surgery, Chicago*, **34,** 1105 (1937)
12. Gibbon, J. H., Miller, B. J. and Feinberg, C. 'An improved mechanical heart and lung apparatus.' *Medical Clinics of North America*, **37,** 1603 (1953)
13. Hill, J. D., Rodvien, R., Snider, M. T. and Bartlett, R. H. 'Clinical extracorporeal membrane oxygenation for acute respiratory insufficiency.' *Transactions of the American Society for Artificial Internal Organs*, **24,** 753 (1978)

14. Jarvik, R. K., Smith, L. M., Lawson, J. H., Sandgrist, G. M., Fukumasu, H., Olsen, D. B., Iwaya, F. and Kolff, W. J. 'Comparison of pneumatic and electrically powered total artificial hearts *in vivo*.' *Transactions of the American Society for Artificial Internal Organs*, **24,** 593 (1978)
15. Kessler, T. R., Pons, A. B., Jarvik, R. K., Lawson, J. H., Rawzenca, K. J. and Kolff, W. J. 'Elimination of predilection sites for thrombus formation in the total artificial heart.' *Transactions of the American Society for Artificial Internal Organs*, **24,** 532 (1970)
16. Kolff, W. J. and Berk, H. T. J. 'Artificial kidney: dialyzer with great area.' *Acta medica Scandinavica*, **117,** 121 (1944)
17. Kralios, A. C. and Zwart, H. H. J. 'Transpulmonary decompression of left ventricle.' (Abstract), *Sixth World Congress on Cardiology*, London (1970)
18. Kuhn, L. A. 'Shock in myocardial infarction.' *American Journal of Cardiology*, **26,** 578 (1970)
19. Landé, A. J. 'Assisted circulation with membrane oxygenators.' In *Artificial Organs and Cardiopulmonary Support Systems*. Ed. F. T. Rapaport. p. 85. New York: Grune and Stratton (1972)
20. Landé, A. J., Edwards, L., Bloch, J. H., Carlson, R. G., Subramanian, V., Ascheim, R. S., Scheidt, S., Fillore, S., Killip, T. and Lillehei, C. W. 'Prolonged cardiopulmonary support with a practical membrane oxygenator.' *Transactions of the American Society for Artificial Internal Organs*, **16,** 352 (1970)
21. Lefemine, A. A. and Harken, D. E. 'Extracorporeal support of the circulation by means of veno-arterial bypass with an oxygenator: case study of eight patients in shock.' *Journal of Thoracic and Cardiovascular Surgery*, **62,** 769 (1971)
22. LeGallois, J. J. C. *Experiences sur le Principe de la Vie*. Paris: D'Hautel (1812) (*Experiments on the Principle of Life*. Transls. M. C. and J. C. Nancrede. Philadelphia: Thomas (1813)
23. McLean, J. 'The discovery of heparin.' *Circulation*, **19,** 75 (1959)
24. Morse, J. C., Eversten, J. M., Faeser, R. J. and Mellwig, J. W. 'Development of compact thermal and electrical energy converters for left heart assist systems.' *Transactions of the American Society for Artificial Internal Organs*, **24,** 77 (1978)
25. Patt, H. H., Clift, J. W., Loh, P. B., Roa, J. C., Wexler, J. and Seligman, A. M. 'Veno-arterial pumping in normal dogs and dogs with coronary occlusion.' *Journal of Thoracic and Cardiovascular Surgery*, **39,** 464 (1960)
26. Peters, J. L., Fukumasu, H., McRea, J. C., Nakagaki, M., Iwaya, F., Owen, D., Kolff, J. and Kolff, W. J. 'Prolonged, transapical left ventricular bypass (TALVB) in sheep and man.' *Transactions of the American Society for Artificial Internal Organs*, **24,** 113 (1978)
27. Rapaport, F. T. and Merrill, J. P. *Artificial Organs and Cardiopulmonary Support Systems*. New York: Grune and Stratton (1972)
28. Scheidt, S., 'Physiologic effects of intra-aortic balloon pumping in cardiogenic shock.' (Abstract). *American Journal of Cardiology*, **29,** 290 (1972)
29. Scheidt, S., Alonso, D. R. and Killip, T. 'Quantification of myocardial damage in cardiogenic shock.' *Circulation*, **63 (Suppl. II)**, 46 (1971)
30. Stuckey, J. H., Newman, M. M., Dennis, C., Berg, E., Goodman, S. E., Fries, C. C., Karlson, K. E., Blumenfeld, M., Weitzner, S. W., Binder, L. S. and Winston, A. 'Partial perfusion in the treatment of selected cases of myocardial infarction.' *Transactions of the American Society for Artificial Internal Organs*, **3,** 30 (1957)
31. von Frey, M. and Gruber, M. 'Untersuchungen über den Stoffwechsel isolierter Organe. Ein Respirations-Apparat fur isolierte Organe.' (Studies on the metabolism of isolated organs. An oxygenator for isolated organs.) *Virchow's Archives of Pathological Anatomy and Physiology*, **9,** 519 (1885)

32. Zwart, H. H. J. 'Complete left heart bypass without thoracotomy.' *Thesis, SOL Offsetdruk, Ameterdam* (1966)
33. Zwart, H. H. J., Kralios, A., Kwan-Gett, C. S., Backman, D. K., Foote, J. and Kolff, W. J. 'Mechanical devices for cardiopulmonary assistance: transarterial closed-chest left ventricular bypass.' *Fortschritte fur Kardiologie*, **6,** 157 (1971)
34. Zwart, H. H. J., Kralios, A., Kwan-Gett, C. S., Carlton, F. and Kolff, W. J. 'First clinical application of transarterial closed-chest left ventricular (taCLV) bypass.' *Transactions of the American Society for Artificial Internal Organs*, **16,** 386 (1970)

Index

dum tacent, clamant